PHYSICIANS'
CANCER CHEMOTHERAPY
DRUG MANUAL

2024

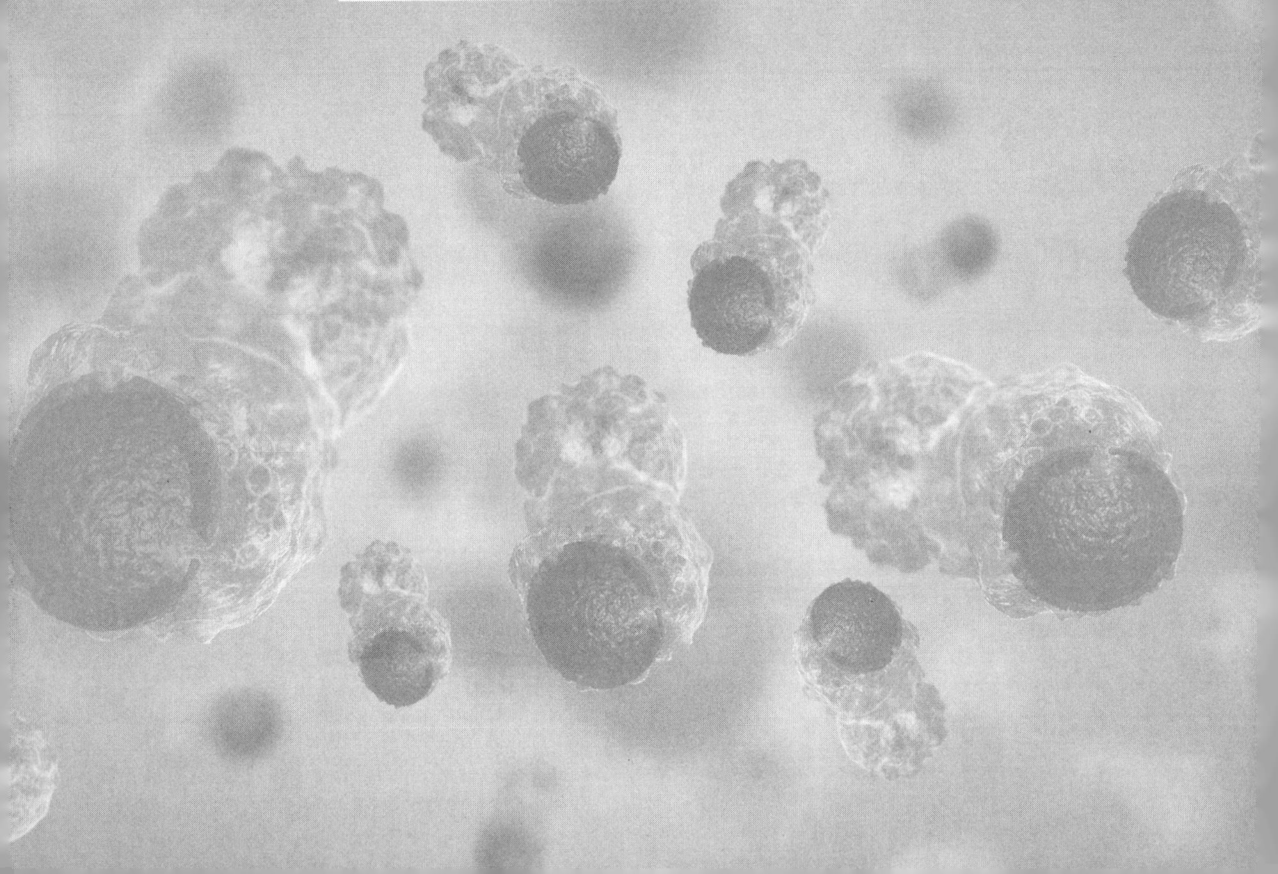

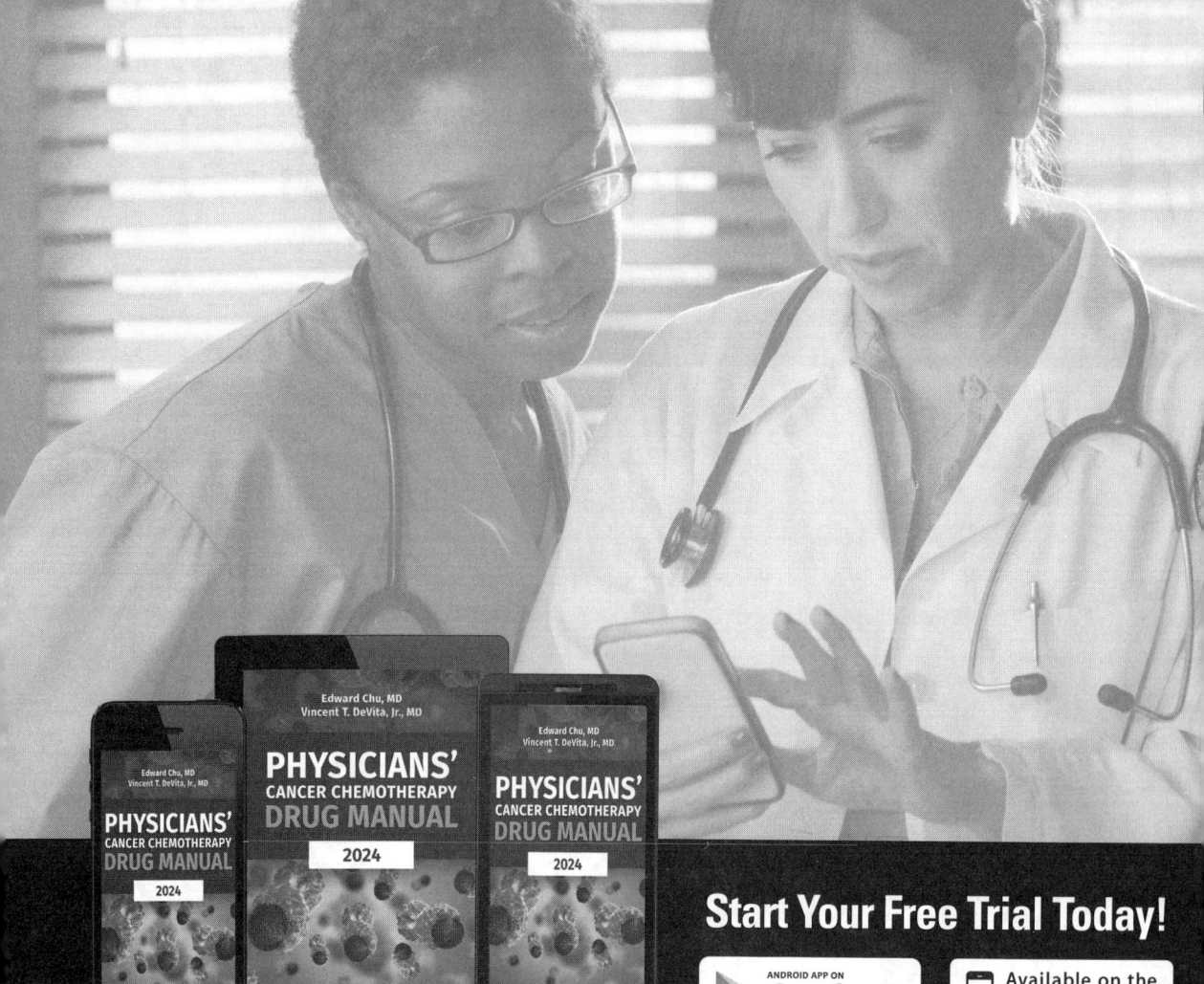

PHYSICIANS'
CANCER CHEMOTHERAPY
DRUG MANUAL

2024

Edward Chu, MD, MMS, FACP

Director, Montefiore Einstein
Comprehensive Cancer Center

Vice-President for Cancer Medicine,
Montefiore Medicine

Professor of Oncology, Medicine, and
Molecular Pharmacology

Carol and Roger Einiger Professor of
Cancer Medicine

Albert Einstein College of Medicine

Bronx, New York

Vincent T. DeVita, Jr., MD

Amy and Joseph Perella Professor of
Medicine

Professor of Epidemiology and Public
Health

Yale Cancer Center

Yale University School of Medicine

New Haven, Connecticut

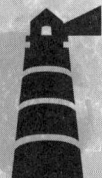

JONES & BARTLETT
LEARNING

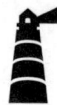

World Headquarters
Jones & Bartlett Learning
25 Mall Road
Burlington, MA 01803
978-443-5000
info@jblearning.com
www.jblearning.com

Jones & Bartlett Learning books and products are available through most bookstores and online booksellers. To contact Jones & Bartlett Learning directly, call 800-832-0034, fax 978-443-8000, or visit our website, www.jblearning.com.

Substantial discounts on bulk quantities of Jones & Bartlett Learning publications are available to corporations, professional associations, and other qualified organizations. For details and specific discount information, contact the special sales department at Jones & Bartlett Learning via the above contact information or send an email to specialsales@jblearning.com.

Production Credits
Vice President, Product Management: Marisa R. Urbano
Vice President, Content Strategy and Implementation: Christine Emerton
Director, Product Management: Matthew Kane
Product Manager: Marc Bove
Director, Content Management: Donna Gridley
Manager, Content Strategy: Orsolya Gall
Content Strategist: Christina Freitas
Director, Project Management and Content Services: Karen Scott
Manager, Program Management: Kristen Rogers
Program Manager: Dan Stone
Senior Digital Project Specialist: Angela Dooley
Director, Marketing: Andrea DeFronzo
Senior Product Marketing Manager: Lindsay White
Content Services Manager: Colleen Lamy
Senior Director of Supply Chain: Ed Schneider
Procurement Manager: Wendy Kilborn
Composition: S4Carlisle Publishing Services
Cover Design: Michael O'Donnell
Senior Media Development Editor: Troy Liston
Rights & Permissions Manager: John Rusk
Rights Specialist: Maria Leon Maimone
Cover Image (Title Page, Chapter Opener): © crystal light/Shutterstock
Printing and Binding: Sheridan Saline

ISBN: 978-1-284-00000-9

6048

Printed in the United States of America
27 26 25 24 23   10 9 8 7 6 5 4 3 2 1

Contents

Editors

Edward Chu, MD, MMS, FACP
Director, Montefiore Einstein Comprehensive Cancer Center
Vice-President for Cancer Medicine, Montefiore Medicine
Professor of Oncology, Medicine, and Molecular Pharmacology
Carol and Roger Einiger Professor of Cancer Medicine
Albert Einstein College of Medicine
Bronx, NY

Vincent T. DeVita, Jr., MD
Amy and Joseph Perella Professor of Medicine
Professor of Epidemiology and Public Health
Yale Cancer Center
Yale University School of Medicine
New Haven, CT

Contributing Authors

Fernand Bteich, MD
Assistant Professor of Oncology
Department of Oncology
Montefiore Einstein Comprehensive Cancer Center
Albert Einstein College of Medicine
Bronx, NY

M. Sitki Copur, MD, FACP
Adjunct Professor of Medicine
University of Nebraska
Medical Director, Morrison Cancer Center
Mary Lanning Healthcare
Hastings, NE

Laurie J. Harrold, MD
Staff Medical Oncologist
Clinical Assistant Professor of Medicine
VA Pittsburgh Healthcare System
University of Pittsburgh School of Medicine
Pittsburgh, PA

Chaoyuan Kuang, MD, PhD
Assistant Professor of Oncology and Medicine
Department of Oncology and Medicine
Montefiore Einstein Comprehensive Cancer Center
Albert Einstein College of Medicine
Bronx, NY

Matthew Lee, MD, MPH
Assistant Professor of Oncology
Department of Oncology
Montefiore Einstein Comprehensive Cancer Center
Albert Einstein College of Medicine
Bronx, NY

Amalia Sofianidi
Senior Medical Student
School of Medicine, National and Kapodistrian University of Athens
Athens, Greece

Preface

The development of effective drugs for the treatment of cancer represents a significant achievement beginning with the discovery of the antimetabolites and alkylating agents in the 1940s and 1950s. The success of that effort can be attributed in large measure to the close collaboration and interaction between basic scientists, synthetic organic chemists, pharmacologists, and clinicians. This tradition continues to flourish, especially as we now enter the world of pharmacogenomics, genomics, proteomics, and other omics science along with the rapid identification of new molecular targets for drug design and development.

In this, the *Twenty-Fourth Edition*, we have condensed and summarized a wealth of information on chemotherapeutic and biologic agents in current clinical practice into a reference guide that presents essential information in a practical and readable format. The primary indications, drug doses and schedules, toxicities, and special considerations for each agent have been expanded and revised to take into account new information that has been gathered over the past year. In this edition, we have included 12 new agents and several new supplemental indications that have all been approved by the FDA for previously approved agents within the past year.

This drug manual is divided into five chapters. Chapter 1 provides a brief overview of the main principles of cancer chemotherapy and reviews the clinical settings where chemotherapy is used. Chapter 2 reviews individual chemotherapeutic and biologic agents that are in current clinical use; these agents are presented in alphabetical order according to their generic name. Specific details are provided regarding drug classification and category, key mechanisms of action and resistance, critical aspects of clinical pharmacology and pharmacokinetics, clinical indications, special precautions and considerations, and toxicity. Chapter 3 includes recommendations for dose modifications that are required in the setting of myelosuppression and/or liver and renal dysfunction. Relevant information is also provided highlighting the teratogenic potential of various agents. Chapter 4 presents a review of the combination drug regimens and selected single-agent regimens for solid tumors and hematologic malignancies that are used commonly in daily clinical practice. This section is organized alphabetically by specific cancer type. Finally, Chapter 5 reviews commonly used antiemetic agents and regimens used to treat chemotherapy-induced nausea and vomiting, which is a significant toxicity observed with many of the anticancer agents in current practice.

Our hope remains for this book to continue to serve as both an in-depth reference and an immediate source of practical information that can be used by physicians and other healthcare professionals actively involved in the daily care of cancer patients. This drug manual continues to be a work in progress, and our goal is to continue to provide new updates on an annual basis and to incorporate new drugs and treatment regimens that reflect the rapid advances in the field of cancer drug development.

Edward Chu, MD, MMS, FACP
Vincent T. DeVita, Jr., MD

Acknowledgments

This book represents the efforts of many dedicated people. It reflects my own personal and professional roots in the field of cancer pharmacology and cancer drug development. It also reaffirms the teaching and support of my colleagues and mentors at Brown University, the National Cancer Institute (NCI), and the Yale Cancer Center. In particular, Bruce Chabner, Paul Calabresi, Robert Parks, Joseph Bertino, and Vince DeVita each had a major influence on my development as a cancer pharmacologist and medical oncologist. While at the NCI, I was fortunate to have been trained under the careful mentorship of Carmen Allegra, Bob Wittes, and Bruce Chabner. At Yale, I was privileged to work with a group of extraordinarily talented individuals including Yung-chi Cheng, William Prusoff, Alan Sartorelli, and Vince DeVita, all of whom graciously shared their scientific insights, wisdom, support, and friendship. I would also like to thank my co-author, colleague, mentor, and friend, Vince DeVita, who recruited me to the Yale Cancer Center and who has been so tremendously supportive of my professional and personal career. Special thanks go to my colleagues at Jones & Bartlett Learning for giving me the opportunity to develop this book and for their continued encouragement, support, and patience throughout this entire process.

I wish to thank my wife, Laurie Harrold, for her love and patience, for her insights as a practicing medical oncologist, and for her help in writing and reviewing various sections of this book. I would also like to thank our two dogs, Mika and Lexi, who are no longer with us, but who live in our hearts forever; to our two new dogs, Rosie and Allie; and to our two beautiful children, Ashley and Joshua, who have brought great joy and pride to our family. Finally, this book is dedicated to my parents, Ming and Shih-Hsi Chu, for their constant and unconditional loyalty and love, support, and encouragement, and for instilling in me the desire, joy, and commitment to become a medical oncologist and cancer pharmacologist and who have shown me the way to be a better physician, scientist, and person. While they are no longer here with us, their spirit lives in our hearts forever.

Edward Chu, MD, MMS, FACP

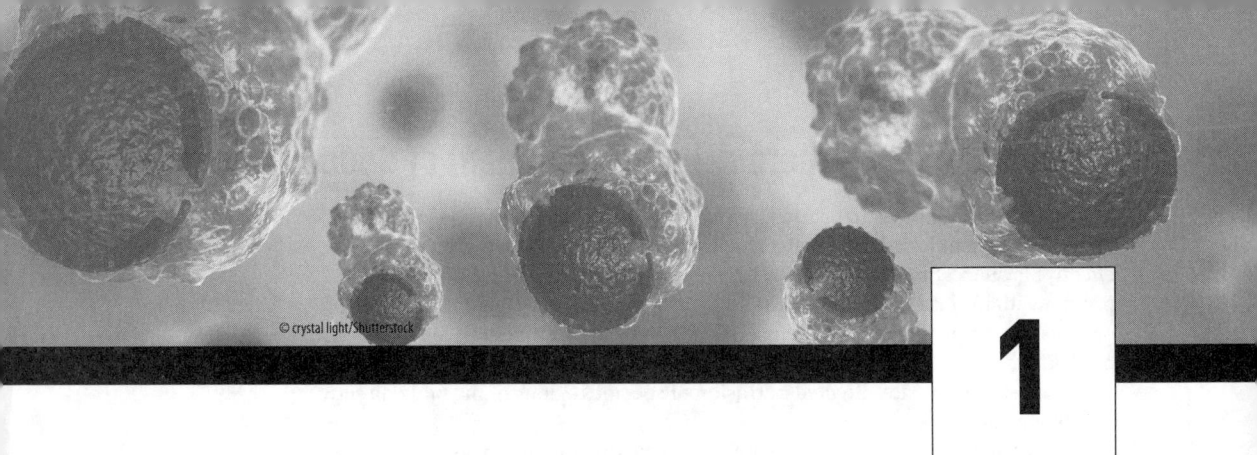

1

Principles of Cancer Chemotherapy

Vincent T. DeVita, Jr., and Edward Chu

Introduction

The development of chemotherapy in the 1950s and 1960s resulted in curative therapeutic strategies for patients with hematologic malignancies and a small number of advanced solid tumors. These advances confirmed the principle that chemotherapy could indeed cure cancer and provided the rationale for integrating chemotherapy into combined-modality programs with surgery and radiation therapy in the early stages of disease to provide clinical benefit. Since its early days, the principal obstacles to the clinical efficacy of chemotherapy have been toxicity to the normal tissues of the body, tumor heterogeneity, and the development of cellular drug resistance. The development and application of molecular technologies to analyze the expression of normal and malignant cells at the level of DNA, RNA, and/or protein have greatly facilitated the identification of some of the critical mechanisms through which chemotherapy exerts its antitumor effects and activates the program of cell death. The newer advances in molecular diagnostics, which now include next-generation sequencing, whole exome sequencing, and whole genome sequencing, have provided important new insights into the molecular events in cancer cells that confer chemosensitivity to drug treatment as well as identified potential new therapeutic targets. This enhanced understanding of the key molecular and signaling pathways by which chemotherapy, targeted therapies, biological therapies, and immunotherapy exert their antitumor activity, and by which genetic alterations result in resistance to drug therapy, has provided the rational basis for developing innovative therapeutic strategies.

The Role of Chemotherapy in the Treatment of Cancer

Chemotherapy continues to be used in four main clinical settings: (1) primary induction treatment for advanced disease or for cancers for which there are no other effective local treatment approaches; (2) neoadjuvant treatment for patients who present with localized disease, for whom local forms of therapy, such as surgery and/or radiation, are inadequate by themselves; (3) adjuvant treatment to local treatment modalities, including surgery and/or radiation therapy; and (4) direct instillation into sanctuary sites or by site-directed perfusion of specific regions of the body directly affected by the cancer.

Primary induction chemotherapy refers to drug therapy administered as the primary treatment for patients who present with advanced cancer for which no alternative treatment exists. This has been the main approach to treat patients with advanced, metastatic disease. In most cases, the goals of therapy are to palliate tumor-related symptoms, improve overall quality of life, and prolong time to tumor progression (TTP) and overall survival (OS). Despite the tremendous advances that have been made over the past 25 years, cancer chemotherapy is curative in only a very small subset of patients who present with advanced disease. In adults, these potentially curable cancers include Hodgkin's and non-Hodgkin's lymphoma, germ cell cancer, acute leukemias, and choriocarcinoma. For pediatric patients, the curable childhood cancers include acute lymphoblastic leukemia, Burkitt's lymphoma, Wilms' tumor, and embryonal rhabdomyosarcoma.

Neoadjuvant chemotherapy refers to the use of chemotherapy in patients who present with locally advanced cancer for which local therapies, such as surgery and radiation therapy, exist but are less than completely effective. The diseases for which a neoadjuvant approach is usually considered include anal cancer, bladder cancer, breast cancer, esophageal cancer, laryngeal cancer, locally advanced non–small cell lung cancer (NSCLC), and osteogenic sarcoma. For neoadjuvant therapy, chemotherapy is administered concurrently with radiation therapy with the goal of reducing the size of the tumor to where it is more easily removed by surgery. This combined modality approach is particularly relevant for anal cancer, gastroesophageal cancer, rectal cancer, laryngeal cancer, and NSCLC.

One of the most important roles for systemic chemotherapy is in follow-up to local treatment modalities such as surgery and/or radiation therapy; this has been termed *adjuvant chemotherapy*. The development of disease recurrence, either locally or systemically, following surgery and/or radiation is mainly due to the spread of occult micrometastases. The goal of adjuvant therapy is to reduce the incidence of both local and systemic recurrence and to improve the OS of patients. In general, chemotherapy regimens with clinical activity against advanced disease may have curative potential following surgical resection of the primary tumor, provided the appropriate dose and schedule are administered. It is now well-established that adjuvant chemotherapy is effective in prolonging both disease-free survival (DFS) and OS in patients with breast cancer, colorectal cancer (CRC), gastric cancer, NSCLC, Wilms' tumor, osteogenic sarcoma, and anaplastic astrocytoma. Patients with primary malignant melanoma at high risk of developing metastases derive benefit in terms of improved DFS and OS from adjuvant treatment with the immune checkpoint inhibitors ipilimumab, nivolumab, and pembrolizumab as they provide clinical benefit in the adjuvant treatment of surgically resected melanoma with lymph node involvement.

Principles of Combination Chemotherapy

With rare exceptions (e.g., choriocarcinoma), single drugs, when used at clinically tolerable doses, have been unable to cure cancer. In the 1960s and early 1970s, drug combination regimens were developed based on known biochemical actions of available anticancer drugs rather than on their clinical efficacy. Such regimens were, however, largely ineffective. The era of combination chemotherapy began when several active drugs from different classes became available for use in combination in the treatment of the acute leukemias and lymphomas. Following the initial success with hematologic malignancies, combination chemotherapy was subsequently extended to the treatment of solid tumors.

Combination chemotherapy with conventional cytotoxic agents accomplishes several key objectives not possible with single-agent therapy. First, it provides maximal cell kill within the range of toxicity tolerated by the host for each drug as long as dosing is not compromised. Second, it provides a broader range of interaction between drugs and tumor cells with different genetic abnormalities in a heterogeneous tumor population. Finally, it may prevent and/or slow the subsequent development of cellular drug resistance.

Certain principles have guided the selection of drugs in the most effective drug combinations, and they provide a paradigm for the development of new drug therapeutic regimens. First, only drugs known to be partially effective against the same tumor when used alone should be selected for use in combination. If available, drugs that produce some fraction of complete remission are preferred to those that produce only partial responses. Second, when several drugs of a class are available and are equally effective, a drug should be selected on the basis of toxicity that does not overlap with the toxicity of other drugs to be used in the combination. Although such selection leads to a wider range of side effects, it minimizes the risk of a potentially lethal effect caused by multiple insults to the same organ system by different drugs. Moreover, this approach allows dose intensity to be maximized. In addition, drugs should be used in their optimal dose and schedule, and drug combinations should be given at consistent intervals. The treatment-free interval between cycles should be the shortest possible time necessary for recovery of the most sensitive normal target tissue, which is usually the bone marrow. The biochemical, molecular, and pharmacologic mechanisms of interaction between individual drugs in a given combination should be understood to allow for maximal effect. Finally, arbitrary reduction in the dose of an effective drug to allow for the addition of other, less effective drugs may dramatically reduce the clinical activity of the most effective agent below the threshold of effectiveness and reduce the capacity of the combination regimen to cure disease in a given patient.

One final issue relates to the optimal duration of drug administration. The antihormonal agents tamoxifen, anastrozole, and letrozole are effective in the adjuvant therapy of postmenopausal women whose breast tumors express the estrogen receptor. These agents are administered on a long-term basis, with treatment usually given for up to 5 years. Several randomized trials in the adjuvant treatment of breast cancer have shown that 6 months of treatment is as effective as long-course therapy (12 months). International Duration Evaluation of Adjuvant Therapy (IDEA) was a multinational collaborative effort that showed that a shorter course of 3 months of adjuvant oxaliplatin-based chemotherapy yields the same level of clinical benefit as 6 months of treatment of stage III colon cancer. However, optimal treatment duration may depend on the particular tumor type, as it is now well established that prolonged duration of adjuvant therapy in patients with surgically resected gastrointestinal stromal tumor (GIST), 3 years versus 1 year, results in improved clinical benefit.

While progressive disease during chemotherapy is a clear indication to stop treatment in the advanced disease setting, the optimal duration of chemotherapy for patients without disease progression has not been well defined. With the development of novel and more potent drug regimens, the potential risk of cumulative adverse events, such as cardiotoxicity secondary to the anthracyclines and neurotoxicity secondary to the taxanes and the platinum analogs, must be factored into the decision-making process. There is, however, no evidence of clinical benefit in continuing therapy indefinitely until disease progression. A randomized study in metastatic CRC comparing continuous versus intermittent palliative chemotherapy showed that a policy of stopping and re-challenging with the same chemotherapy may provide a reasonable treatment option for certain patients. Similar observations have been observed in the treatment of metastatic disease of other tumor types, including NSCLC, breast cancer, germ cell cancer, ovarian cancer, and small cell lung cancer (SCLC).

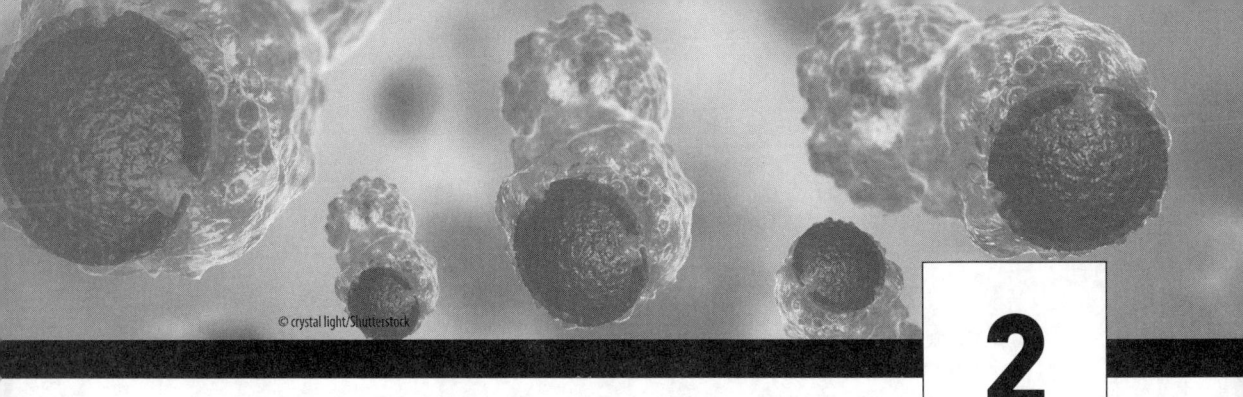
© crystal light/Shutterstock

2

Chemotherapeutic and Biologic Drugs

Edward Chu, Amalia Sofianidi, Laurie J. Harrold, and M. Sitki Copur

Abemaciclib

TRADE NAME	Verzenio, PD 0332991	CLASSIFICATION	Signal transduction inhibitor, CDK inhibitor
CATEGORY	Targeted agent	DRUG MANUFACTURER	Eli Lilly

MECHANISM OF ACTION
- Inhibitor of cyclin-dependent kinase (CDK) 4 and 6.
- Inhibition of CDK4 and CDK6 leads to inhibition of cell proliferation and growth by blocking progression of cells from G1 to the S-phase of the cell cycle.
- Decreased expression of retinoblastoma protein phosphorylation (pRB) results in reduced E2F expression and signaling.
- Induces cell senescence.

MECHANISM OF RESISTANCE
- Acquired CDK6 amplification resulting in increased CDK6 expression.
- Increased expression of CDK2 and CDK4.
- Loss of pRb expression.
- Overexpression of cyclins A and E.
- Increased expression of 3-phosphoinositide-dependent protein kinase 1 (PDK1) with activation of AKT pathway and other AGC kinases.

ABSORPTION
Oral bioavailability is on the order of 46%. High-fat, high-calorie meal increases the AUC (area under the curve) of parent drug and its active metabolites by 9% and increases C_{max} (maximum concentration) by 26%.

DISTRIBUTION
Significant binding (96.3%) to plasma proteins, serum albumin, and α1-acid glycoprotein with extensive tissue distribution. Steady-state drug levels are achieved within 5 days following repeat daily dosing.

METABOLISM
Extensively metabolized in the liver primarily by CYP3A4 microsomal enzymes, with formation of the major metabolite N-desethylabemaciclib (M2) and other additional metabolites, including M20, M18, and an oxidative metabolite (M1). These metabolites have similar biologic activity as the parent drug. Acylation and glucuronidation play only minor roles in drug metabolism. Nearly 81% of drug is recovered in feces and only 3% in urine, with the majority of eliminated drug being in metabolite form. The elimination half-life of the drug is 18.3 hours.

INDICATIONS
1. Approved by the Food and Drug Administration (FDA) in combination with an aromatase inhibitor for patients with hormone receptor (HR)-positive, HER2-negative advanced or metastatic breast cancer as initial endocrine-based therapy in postmenopausal women.
2. FDA-approved in combination with fulvestrant for patients with HR-positive, HER2-negative advanced or metastatic breast cancer in women with disease progression following endocrine therapy.
3. FDA-approved as monotherapy for patients with HR-positive, HER2-negative advanced or metastatic breast cancer in women with disease progression following endocrine therapy and prior chemotherapy in the metastatic setting.

4. FDA-approved in combination with endocrine therapy (tamoxifen or an aromatase inhibitor) for the adjuvant treatment of adult patients with hormone receptor (HR)-positive, HER2-negative, node-positive early breast cancer at high risk of recurrence.

DOSAGE RANGE
1. Combination therapy with fulvestrant, tamoxifen, or an aromatase inhibitor—150 mg PO bid.
2. Monotherapy—200 mg PO bid.

DRUG INTERACTION 1
Drugs that stimulate liver microsomal CYP3A4 enzymes, including phenytoin, carbamazepine, rifampin, phenobarbital, and St. John's Wort—These drugs may increase the metabolism of abemaciclib, resulting in lower drug levels and potentially reduced clinical activity.

DRUG INTERACTION 2
Drugs that inhibit liver microsomal CYP3A4 enzymes, including ketoconazole, itraconazole, erythromycin, and clarithromycin—These drugs may reduce the metabolism of abemaciclib, resulting in increased drug levels and potentially increased toxicity.

SPECIAL CONSIDERATIONS
1. Dose reduction is not required in the setting of mild or moderate hepatic impairment (Child-Pugh Class A or B). Use with caution in patients with severe hepatic impairment, and dose reduction is recommended.
2. Dose reduction is not required in the setting of mild or moderate renal impairment. Has not been studied in the setting of severe renal impairment, end-stage renal disease, or in patients on dialysis.
3. Monitor complete blood count (CBC) and platelet count every 2 weeks during the first 2 months of therapy and at monthly intervals thereafter.
4. Monitor liver function tests (LFTs) at baseline and periodically while on therapy. LFTs should be monitored every 2 weeks for the first 2 months, monthly for the next 2 months, and then as clinically indicated.
5. Monitor for signs and symptoms of infection.
6. Monitor for signs and symptoms of venous thromboembolism.
7. Pregnancy category D.

TOXICITY 1
Myelosuppression with neutropenia, anemia, and thrombocytopenia.

TOXICITY 2
Fatigue, asthenia, and anorexia.

TOXICITY 3
Increased risk of infections, with upper respiratory infection being most common.

TOXICITY 4
Nausea/vomiting, abdominal pain, and diarrhea.

TOXICITY 5
Increased risk of venous thromboembolic events, including deep vein thrombosis (DVT) and pulmonary embolism (PE).

TOXICITY 6
Hepatotoxicity with elevated SGOT and SGPT.

Abiraterone Acetate

TRADE NAME	Zytiga	**CLASSIFICATION**	Steroid inhibitor
CATEGORY	Hormonal drug	**DRUG MANUFACTURER**	Janssen Biotech, Johnson & Johnson

MECHANISM OF ACTION
- Prodrug of abiraterone.
- Selective inhibition of 17α-hydroxylase/C17, 20-lyase (CYP17). This enzyme is expressed in testicular, adrenal, and prostatic tumor tissues and is required for androgen biosynthesis.
- Inhibition of CYP17 leads to inhibition of the conversion of pregnenolone and progesterone to their 17α-hydroxy derivatives.
- Inhibition of CYP17 leads to inhibition of subsequent formation of dehydroepiandrosterone (DHEA) and androstenedione.
- Associated with a rebound increase in mineralocorticoid production by the adrenals.

MECHANISM OF RESISTANCE
- Upregulation of CYP17.
- Induction of androgen receptor (AR) and AR splice variants that result in ligand-independent AR transactivation.
- Expression of truncated androgen receptors.

ABSORPTION

Following oral administration, maximum drug levels are reached within 1.5–4 hours. Oral absorption is increased with food and, in particular, food with high fat content.

DISTRIBUTION

Highly protein bound (>99%) to albumin and α1-acid glycoprotein.

METABOLISM

Following oral administration, abiraterone acetate is rapidly hydrolyzed to abiraterone, the active metabolite. The two main circulating metabolites of abiraterone are abiraterone sulphate and N-oxide abiraterone sulphate, both of which are inactive. Nearly 90% of an administered dose is recovered in feces, while only 5% is eliminated in urine. The terminal half-life of abiraterone ranges from 5 to 14 hours, with a median half-life of 12 hours.

INDICATIONS

1. FDA-approved in combination with prednisone for patients with metastatic, castration-resistant prostate cancer (CRPC) who have received prior chemotherapy containing docetaxel.
2. FDA-approved in combination with prednisone for patients with metastatic high-risk castration-sensitive prostate cancer (CSPC).

DOSAGE RANGE

Recommended dose is 1,000 mg PO once daily in combination with prednisone 5 mg PO bid.

DRUG INTERACTIONS

*   Use with caution in the presence of CYP2D6 substrates.
*   Use with caution in the presence of CYP3A4 inhibitors and inducers.

SPECIAL CONSIDERATIONS

1. No dosage adjustment is necessary for patients with mild hepatic impairment. In patients with moderate hepatic impairment (Child-Pugh Class B), reduce dose to 250 mg once daily. If elevations in ALT or AST >5 × upper limit of normal (ULN) or total bilirubin >3 × ULN occur in patients, discontinue treatment. Avoid use in patients with severe hepatic impairment, as the drug has not been tested in this patient population.
2. No dosage adjustment is necessary for patients with renal impairment.
3. Abiraterone acetate should be taken on an empty stomach with no food being consumed for at least 2 hours before and for at least 1 hour after an oral dose. Tablets should be swallowed whole with water.
4. Closely monitor for adrenal insufficiency, especially if patients are withdrawn from prednisone, undergo a reduction in prednisone dose, or experience concurrent infection or stress.
5. Pregnancy category X. Breastfeeding should be avoided.

TOXICITY 1
Fatigue.

TOXICITY 2
Mild nausea and vomiting.

TOXICITY 3
Mild elevations in SGOT/SGPT.

TOXICITY 4
Hypertension.

TOXICITY 5
Peripheral edema.

TOXICITY 6
Hypokalemia.

TOXICITY 7
Arthralgias, myalgias, and muscle spasms.

TOXICITY 8
Hot flashes.

Acalabrutinib

TRADE NAME	Calquence, ACP-196	CLASSIFICATION	Signal transduction inhibitor, BTK inhibitor
CATEGORY	Targeted agent	DRUG MANUFACTURER	Acerta and AstraZeneca

MECHANISM OF ACTION
- Irreversible second-generation, small-molecule inhibitor of Bruton's tyrosine kinase (BTK).
- Parent drug and its active metabolite, ACP-5862, form a covalent bond with a cysteine residue in the BTK active site, leading to enzymatic inhibition.
- BTK is a key signaling protein of the B-cell antigen receptor (BCR) and cytokine receptor pathways.

MECHANISM OF RESISTANCE
- Mutations in the Cys481 residue in the BTK active site with reduced binding affinity to acalabrutinib.
- Mutations in the gene encoding phospholipase C-γ2 (PLCG2).
- Increased expression of kinases SYK and LYN, which are critical for activation of mutant PLCG2.

ABSORPTION
Absolute oral bioavailability is approximately 25%. Peak plasma drug levels are achieved in 0.75 hour after ingestion, and food does not appear to alter bioavailability.

DISTRIBUTION
Extensive binding (97.5%) to plasma proteins. Steady-state drug levels are reached in approximately 8 days.

METABOLISM
Metabolism in the liver primarily by CYP3A4 and to a minor extent by glutathione conjugation and amide hydrolysis. ACP-5862 is the major active metabolite, with 50% inhibitory activity against BTK when compared to parent drug. Elimination is mainly hepatic (84%), with excretion in feces. Renal elimination accounts for only 12% of an administered dose. Most of the drug is eliminated in metabolite form, as only <1% is excreted as unchanged drug. Short terminal half-life of the parent drug approaching 1 hour.

INDICATIONS
FDA-approved under accelerated approval based on overall response rate for patients with mantle cell lymphoma (MCL) who have received at least one prior therapy.

DOSAGE RANGE
Recommended dose is 100 mg PO bid. Should be swallowed whole with or without food.

DRUG INTERACTION 1
Phenytoin and other drugs that stimulate the liver microsomal CYP3A4 enzymes, including carbamazepine, rifampin, phenobarbital, and St. John's Wort—These drugs may increase the metabolism of acalabrutinib, resulting in its inactivation and lower effective drug levels.

DRUG INTERACTION 2

Drugs that inhibit the liver microsomal CYP3A4 enzymes, including ketoconazole, itraconazole, erythromycin, and clarithromycin—These drugs may decrease the metabolism of acalabrutinib, resulting in increased drug levels and potentially increased toxicity.

DRUG INTERACTION 3

Warfarin—Patients receiving warfarin should be closely monitored for alterations in their clotting parameters, prothrombin time (PT) and international normalized ratio (INR), and/or bleeding, as acalabrutinib may inhibit the metabolism of warfarin by the liver P450 system. Dose of warfarin may require careful adjustment in the presence of acalabrutinib therapy.

DRUG INTERACTION 4

Proton pump inhibitors—Proton pump inhibitors may reduce oral bioavailability and concomitant use may lead to reduced drug plasma concentrations. If treatment with a gastric acid–reducing agent is required, an antacid or an H2-antagonist should be considered.

SPECIAL CONSIDERATIONS

1. Dose reduction is not required in the setting of mild or moderate hepatic impairment (Child-Pugh Class A or B). Use with caution in patients with severe hepatic impairment, as the drug has not been studied in this setting.
2. Dose reduction is not required in the setting of mild or moderate renal impairment. Has not been studied in the setting of severe renal impairment, end-stage renal disease, or in patients on dialysis.
3. Acalabrutinib capsules should be swallowed whole with water.
4. Closely monitor CBCs on a monthly basis.
5. Acalabrutinib may increase the risk of bleeding in patients on antiplatelet or anticoagulant therapies.
6. Consider holding acalabrutinib for 3–7 days pre- and post-surgery to reduce the potential risk for bleeding.
7. Closely monitor patients for fever and signs of infection.
8. Patients should be advised to protect against sun exposure.
9. Pregnancy category D. Breastfeeding should be avoided.

TOXICITY 1

Bleeding in the form of ecchymoses, gastrointestinal (GI) bleeding, and hematuria.

TOXICITY 2

Infections with pneumonia are most common. Hepatitis B virus reactivation and progressive multifocal leukoencephalopathy (PML) have been reported.

TOXICITY 3

Myelosuppression with neutropenia, thrombocytopenia, and anemia.

TOXICITY 4
Abdominal pain, diarrhea, and nausea/vomiting are the most common GI side effects.

TOXICITY 5
Second primary cancers with skin cancer and other solid tumors.

TOXICITY 6
Fatigue, headache, and myalgias.

TOXICITY 7
Rare instances of atrial fibrillation/atrial flutter.

Adagrasib

TRADE NAME	Krazati, MRTX849	CLASSIFICATION	Signal transduction inhibitor, KRAS G12C inhibitor
CATEGORY	Targeted agent	DRUG MANUFACTURER	Mirati Therapeutics

MECHANISM OF ACTION
- Selective and irreversible small molecule inhibitor of KRAS G12C mutation.
- Forms a covalent bond with the unique cysteine of the KRAS G12C protein, which locks the protein in an inactive GDP-bound state that prevents downstream signaling without affecting wild-type KRAS.

- KRAS G12C mutation present in 14% of NSCLC and 3%–4% of CRC, 2% of pancreatic cancer and other solid tumors.
- Results in a pro-inflammatory tumor microenvironment that drives antitumor immunity.

MECHANISM OF RESISTANCE
- Secondary KRAS mutation in the adagrasib-binding pocket.
- High-level amplification of the KRAS G12C allele.
- Polyclonal RAS-MAPK reactivation with activation/induction of downstream cellular signaling pathways, such as RAS/RAF, PI3K/AKT, and MAPK.
- Secondary MET mutations and MET amplification.
- Oncogenic fusions involving ALK, TET, BRAF, RAF1, and FGFR3.

ABSORPTION
Median time to peak drug levels is 6 hours. Food does not affect oral absorption.

DISTRIBUTION
Extensive protein binding (98%) to human plasma proteins. Steady-state drug levels reached in 8 days.

METABOLISM
Metabolized mainly by liver CYP3A4 microsomal enzymes. Elimination of drug is mainly in feces (75%), the majority of which is in parent form. Renal clearance of parent drug and metabolites account for only about 5% of an administered dose. Relatively long half-life on the order of 23 hours.

INDICATIONS
FDA-approved for the treatment of KRAS G12C-mutated locally advanced or metastatic non–small cell lung cancer (NSCLC). Approved under accelerated approval based on overall response rate and duration of response.

DOSAGE RANGE
Recommended dose is 600 mg PO bid with or without food.

DRUG INTERACTION 1
Drugs such as ketoconazole, itraconazole, erythromycin, clarithromycin, atazanavir, indinavir, nefazodone, nelfinavir, ritonavir, saquinavir, telithromycin, and voriconazole may decrease the metabolism of adagrasib, resulting in increased drug levels and potentially increased toxicity.

DRUG INTERACTION 2
Phenytoin and other drugs that stimulate the liver microsomal CYP3A4 enzymes, including carbamazepine, rifampin, phenobarbital, and St. John's Wort—These drugs may increase the metabolism of adagrasib, resulting in lower effective drug levels and potentially reduced activity.

DRUG INTERACTION 3

CYP2C9 and CYP2D6 substrates—Avoid concomitant use of adagrasib with CYP2C9 and CYP2D6 substrates, as this may lead to increased drug levels and potentially increased toxicity.

DRUG INTERACTION 4

Certain P-gp substrates—Avoid concomitant use of adagrasib with certain P-gp substrates, such as digoxin, verapamil, diltiazem, dabigatran, and fexofenadine.

DRUG INTERACTION 5

Avoid concomitant use of adagrasib with other drugs known to prolong the QTc interval.

SPECIAL CONSIDERATIONS

1. No need for dose reduction in setting of mild to severe hepatic impairment.
2. No need for dose reduction in setting of mild to severe renal impairment. Has not been studied in the setting of end-stage renal disease or in patients on dialysis.
3. Monitor liver function tests every month for the first 3 months of treatment and then as clinically indicated. Need to monitor more frequently in patients who develop hepatotoxicity.
4. Monitor patients for GI symptoms, especially nausea/vomiting and diarrhea.
5. Baseline and periodic evaluations of ECG and electrolyte status should be performed while on therapy. Use with caution in patients at risk of developing QT prolongation, including hypokalemia, hypomagnesemia, congenital long QT syndrome, and in patients taking antiarrhythmic medications or any other drugs that may cause QT prolongation.
6. Monitor patients for pulmonary symptoms. Therapy should be held in patients presenting with new or progressive pulmonary symptoms and should be permanently stopped if treatment-related pneumonitis or interstitial lung disease (ILD) is confirmed.
7. No data currently available on the risk of adagrasib in pregnant women. Breastfeeding should be avoided while on treatment and for 1 week after the last dose.

TOXICITY 1

GI side effects with diarrhea and nausea/vomiting.

TOXICITY 2

Pulmonary toxicity with increased cough, dyspnea, and pulmonary infiltrates. Interstitial lung disease (ILD) and pneumonitis are the more serious events.

TOXICITY 3

Hepatotoxicity with elevations in SGOT/SGPT and serum bilirubin.

TOXICITY 4
Fatigue and anorexia.

TOXICITY 5
QTc prolongation.

TOXICITY 6
Arthralgias and musculoskeletal pain.

Ado-trastuzumab emtansine

MCC linker

DM1

n

Where n ~ 3.5
DM1/Mab

TRADE NAME	Kadcyla, T-DM1	**CLASSIFICATION**	Antibody-drug conjugate
CATEGORY	Biologic response modifier agent/ chemotherapy drug	**DRUG MANUFACTURER**	Genentech/ Roche

MECHANISM OF ACTION
- HER2-targeted antibody-drug conjugate that is made up of trastuzumab and the small-molecule microtubule inhibitor DM1.
- Upon binding to the HER2 receptor, ado-trastuzumab emtansine undergoes receptor-mediated internalization and lysosomal degradation, leading to intracellular release of the DM1 molecule.
- Binding of DM1 to tubulin leads to disruption of the microtubule network, resulting in cell-cycle arrest and apoptosis.
- Inhibits HER2 downstream signaling pathways.
- Immunologic-mediated mechanisms, such as antibody-dependent cell-mediated cytotoxicity (ADCC), may also be involved in antitumor activity.

MECHANISM OF RESISTANCE
- Reduced expression of HER2 receptor.
- Poor internalization of the HER2-T-DM1 complexes.
- Impaired lysosomal proteolytic, activity leading to reduced intracellular levels of the DM1 molecule.
- Defective intracellular and endosomal trafficking of the HER2-T-DM1 complex.
- Increased expression of p95HER2.
- Activation of the neuregulin-HER3 signaling pathway.
- Alterations in tubulin resulting in reduced affinity to DM1.
- Multidrug-resistant phenotype with increased expression of the P170 glycoprotein, leading to enhanced DM1 efflux.

ABSORPTION
Administered only via the intravenous (IV) route.

DISTRIBUTION
Extensive binding (93%) of ado-trastuzumab emtansine to plasma proteins.

METABOLISM
DM1 is metabolized by the liver microsomal enzymes CYP3A4/5. The median terminal half-life of ado-trastuzumab emtansine is on the order of 4 days.

INDICATIONS
1. FDA-approved for patients with HER2-positive metastatic breast cancer who have received prior treatment with trastuzumab and a taxane chemotherapy.
2. FDA-approved for patients with HER2-positive disease who developed recurrence during or within 6 months after completion of adjuvant therapy.
3. FDA-approved for the adjuvant treatment of patients with HER2-positive early breast cancer who have residual disease after neoadjuvant taxane and trastuzumab-based therapy.

DOSAGE RANGE
Recommended dose is 3.6 mg/kg IV every 3 weeks.

DRUG INTERACTIONS
None well characterized to date.

SPECIAL CONSIDERATIONS
1. Ado-trastuzumab emtansine can **NOT** be substituted for or with trastuzumab.
2. Baseline and periodic evaluations of left ventricular ejection fraction (LVEF) should be performed while on therapy. Treatment should be held if the LVEF drops <40% or is between 40% and 45% with a 10% or greater absolute reduction from pretreatment baseline. Therapy should be permanently stopped if the LVEF function has not improved or has declined further. This is a black-box warning.

3. Monitor LFTs and serum bilirubin levels closely, as serious hepatotoxicity has been observed. This is a black-box warning.
4. Monitor for infusion-related reactions, especially during the first infusion.
5. Monitor patients for pulmonary symptoms. Therapy should be held in patients presenting with new or progressive pulmonary symptoms and should be terminated in patients diagnosed with treatment-related pneumonitis or interstitial lung disease (ILD).
6. Monitor CBC and specifically platelet counts.
7. HER2 testing using an FDA-approved diagnostic test to confirm the presence of HER2 protein overexpression or gene amplification is required for determining which patients should receive ado-trastuzumab emtansine therapy.
8. No dose adjustment is recommended for patients with mild or moderate hepatic dysfunction. Use with caution in patients with severe hepatic dysfunction as the drug has not been studied in this setting.
9. No dose adjustment is recommended for patients with mild or moderate renal dysfunction. Use with caution in patients with severe renal dysfunction, as there is only very limited information about the drug in this setting.
10. Embryo-fetal toxicity. Breastfeeding should be avoided.

TOXICITY 1
Cardiac toxicity with cardiomyopathy.

TOXICITY 2
Infusion-related reactions.

TOXICITY 3
Hepatotoxicity with transient elevations in LFTs. Severe drug-induced liver injury and hepatic encephalopathy have been reported rarely. Rare cases of nodular regenerative hyperplasia of the liver have also been reported.

TOXICITY 4
Myelosuppression with thrombocytopenia.

TOXICITY 5
Pulmonary toxicity presenting as cough, dyspnea, and infiltrates. Observed rarely in about 1% of patients.

TOXICITY 6
Neurotoxicity with peripheral sensory neuropathy.

TOXICITY 7
Asthenia, fatigue, and pyrexia.

Afatinib

TRADE NAME	Gilotrif	CLASSIFICATION	Signal transduction inhibitor, pan-ErB inhibitor
CATEGORY	Targeted agent	DRUG MANUFACTURER	Boehringer Ingelheim

MECHANISM OF ACTION
- Potent and selective small-molecule inhibitor of the kinase domains of EGFR, HER2, and HER4, resulting in inhibition of autophosphorylation and inhibition of downstream ErbB signaling.
- Inhibition of the ErbB tyrosine kinases results in inhibition of critical mitogenic and antiapoptotic signals involved in proliferation, growth, invasion/metastasis, angiogenesis, and response to chemotherapy and/or radiation therapy.

MECHANISM OF RESISTANCE
- Mutations in ErbB tyrosine kinases leading to decreased binding affinity to afatinib.
- Presence of KRAS mutations.
- Presence of BRAF mutations.
- Activation/induction of alternative cellular signaling pathways such as PI3K/Akt, IGF-1R, and c-Met.
- Increased expression/activation of mTORC1 signaling pathway.

ABSORPTION
Oral bioavailability is on the order of 92%. Peak plasma drug levels are achieved in 2–5 hours after ingestion.

DISTRIBUTION
Extensive binding (95%) to plasma proteins. Steady-state drug levels are reached in approximately 8 days.

METABOLISM

Metabolism in the liver primarily by CYP3A4 microsomal enzymes. Elimination is mainly hepatic (85%), with excretion in the feces. Renal elimination of parent drug and its metabolites accounts for only about 4% of an administered dose. The terminal half-life of the parent drug is 37 hours.

INDICATIONS

1. FDA-approved as first-line treatment of metastatic non–small cell lung cancer (NSCLC) with EGFR exon 19 deletion or exon 21 (L858R) substitution mutations as detected by an FDA-approved test.
2. FDA-approved for metastatic, squamous NSCLC progressing after platinum-based chemotherapy.

DOSAGE RANGE

Recommended dose is 40 mg/day PO.

DRUG INTERACTION 1

Phenytoin and other drugs that stimulate the liver microsomal CYP3A4 enzymes, including carbamazepine, rifampin, phenobarbital, and St. John's Wort—These drugs may increase the metabolism of afatinib, resulting in its inactivation and lower effective drug levels.

DRUG INTERACTION 2

Drugs that inhibit the liver microsomal CYP3A4 enzymes, including ketoconazole, itraconazole, erythromycin, and clarithromycin—These drugs may decrease the metabolism of afatinib, resulting in increased drug levels and potentially increased toxicity.

DRUG INTERACTION 3

Warfarin—Patients receiving warfarin should be closely monitored for alterations in their clotting parameters (PT and INR) and/or bleeding, as afatinib may inhibit the metabolism of warfarin by the liver P450 system. Dose of warfarin may require careful adjustment in the presence of afatinib therapy.

SPECIAL CONSIDERATIONS

1. Dose reduction is not recommended in patients with mild or moderate hepatic impairment. Has not been studied in patients with severe hepatic dysfunction and should be used with caution in this setting.
2. Monitor patients for new or progressive pulmonary symptoms, including cough, dyspnea, and fever. Afatinib therapy should be interrupted pending further diagnostic evaluation.
3. In patients who develop a skin rash, topical antibiotics such as Cleocin (clindamycin) gel or erythromycin cream/gel or oral clindamycin, oral doxycycline, or oral minocycline may help.
4. Patients should be warned to avoid sunlight exposure.
5. Monitor patients with a history of keratitis, ulcerative keratitis, or severe dry eye and in those who wear contact lenses.

6. Avoid Seville oranges, starfruit, pomelos, grapefruit, and grapefruit juice while on afatinib therapy.
7. Pregnancy category D. Breastfeeding should be avoided.

TOXICITY 1
Skin toxicity in the form of rash, erythema, and acneiform skin rash occurs in 90% of patients. Pruritus, dry skin, and nail bed changes are also observed. Grade 3 skin toxicity occurs in nearly 20% of patients, with bullous, blistering, and exfoliating lesions occurring rarely.

TOXICITY 2
Diarrhea is the most common GI toxicity. Mild nausea/vomiting and mucositis.

TOXICITY 3
Pulmonary toxicity in the form of ILD manifested by increased cough, dyspnea, fever, and pulmonary infiltrates. Observed in 1.5% of patients, and incidence appears to be higher in Asian patients.

TOXICITY 4
Hepatotoxicity with mild to moderate elevations in serum transaminases. Usually transient and clinically asymptomatic.

TOXICITY 5
Fatigue and anorexia.

TOXICITY 6
Keratitis presenting as acute eye inflammation, lacrimation, light sensitivity, blurred vision, eye pain, and/or red eye.

Albumin-Bound Paclitaxel

TRADE NAME	Abraxane, Nab-paclitaxel	CLASSIFICATION	Taxane, antimicrotubule agent
CATEGORY	Chemotherapy drug	DRUG MANUFACTURER	Celgene

MECHANISM OF ACTION
- Albumin-bound form of paclitaxel with a mean particle size of about 130 nm. Selective binding of albumin-bound paclitaxel to specific albumin receptors present on tumor cells versus normal cells.
- Active moiety is paclitaxel, which is isolated from the bark of the Pacific yew tree, *Taxus brevifolia*.

- Cell cycle specific, active in the mitosis (M) phase of the cell cycle.
- High-affinity binding to microtubules enhances tubulin polymerization. Normal dynamic process of microtubule network is inhibited, leading to inhibition of mitosis and cell division.

MECHANISM OF RESISTANCE
- Alterations in tubulin with decreased binding affinity for drug.
- Multidrug-resistant phenotype with increased expression of P170 glycoprotein. Results in enhanced drug efflux with decreased intracellular accumulation of drug. Cross-resistant to other natural products, including vinca alkaloids, anthracyclines, taxanes, and etoposide.

ABSORPTION
Administered only via the IV route.

DISTRIBUTION
Distributes widely to all body tissues. Extensive binding (<90%) to plasma and cellular proteins.

METABOLISM
Metabolized extensively by the hepatic P450 microsomal system. About 20% of the drug is excreted via fecal elimination. Less than 10% is eliminated as the parent form, with the majority being eliminated as metabolites. Renal clearance is relatively minor, with less than 1% of the drug cleared via the kidneys. The clearance of nab-paclitaxel is 43% greater than paclitaxel, and the volume of distribution is about 50% higher than paclitaxel. Terminal elimination half-life is on the order of 27 hours.

INDICATIONS
1. FDA-approved for the treatment of breast cancer after failure of combination chemotherapy for metastatic disease or relapse within 6 months of adjuvant chemotherapy.
2. FDA-approved for the treatment of locally advanced or metastatic NSCLC, in combination with carboplatin, in patients who are not candidates for curative surgery or radiation therapy.
3. FDA-approved for the treatment of locally advanced or metastatic pancreatic cancer in combination with gemcitabine.

DOSAGE RANGE
1. Recommended dose for metastatic breast cancer is 260 mg/m^2 IV on day 1 every 21 days.
2. An alternative regimen is a weekly schedule of 125 mg/m^2 IV on days 1, 8, and 15 every 28 days.
3. Recommended dose for NSCLC is 100 mg/m^2 IV on days 1, 8, and 15 every 21 days.
4. Recommended dose for pancreatic cancer is 125 mg/m^2 IV on days 1, 8, and 15 every 28 days.

DRUG INTERACTIONS
None well characterized to date.

SPECIAL CONSIDERATIONS
1. Contraindicated in patients with baseline neutrophil counts <1,500 cells/mm^3.
2. Monitor CBCs on a periodic basis.
3. Has not been studied in patients with renal dysfunction.
4. Use with caution in patients with abnormal liver function, as patients with abnormal liver function may be at higher risk for toxicity. The drug should **NOT** be given to patients with metastatic pancreatic cancer who have moderate to severe liver dysfunction. For diseases other than metastatic pancreatic cancer, dose reduction is recommended in patients with moderate or severe hepatic dysfunction.
5. In contrast to paclitaxel, no premedication is required to prevent hypersensitivity reactions prior to administration of the drug.
6. Abraxane can **NOT** be substituted for or with other paclitaxel formulations, as the albumin form of paclitaxel may significantly alter the drug's clinical activity.
7. Closely monitor infusion site for infiltration during drug administration, as injection site reactions have been observed.
8. Use with caution when administering with known substrates or inhibitors of CYP2C8 and CYP3A4.
9. Pregnancy category D. Breastfeeding should be avoided.

TOXICITY 1
Myelosuppression with dose-limiting neutropenia and anemia. Thrombocytopenia relatively uncommon.

TOXICITY 2
Neurotoxicity mainly in the form of sensory neuropathy with numbness and paresthesias. Dose-dependent effect. In contrast to paclitaxel, Abraxane-mediated neuropathy appears to be more readily reversible.

TOXICITY 3
Ocular and visual disturbances seen in 13% of patients, with severe cases seen in 1%.

TOXICITY 4
Asthenia, fatigue, and weakness.

TOXICITY 5
Alopecia with loss of total body hair.

TOXICITY 6
Nausea/vomiting, diarrhea, and mucositis are the main GI toxicities. Mucositis is generally mild (seen in less than 10%). Mild-to-moderate nausea and vomiting, usually of brief duration.

TOXICITY 7
Transient elevations in serum transaminases, bilirubin, and alkaline phosphatase.

TOXICITY 8
Cardiac toxicity with chest pain, supraventricular tachycardia, hypertension, pulmonary embolus, peripheral edema, and rare cases of cardiac arrest.

Aldesleukin

TRADE NAME	Interleukin-2, IL-2, Proleukin	CLASSIFICATION	Immunotherapy, cytokine
CATEGORY	Biologic response modifier agent	DRUG MANUFACTURER	Prometheus

MECHANISM OF ACTION
- Glycoprotein cytokine that functions as a T-cell growth factor.
- Biologic effect of interleukin-2 (IL-2) is mediated by specific binding to the interleukin-2 receptor (IL-2R).
- Precise mechanism by which IL-2 mediates its anticancer activity remains unknown but appears to require an intact immune system.
- Enhances lymphocyte mitogenesis and lymphocyte cytotoxicity.
- Induces lymphokine-activated killer (LAK) and natural killer (NK) cell activity.
- Induces interferon-γ production.

MECHANISM OF RESISTANCE
- Up to 75% of patients may develop anti–IL-2 antibodies.
- Increased expression of counter-regulatory factors, such as glucocorticoids, which act to reduce the efficacy of interleukin-2.

ABSORPTION
Administered only via the parenteral route. Peak plasma levels are achieved in 5 hours after subcutaneous (SC) administration.

DISTRIBUTION
After short IV infusion, high plasma concentrations of IL-2 are achieved followed by rapid distribution into the extravascular space.

METABOLISM
IL-2 is catabolized to amino acids. The major route of elimination is through the kidneys by both glomerular filtration and tubular secretion. The elimination half-life is 85 minutes.

INDICATIONS
1. Metastatic renal cell cancer.
2. Metastatic malignant melanoma.

DOSAGE RANGE
Renal cell cancer—600,000 IU/kg IV every 8 hours for a maximum of 14 doses. Following 9 days of rest, the schedule is repeated for another 14 doses, for a maximum of 28 doses per course.

DRUG INTERACTION 1
Corticosteroids—May decrease the antitumor efficacy of IL-2 due to its inhibitory effect on the immune system.

DRUG INTERACTION 2
Nonsteroidal anti-inflammatory drugs (NSAIDs)—May enhance the capillary leak syndrome observed with IL-2.

DRUG INTERACTION 3
Antihypertensives—IL-2 potentiates the effect of antihypertensive medications. For this reason, all antihypertensives should be stopped at least 24 hours before IL-2 treatment.

SPECIAL CONSIDERATIONS
1. Use with caution in patients with pre-existing cardiac, pulmonary, central nervous system (CNS), hepatic, and/or renal impairment, as there is an increased risk for developing serious and sometimes fatal reactions.
2. Pretreatment evaluation should include CBC; serum chemistries, including LFTs, renal function, and electrolytes; pulmonary function tests (PFTs); and stress thallium.
3. Patients should be monitored closely throughout the entire treatment, including vital signs every 2–4 hours, strict input and output, and daily weights. Continuous cardiopulmonary monitoring is important during therapy.
4. Monitor for capillary leak syndrome (CLS), which begins almost immediately after initiation of therapy. Manifested by hypotension, peripheral edema, ascites, pleural and/or pericardial effusions, weight gain, and altered mental status.
5. Early administration of dopamine (1–5 mg/kg/min) in the setting of CLS may maintain perfusion to the kidneys and preserve renal function.
6. Use with caution in the presence of concurrent medications known to be nephrotoxic and hepatotoxic, as IL-2 therapy is associated with both nephrotoxicity and hepatotoxicity.
7. Use with caution in patients with known autoimmune disease, as treatment with IL-2 is associated with autoimmune thyroiditis, leading to thyroid function impairment.
8. Allergic reactions have been reported in patients receiving iodine contrast media up to 4 months following IL-2 therapy.
9. Pregnancy category C. Breastfeeding should be avoided.

TOXICITY 1
Flu-like symptoms, including fever, chills, malaise, myalgias, and arthralgias.

TOXICITY 2
Vascular leak syndrome. Usual dose-limiting toxicity, characterized by weight gain, arrhythmias, tachycardia, hypotension, edema, oliguria and renal insufficiency, pleural effusion, and pulmonary congestion.

TOXICITY 3
Myelosuppression with anemia, thrombocytopenia, and neutropenia.

TOXICITY 4
Hepatotoxicity presenting as increases in serum bilirubin levels along with changes in serum transaminases. Usually reversible within 4–6 days after discontinuation of IL-2 therapy.

TOXICITY 5
Neurologic and neuropsychiatric findings can develop both acutely and chronically during treatment. Somnolence, delirium, and confusion are common but generally resolve after drug termination. Alterations in cognitive function and impaired memory more common with continuous-infusion IL-2.

TOXICITY 6
Erythema, skin rash, urticaria, and generalized erythroderma may occur within a few days of starting therapy.

TOXICITY 7
Alterations in thyroid function, including hyperthyroidism and hypothyroidism.

Alectinib

TRADE NAME	Alecensa	CLASSIFICATION	Signal transduction inhibitor, ALK inhibitor
CATEGORY	Targeted agent	DRUG MANUFACTURER	Genentech/Roche

MECHANISM OF ACTION
- Inhibits multiple receptor tyrosine kinases (RTKs), including anaplastic lymphoma kinase (ALK) and RET, which leads to inhibition of downstream signaling proteins, such as STAT3 and Akt.
- Pre-clinical studies show that it inhibits tumor cell lines that have ALK fusions, amplifications, or activating mutations. Major active metabolite of alectinib is M4, which displays similar in vitro potency and activity as the parent drug.
- Retains activity in NSCLC tumors resistant to crizotinib.

MECHANISM OF RESISTANCE
- Development of ALK mutations, including V1180L gatekeeper mutation, and I1171T and I1171N mutations. These mutations result in reduced binding of alectinib to the ALK fusion protein.
- Amplification of the MET gene, resulting in activation of the hepatocyte growth factor (HGF)-MET signaling pathway.
- Increased activation of the neuregulin 1 (NRG1)-HER3-EGFR signaling axis.

ABSORPTION
Rapidly absorbed after an oral dose, with peak plasma levels achieved within 4 hours. Absolute oral bioavailability is approximately 37%. Food with high fat content can significantly increase drug concentrations by up to threefold.

DISTRIBUTION
Extensive binding of alectinib and M4 metabolite (>99%) to plasma proteins.

METABOLISM
Metabolized in the liver primarily by CYP3A4 microsomal enzymes, with formation of the major active metabolite M4. Elimination is mainly hepatic, with excretion in feces (98%), with 84% as unchanged parent drug and 6% as M4 metabolite. Renal elimination is relatively minor, with <0.5% of an administered dose being recovered in the urine. Steady-state drug levels of parent alectinib and the M4 metabolite are achieved in approximately 7 days. The terminal half-life of alectinib is approximately 33 hours and 31 hours for the M4 metabolite.

INDICATIONS
FDA-approved for the treatment of patients with ALK-positive metastatic NSCLC who have progressed on or are intolerant to crizotinib as detected by an FDA-approved test.

DOSAGE RANGE
Recommended dose is 600 mg PO daily with food.

DRUG INTERACTION 1
Drugs such as ketoconazole, itraconazole, erythromycin, clarithromycin, atazanavir, indinavir, nefazodone, nelfinavir, ritonavir, saquinavir, telithromycin, and voriconazole may decrease the metabolism of alectinib, resulting in increased drug levels and potentially increased toxicity.

DRUG INTERACTION 2
Drugs such as rifampin, phenytoin, phenobarbital, carbamazepine, and St. John's Wort may increase the metabolism of alectinib, resulting in its inactivation and lower effective drug levels.

SPECIAL CONSIDERATIONS
1. No dose adjustment is needed for patients with mild hepatic dysfunction. The drug has not been evaluated in patients with moderate or severe hepatic dysfunction.
2. No dose reduction is needed for patients with mild or moderate renal dysfunction. The drug has not been evaluated in patients with severe renal dysfunction or end-stage renal disease.
3. Patients receiving alectinib along with oral warfarin anticoagulant therapy should have their coagulation parameters (PT and INR) monitored frequently.
4. Monitor LFTs and serum bilirubin every 2 weeks for the first 2 months of treatment and then periodically, as alectinib may cause hepatotoxicity. More frequent testing is required in patients who develop LFT elevations. May need to suspend, dose-reduce, or permanently stop alectinib with the development of drug-induced hepatotoxicity.
5. Monitor patients for new or progressive pulmonary symptoms, including cough, dyspnea, and fever.
6. Monitor hemodynamic status with heart rate and blood pressure.
7. Monitor creatine phosphokinase (CPK) levels every 2 weeks during the first month of treatment and in patients with unexplained muscle pain, tenderness, or weakness.
8. ALK testing using an FDA-approved test is required to confirm the presence of ALK-positive NSCLC for determining which patients should receive alectinib therapy.
9. Pregnancy category D. Breastfeeding should be avoided.

TOXICITY 1
Hepatotoxicity with elevations in serum transaminases (SGOT, SGPT).

TOXICITY 2
Nausea/vomiting, constipation, diarrhea, and abdominal pain are the most common GI side effects.

TOXICITY 3
Pulmonary toxicity with increased cough, dyspnea, fever, and pulmonary infiltrates.

TOXICITY 4
Constitutional side effects with fatigue, asthenia, and anorexia.

TOXICITY 5
Bradycardia.

TOXICITY 6
Myalgia or musculoskeletal pain with CPK elevation.

TOXICITY 7
Skin rash.

Alemtuzumab

TRADE NAME	Campath	**CLASSIFICATION**	Anti-CD52 monoclonal antibody
CATEGORY	Biologic response modifier agent	**DRUG MANUFACTURER**	Genzyme

MECHANISM OF ACTION
- Recombinant humanized monoclonal antibody (Campath-1H) directed against the 21- to 28-kDa cell-surface glycoprotein CD52 that is expressed on most normal and malignant B and T lymphocytes, NK cells, monocytes, and macrophages.
- CD52 antigen is not expressed on the surface of hematopoietic stem cells and mature plasma cells.
- Immunologic mechanisms involved in antitumor activity, including ADCC and/or complement-mediated cell lysis.

MECHANISM OF RESISTANCE
None well characterized to date.

ABSORPTION
Administered only via the IV route.

DISTRIBUTION
Peak and trough levels rise during the first few weeks of therapy and approach steady-state levels by week 6. However, there is marked variability, and drug levels correlate roughly with the number of circulating CD52+ B cells.

METABOLISM
Metabolism has not been extensively characterized. Half-life is on the order of 12 days, with minimal clearance by the liver and kidneys.

INDICATIONS

1. Relapsed and/or refractory B-cell chronic lymphocytic leukemia (B-CLL)—Indicated in patients who have been treated with alkylating agents and who have failed fludarabine therapy.
2. T-cell prolymphocytic leukemia—Clinical activity in patients who failed first-line therapy.

DOSAGE RANGE

Recommended dose is 30 mg/day IV three times per week for a maximum of 12 weeks.

DRUG INTERACTIONS

None well characterized to date.

SPECIAL CONSIDERATIONS

1. Contraindicated in patients with active systemic infections, underlying immunodeficiency (HIV-positive, AIDS, etc.), or known type I hypersensitivity or anaphylactic reactions to alemtuzumab or any of its components.
2. Patients should be premedicated with acetaminophen, 650 mg PO, and diphenhydramine, 50 mg PO, 30 minutes before drug infusion to reduce the incidence of infusion-related reactions.
3. Alemtuzumab should be initiated at a dose of 3 mg, administered daily as a 2-hour IV infusion. When this daily dose of 3 mg is tolerated, the daily dose can then be increased to 10 mg. Once the 10-mg daily dose is tolerated, a maintenance dose of 30 mg daily can then be initiated. This maintenance dose of 30 mg/day is administered three times each week on alternate days (Monday, Wednesday, and Friday) for a maximum of 12 weeks. Dose escalation to the 30-mg daily dose usually can be accomplished within 7 days. Alemtuzumab should **NOT** be given by IV push or bolus.
4. Monitor closely for infusion-related events, which usually occur within the first 30–60 minutes after the start of the infusion and most commonly during the first week of therapy. Pulse, blood pressure, and oral temperature should be measured every 15–30 minutes. Immediate institution of diphenhydramine (50 mg IV), acetaminophen (625 mg PO), hydrocortisone (200 mg IV), and/or vasopressors may be required. Resuscitation equipment should be readily available at bedside.
5. Patients should be placed on anti-infective prophylaxis upon initiation of therapy to reduce the risk of serious opportunistic infections. This should include Bactrim DS, 1 tablet PO bid three times per week, and famciclovir or equivalent, 250 mg PO bid. Fluconazole may also be included in the regimen to reduce the incidence of fungal infections. If a serious infection occurs while on therapy, alemtuzumab should be stopped immediately and only reinitiated following the complete resolution of the underlying infection.
6. Monitor CBC and platelet counts on a weekly basis during alemtuzumab therapy. Treatment should be stopped for severe hematologic toxicity

or in any patient with evidence of autoimmune anemia and/or thrombocytopenia.

7. Most significant antitumor effects of alemtuzumab are observed in peripheral blood, bone marrow, and spleen. Tumor cells usually cleared from blood within 1–2 weeks of initiation of therapy, while normalization in bone marrow may take up to 6–12 weeks. Lymph nodes, especially those that are large and bulky, seem to be less responsive to therapy.

8. Pregnancy category C. Should be given to a pregnant woman only if clearly indicated. Breastfeeding should be avoided during treatment and for at least 3 months following the last dose of drug.

TOXICITY 1

Infusion-related symptoms, including fever, chills, nausea and vomiting, urticaria, skin rash, fatigue, headache, diarrhea, dyspnea, and/or hypotension. Usually occur within the first week of initiation of therapy.

TOXICITY 2

Significant immunosuppression with an increased incidence of opportunistic infections, including Pneumocystis jiroveci (PJP; formerly PCP), cytomegalovirus (CMV), herpes zoster, Candida, Cryptococcus, and Listeria meningitis. Prophylaxis with anti-infective agents is indicated as outlined previously. Recovery of CD4 and CD8 counts is slow and may take over 1 year to return to normal.

TOXICITY 3

Myelosuppression with neutropenia most common, but anemia and thrombocytopenia also observed. In rare instances, pancytopenia with marrow hypoplasia occurs, which can be fatal.

Alpelisib

TRADE NAME	Piqray	CLASSIFICATION	Signal transduction inhibitor, PI3K inhibitor
CATEGORY	Targeted agent	DRUG MANUFACTURER	Novartis

MECHANISM OF ACTION

- Phosphatidylinositol-3-kinase (PI3K) inhibitor with specific activity against the p110α isoform.
- Inhibits several key signaling pathways, including AKT.
- The combination of alpelisib and fulvestrant has enhanced antitumor activity compared to either treatment alone in in vivo models of ER+, PIK3CA mutated breast cancer.

MECHANISM OF RESISTANCE

- Activation of alternative pathways, including MAPK, ER, HER2, AXL, PIM-1, and FOXO transcription factors.
- Signaling via other PI3K isoforms.
- Activation of downstream effectors in PI3K pathway, such as AKT and mTOR.
- Loss of PTEN expression.
- Cross-talk between PI3K and ER pathways.

ABSORPTION

Oral bioavailability is approximately 25%. Peak plasma drug levels are achieved in 2–4 hours after ingestion, and there is no food effect on oral absorption.

DISTRIBUTION

Extensive binding (89%) to plasma proteins. Steady-state drug levels are reached in approximately 3 days.

METABOLISM

Metabolism primarily by chemical and enzymatic hydrolysis to form the BZG791 metabolite. Also metabolized by CYP3A4 but to a lesser extent. Elimination is mainly hepatic (81%), with excretion in the feces. Renal elimination accounts for 14% of an administered dose. Approximately 36% of an administered dose is eliminated in feces as unchanged parent form, and 32% is eliminated as the BZG791 metabolite. The terminal half-life of the parent drug is 8–9 hours.

INDICATIONS

FDA-approved in combination with fulvestrant for post-menopausal women and men with HR-positive, HER2-negative, PIK3CA-mutated, advanced, or metastatic breast cancer as detected by an FDA-approved test following progression on or after an endocrine-based regimen.

DOSAGE RANGE

Recommended dose is 300 mg PO once daily.

DRUG INTERACTION 1

Phenytoin and other drugs that stimulate the liver microsomal CYP3A4 enzymes, including carbamazepine, rifampin, phenobarbital, and St. John's Wort—These drugs may increase the metabolism of alpelisib, resulting in lower effective drug levels.

DRUG INTERACTION 2

Drugs that inhibit the liver microsomal CYP3A4 enzymes, including ketoconazole, itraconazole, erythromycin, and clarithromycin—These drugs may decrease the metabolism of alpelisib, resulting in increased drug levels and potentially increased toxicity.

DRUG INTERACTION 3

Warfarin—Patients receiving warfarin should be closely monitored for alterations in their clotting parameters (PT and INR) and/or bleeding, as alpelisib may inhibit warfarin metabolism by the liver P450 system. Dose of warfarin may require careful adjustment in the presence of alpelisib therapy.

SPECIAL CONSIDERATIONS

1. Dose reduction is not required in the setting of mild to severe hepatic impairment (Child-Pugh Class A, B, and C).
2. Dose reduction is not required in the setting of mild or moderate renal impairment. Has not been studied in the setting of severe renal impairment, in end-stage renal disease, or in patients on dialysis.
3. Monitor for signs and symptoms of severe hypersensitivity reactions. Drug therapy should be permanently discontinued in the event of severe hypersensitivity.
4. Monitor blood glucose levels at least once per week for the first 8 weeks of treatment, followed by once every 2 weeks, and then as clinically indicated. Patients with diabetes mellitus should have their blood glucose levels under control before starting therapy.
5. Patients should be educated on the signs and symptoms of severe skin reactions. Patients with a prior history of Stevens-Johnson syndrome, erythema multiforme, or toxic epidermal necrolysis should not be treated with alpelisib.
6. Monitor patients for diarrhea and any symptoms of colitis, including abdominal pain or blood in stool. Patients should start on anti-diarrheal medication, increase oral fluid intake, and notify their physician if diarrhea should occur while on therapy.
7. Monitor patients for new or worsening respiratory symptoms. Therapy should be discontinued in any patient with confirmed pneumonitis.
8. May cause fetal harm when administered to a pregnant woman. Breastfeeding should be avoided.

TOXICITY 1

Hyperglycemia.

TOXICITY 2

Hypersensitivity reactions with dyspnea, flushing, rash, fever, or tachycardia. Anaphylaxis and anaphylactic shock have been observed.

TOXICITY 3

Maculopapular skin rash and more serious reactions, including Stevens-Johnson syndrome, erythema multiforme, and toxic epidermal necrolysis.

TOXICITY 4
Non-infectious pneumonitis with cough, dyspnea, pulmonary infiltrates, and hypoxia.

TOXICITY 5
Diarrhea, nausea/vomiting, and mucositis.

TOXICITY 6
Fatigue, asthenia, and anorexia.

TOXICITY 7
Skin reactions, including maculopapular rash, pruritus, and exfoliative rash.

Altretamine

TRADE NAME	Hexalen, Hexamethylmelamine, HMM	CLASSIFICATION	Nonclassic alkylating agent
CATEGORY	Chemotherapy drug	DRUG MANUFACTURER	MGI Pharma

MECHANISM OF ACTION
- Triazine derivative that requires biochemical activation in the liver for its antitumor activity.
- Exact mechanism(s) of action unclear but appears to act like an alkylating agent. Forms cross-links with DNA, resulting in inhibition of DNA synthesis and function.
- May also inhibit RNA synthesis.

MECHANISM OF RESISTANCE
- Mechanisms of resistance have not been well characterized.
- Does not exhibit cross-resistance to other classic alkylating agents and does not exhibit multidrug-resistant phenotype.

ABSORPTION

Oral absorption is extremely variable secondary to extensive first-pass metabolism in the liver. Peak plasma levels are achieved 0.5–3 hours after an oral dose.

DISTRIBUTION

Widely distributed throughout the body, with highest concentrations found in tissues with high fat content. About 90% of drug is bound to plasma proteins.

METABOLISM

Extensively metabolized in the liver by the microsomal P450 system. Less than 1% of parent compound is excreted in urine. About 60% of drug is eliminated in urine as demethylated metabolites (pentamethylmelamine and tetramethylmelamine) within the first 24 hours. The terminal elimination half-life is on the order of 4–10 hours.

INDICATIONS

Ovarian cancer—Active in advanced disease and in persistent and/or recurrent tumors following first-line therapy with a cisplatin- and/or alkylating agent–based regimen.

DOSAGE RANGE

Usual dose is 260 mg/m^2/day PO for either 14 or 21 days on a 28-day schedule. Total daily dose is given in four divided doses after meals and at bedtime.

DRUG INTERACTION 1

Cimetidine—Cimetidine increases the half-life and subsequent toxicity of altretamine. In contrast, ranitidine does not affect drug metabolism.

DRUG INTERACTION 2

Phenobarbital—Phenobarbital may decrease the half-life and toxicity of altretamine.

DRUG INTERACTION 3

Monoamine oxidase (MAO) inhibitors—Concurrent use of MAO inhibitors with altretamine may result in significant orthostatic hypotension.

SPECIAL CONSIDERATIONS

1. Closely monitor patient for signs of neurologic toxicity.
2. Vitamin B6 (pyridoxine) may be used to decrease the incidence and severity of neurologic toxicity. However, antitumor activity may be compromised with vitamin B6 treatment.
3. Pregnancy category D. Breastfeeding should be avoided.

TOXICITY 1

Nausea and vomiting. Usually mild to moderate, observed in 30% of patients, and worsens with increasing cumulative doses of drug.

TOXICITY 2
Myelosuppression. Dose-limiting toxicity. Leukocyte and platelet nadirs occur at 3–4 weeks, with recovery by day 28. Anemia occurs in 20% of patients.

TOXICITY 3
Neurotoxicity in the form of somnolence, mood changes, lethargy, depression, agitation, hallucinations, and peripheral neuropathy. Observed in about 25% of patients.

TOXICITY 4
Hypersensitivity skin rash.

TOXICITY 5
Elevations in LFTs, mainly alkaline phosphatase.

TOXICITY 6
Flu-like syndrome in the form of fever, malaise, arthralgias, and myalgias.

TOXICITY 7
Abdominal cramps and diarrhea are occasionally observed.

Aminoglutethimide

TRADE NAME	Cytadren	CLASSIFICATION	Adrenal steroid inhibitor
CATEGORY	Hormonal agent	DRUG MANUFACTURER	Novartis

MECHANISM OF ACTION
- Nonsteroidal inhibitor of corticosteroid biosynthesis.
- Produces a chemical adrenalectomy with a decreased synthesis of estrogens, androgens, glucocorticoids, and mineralocorticoids.

ABSORPTION
Excellent bioavailability via the oral route. Peak plasma concentrations occur within 1–1.5 hours after ingestion.

DISTRIBUTION
Approximately 25% of the drug is bound to plasma proteins. Significant reduction in distribution with prolonged treatment.

METABOLISM
Metabolized in the liver by the cytochrome P450 system, with N-acetylaminoglutethimide being the major metabolite. Metabolism is under genetic control, and acetylator status of patients is important. About 40%–50% of the drug is excreted unchanged in the urine. Initial half-life of drug is about 13 hours but decreases to 7 hours with chronic treatment, suggesting that the drug may accelerate its own rate of degradation.

INDICATIONS
1. Breast cancer—Hormone-responsive, advanced disease.
2. Prostate cancer—Hormone-responsive, advanced disease.

DOSAGE RANGE
Usual dose is 250 mg PO qid (1,000 mg total).

DRUG INTERACTION 1
Warfarin, phenytoin, phenobarbital, theophylline, medroxyprogesterone, and digoxin—Aminoglutethimide enhances the metabolism of warfarin, phenytoin, phenobarbital, theophylline, medroxyprogesterone, and digoxin, thereby decreasing their clinical activity.

DRUG INTERACTION 2
Dexamethasone—Aminoglutethimide enhances the metabolism of dexamethasone but not hydrocortisone.

SPECIAL CONSIDERATIONS
1. Administer hydrocortisone along with aminoglutethimide to prevent adrenal insufficiency. The use of higher doses during the initial 2 weeks of therapy reduces the frequency of adverse events. For example, start at 100 mg PO daily for the first 2 weeks, then 40 mg PO daily in divided doses. Higher doses of steroid replacement may be required under conditions of stress, such as surgery, trauma, or acute infection.
2. Closely monitor patient for signs and symptoms of hypothyroidism. Monitor thyroid function tests on a regular basis.
3. Monitor for signs and symptoms of orthostatic hypotension. May need to add fludrocortisone (Florinef) 0.1–0.2 mg PO qd.
4. Monitor patient for signs of somnolence and lethargy. Severe cases may warrant immediate discontinuation of drug.
5. Discontinue drug if skin rash persists for more than 1 week.
6. Pregnancy category D. Breastfeeding should be avoided.

TOXICITY 1
Maculopapular skin rash. Usually seen in the first week of therapy. Self-limited, with resolution in 5–7 days, and discontinuation of therapy not necessary.

TOXICITY 2
Fatigue, lethargy, and somnolence. Occur in 40% of patients, and onset is within the first week of therapy. Dizziness, nystagmus, and ataxia are less common (10% of patients).

TOXICITY 3
Mild nausea and vomiting.

TOXICITY 4
Hypothyroidism.

TOXICITY 5
Adrenal insufficiency. Occurs in the absence of hydrocortisone replacement. Presents as postural hypotension, hyponatremia, and hyperkalemia.

TOXICITY 6
Myelosuppression. Leukopenia and thrombocytopenia rarely occur.

Amivantamab-vmjw

TRADE NAME	Rybrevant, JNJ-61186372	CLASSIFICATION	Anti-EGFR-MET bispecific monoclonal antibody
CATEGORY	Targeted agent	DRUG MANUFACTURER	Janssen, Johnson & Johnson

MECHANISM OF ACTION
- IgG1 bispecific monoclonal antibody directed against the EGFR and MET receptors. The antibody binds to cells that highly express both receptors, which is a feature of tumor tissue and not normal tissue.
- Inhibitory activity in activating and resistant EGFR mutations, MET mutations, and MET gene amplification.
- First molecule to show inhibitory activity in NSLC with EGFR exon 20 insertion mutations.
- Inhibition of the EGFR and MET signaling pathway results in inhibition of critical mitogenic and anti-apoptotic signals involved in proliferation, growth, invasion/metastasis, and angiogenesis.

- Antibody treatment also associated with receptor downregulation through receptor internalization and lysosomal degradation.
- Modified Fc region engineered to increase affinity for the activating Fcγ receptor CD16A (FCγRIIIa) on immune cells. This engineered antibody can then mediate immunologic-mediated functions, including antibody-dependent cellular cytotoxicity (ADCC) and/or complement-mediated cytotoxicity (CDC).
- Other immunologic-mediated mechanisms that are activated include antibody-dependent cellular phagocytosis (ADCP) and antibody-dependent cellular trogocytosis (ADCT), the latter process being mediated by monocytes and macrophages.

MECHANISM OF RESISTANCE
- Increased expression of Shc 1 and Gab 1.
- Increased activation and expression of Src family kinases.
- Activation/induction of downstream cellular signaling pathways, such as PI3K/Akt and MAPK.

ABSORPTION
Administered only via the IV route.

DISTRIBUTION
Distribution in the body is not well characterized.

METABOLISM
Metabolism of amivantamab has not been extensively characterized. Half-life is on the order of 11 days.

INDICATIONS
FDA-approved for the treatment of locally advanced or metastatic non-small cell lung cancer (NSCLC) with epidermal growth factor receptor (EGFR) exon 20 insertion mutations.

DOSAGE RANGE
Recommended dose for patients with body weight <80 kg is 1,050 mg IV to be given as a split infusion in Week 1 on Days 1 and 2 on a weekly schedule for 4 weeks and then every 2 weeks thereafter.

Recommended dose for patients with body weight >80 mg is 1,400 mg IV to be given as a split infusion in Week 1 on Days 1 and 2 on a weekly schedule for 4 weeks and then every 2 weeks thereafter.

DRUG INTERACTIONS
No formal drug interactions have been characterized to date.

SPECIAL CONSIDERATIONS
1. Carefully monitor for infusion-related reactions, which are most frequently seen with the first infusion. The infusion rate should be reduced or permanently discontinued based on the severity of the

infusion reaction. Premedication with antihistamines (diphenhydramine), antipyretics (acetaminophen), and glucocorticoids (dexamethasone or methylprednisolone) can prevent and/or reduce the severity of the infusion reaction.

2. Monitor patients for pulmonary symptoms. Therapy should be held in patients presenting with new or progressive pulmonary symptoms and should be permanently stopped if treatment-related pneumonitis or interstitial lung disease (ILD) is confirmed.

3. Patients should be instructed to limit sun exposure and to use broad-spectrum sunscreen and protective clothing during and for 2 months after completion of treatment.

4. Topical corticosteroids as well as topical and/or oral antibiotics should be considered in patients who develop a skin rash.

5. Monitor patients for new eye symptoms and promptly refer to an opthalmologist.

6. Embryo-fetal toxicity. Females of reproductive potential should use effective contraception during drug therapy and for 3 months after the final dose. Breastfeeding should be avoided.

TOXICITY 1
Acneiform skin rash, dry skin, and pruritus.

TOXICITY 2
Infusion-related symptoms with fever, chills, urticaria, flushing, and headache.

TOXICITY 3
Pulmonary toxicity with increased cough, dyspnea, and pulmonary infiltrates. Interstitial lung disease (ILD) and pneumonitis are more serious events.

TOXICITY 4
Ocular toxicity with keratitis, dry eye, conjunctival redness, blurred vision, and uveitis.

TOXICITY 5
Mild nausea/vomiting and diarrhea.

TOXICITY 6
Fatigue and anorexia.

TOXICITY 7
Paronychial inflammation.

Anastrozole

TRADE NAME	Arimidex	**CLASSIFICATION**	Nonsteroidal aromatase inhibitor
CATEGORY	Hormonal agent	**DRUG MANUFACTURER**	AstraZeneca

MECHANISM OF ACTION
- Potent and selective nonsteroidal inhibitor of aromatase.
- Inhibits the synthesis of estrogens by inhibiting the conversion of adrenal androgens (androstenedione and testosterone) to estrogens (estrone, estrone sulfate, and estradiol). Serum estradiol levels are suppressed by 90% within 14 days and nearly completely suppressed after 6 weeks of therapy.
- No inhibitory effect on adrenal corticosteroid or aldosterone biosynthesis.

MECHANISM OF RESISTANCE
- Decreased expression of estrogen receptors (ER).
- Mutations in ER leading to decreased binding affinity to anastrozole.
- Overexpression of growth factor receptors, such as EGFR, HER2/neu, IGF-1R, or TGF-β, that counteract the inhibitory effects of anastrozole.
- Presence of ESR1 mutations.

ABSORPTION
Excellent bioavailability via the oral route, with 85% of a dose absorbed within 2 hours of ingestion. Absorption is not affected by food.

DISTRIBUTION
Widely distributed throughout the body. About 40% of drug is bound to plasma proteins.

METABOLISM
Extensively metabolized in the liver (up to 85%), by N-dealkylation, hydroxylation, and glucuronidation, to inactive forms. Half-life of drug is about 50 hours. Steady-state levels of drug are achieved after 7 days of a once-daily administration. The major route of elimination is via the hepatobiliary route with excretion in stool, with renal excretion accounting for only 10% of drug clearance.

INDICATIONS

1. Metastatic breast cancer—FDA-approved for the first-line treatment of post-menopausal women with hormone-receptor-positive or hormone-receptor-unknown disease.
2. Metastatic breast cancer—Post-menopausal women with hormone-receptor-positive, advanced disease, and progression while on tamoxifen therapy.
3. Adjuvant treatment of post-menopausal women with hormone-receptor-positive, early-stage breast cancer; FDA-approved.

DOSAGE RANGE

1. Metastatic breast cancer—Recommended dose is 1 mg PO qd for both first- and second-line therapy.
2. Early-stage breast cancer—Recommended dose is 1 mg PO qd for adjuvant therapy. The optimal duration of therapy is unknown. In the ATAC trial, anastrozole was given for 5 years.

DRUG INTERACTIONS

None have been well characterized.

SPECIAL CONSIDERATIONS

1. No dose adjustments are required for patients with either hepatic or renal dysfunction.
2. Caution patients about the risk of hot flashes.
3. No need for glucocorticoid and/or mineralocorticoid replacement.
4. Closely monitor women with osteoporosis or at risk of osteoporosis by performing bone densitometry at the start of therapy and at regular intervals. Treatment or prophylaxis for osteoporosis should be initiated when appropriate.
5. Pregnancy category D. Breastfeeding should be avoided.

TOXICITY 1

Asthenia is most common toxicity and occurs in up to 20% of patients.

TOXICITY 2

Mild nausea and vomiting. Constipation or diarrhea can also occur.

TOXICITY 3

Hot flashes occur in 10% of patients.

TOXICITY 4

Dry, scaling skin rash.

TOXICITY 5

Arthralgias occur in 10%–15% of patients, involving hands, knees, hips, lower back, and shoulders. Early morning stiffness is usual presentation.

TOXICITY 6
Headache.

TOXICITY 7
Peripheral edema in 7% of patients.

TOXICITY 8
Flu-like syndrome in the form of fever, malaise, and myalgias.

Apalutamide

TRADE NAME	Erleada	CLASSIFICATION	Antiandrogen
CATEGORY	Hormonal drug	DRUG MANUFACTURER	Janssen

MECHANISM OF ACTION
- Nonsteroidal antiandrogen agent that binds to androgen receptor (AR) and inhibits AR translocation, inhibits DNA binding, and inhibits AR-mediated transcription.

MECHANISM OF RESISTANCE
- Decreased expression of AR.
- Mutation in AR leading to decreased binding affinity to drug.

ABSORPTION
Well absorbed by the GI tract with 100% bioavailability. Peak plasma levels observed 2 hours after oral administration. Food delays absorption by about 2 hours. Steady-state levels are achieved in 4 weeks.

DISTRIBUTION
Extensively bound to plasma proteins (96%).

METABOLISM
Extensive metabolism occurs in the liver by CYP3A4 and CYP2C8 to form the active metabolite N-desmethyl apalutamide as well as inactive metabolites.

About 65% of an administered dose is eliminated in urine and 24% eliminated in feces. Only a small fraction (1.5–2%) of parent drug and its active metabolite, respectively, are cleared in urine and feces. The elimination half-life is on the order of 3 days.

INDICATIONS
FDA-approved for nonmetastatic castration-resistant prostate cancer.

DOSAGE RANGE
Recommended dose is 240 mg PO once daily, either alone or in combination with a luteinizing hormone–releasing hormone (LHRH) analog.

DRUG INTERACTION 1
Phenytoin and other drugs that stimulate the liver microsomal CYP3A4 enzymes, including carbamazepine, rifampin, phenobarbital, and St. John's Wort—These drugs may increase the metabolism of apalutamide, resulting in reduced drug levels.

DRUG INTERACTION 2
Drugs that inhibit the liver microsomal CYP3A4 enzymes, including ketoconazole, itraconazole, erythromycin, and clarithromycin—These drugs may decrease the metabolism of apalutamide, resulting in increased drug levels and potentially increased toxicity.

SPECIAL CONSIDERATIONS
1. Dose reduction is not required in the setting of mild or moderate hepatic impairment (Child-Pugh Class A or B). Has not been studied in the setting of severe hepatic impairment.
2. Dose reduction is not required in the setting of mild or moderate renal impairment. Has not been studied in the setting of severe renal impairment, in end-stage renal disease, or in patients on dialysis.
3. Monitor patients for fracture and fall risk.
4. Caution patients about the risk for seizures. Apalutamide treatment should be permanently discontinued in patients who develop a seizure while on therapy.
5. Caution patients about the potential for hot flashes. Consider the use of clonidine 0.1–0.2 mg PO daily, megestrol acetate 20 mg PO bid, or soy tablets 1 tablet PO tid for prevention and/or treatment.
6. Instruct patients on the potential risk of altered sexual function and impotence.
7. Pregnancy category D.

TOXICITY 1
Hot flashes, decreased libido, impotence, gynecomastia, nipple pain, and galactorrhea.

TOXICITY 2
Fall and fracture.

TOXICITY 3
Skin rash.

TOXICITY 4
Fatigue and anorexia.

TOXICITY 5
Arthralgias.

Arsenic trioxide (As$_2$O$_3$)

TRADE NAME	Trisenox	CLASSIFICATION	Natural product
CATEGORY	Chemotherapy and differentiating agent	DRUG MANUFACTURER	Cephalon, Teva

MECHANISM OF ACTION
- Precise mechanism of action has not been fully elucidated.
- Induces differentiation of acute promyelocytic leukemic cells by degrading the chimeric PML/RAR-α protein, resulting in release of the maturation block at the promyelocyte stage of myelocyte differentiation.
- Induces apoptosis through a mitochondrial-dependent pathway, resulting in release of cytochrome C and subsequent caspase activation.
- Direct antiproliferative activity by arresting cells at either the G1-S or G2-M checkpoints.
- Inhibits the process of angiogenesis through apoptosis of endothelial cells and/or inhibition of production of critical angiogenic factors, including vascular endothelial growth factor.

MECHANISM OF RESISTANCE
None well characterized to date.

ABSORPTION
Administered only via the IV route.

DISTRIBUTION
Widely distributes in liver, kidneys, heart, lung, hair, nails, and skin.

METABOLISM
The clinical pharmacology of arsenic trioxide has not been well characterized. Metabolism occurs via reduction of pentavalent arsenic to trivalent arsenic and methylation reactions mediated by methyltransferase enzymes that occur primarily in the liver. However, the methyltransferases appear to be distinct from the liver microsomal P450 system. The methylated trivalent arsenic metabolite is excreted mainly in the urine.

INDICATIONS

1. Acute promyelocytic leukemia (APL)—FDA-approved in combination with tretinoin for adults with newly diagnosed low-risk APL whose APL is characterized by the presence of the t(15;17) translocation or PML/RAR-α gene expression.
2. Acute promyelocytic leukemia (APL)—FDA-approved for induction of remission and consolidation in patients with APL who are refractory to or have relapsed following first-line therapy with all-trans retinoic acid (ATRA) and anthracycline-based chemotherapy and whose APL is characterized by the presence of the t(15;17) translocation or PML/RAR-α gene expression.

DOSAGE RANGE

1. Newly diagnosed low-risk APL: treatment course consists of 1 induction cycle and 4 consolidation cycles
   - Induction therapy—0.15 mg/kg/day IV for a maximum of 60 days in combination with tretinoin.
   - Consolidation therapy—0.15 mg/kg/day IV for 5 days/week on weeks 1–4 of an 8-week cycle for a total of 4 cycles in combination with tretinoin.
2. Relapsed or refractory APL: treatment course consists of 1 induction cycle and 1 consolidation cycle
   - Induction therapy—0.15 mg/kg/day IV for a maximum of 60 days.
   - Consolidation therapy—Should be initiated 3–6 weeks after completion of induction treatment and only in those patients who achieve a complete bone marrow remission. The recommended dose is 0.15 mg/kg/day IV for 5 days/week for a total of 5 weeks.

DRUG INTERACTION 1

Medications that can prolong the QT interval, such as antiarrhythmics—Increased risk of prolongation of the QT interval and subsequent arrhythmias when arsenic trioxide is administered concomitantly.

DRUG INTERACTION 2

Amphotericin B—Increased risk of prolonged QT interval and Torsades de Pointes ventricular arrhythmia in patients receiving amphotericin and induction therapy with arsenic trioxide.

SPECIAL CONSIDERATIONS

1. Contraindicated in patients who are hypersensitive to arsenic.
2. Use with caution in patients who are on drugs that prolong the QT interval; in those who have a history of Torsades de Pointes, pre-existing QT interval prolongation, untreated sinus node dysfunction, high-degree atrioventricular block; or in those who may be severely dehydrated or malnourished at baseline.
3. Use with caution in patients with renal impairment, as renal excretion is the main route of elimination of arsenic.
4. Use with caution in patients with severe hepatic impairment, as the drug has not been studied in this setting.

5. Before initiation of therapy, all patients should have a baseline electrocardiogram (ECG) performed, and serum electrolytes, calcium, magnesium, blood urea nitrogen (BUN), and creatinine should be evaluated. Any pre-existing electrolyte abnormalities should be corrected before starting therapy.

6. Serum electrolytes and magnesium should be closely monitored during therapy. Serum potassium concentrations should be maintained above 4 mEq/L and magnesium concentrations above 1.8 mg/dL.

7. Therapy should be stopped when the QT interval >500 milliseconds (msec) and only resumed when the QT interval drops to below 460 msec, all electrolyte abnormalities are corrected, and cardiac monitoring shows no evidence of arrhythmias. This is a black-box warning.

8. Monitor closely for new-onset fever, dyspnea, weight gain, abnormal respiratory symptoms and/or physical findings, or chest x-ray abnormalities because 30% of patients will develop the APL differentiation syndrome. This syndrome can be fatal, and high-dose steroids with dexamethasone 10 mg IV bid should be started immediately and continued for 3–5 days. While this syndrome more commonly occurs with median baseline white blood cell counts of 5,000/mm^3, it can occur in the absence of leukocytosis. In most cases, therapy can be resumed once the syndrome has completely resolved. This is a black-box warning.

9. Prophylaxis with prednisone 0.5 mg/kg daily from Day 1 until the end of induction therapy is recommended to prevent the APL differentiation syndrome.

10. Monitor patients for neurologic symptoms while on therapy. Patients are at risk for developing Wernicke's encephalopathy, which is a neurologic emergency that can be prevented and treated with parenteral thiamine. This is a black-box warning.

11. Monitor CBC every other day and bone marrow cytology every 10 days during induction therapy.

12. Pregnancy category D. Breastfeeding should be avoided, as arsenic is excreted in breast milk.

TOXICITY 1
Fatigue.

TOXICITY 2
Prolonged QT interval (>500 msec) on ECG seen in 40%–50% of patients. Does not usually increase upon repeat exposure to arsenic trioxide, and QT interval returns to baseline following termination of therapy. Torsades de Pointes ventricular arrhythmia and/or complete AV block can be observed.

TOXICITY 3
APL differentiation syndrome. Occurs in about 30% of patients and is characterized by fever, dyspnea, skin rash, fluid retention and weight gain, and pleural and/or pericardial effusions. This syndrome is identical to the retinoic acid syndrome observed with retinoid therapy.

TOXICITY 4

Leukocytosis is observed in 50%–60% of patients with a gradual increase in white blood cells (WBCs) that peaks between 2 and 3 weeks after starting therapy. Usually resolves spontaneously without treatment and/or complications.

TOXICITY 5

Light-headedness most commonly observed during drug infusion.

TOXICITY 6

Mild nausea and vomiting, abdominal pain, and diarrhea.

TOXICITY 7

Musculoskeletal pain.

TOXICITY 8

Mild hyperglycemia.

TOXICITY 9

Neurologic symptoms with confusion, decreased level of consciousness, cognitive changes, ataxia, visual symptoms, seizures, and ocular motor dysfunction. Wernicke's encephalopathy is a neurologic emergency.

TOXICITY 10

Carcinogen and teratogen.

Asciminib

TRADE NAME	Scemblix	CLASSIFICATION	Signal transduction inhibitor, Bcr-Abl inhibitor
CATEGORY	Targeted agent	DRUG MANUFACTURER	Novartis

MECHANISM OF ACTION

- Selective allosteric inhibitor that targets the myristoyl pocket of BCR-ABL1. Induces and stabilizes an inactive conformation of the kinase.
- Referred to as a STAMP inhibitor.
- Different than other conventional TKIs, which bind to the catalytic ATP-binding site.
- Inactive against other tyrosine kinases and much less off-target activity, including SRC.

MECHANISM OF RESISTANCE

- Mutations within and beyond the BCR-ABL1 myristoyl-binding site leading to reduced binding affinity.
- Induction of ABCB1 and ABCG2 efflux pump with reduced intracellular drug accumulation.

ABSORPTION

Peak plasma drug levels achieved in 2–3 hours. Food with high fat content reduces AUC and Cmax.

DISTRIBUTION

Extensive binding (97%) to plasma proteins. Steady-state drug levels reached in 3 days.

METABOLISM

Metabolism in the liver, primarily by CYP3A4 microsomal enzymes and by glucuronidation via UGT2B7 and UGT2B17 enzymes. Elimination is mainly in the feces, via the hepatobiliary route. Approximately 80% (57% unchanged) and 11% (2.5% unchanged) of an administered dose of drug recovered in feces and urine. The terminal half-life of the parent drug is 5.5 hours at the dosing schedule of 40 mg PO bid or 80 mg PO daily and 9 hours at the 200 mg PO bid dosing schedule.

INDICATIONS

1. FDA-approved in adult patients with Ph+ chronic phase CML, previously treated with two or more TKIs. This indication is approved under accelerated approval based on major molecular response.
2. FDA-approved in adult patients with Ph+ chronic phase CML with the T315I mutation.

DOSAGE RANGE

1. Ph+ chronic phase CML–80 mg PO once daily or 40 mg PO bid
2. Ph+ chronic phase CML with T315I mutation–200 mg PO bid

DRUG INTERACTION 1

Phenytoin and other drugs that stimulate the liver microsomal CYP3A4 enzymes, including carbamazepine, rifampin, phenobarbital, and St. John's Wort—These drugs increase the metabolism of asciminib, resulting in its inactivation and lower effective drug levels.

DRUG INTERACTION 2

Drugs that inhibit the liver microsomal CYP3A4 enzymes, including ketoconazole, itraconazole, erythromycin, and clarithromycin—These drugs decrease the metabolism of asciminib, resulting in increased drug levels and potentially increased toxicity.

DRUG INTERACTION 3

Itraconazole oral solution—Avoid concomitant use with itraconazole oral solution as it may reduce the asciminib Cmax and AUC, leading to reduced clinical efficacy.

DRUG INTERACTION 4

CYP2C9 substrates—Asciminib is a CYP2C9 inhibitor, and concomitant use of ascminib increases the Cmax and AUC of CYP2C9 substrates, which may increase toxicity associated with these agents.

SPECIAL CONSIDERATIONS

1. Monitor CBC every 2 weeks for the first 3 months and monthly thereafter.
2. Monitor serum amylase and lipase levels monthly while on treatment.
3. Dose adjustment is not required in patients with mild to severe hepatic impairment.
4. Dose adjustment is not required in patients with mild to severe renal impairment.
5. Monitor blood pressure and treat hypertension with standard anti-hypertensive medication when indicated. In the presence of >grade 3 hypertension, therapy should be withheld, dose reduced, or permanently discontinued depending on level and persistence of hypertension.
6. Monitor for symptoms and signs of hypersensitivity.
7. Patients with history of cardiovascular disease should be monitored for any evidence of cardiovascular symptoms and signs.
8. Advise females of potential of increased risk to a fetus and to use effective contraception during treatment and for one week after the last dose of drug.

TOXICITY 1

Myelosuppression with thrombocytopenia and neutropenia.

TOXICITY 2

Hypersensitivity reactions.

TOXICITY 3

Hypertension.

TOXICITY 4

Cardiovascular toxicity with ischemic heart disease, arterial thrombotic and embolic conditions, and CHF.

TOXICITY 5
Pancreatitis.

TOXICITY 6
Fatigue and anorexia.

TOXICITY 7
Mild nausea and vomiting.

TOXICITY 8
Myalgias and arthralgias.

Asparaginase ewinia chrysantemi-rywn

TRADE NAME	Rylaze, L-Asparaginase	CLASSIFICATION	Enzyme
CATEGORY	Chemotherapy drug	DRUG MANUFACTURER	Jazz Pharmaceuticals

MECHANISM OF ACTION
- Recombinant enzyme isolated from Erwinia chrysanthemi.
- Tumor cells lack asparagine synthetase and thus require exogenous sources of L-asparagine.
- Asparaginase hydrolyzes circulating L-asparagine to aspartic acid and ammonia.
- Depletion of the essential amino acid L-asparagine results in rapid inhibition of protein synthesis. Cytotoxicity of drug correlates with inhibition of protein synthesis.

MECHANISM OF RESISTANCE
- Increased expression of the L-asparagine synthetase gene, which facilitates the cellular production of L-asparagine from endogenous sources.
- Formation of antibodies against L-asparaginase, resulting in inhibition of function.

ABSORPTION
Not orally bioavailable and is administered via the intramuscular (IM) route. The mean absolute bioavailability is 37%.

DISTRIBUTION
After IM injection, peak plasma levels are reached within 10 hours. The apparent volume of distribution is about 49% of the plasma volume.

METABOLISM
Metabolism is expected to be mediated via catabolic pathways into small peptides and amino acids. The terminal half-life is about 18 hours.

INDICATIONS
FDA-approved for treatment of adult and pediatric patients 1 month or older with acute lymphoblastic leukemia (ALL) and lymphoblastic lymphoma (LBL) who have developed hypersensitivity to *E. coli*–derived asparaginase.

DOSAGE RANGE
Recommended dose is 25 mg/m^2 IM every 48 hours.

DRUG INTERACTION 1
Methotrexate—Asparaginase can inhibit the cytotoxic effects of methotrexate and thus reduce methotrexate antitumor activity and toxicity. It is recommended that these drugs be administered 24 hours apart.

DRUG INTERACTION 2
Vincristine—Asparaginase inhibits the clearance of vincristine, resulting in increased toxicity, especially neurotoxicity. Vincristine should be administered 12–24 hours before Asparaginase.

SPECIAL CONSIDERATIONS
1. Monitor patient for allergic reactions and/or anaphylaxis. The drug should administered in a setting with resuscitation equipment and medications to treat anaphylaxis, including oxygen, epinephrine, intravenous steroids, and antihistamines.
2. Induction treatment of acute lymphoblastic leukemia with asparaginase may induce rapid lysis of blast cells. Prophylaxis against tumor lysis syndrome with vigorous IV hydration, urinary alkalinization, and allopurinol is recommended for all patients.
3. Monitor for signs and symptoms of pancreatitis. Contraindicated in patients with either active pancreatitis or a history of pancreatitis. If pancreatitis develops while on therapy, asparaginase should be stopped immediately.
4. Monitor LFTs and serum bilirubin at baseline and every 2–3 weeks.
5. Monitor for evidence of bleeding complications, and monitor coagulation parameters (PT, PTT, INR) and fibrinogen levels.
6. Asparaginase can interfere with thyroid function tests. This effect is probably due to a marked reduction in serum concentration of thyroxine-binding globulin, which is observed within 2 days after the first dose. Levels of thyroxine-binding globulin return to normal within 4 weeks of the last dose.
7. The effect of hepatic and renal impairment on asparaginase erwinia chrysanthemi has not been studied.

8. May cause fetal harm. Females of reproductive potential should use effective non-hormonal contraception during drug therapy and for 3 months after the final dose. Breastfeeding should be avoided.

TOXICITY 1
Hypersensitivity reactions occu in up to 25% of patients. Mild form manifested by skin rash and urticaria. Anaphylactic reaction may be life-threatening and presents as bronchospasm, respiratory distress, and hypotension.

TOXICITY 2
Pancreatitis with transient increases in serum amylase and lipase levels.

TOXICITY 3
Hepatotoxicity with mild elevation in LFTs, including serum bilirubin, alkaline phosphatase, and SGOT/SGPT.

TOXICITY 4
Increased risk of both bleeding and clotting. Alterations in clotting with decreased levels of clotting factors, including fibrinogen, factors IX and XI, antithrombin III, proteins C and S, plasminogen, and α-2-antiplasmin. Observed in over 50% of patients.

TOXICITY 5
Fatigue and anorexia.

Atezolizumab

TRADE NAME	Tecentriq	CLASSIFICATION	Anti PD-L1 antibody
CATEGORY	Immune checkpoint inhibitor, immunotherapy	DRUG MANUFACTURER	Genentech/ Roche

MECHANISM OF ACTION
- Humanized IgG4 antibody that binds to the programmed death-ligand 1 (PD-L1) ligand expressed on tumor cells and/or tumor infiltrating cells, which then blocks the interaction between the PD-L1 ligand and the programmed cell death 1 (PD-1) and B7.1 receptors found on T cells and antigen-presenting cells.
- Blockade of the PD-1 pathway-mediated immune checkpoint overcomes immune escape mechanisms and enhances T-cell immune response, leading to T-cell activation and proliferation.

MECHANISM OF RESISTANCE

- Increased expression and/or activity of other immune checkpoint pathways (e.g., TIGIT, TIM3, and LAG3).
- Increased expression of other immune escape mechanisms.
- Increased infiltration of immune suppressive populations within the tumor microenvironment, which include Tregs, myeloid-derived suppressor cells (MDSCs), and M2 macrophages.
- Release of various cytokines, chemokines, and metabolites within the tumor microenvironment, including CSF-1, tryptophan metabolites, TGF-β, and adenosine.

DISTRIBUTION

Distribution in body is not well characterized. Steady-state levels are achieved by 6–9 weeks.

METABOLISM

Metabolism of atezolizumab has not been extensively characterized. The terminal half-life is on the order of 27 days.

INDICATIONS

1. FDA-approved as adjuvant treatment of Stage II to IIIA NSCLC following surgical resection and platinum-based chemotherapy whose tumors have PD-L1 expression on >1% of tumor cells.
2. FDA-approved for metastatic non–small cell lung cancer (NSCLC) with disease progression during or following platinum-based chemotherapy. Patients with EGFR or ALK genetic alterations should have disease progression on FDA-approved targeted therapy for these genetic alterations prior to treatment with atezolizumab.
3. FDA-approved for first-line treatment of metastatic NSCLC whose tumors have high PD-L1 expression (PD-L1 stained >50% of tumor cells or PD-L1 stained tumor-infiltrating immune cells covering >10% of the tumor area) with no EGFR or ALK alterations.
4. FDA-approved in combination with bevacizumab, paclitaxel, and carboplatin for first-line treatment of metastatic non-squamous NSCLC with no EGFR or ALK genomic alterations.
5. FDA-approved in combination with nab-paclitaxel and carboplatin for first-line treatment of metastatic non-squamous NSCLC with no EGFR or ALK genomic alterations.
6. FDA-approved in combination with carboplatin and etoposide for first-line treatment of extensive-stage small cell lung cancer (SCLC).
7. FDA-approved in combination with bevacizumab for unresectable or metastatic hepatocellular cancer (HCC) with no prior systemic therapy.
8. FDA-approved in combination with cobimetinib and vemurafenib for advanced BRAF V600 mutation-positive unresectable or metastatic melanoma.
9. FDA-approved for unresectable or metastatic alveolar soft part sarcoma (ASPS).

DOSAGE RANGE

1. Early-stage NSCLC (adjuvant therapy): 840 mg IV every 2 weeks, 1,200 mg IV every 3 weeks, or 1,680 mg IV every 4 weeks for up to 1 year.
2. Metastatic NSCLC monotherapy: 840 mg IV every 2 weeks, 1,200 mg IV every 3 weeks, or 1,680 mg IV every 4 weeks when used in combination with paclitaxel, carboplatin, and bevacizumab.
3. Metastatic NSCLC combination therapy: 840 mg IV every 2 weeks, 1,200 mg IV every 3 weeks, or 1,680 mg IV every 4 weeks when used in combination with paclitaxel, carboplatin, and bevacizumab.
4. SCLC: 840 mg IV every 2 weeks, 1,200 mg IV every 3 weeks, or 1,680 mg IV every 4 weeks with carboplatin and etoposide. Following the completion of 4 cycles of chemotherapy, atezolizumab is administered 840 mg IV every 2 weeks, 1,200 mg IV every 3 weeks, or 1,680 mg IV every 4 weeks.
5. Hepatocellular cancer: 840 mg IV every 2 weeks, 1,200 mg IV every 3 weeks, or 1,680 mg IV every 4 weeks followed by bevacizumab 15 mg/kg IV every 3 weeks.
6. Melanoma: 840 mg IV every 2 weeks, 1,200 mg IV every 3 weeks, or 1,680 mg IV every 4 weeks with cobimetinib 60 mg PO (21 days on, 7 days off) and vemurafenib 720 mg PO bid.
7. ASPS: Adults—840 mg IV every 2 weeks, 1,200 mg IV every 3 weeks, or 1,680 mg IV every 4 weeks
8. Pediatric patients 2 years of age and older—15 mg/kg (up to maximum of 1,200 mg) IV every 3 weeks

DRUG INTERACTIONS

None well characterized to date.

SPECIAL CONSIDERATIONS

1. Atezolizumab associated with significant immune-mediated adverse reactions due to T-cell activation and proliferation. These immune-mediated reactions may involve any organ system, with the most common reactions being pneumonitis, hepatitis, colitis, hypophysitis, pancreatitis, neurological disorders, and adrenal and thyroid dysfunction.
2. Atezolizumab should be withheld for any of the following:
   - Grade 2 pneumonitis
   - Grade 2 or 3 colitis
   - SGOT/SGPT > 3 × ULN and up to 5 × ULN or total bilirubin > 1.5 × ULN and up to 3 × ULN
   - Symptomatic hypophysitis, adrenal insufficiency, hypothyroidism, hyperthyroidism, or grade 3 or 4 hyperglycemia
   - Grade 2 ocular inflammatory toxicity
   - Grade 2 or 3 pancreatitis or grade 3 or 4 increases in serum amylase or lipase levels
   - Grade 3 or 4 infection
   - Grade 2 infusion-related reactions
   - Grade 3 skin rash

3. Atezolizumab should be permanently discontinued for any of the following:
    -   Grade 3 or 4 pneumonitis
    -   SGOT/SGPT > 5 × ULN or total bilirubin > 3 × ULN
    -   Grade 4 colitis
    -   Grade 4 hypophysitis
    -   Myasthenic syndrome/myasthenia gravis, Guillain-Barré syndrome, or meningoencephalitis (all grades)
    -   Grade 3 or 4 ocular inflammatory toxicity
    -   Grades 2, 3, or 4 myocarditis
    -   Grade 4 nephritis with renal dysfunction
    -   Grade 4 or any grade of recurrent pancreatitis
    -   Grade 3 or 4 infusion-related reactions
    -   Grade 4 skin rash
4. The first infusion should be administered over 60 minutes. If the first infusion is well tolerated, all subsequent infusions may be administered over 30 minutes.
5. Monitor for symptoms and signs of infection.
6. Monitor thyroid and adrenal function prior to and during therapy.
7. Dose modification is not needed for patients with renal dysfunction.
8. Dose modification is not needed for patients with mild hepatic dysfunction. Atezolizumab has not been studied in patients with moderate or severe hepatic dysfunction.
9. Pregnancy category D.

TOXICITY 1
Infusion-related reactions.

TOXICITY 2
Colitis with diarrhea and abdominal pain.

TOXICITY 3
Pneumonitis with dyspnea and cough.

TOXICITY 4
Hepatotoxicity with elevations in SGOT/SGPT and serum bilirubin.

TOXICITY 5
GI side effects with nausea/vomiting and dry mouth.

TOXICITY 6
Endocrinopathies, including hypophysitis, thyroid disorders, adrenal insufficiency, and diabetes.

TOXICITY 7
Pancreatitis.

TOXICITY 8
Neurologic toxicity with neuropathy, myositis, myasthenia gravis, Guillain-Barré syndrome, or meningoencephalitis.

TOXICITY 9
Musculoskeletal symptoms with arthralgias, oligoarthritis, polyarthritis, tenosynovitis, polymyalgia rheumatica, and myalgias.

TOXICITY 10
Infections with sepsis, herpes encephalitis, and mycobacterial infections. All-grade infections observed in up to 38% of patients and >grade 3 infections in 11% of patients, with urinary tract infections being the most common cause of >grade 3 infections.

TOXICITY 11
Ocular toxicity.

TOXICITY 12
Maculopapular skin rash, erythema, dermatitis, and pruritus.

TOXICITY 13
Fatigue, anorexia, and asthenia.

Avapritinib

TRADE NAME	Ayvakit, BLU-285	CLASSIFICATION	Signal transduction inhibitor, PDGFR-α and KIT inhibitor
CATEGORY	Targeted agent	DRUG MANUFACTURER	Blueprint Medicines

MECHANISM OF ACTION
- Potent and selective type I inhibitor of KIT and platelet-derived growth factor receptor-α (PDGFRA) activation loop mutant proteins.
- Inhibits wild-type KIT, PDGFRA, PDGFRB, and CSFR1.

MECHANISM OF RESISTANCE
- Mutations in the KIT kinase domain, including the T670I gatekeeper mutation.
- Mutations in PDGFR exons 13, 14, and 15, including V658A, N659K, Y676C, and G680R.
- Distant conformational changes in the phosphate-binding loop of KIT.

ABSORPTION
Rapidly absorbed with a median time to peak drug levels of 2–4 hours after oral ingestion. Steady-state drug levels are achieved in 15 days. Food with high fat content increases C_{max} and AUC.

DISTRIBUTION
Extensive binding (98.8%) of drug to plasma proteins.

METABOLISM
Metabolized in the liver primarily by CYP3A4 microsomal enzymes and to a lesser extent by CYP2C9. The 2 major metabolites are M690 (hydroxyglucuronide) and M499, which is formed via oxidative deamination. Approximately 70% of an administered dose is eliminated in feces (11% in parent form) and 18% is eliminated in urine (0.23% in parent form). The terminal half-life of avapritinib is approximately 57 hours.

INDICATIONS
1. FDA-approved for patients with unresectable or metastatic gastrointestinal stromal tumor (GIST) harboring a PDGFRA exon 18 mutation, including PDGFRA D842V mutation.
2. FDA-approved for advanced systemic mastocytosis.

DOSAGE RANGE
GIST: Recommended dose is 300 mg PO once daily.
Systemic mastocytosis: Recommended dose is 200 mg PO once daily.

DRUG INTERACTION 1
Drugs such as ketoconazole, itraconazole, erythromycin, clarithromycin, atazanavir, indinavir, nefazodone, nelfinavir, ritonavir, saquinavir, telithromycin, and voriconazole may decrease the metabolism of avapritinib, resulting in increased drug levels and potentially increased toxicity.

DRUG INTERACTION 2
Phenytoin and other drugs that stimulate the liver microsomal CYP3A4 enzymes, including carbamazepine, rifampin, phenobarbital, and St. John's Wort—These drugs may increase the metabolism of avapritinib, resulting in lower effective drug levels.

SPECIAL CONSIDERATIONS

1. Dose reduction is not required in the setting of mild to moderate hepatic impairment. Has not been studied in the setting of severe hepatic impairment.
2. Dose reduction is not required in the setting of mild to moderate renal impairment. Has not been studied in patients with severe renal impairment or in those with end-stage renal disease.
3. Monitor patients for CNS effects, including cognitive impairment, dizziness, mood disorders, sleep disorders, speech disorders, and hallucinations.
4. Monitor patients for a sudden change in mental status, as avapritinib is associated with an increased risk of intracranial hemorrhage, including subdural hematoma and cerebral hemorrhage.
5. Avoid concomitant use of a moderate or strong CYP3A inhibitor. If these agents can not be avoided, the dose of avapritinib should be reduced from 300 mg once daily to 100 mg once daily.
6. Concomitant use of a moderate or strong CYP3A inducer should be avoided.
7. Can cause fetal harm when administered to a pregnant woman. Females of reproductive potential should use effective contraception during therapy and for 6 weeks after the final dose. Breastfeeding should be avoided while on therapy and for 2 weeks following the final dose.

TOXICITY 1
Fatigue, asthenia, and anorexia.

TOXICITY 2
CNS toxicity with cognitive impairment, dizziness, mood disorders, sleep disorders, speech disorders, and hallucinations.

TOXICITY 3
Nausea/vomiting, diarrhea, and abdominal pain.

TOXICITY 4
Myelosuppression with anemia and neutropenia.

TOXICITY 5
Intracranial hemorrhage with subdural hematoma and cerebral hemorrhage.

TOXICITY 6
Fluid retention with peripheral edema and periorbital edema.

TOXICITY 7
Hair color changes.

Avelumab

TRADE NAME	Bavencio	CLASSIFICATION	Anti-PD-L1 monoclonal antibody
CATEGORY	Immune checkpoint inhibitor, immunotherapy	DRUG MANUFACTURER	EMD Serono/ Pfizer

MECHANISM OF ACTION
- Human IgG1 antibody that binds to the PD-L1 ligand expressed on tumor cells and/or tumor infiltrating cells, which then blocks the interaction between the PD-L1 ligand and the PD-1 and B7.1 receptors found on T cells and antigen-presenting cells.
- Blockade of the PD-1 pathway-mediated immune checkpoint overcomes immune escape mechanisms and enhances T-cell immune response, leading to T-cell activation and proliferation.
- Differs from other PD-L1/PD-1 immune checkpoint-blocking antibodies in that it may also induce ADCC.

MECHANISM OF RESISTANCE
- Increased expression and/or activity of other immune checkpoint pathways (e.g., TIGIT, TIM3, and LAG3).
- Increased expression of other immune escape mechanisms.
- Increased infiltration of immune suppressive populations within the tumor microenvironment, which include Tregs, myeloid-derived suppressor cells (MDSCs), and M2 macrophages.
- Release of various cytokines, chemokines, and metabolites within the tumor microenvironment, including CSF-1, tryptophan metabolites, TGF-β, and adenosine.

DISTRIBUTION
Mean volume of distribution in the body is 4.72 L. Steady-state levels are achieved by 4–6 weeks.

METABOLISM
Metabolism of avelumab is mediated by proteolytic degradation. The terminal half-life is on the order of 6 days.

INDICATIONS
1. FDA-approved for adult and pediatric patients 12 years and older with metastatic Merkel cell cancer (MCC). This indication is approved under accelerated approval based on tumor response rate and duration of response.
2. FDA-approved for locally advanced or metastatic bladder cancer with disease progression during or following platinum-based chemotherapy

or with disease progression within 12 months of neoadjuvant or adjuvant therapy with platinum-based chemotherapy.
3. FDA-approved for maintenance treatment of locally advanced or metastatic bladder cancer that has not progressed with first-line platinum-based chemotherapy.
4. FDA-approved in combination with axitinib for first-line treatment of advanced renal cell carcinoma (RCC).

DOSAGE RANGE
Recommended dose for bladder cancer, MCC, and RCC is 800 mg IV every 2 weeks.

DRUG INTERACTIONS
None well characterized to date.

SPECIAL CONSIDERATIONS
1. Avelumab can result in significant immune-mediated adverse reactions due to T-cell activation and proliferation. These immune-mediated reactions may involve any organ system, with the most common reactions being pneumonitis, hepatitis, colitis, hypophysitis, pancreatitis, neurological disorders, and adrenal and thyroid dysfunction.
2. Monitor for infusion-related reactions. Patients should be pre-medicated with an antihistamine and acetaminophen prior to the first 4 infusions. For mild or moderate infusion reactions, need to interrupt or slow the rate of infusion. For severe or life-threatening infusion reactions, the infusion should be stopped and permanently discontinued.
3. Monitor thyroid and adrenal function prior to and during therapy.
4. Monitor patients for hyperglycemia and/or other signs and symptoms of diabetes.
5. Dose modification is not needed for patients with renal dysfunction.
6. Dose modification is not needed for patients with mild or moderate hepatic dysfunction. Has not been studied in patients with severe hepatic dysfunction.
7. Pregnancy category D.

TOXICITY 1
Fatigue and asthenia.

TOXICITY 2
Infusion-related reactions.

TOXICITY 3
Nausea, vomiting, decreased appetite.

TOXICITY 4
Musculoskeletal symptoms with arthralgias, oligoarthritis, polyarthritis, tenosynovitis, polymyalgia rheumatica, and myalgias.

TOXICITY 5

Colitis with diarrhea and abdominal pain.

TOXICITY 6

Endocrinopathies, including hypophysitis, thyroid disorders, adrenal insufficiency, and diabetes.

TOXICITY 7

Neurologic toxicity with neuropathy, myositis, myasthenia gravis, Guillain-Barré syndrome, or meningoencephalitis.

TOXICITY 8

Skin rash and pruritus.

TOXICITY 9

Dyspnea and cough.

TOXICITY 10

Hepatotoxicity with elevations in liver function tests (SGOT, SGPT) and serum bilirubin.

TOXICITY 11

Anemia, thrombocytopenia, lymphopenia, and neutropenia.

TOXICITY 12

Elevations in serum lipase and serum amylase.

Axicabtagene ciloleucel

TRADE NAME	Yescarta, axi-cel	**CLASSIFICATION**	CAR T-cell therapy
CATEGORY	Cellular therapy, immunotherapy	**DRUG MANUFACTURER**	Kite, Gilead

MECHANISM OF ACTION

- Axicabtagene ciloleucel is a CD19-directed genetically modified autologous T-cell immunotherapy that binds to CD19-expressing target cells and normal B cells.
- Axicabtagene ciloleucel is prepared from the patient's own peripheral blood mononuclear cells, which are enriched for T cells, and then genetically modified ex vivo by retroviral transduction to express a chimeric antigen receptor (CAR) made up of a murine anti-CD19

single-chain variable fragment linked to CD28 and CD3-zeta co-stimulatory domains. The anti-CD19 CAR T cells are expanded ex vivo and infused back to the patient, where they target CR19-expressing cells.

- Lymphocyte depletion conditioning regimen with cyclophosphamide and fludarabine leads to increased systemic levels of IL-15 and other pro-inflammatory cytokines and chemokines that enhance CAR T-cell activity.
- The conditioning regimen may also decrease immunosuppressive regulatory T cells, activate antigen-presenting cells, and induce pro-inflammatory tumor cell damage.
- Clinical studies have shown an association between higher CAR T-cell levels in peripheral blood and clinical response.

MECHANISM OF RESISTANCE

- Selection of alternatively spliced CD19 isoforms that lack the CD19 epitope recognized by the CAR T cells.
- Antigen loss or modulation.
- Insufficient reactivity against tumors cells with low antigen density.
- Emergence of an antigen-negative clone.
- Lineage switching from lymphoid to myeloid leukemia phenotype.

ABSORPTION

Administered only via the IV route.

DISTRIBUTION

Peak levels of anti-CD19 CAR T cells are observed within the first 1–2 weeks after infusion.

METABOLISM

Metabolism of axicabtagene ciloleucel has not been well characterized.

INDICATIONS

1. FDA-approved for relapsed or refractory large B-cell lymphoma after two or more lines of systemic therapy, including diffuse large B-cell lymphoma (DLBCL), primary mediastinal large B-cell lymphoma, high-grade B-cell lymphoma, and DLBCL arising from follicular lymphoma.
2. FDA-approved for large B-cell lymphoma that is refractory to first-line chemoimmunotherapy or that relapses within 12 months of first-line chemoimmunotherapy.

DOSAGE RANGE

- A lymphodepleting chemotherapy regimen of cyclophosphamide 500 mg/m^2 IV and fludarabine 30 mg/m^2 IV on the fifth, fourth, and third day should be administered before infusion of axicabtagene ciloleucel.
- Patients should be pre-medicated with acetaminophen 650 mg PO and diphenhydramine 12.5 mg IV 1 hour before infusion of axicabtagene ciloleucel.
- Dosing of axicabtagene ciloleucel is based on a target dose of 2×10^6 CAR-positive viable T cells per kilogram of body weight, with a maximum of 2×10^8 CAR-positive viable T cells.

DRUG INTERACTIONS

None well characterized to date.

SPECIAL CONSIDERATIONS

1. Axicabtagene ciloleucel is available only through a restricted program under a Risk Evaluation and Mitigation Strategy (REMS).
2. Monitor for hypersensitivity infusion reactions. Patients should be pre-medicated with acetaminophen 650 mg PO and diphenhydramine 12.5 mg IV at 1 hour prior to CAR T-cell infusion. Prophylactic use of systemic corticosteroids should be avoided, as they may interfere with the clinical activity of axicabtagene ciloleucel.
3. Monitor patients at least daily for 7 days following infusion for signs and symptoms of cytokine release syndrome (CRS), which may be fatal or life-threatening in some cases. Patient need to be monitored for up to 4 weeks after infusion. Please see package insert for complete guidelines regarding the appropriate management for CRS. This is a black-box warning.
4. Monitor for signs and symptoms of neurologic toxicities, which may be fatal or life-threatening in some cases. This is a black-box warning.
5. Monitor for signs and symptoms of infection.
6. Monitor CBCs periodically after infusion.
7. Immunoglobulin levels should be monitored after treatment with axicabtagene ciloleucel. Infection precautions, antibiotic prophylaxis, and immunoglobulin replacement may need to be instituted.
8. Patients should be advised not to drive and not to engage in operating heavy or potentially dangerous machinery for at least 8 weeks after receiving axicabtagene ciloleucel.
9. Patients will require lifelong monitoring for secondary malignancies.
10. This therapy is **NOT** indicated for the treatment of primary CNS lymphoma.
11. Pregnancy category D. Breastfeeding should be avoided.

TOXICITY 1

Hypersensitivity infusion reactions.

TOXICITY 2

CRS with fever, hypotension, tachycardia, chills, and hypoxia. More serious events include cardiac arrhythmias (both atrial and ventricular), decreased cardiac ejection fraction, cardiac arrest, capillary leak syndrome, hepatotoxicity, renal failure, and prolongation of coagulation parameters PT and partial thromboplastin time (PTT).

TOXICITY 3

Neurologic toxicity, which includes headache, delirium, encephalopathy, tremors, dizziness, aphasia, imbalance and gait instability, and seizures.

TOXICITY 4
Myelosuppression with thrombocytopenia and neutropenia, which in some cases can be prolonged for several weeks after infusion.

TOXICITY 5
Infections with non-specific pathogen, bacterial, and viral infections most common.

TOXICITY 6
Hypogammaglobulinemia.

TOXICITY 7
Hepatitis B reactivation.

TOXICITY 8
Secondary malignancies.

Axitinib

TRADE NAME	Inlyta, AG-13736	**CLASSIFICATION**	Signal transduction inhibitor, anti-angiogenesis agent
CATEGORY	Targeted agent	**DRUG MANUFACTURER**	Pfizer

MECHANISM OF ACTION
- Small-molecule inhibitor of the ATP-binding domains of VEGFR-1, VEGFR-2, and VEGFR-3 tyrosine kinases.
- Shows limited effects on platelet-derived growth factor (PDGFR) and c-Kit (CD117).
- Interferes with processes involved in tumor growth and proliferation, metastasis, and angiogenesis.

MECHANISM OF RESISTANCE
- Increased expression of VEGFR-1, VEGFR-2, and VEGFR-3.
- Activation of angiogenic switch with increased expression of alternative pro-angiogenic pathways.
- Increased pericyte coverage to tumor vessels with increased expression of VEGF and other pro-angiogenic factors.
- Recruitment of pro-angiogenic inflammatory cells from bone marrow, such as tumor-associated macrophages, monocytes, and myeloid-derived suppressor cells (MDSCs).

ABSORPTION
Rapid oral absorption when given with food, with a mean absolute bioavailability of approximately 60%. Peak plasma concentrations are reached 2–6 hours after oral ingestion, and steady state is achieved within 2–3 days of dosing.

DISTRIBUTION
Extensively bound (>99%) to albumin and to α1-acid glycoprotein.

METABOLISM
Metabolism is primarily in the liver by CYP3A4 and CYP3A5 enzymes and to a lesser extent by CYP1A2, CYP2C19, and UGT1A1. Sulfoxide and N-glucuronide metabolites are significantly less potent against VEGFR-2 compared to parent drug. Hepatobiliary excretion is the main route of drug elimination. Approximately 40% is eliminated in feces, of which 12% as unchanged drug, and 23% in the urine as metabolites. The terminal half-life is 2–5 hours.

INDICATIONS
1. FDA-approved for the treatment of advanced renal cell carcinoma after failure of one prior systemic therapy.
2. FDA-approved in combination with avelumab for the first-line treatment of renal cell carcinoma (RCC).

DOSAGE RANGE
Recommended starting dose for RCC is 5 mg PO bid. Dose can be increased or decreased based on tolerability or safety. Dose increase—If dose is tolerated for at least 2 consecutive weeks, dose can be increased to 7 mg PO bid, then up to 10 mg PO bid. Dose reduction—To minimize the risk of adverse events, the dose can be decreased to 3 mg PO bid, then to 2 mg PO bid.

DRUG INTERACTION 1
Drugs such as ketoconazole, itraconazole, erythromycin, clarithromycin, atazanavir, indinavir, nefazodone, nelfinavir, ritonavir, saquinavir, telithromycin, and voriconazole may decrease the metabolism of axitinib, resulting in increased drug levels and potentially increased toxicity.

DRUG INTERACTION 2

Drugs such as rifampin, phenytoin, phenobarbital, carbamazepine, and St. John's Wort may increase the metabolism of axitinib, resulting in its inactivation and lower effective drug levels.

DRUG INTERACTION 3

Proton pump inhibitors, H2-receptor inhibitors, and antacids—Drugs that alter the pH of the upper GI tract may alter axitinib solubility, thereby reducing drug bioavailability and decreasing systemic drug exposure.

SPECIAL CONSIDERATIONS

1. No dose adjustment is needed for patients with creatinine clearance (CrCl) > 15 mL/min. However, caution should be used in patients with end-stage renal disease.
2. Dose adjustment is not required in patients with mild hepatic impairment. The dose of axitinib should be reduced by 50% in patients with moderate impairment (Child-Pugh Class B). Axitinib has not been studied in patients with severe hepatic impairment (Child-Pugh Class C).
3. Axitinib should be taken approximately 12 hours apart with or without food and should be taken with water.
4. Patients should be warned of the increased risk of arterial thromboembolic events, including myocardial ischemia and stroke.
5. Patients should be warned of the increased risk of venous thromboembolic events, including DVT and PE.
6. Blood pressure should be well controlled prior to starting axitinib therapy. Closely monitor blood pressure while on therapy and treat as needed with standard oral antihypertensive medication.
7. Axitinib therapy should be stopped at least 24 hours prior to scheduled surgery.
8. Closely monitor thyroid function tests and thyroid-stimulating hormone (TSH), as axitinib therapy results in hypothyroidism.
9. Closely monitor LFTs and serum bilirubin while on therapy.
10. Avoid Seville oranges, starfruit, pomelos, grapefruit, and grapefruit products while on therapy.
11. Pregnancy category D. Breastfeeding should be avoided.

TOXICITY 1

Hypertension occurs in 40% of patients.

TOXICITY 2

Increased risk of arterial and venous thromboembolic events.

TOXICITY 3

Bleeding complications.

TOXICITY 4

GI perforations and wound-healing complications.

TOXICITY 5
Diarrhea, nausea/vomiting, and constipation.

TOXICITY 6
Proteinuria develops in up to 10% of patients.

TOXICITY 7
Hypothyroidism.

TOXICITY 8
Elevations in SGOT/SGPT and serum bilirubin.

TOXICITY 9
Reversible posterior leukoencephalopathy syndrome (RPLS) occurs rarely (<1%) and presents with headache, seizure, lethargy, confusion, blindness, and other visual disturbances.

Azacitidine

TRADE NAME	Vidaza	CLASSIFICATION	Antimetabolite, hypomethylating agent
CATEGORY	Chemotherapy drug	DRUG MANUFACTURER	Celgene

MECHANISM OF ACTION
- Cytidine analog.
- Cell cycle–specific with activity in the S-phase.
- Requires activation to the nucleotide metabolite azacitidine triphosphate.
- Incorporation of azacitidine triphosphate into RNA, resulting in inhibition of RNA processing and function.
- Incorporation of azacitidine triphosphate into DNA, resulting in inhibition of DNA methyltransferases, which then leads to loss of DNA methylation and gene reactivation. Aberrantly silenced genes, such as tumor suppressor genes, are reactivated and expressed.

MECHANISM OF RESISTANCE
- Reduced activation of azacitidine resulting from mutations in the uridine-cytidine kinase 2 gene with reduced expression of UCK2 protein.
- Reduced expression of lysosome-mediated protein 2 (LAMP2), leading to defects in chaperone-mediated autophagy (CMA).

ABSORPTION
Administered only via the SC and IV route. The bioavailability of SC azacitidine is 89% relative to IV azacitidine.

DISTRIBUTION
Distribution in humans has not been fully characterized. The drug is able to cross the blood-brain barrier.

METABOLISM
Precise route of elimination and metabolic fate of azacitidine are not well characterized in humans. In vitro studies suggest that azacitidine may be metabolized by the liver. One of the main elimination pathways is via deamination by cytidine deaminase, found principally in the liver but also in plasma, granulocytes, intestinal epithelium, and peripheral tissues. Urinary excretion is the main route of elimination of the parent drug and its metabolites. The half-lives of azacitidine and its metabolites are approximately 4 hours.

INDICATIONS
1. FDA-approved for treatment of patients with myelodysplastic syndromes (MDS), including refractory anemia, refractory anemia with ringed sideroblasts, refractory anemia with excess blasts, refractory anemia with excess blasts in transformation, and chronic myelomonocytic leukemia.
2. FDA-approved in combination with ivosidenib for newly diagnosed AML with an IDH1 mutation in patients who are >75 years of age or who have comorbidities that preclude the use of intensive induction chemotherapy.

DOSAGE RANGE
1. MDS: 75 mg/m^2 SC or IV daily for 7 days. Cycles are repeated every 4 weeks.
2. AML: 75 mg/m^2 IV daily on days 1–7 or on days 1–5 and 8 and 9. Cycles are repeated every 4 weeks.

DRUG INTERACTIONS
None well characterized to date.

SPECIAL CONSIDERATIONS
1. Patients should be treated for a minimum of 4 cycles, as it may take longer than 4 cycles for clinical benefit.
2. Patients should be pre-treated with effective antiemetics to prevent nausea/vomiting.
3. Monitor complete blood counts on a regular basis during therapy.

4. Use with caution in patients with underlying kidney dysfunction. If unexplained elevations in BUN or serum creatinine occur, the next cycle should be delayed, and the subsequent dose should be reduced by 50%. If unexplained reductions in serum bicarbonate levels to <20 mEq/L occur, the subsequent dose should be reduced by 50%.
5. Pregnancy category D. Breastfeeding should be avoided.

TOXICITY 1

Myelosuppression with neutropenia and thrombocytopenia.

TOXICITY 2

Fatigue and anorexia.

TOXICITY 3

GI toxicity in the form of nausea/vomiting, constipation, and abdominal pain.

TOXICITY 4

Renal toxicity with elevations in serum creatinine, renal tubular acidosis, and hypokalemia.

TOXICITY 5

Peripheral edema.

Belantamab mafodotin-blmf

mcMMAF

mAb

Where n ~4 mcMMAF per mAb

TRADE NAME	Blenrep	**CLASSIFICATION**	Antibody-drug conjugate
CATEGORY	Biologic response modifier agent, chemotherapy drug	**DRUG MANUFACTURER**	GlaxoSmithKline

MECHANISM OF ACTION

- First-in-class antibody-drug conjugate composed of an afucosylated, humanized IgG1 anti-B cell maturation antigen (BCMA) monoclonal antibody conjugated to a microtubule-disrupting agent, monomethyl auristatin F (MMAF).
- BCMA is a cell surface receptor that is expressed on multiple myeloma cells but absent on naïve and memory B cells.
- Inhibits BCMA-expressing multiple myeloma cells via multiple mechanisms, including inhibition of mitosis with induction of apoptosis, antibody-dependent cellular cytotoxicity (ADCC), antibody-dependent cellular phagocytosis (ADCP), and immunogenic cell death.

MECHANISM OF RESISTANCE

None well characterized to date.

ABSORPTION

Administered only via the IV route.

DISTRIBUTION

Maximum plasma concentrations of belantamab mafodotin are observed at or shortly after the end of the infusion. The time to reach steady-state levels is approximately 70 days.

METABOLISM

Metabolism of the monoclonal antibody part of belantamab mafodotin is mediated by catabolic pathways to small peptides and amino acids.

INDICATIONS
FDA-approved for the treatment of relapsed or refractory multiple myeloma after 4 or more lines of systemic therapy, including an immunomodulatory agent, a proteasome inhibitor, and an anti-CD38 monoclonal antibody.

DOSAGE RANGE
Recommended dose is 2.5 mg/kg IV every 3 weeks.

DRUG INTERACTIONS
None well characterized to date.

SPECIAL CONSIDERATIONS
1. Available only through a restricted program under a Risk Evaluation and Mitigation Strategy (REMS).
2. No need for dose reduction in setting of mild hepatic impairment. Has not been studied in the setting of moderate or severe hepatic impairment (total bilirubin >1/5 × ULN and any AST).
3. No need for dose reduction in setting of mild or moderate renal impairment (CrCl, 30–89 mL/min). Has not been studied in the setting of severe renal impairment or end-stage renal disease.
4. Monitor for infusion reactions. May consider pre-medication with acetaminophen 650 mg PO and diphenhydramine 12.5 mg IV at 30–60 minutes prior to infusion.
5. Monitor CBC at baseline and periodically during treatment as myelosuppression with thrombocytopenia is observed in up to 70% of patients.
6. Monitor patients for ocular symptoms. This is a black-box warning. Eye exams with visual acuity and slit lamp should be performed at baseline, prior to each dose, and for any worsening symptoms. In the presence of new ocular symptoms, treatment should be withheld until improvement and resumed at the same or reduced dose, or consider permanent discontinuation based on severity.
7. Patients should be instructed to use preservative-free lubricant eye drops at least 4 times a day starting with the first infusion and to continue until the end of treatment. Patients should also be advised to avoid the use of contact lenses unless directed by an ophthalmologist.
8. Advise patients to use caution when driving or when operating machinery.
9. May cause fetal harm when administered to pregnant women. Effective contraception should be used in women during treatment and for 4 months after the last dose. Breastfeeding should be avoided.

TOXICITY 1
Infusion reactions.

TOXICITY 2
Ocular toxicity with keratopathy, changes in visual acuity, blurred vision, and dry eye.

TOXICITY 3
Myelosuppression with thrombocytopenia.

TOXICITY 4
Nausea/vomiting, constipation, and diarrhea.

TOXICITY 5
Fatigue and anorexia.

TOXICITY 6
Arthralgias and back pain.

Belinostat

TRADE NAME	Beleodaq, PXD101	CLASSIFICATION	Histone deacetylase (HDAC) inhibitor
CATEGORY	Chemotherapy drug	DRUG MANUFACTURER	Spectrum Pharmaceuticals

MECHANISM OF ACTION
- Potent inhibitor of class I, II, and IV histone deacetylase enzymes.
- Inhibition of HDAC activity leads to accumulation of acetyl groups on the histone lysine residues, resulting in open chromatin structure and transcriptional activation.
- HDAC inhibition activates differentiation, inhibits the cell cycle, and induces cell-cycle arrest and apoptosis.
- Preferential cytotoxicity toward tumor cells compared to normal cells.
- Exhibits stimulation of the immune system and blockage of angiogenesis in in vivo studies.

MECHANISM OF RESISTANCE
- Increased expression of target HDACs.
- Mutations in the target HDACs, leading to reduced binding affinity to drug.
- Increased expression/activity of the IGF2/IGF-1R signaling pathway.
- Increased activation of MAPK signaling.
- Reduced expression of the pro-apoptotic protein Bim.

DISTRIBUTION
Limited body tissue distribution. Approximately 92.9%–95.8% of drug is bound to plasma proteins.

METABOLISM
Extensively metabolized in the liver by hepatic UGT1A1, with the belinostat glucuronide being the main metabolite. Also undergoes metabolism by CYP2A6, CYP2C9, and CYP3A4 enzymes to form belinostat amide and belinostat acid metabolites. Approximately 40% of belinostat is excreted renally, with less than 2% of the dose recovered unchanged in urine. All major metabolites are excreted in urine within the first 24 hours after dose administration. The elimination half-life is on the order of 1 hour.

INDICATIONS
FDA-approved for the treatment of patients with relapsed or refractory peripheral T-cell lymphoma (PTCL).

DOSAGE RANGE
Recommended dose is 1,000 mg/m^2 IV on days 1 through 5 with cycles repeated every 21 days.

DRUG INTERACTION 1
Atazanavir—Avoid concomitant administration of belinostat with atazanavir, a strong UGT1A1 inhibitor. Concomitant administration with atazanavir may increase belinostat exposure.

DRUG INTERACTION 2
Gemfibrozil—Avoid concomitant administration with gemfibrozil, a UGT1A1 inhibitor.

SPECIAL CONSIDERATIONS
1. Use with caution in patients with hepatic impairment, especially in those with moderate and severe hepatic impairment, as belinostat has not been studied in these settings.
2. Belinostat can be used safely in patients with CrCL >39 mL/min. Use with caution in patients whose CrCl <39 mL/min, as the drug has not been studied in this setting, and dose reduction may be required.
3. Serious and sometimes fatal infections, including pneumonia and sepsis, have occurred. Patients with a history of extensive or intensive chemotherapy may be at higher risk of life-threatening infections.
4. Closely monitor CBCs during therapy.
5. Monitor patients with advanced-stage disease and/or high tumor burden, as belinostat therapy can result in tumor lysis syndrome.
6. Fatal hepatotoxicity and liver function test abnormalities may occur. Monitor liver function tests before treatment and before the start of each cycle. Interrupt and/or adjust dosage until recovery, or permanently discontinue based on the severity of the hepatic toxicity.

7. Monitor ECG with QTc measurement at baseline and periodically during therapy, as QTc prolongation has been observed, albeit not as frequently as with vorinostat and romidepsin.
8. Patients with the UGT1A1*28 allele are at increased risk for developing side effects, given the importance of UGT1A1 in drug metabolism. In this setting, the starting dose of belinostat should be reduced to 750 mg/m^2.
9. Pregnancy category D.

TOXICITY 1
GI toxicity with nausea/vomiting and diarrhea.

TOXICITY 2
Myelosuppression with thrombocytopenia and anemia more common than neutropenia.

TOXICITY 3
Fatigue and anorexia.

TOXICITY 4
Hepatotoxicity.

TOXICITY 5
Tumor lysis syndrome.

TOXICITY 6
Increased risk of infections.

TOXICITY 7
QTc prolongation.

Bendamustine

TRADE NAME	Treanda	CLASSIFICATION	Alkylating agent
CATEGORY	Chemotherapy drug	DRUG MANUFACTURER	Cephalon, Teva

MECHANISM OF ACTION
- Bifunctional alkylating agent consisting of a purine benzimidazole ring and a nitrogen mustard moiety.
- Forms cross-links with DNA resulting in single- and double-strand breaks and inhibition of DNA synthesis and function.
- Inhibits mitotic checkpoints and induces mitotic catastrophe, leading to cell death.
- Cell cycle–nonspecific. Active in all phases of the cell cycle.

MECHANISM OF RESISTANCE
- Increased activity of DNA repair enzymes.
- Increased expression of sulfhydryl proteins, including glutathione and glutathione-related enzymes.
- Cross-resistance between bendamustine and other alkylating agents is only partial.

ABSORPTION
Administered only via the IV route.

DISTRIBUTION
Highly protein bound (>95%), mainly to albumin. Protein binding is not affected by age or low serum albumin levels.

METABOLISM
Metabolized in the liver via hydrolysis to both active and inactive forms. Two active minor metabolites, M3 and M4, are mainly formed by CYP1A2 enzymes. Parent drug and its metabolites are eliminated to a large extent by the kidneys, and 45% of the parent drug is excreted in urine. The elimination half-life of the parent compound is approximately 40 minutes.

INDICATIONS
1. FDA-approved for the treatment of chronic lymphocytic leukemia (CLL).
2. FDA-approved for the treatment of indolent B-cell non-Hodgkin's lymphoma that has progressed during or within 6 months of treatment with rituximab or a rituximab-containing regimen.

DOSAGE RANGE
1. CLL treatment-naïve—100 mg/m^2 IV on days 1 and 2 every 28 days. May give up to a total of 6 cycles.
2. Non-Hodgkin's lymphoma—120 mg/m^2 IV on days 1 and 2 every 21 days. May give up to a total of 8 cycles.

DRUG INTERACTIONS
Inhibitors or inducers of CYP1A2—Concurrent use of bendamustine with CYP1A2 inhibitors (ciprofloxacin, fluvoxamine) or CYP1A2 inducers (omeprazole, smoking) may alter bendamustine metabolism and subsequent drug levels.

SPECIAL CONSIDERATIONS

1. Use with caution in patients with mild or moderate renal impairment. Bendamustine should not be used in patients with CrCl <40 mL/min.
2. Use with caution in patients with mild hepatic impairment. Should not be used in the setting of moderate (SGOT or SGPT 2.5–10 × ULN and total bilirubin 1.5–3 × ULN) or severe (total bilirubin >3 × ULN) hepatic impairment.
3. Monitor for tumor lysis syndrome, especially within the first treatment cycle. Consider using allopurinol during the first 1 to 2 weeks of bendamustine therapy in patients at high risk.
4. Monitor CBCs on a periodic basis. Treatment delays and/or dose reduction may be warranted. Prior to starting the next cycle of therapy, the ANC should be ≥1,000/mm^3 and the platelet count ≥75,000/mm^3.
5. Monitor for hypersensitivity infusion reactions, and discontinuation of therapy should be considered in patients who experience grades 3 or 4 infusion reactions.
6. Bendamustine therapy should be held or discontinued in the setting of severe or progressive skin reactions.
7. Pregnancy category D. Breastfeeding should be avoided.

TOXICITY 1
Myelosuppression with neutropenia and thrombocytopenia is dose-limiting.

TOXICITY 2
Mild nausea and vomiting.

TOXICITY 3
Hypersensitivity reactions presenting with fever, chills, pruritus, and rash. Anaphylactoid and severe anaphylactic reactions have occurred rarely.

TOXICITY 4
Pyrexia, fatigue, and asthenia.

TOXICITY 5
Tumor lysis syndrome typically occurs within the first treatment cycle and in high-risk patients.

TOXICITY 6
Skin rash, toxic skin reactions, and bullous exanthema occur in <10% of patients.

Bevacizumab

TRADE NAME	Avastin	**CLASSIFICATION**	Anti-VEGF monoclonal antibody
CATEGORY	Biologic response modifier agent	**DRUG MANUFACTURER**	Genentech/Roche

MECHANISM OF ACTION
- Recombinant humanized monoclonal antibody directed against the vascular endothelial growth factor-A (VEGF-A) and binds to all VEGF-A isoforms. VEGF is a pro-angiogenic growth factor that is overexpressed in a wide range of solid human cancers, including colorectal cancer.
- Precise mechanism(s) of action remain(s) unknown.
- Binding of the antibody to VEGF prevents its subsequent interaction with VEGF receptors (VEGFRs) on the surface of endothelial cells and tumors, and in so doing, results in inhibition of VEGFR-mediated signaling.
- Inhibits formation of new blood vessels in primary tumor and metastatic tumors.
- Inhibits tumor blood vessel permeability and reduces interstitial tumoral pressures and, in so doing, may enhance blood flow delivery within tumor.
- Restores antitumor response by enhancing dendritic cell function.
- Immunologic mechanisms may also be involved in antitumor activity, and they include recruitment of ADCC and/or complement-mediated cell lysis.

MECHANISM OF RESISTANCE
- Increased expression of other VEGF ligands, including VEGF C, VEGF D, and PlGF
- Increased expression of pro-angiogenic factor ligands, such as PlGF, bFGF, and hepatocyte growth factor (HGF).
- Recruitment of bone marrow–derived cells, which circumvents the requirement of VEGF signaling and restores neovascularization and tumor angiogenesis.
- Increased pericyte coverage of the tumor vasculature, which serves to support its integrity and reduces the need for VEGF-mediated survival signaling.
- Activation and enhancement of invasion and metastasis to provide access to normal tissue vasculature without obligate neovascularization.

DISTRIBUTION
Distribution in body is not well characterized. The time to reach steady-state levels is on the order of 100 days.

METABOLISM
Metabolism of bevacizumab has not been extensively characterized. Peripheral half-life is on the order of 17–21 days, with minimal clearance by the liver or kidneys. Tissue half-life has not been well characterized.

INDICATIONS

1. Metastatic colorectal cancer—FDA-approved for use in combination with any intravenous 5-fluorouracil (5-FU)–based chemotherapy in first-line therapy.
2. Metastatic colorectal cancer—FDA-approved for use in the second-line setting in combination with fluoropyrimidine-based chemotherapy after progression on first-line treatment that includes bevacizumab.
3. NSCLC—FDA-approved for non-squamous NSCLC in combination with carboplatin/paclitaxel.
4. Glioblastoma—FDA-approved as a single agent for glioblastoma with progressive disease following prior therapy.
5. Renal cell cancer—FDA-approved in combination with interferon-α for metastatic renal cell cancer.
6. Cervical cancer—FDA-approved in combination with cisplatin/paclitaxel or paclitaxel/topotecan for persistent, recurrent, or metastatic cervical cancer.
7. Ovarian, fallopian tube, or primary peritoneal cancer—FDA-approved in combination with paclitaxel, pegylated liposomal doxorubicin, or topotecan for platinum-resistant recurrent disease.
8. Ovarian, fallopian tube, or primary peritoneal cancer—FDA-approved in combination with carboplatin and paclitaxel or carboplatin and gemcitabine, followed by bevacizumab as a single agent, for platinum-sensitive recurrent disease.
9. Ovarian, fallopian tube, or primary peritoneal cancer—FDA-approved in combination with carboplatin and paclitaxel followed by bevacizumab as a single agent for stage III or IV disease following initial surgical resection.
10. Hepatocellular cancer (HCC)—FDA-approved in combination with atezolizumab for the front-line treatment of unresectable or metastatic HCC.

DOSAGE RANGE

1. Recommended dose for the first-line treatment of advanced colorectal cancer is 5 mg/kg IV in combination with intravenous 5-FU–based chemotherapy on an every-2-week schedule.
2. Recommended dose for the second-line treatment of advanced colorectal cancer in combination with FOLFOX-4 is 10 mg/kg IV on an every-2-week schedule.
3. Can also be administered at 7.5 mg/kg IV every 3 weeks when used in combination with capecitabine-based regimens for advanced colorectal cancer.
4. Recommended dose for advanced NSCLC is 15 mg/kg IV every 3 weeks with carboplatin/paclitaxel.
5. Recommended dose for glioblastoma is 10 mg/kg IV every 2 weeks.
6. Recommended dose for renal cell cancer is 10 mg/kg IV every 2 weeks with interferon-α.
7. Recommended dose for cervical cancer is 15 mg/kg every 3 weeks with cisplatin/paclitaxel or paclitaxel/topotecan.

8. Recommended dose for platinum-resistant ovarian, fallopian tube, or primary peritoneal cancer is 10 mg/kg every 2 weeks with paclitaxel, pegylated liposomal doxorubicin, or weekly topotecan or 15 mg/kg every 3 weeks with topotecan given every 3 weeks.
9. Recommended dose for platinum-sensitive ovarian, fallopian tube, or primary peritoneal cancer is 15 mg/kg every 3 weeks with carboplatin and paclitaxel for 6–8 cycles, followed by 15 mg/kg every 3 weeks as a single agent or 15 mg/kg every 3 weeks with carboplatin and gemcitabine for 6–10 cycles, followed by 15 mg/kg every 3 weeks as a single agent.
10. Recommended dose for stage III or IV ovarian, fallopian tube, or primary peritoneal cancer following initial surgical resection is 15 mg/kg every 3 weeks with carboplatin and paclitaxel for up to 6 cycles, followed by 15 mg/kg every 3 weeks as a single agent for a total of up to 22 cycles.
11. Recommended dose for HCC is 15 mg/kg every 3 weeks with atezolizumab 1,200 mg IV every 3 weeks.

DRUG INTERACTIONS
None well characterized to date.

SPECIAL CONSIDERATIONS
1. Patients should be warned of the increased risk of arterial thromboembolic events, including myocardial infarction and stroke. Risk factors are age ≥65 years and history of angina, stroke, and prior arterial thromboembolic events. This represents a black-box warning.
2. Patients should be warned of the potential for serious and, in some cases, fatal hemorrhage resulting from hemoptysis in patients with NSCLC. These events have been mainly observed in patients with a central, cavitary, and/or necrotic lesion involving the pulmonary vasculature and have occurred suddenly. Patients with recent hemoptysis (≥1/2 tsp of red blood) should not receive bevacizumab. This represents a black-box warning.
3. Bevacizumab treatment can result in the development of GI perforations, which in some cases has resulted in death. This event represents a black-box warning. Use with caution in patients who have undergone recent surgical and/or invasive procedures. Bevacizumab should be given at least 28 days after any surgical and/or invasive intervention.
4. Bevacizumab treatment can result in the development of wound dehiscence, which in some cases can be fatal. This represents a black-box warning. Use with caution in patients who have undergone recent surgical and/or invasive procedures. Bevacizumab should be given at least 28 days after any surgical and/or invasive intervention.
5. Carefully monitor for infusion-related symptoms. May need to treat with diphenhydramine and acetaminophen.
6. Use with caution in patients with uncontrolled hypertension, as bevacizumab can result in grade 3 hypertension in about 10% of patients. Should be permanently discontinued in patients who develop hypertensive crisis. In most cases, however, hypertension is easily managed by increasing the dose of the antihypertensive medication and/or with the addition of another antihypertensive medication.

7. Bevacizumab should be terminated in patients who develop the nephrotic syndrome. Therapy should be interrupted for proteinuria ≥2 grams/24 hours and resumed when <2 grams/24 hours.
8. Bevacizumab treatment can result in reversible posterior leukoencephalopathy syndrome (RPLS), as manifested by headache, seizure, lethargy, confusion, blindness and other visual side effects, as well as other neurologic disturbances. This syndrome can occur from 16 hours to 1 year after initiation of therapy and usually resolves or improves within days, and magnetic resonance imaging is necessary to confirm the diagnosis.
9. There are no recommended dose reductions for bevacizumab. In the setting of adverse events, bevacizumab should be discontinued or temporarily interrupted.
10. Pregnancy category B.

TOXICITY 1
Gastrointestinal perforations and wound-healing complications.

TOXICITY 2
Bleeding complications, with epistaxis being most commonly observed. Serious, life-threatening pulmonary hemorrhage occurs in rare cases in patients with NSCLC, as outlined previously in Special Considerations.

TOXICITY 3
Increased risk of arterial thromboembolic events, including myocardial infarction, angina, and stroke. There is also an increased incidence of venous thromboembolic events.

TOXICITY 4
Hypertension occurs in 5%–18%. Usually well controlled with oral antihypertensive medication.

TOXICITY 5
Proteinuria with nephrotic syndrome <1%.

TOXICITY 6
Infusion-related symptoms with fever, chills, urticaria, flushing, fatigue, headache, bronchospasm, dyspnea, angioedema, and hypotension. Infusion reactions occur in <3% of patients, and severe reactions occur in 0.2% of patients.

TOXICITY 7
CNS events with dizziness and depression. RPLS occurs rarely (incidence of <0.1%) and presents with headache, seizure, lethargy, confusion, blindness, and other visual disturbances.

Bexarotene

TRADE NAME	Targretin	CLASSIFICATION	Retinoid
CATEGORY	Differentiating agent	DRUG MANUFACTURER	Eisai

MECHANISM OF ACTION
- Selectively binds and activates retinoid X receptors (RXRs).
- RXRs form heterodimers with various other receptors, including retinoic acid receptors (RARs), vitamin D receptors, and thyroid receptors. Once activated, these receptors function as transcription factors, which then regulate the expression of various genes involved in controlling cell differentiation, growth, and proliferation.
- Precise mechanism by which bexarotene exerts its antitumor activity in cutaneous T-cell lymphoma (CTCL) remains unknown.

ABSORPTION
Well absorbed by the GI tract. Peak plasma levels observed 2 hours after oral administration.

DISTRIBUTION
Highly bound to plasma proteins (>99%). Distribution is not well characterized.

METABOLISM
Extensive metabolism occurs in the liver via the cytochrome P450 system to both active and inactive metabolites. Both parent drug and its metabolites are eliminated primarily through the hepatobiliary system and in feces. Renal clearance is minimal, accounting for only <1%. The elimination half-life is about 7 hours.

INDICATIONS
Treatment of cutaneous manifestations of CTCL in patients who are refractory to at least one prior systemic therapy.

DOSAGE RANGE
Recommended initial dose is 300 mg/m^2/day PO. Should be taken as a single dose with food.

DRUG INTERACTION 1
Gemfibrozil—Gemfibrozil inhibits metabolism of bexarotene by the liver P450 system, resulting in increased plasma concentrations. Concurrent administration of gemfibrozil with bexarotene is not recommended.

DRUG INTERACTION 2
Inhibitors of cytochrome P450 system—Drugs that inhibit the liver P450 system, such as ketoconazole, itraconazole, and erythromycin, may cause an increase in plasma concentrations of bexarotene.

DRUG INTERACTION 3
Inducers of cytochrome P450 system—Drugs that induce the liver P450 system, such as rifampin, phenytoin, and phenobarbital, may cause a reduction in plasma bexarotene concentrations.

SPECIAL CONSIDERATIONS
1. Use with caution in patients with abnormal liver function. Monitor liver function tests at baseline and during therapy. Treatment should be discontinued when LFTs are 3-fold higher than the upper limit of normal (ULN).
2. Use with caution in diabetic patients who are on insulin, agents enhancing insulin secretion, or insulin sensitizers, as bexarotene therapy can enhance their effects, resulting in hypoglycemia.
3. Use with caution in patients with history of lipid disorders, as significant alterations in lipid profile are observed with bexarotene therapy. Lipid profile should be obtained at baseline, weekly until the lipid response is established, and at 8-week intervals.
4. Thyroid function tests should be obtained at baseline and during therapy, as bexarotene is associated with hypothyroidism.
5. Use with caution in patients with known hypersensitivity to retinoids.
6. Patients should be advised to limit vitamin A supplementation to <1,500 IU/day to avoid potential additive toxic effects with bexarotene.
7. Patients should be advised to avoid exposure to sunlight, as bexarotene is associated with photosensitivity.
8. Patients who experience new-onset visual difficulties should have an ophthalmologic evaluation, as bexarotene is associated with retinal complications, development of new cataracts, and/or worsening of pre-existing cataracts.
9. Pregnancy category X. Must not be given to a pregnant woman or to a woman who intends to become pregnant. If a woman becomes pregnant while on therapy, bexarotene must be stopped immediately.

TOXICITY 1
Hypertriglyceridemia and hypercholesterolemia are common. Reversible upon dose reduction, cessation of therapy, or when antilipemic therapy is begun (gemfibrozil is not recommended; see Drug Interaction 1).

TOXICITY 2
Hypothyroidism develops in 50% of patients.

TOXICITY 3
Headache and asthenia.

TOXICITY 4
Myelosuppression with neutropenia more common than anemia.

TOXICITY 5
Nausea, abdominal pain, and diarrhea.

TOXICITY 6
Skin rash, dry skin, and rarely alopecia.

TOXICITY 7
Dry eyes, conjunctivitis, blepharitis, cataracts, corneal lesions, and visual field defects.

Bezultifan

TRADE NAME	Welireg, MK-6482-	**CLASSIFICATION**		Signal transduction inhibitor, HIF-2 α inhibitor
CATEGORY	Targeted agent	**DRUG MANUFACTURER**		Array BioPharma

MECHANISM OF ACTION
- Oral small molecule inhibitor of hypoxia-inducible factor (HIF)-2α.
- HIF-2 α is part of the transcription factor complex associated with angiogenesis, tumor cell proliferation and growth. This transcription

pathway is activated in the presence of mutations or deletions in the von-Hippel-Lindau (VHL) gene.

- Clear cell renal cancer, CNS hemangioblastoma, and pancreatic neuroendocrine tumors are the cancers most closely associated with VHL mutations or deletions.

MECHANISM OF RESISTANCE
None well characterized to date.

ABSORPTION
Peak plasma drug concentrations are achieved in 1-2 hours after oral ingestion. Food with a high fat content does not affect C_{max} and AUC.

DISTRIBUTION
Moderate binding (45%) to plasma proteins. Steady-state drug levels reached in about 3 days.

METABOLISM
Metabolized in the liver mainly via UGT2B17 glucuronidation and by CYP2C19 and CYP3A4. The mean terminal half-life of belzutifan is 14 hours.

INDICATIONS
FDA-approved for adult patients with VHL disease who require therapy for clear cell renal cell cancer (RCC), CNS hemangioblastoma, or pancreatic neuroendocrine tumors (pNTET) and not requiring immediate surgery.

DOSAGE RANGE
Recommended dose is 120 mg PO once daily with or without food.

DRUG INTERACTIONS
No specific drug interactions have been identified to date.

SPECIAL CONSIDERATIONS
1. Monitor for anemia at baseline and periodically during therapy. Transfuse patients as clinically indicated. The use of erythropoiesis-stimulating agents for anemia is not recommended.
2. Monitor oxygen saturation levels at baseline and periodically during therapy.
3. Patients should be advised to inform their physician and healthcare team on signs and symptoms of hypoxia.
4. Dose reduction is not required in patients with mild hepatic impairment. Has not been studied in setting of moderate or severe hepatic impairment.
5. Dose reduction is not required in patients with mild to moderate renal impairment. Has not been studied in setting of severe renal impairment or end-stage renal disease.
6. May impair fertility in males and females of reproductive potential.

7. Embryo-fetal toxicity with potential risk to fetus. Female patients should use effective non-hormonal contraception while on treatment and for 1 week after the final dose. Non-hormonal contraception should be used as belzutifan can render some hormonal contraceptives ineffective. Breastfeeding should be avoided while on therapy and for 1 week after the final dose.
8. Pregnancy testing should be done prior to initiation of therapy.

TOXICITY 1
Anemia.

TOXICITY 2
Fatigue.

TOXICITY 3
Headache and dizziness.

TOXICITY 4
Mild nausea and vomiting.

TOXICITY 5
Arthralgias and myalgias.

Bicalutamide

$$NH-\overset{O}{\overset{\|}{C}}-\overset{OH}{\underset{CH_3}{\overset{|}{C}}}-CH_2-SO_2-\text{(ring)}-F$$

$C_{18}H_{14}N_2O_4F_4S$

TRADE NAME	Casodex	**CLASSIFICATION**	Antiandrogen
CATEGORY	Hormonal drug	**DRUG MANUFACTURER**	AstraZeneca

MECHANISM OF ACTION
- Nonsteroidal antiandrogen agent that binds to androgen receptor and inhibits androgen uptake as well as inhibiting androgen binding in the nuclei of androgen-sensitive prostate cancer cells.
- Affinity to androgen receptor is 4-fold greater than flutamide.

MECHANISM OF RESISTANCE
- Decreased expression of androgen receptor.
- Mutation in androgen receptor, leading to decreased binding affinity to bicalutamide.

ABSORPTION
Well absorbed by the GI tract. Peak plasma levels observed 1–2 hours after oral administration. Oral absorption is not affected by food.

DISTRIBUTION
Distribution is not well characterized. Extensively bound to plasma proteins (96%).

METABOLISM
Extensive metabolism occurs in the liver via oxidation and glucuronidation by cytochrome P450 enzymes to inactive metabolites. Both parent drug and its metabolites are cleared in urine and feces. The elimination half-life is long, on the order of several days.

INDICATIONS
Stage D2 metastatic prostate cancer.

DOSAGE RANGE
Recommended dose is 50 mg PO once daily, either alone or in combination with a luteinizing hormone–releasing hormone (LHRH) analog.

DRUG INTERACTIONS
Warfarin—Bicalutamide can displace warfarin from its protein-binding sites, leading to increased anticoagulant effect. Coagulation parameters (PT and INR) must be followed closely, and dose adjustments may be needed.

SPECIAL CONSIDERATIONS
1. Use with caution in patients with abnormal liver function. Monitor LFTs at baseline and during therapy.
2. Caution patients about the potential for hot flashes. Consider the use of clonidine 0.1–0.2 mg PO daily, megestrol acetate 20 mg PO bid, or soy tablets 1 tablet PO tid for prevention and/or treatment.
3. Instruct patients on the potential risk of altered sexual function and impotence.
4. Pregnancy category D. Breastfeeding should be avoided.

TOXICITY 1
Hot flashes, decreased libido, impotence, gynecomastia, nipple pain, and galactorrhea. Occur in 50% of patients.

TOXICITY 2
Constipation observed in 10% of patients. Nausea, vomiting, and diarrhea occur rarely.

TOXICITY 3
Transient elevations in serum transaminases are rare.

Binimetinib

TRADE NAME	Mektovi	CLASSIFICATION	Signal transduction inhibitor, MEK inhibitor
CATEGORY	Targeted agent	DRUG MANUFACTURER	Array BioPharma

MECHANISM OF ACTION
- Reversible inhibitor of mitogen-activated extracellular signal-regulated kinase 1 (MEK1) and kinase 2 (MEK2).
- Results in inhibition of downstream regulators of the extracellular signal-regulated kinase (ERK) pathway, leading to inhibition of cellular proliferation.
- Inhibits growth of BRAF-V600 mutation-positive melanoma, such as V600E.
- The combination of binimetinib and encorafenib leads to enhanced growth inhibitory effects in in vitro and in vivo BRAF mutation-positive model systems, such as melanoma and CRC.

MECHANISM OF RESISTANCE
- Increased expression and/or activation of the PI3K/AKT pathway.
- Reactivation of the MAPK signaling pathway.
- Emergence of MEK2 mutations.
- Presence of NRAS mutations.
- Increased expression and/or activation of the HER2-neu pathway.

ABSORPTION
Oral bioavailability is on the order of 50%. Peak plasma drug concentrations are achieved in 1.6 hours after oral ingestion. Food with a high fat content does not affect C_{max} and AUC.

DISTRIBUTION
Extensive binding (97%) to plasma proteins.

METABOLISM
Metabolized in the liver mainly via UGT1A1 glucuronidation with other pathways involved, including N-dealkylation, amide hydrolysis, and loss of ethane-diol from the side chain. An active metabolite, M3, is produced in the liver by CYP1A2 and CYP2C19, and this represents nearly 9% of binimetinib exposure. Elimination is via the hepatobiliary route, with 62% of an administered dose excreted in feces (approximately 30% as parent drug), with renal elimination accounting for only about 31% of an administered dose (6.5% as parent drug). The mean terminal half-life of binimetinib is 3.5 hours.

INDICATIONS
1. FDA-approved in combination with encorafenib for unresectable or metastatic melanoma with a BRAF-V600E or V600K mutation.
2. Clinical activity in combination with encorafenib and cetuximab for metastatic colorectal cancer with a BRAF-V600E mutation.

DOSAGE RANGE
1. Metastatic melanoma: 45 mg PO bid in combination with encorafenib.
2. mCRC: 45 mg PO bid in combination with encorafenib plus cetuximab.

DRUG INTERACTIONS
No specific drug interactions have been identified to date.

SPECIAL CONSIDERATIONS
1. Baseline and periodic evaluations of LVEF, at 1 month after treatment initiation and every 3 months thereafter, should be performed while on therapy. The median time to first onset of LVEF reduction is 4 months. Treatment should be held if the absolute LVEF drops by 10% from pretreatment baseline. Therapy should be permanently stopped for symptomatic cardiomyopathy or persistent, asymptomatic LVEF dysfunction that does not resolve within 4 weeks.
2. Dose reduction is not required in the setting of mild hepatic dysfunction. For patients with moderate or severe hepatic impairment, the dose should be reduced to 30 mg PO bid.
3. Dose reduction is not required in the setting of mild, moderate, or severe renal impairment.
4. Patients should be warned about the possibility of visual disturbances.
5. Careful eye exams should be done at baseline, at regular intervals, and with any new visual changes to rule out the possibility of serous retinopathy or retinal vein occlusion.

6. Monitor patients for symptoms and signs of bleeding.
7. Monitor patients for an increased risk of new primary cancers, both cutaneous and non-cutaneous, while on therapy and for up to 6 months following the last dose of binimetinib.
8. Monitor liver function tests periodically during therapy.
9. Patients should be educated to avoid sun exposure.
10. Baseline and periodic CPK levels while on therapy, as rhabdomyolysis has been observed with binimetinib therapy.
11. BRAF testing using an FDA-approved diagnostic test to confirm the presence of the BRAF-V600E or V600K mutations is required for determining which patients should receive binimetinib therapy.
12. Embryo-fetal toxicity with potential risk to fetus. Female patients should use effective contraception while on treatment and for at least 30 days after the final dose. Breastfeeding should avoided while on therapy and for 3 days after the final dose.

TOXICITY 1
Cardiac toxicity in the form of cardiomyopathy with LV dysfunction.

TOXICITY 2
Ocular side effects, including impaired vision, serous retinopathy, retinal detachment, and retinal vein occlusion.

TOXICITY 3
GI toxicity with diarrhea, nausea/vomiting, and abdominal pain.

TOXICITY 4
Skin toxicity with rash, dermatitis, acneiform rash.

TOXICITY 5
Hepatotoxicity.

TOXICITY 6
Bleeding complications, with rectal hemorrhage, hematochezia, and hemorrhoidal hemorrhage being most common events. Intracranial hemorrhage in the setting of metastatic brain disease has been observed.

TOXICITY 7
Venous thromboembolic events, including DVT and PE.

TOXICITY 8
Elevation of serum CPK levels in 58% of patients. Rhabdomyolysis can occur rarely.

TOXICITY 9
Interstitial lung disease.

Bleomycin

TRADE NAME	Blenoxane	CLASSIFICATION	Antitumor antibiotic
CATEGORY	Chemotherapy drug	DRUG MANUFACTURER	Bristol-Myers Squibb

MECHANISM OF ACTION

- Small peptide with a molecular weight of 1,500.
- Contains a DNA-binding region and an iron-binding region at opposite ends of the molecule.
- Iron is necessary as a cofactor for free radical generation and bleomycin's cytotoxic activity.
- Cytotoxic effects result from the generation of activated oxygen free radical species, which causes single- and double-strand DNA breaks and eventual cell death.

MECHANISM OF RESISTANCE

- Increased expression of DNA repair enzymes, resulting in enhanced repair of DNA damage.
- Decreased drug accumulation through altered uptake of drug.

ABSORPTION

Oral bioavailability of bleomycin is poor. After IM administration, peak levels are obtained in about 60 minutes but reach only one-third the levels achieved after an IV dose. When administered in the intrapleural space for the treatment of malignant pleural effusion (pleurodesis), approximately 45%–50% of the drug is absorbed into the systemic circulation.

DISTRIBUTION
Distributes into intra- and extracellular fluid. Less than 10% of drug bound to plasma proteins.

METABOLISM
After IV administration, there is a rapid, biphasic disappearance from the circulation. The terminal half-life is approximately 3 hours in patients with normal renal function. Bleomycin is rapidly inactivated in tissues, especially the liver and kidney, by the enzyme bleomycin hydrolase. Elimination of bleomycin is primarily via the kidneys, with 50%–70% of an administered dose excreted unchanged in urine. Patients with impaired renal function are at risk for increased toxicity. Dose reductions are recommended in the presence of renal dysfunction.

INDICATIONS
1. Hodgkin's and non-Hodgkin's lymphoma.
2. Germ cell tumors.
3. Head and neck cancer.
4. Squamous cell carcinomas of the skin, cervix, and vulva.
5. Sclerosing agent for malignant pleural effusion and ascites.

DOSAGE RANGE
1. Hodgkin's lymphoma—10 units/m^2 IV on days 1 and 15 every 28 days, as part of the ABVD regimen.
2. Testicular cancer—30 units IV on days 2, 9, and 16 every 21 days, as part of the PEB regimen.
3. Intracavitary instillation into pleural space—60 units/m^2.

DRUG INTERACTION 1
Oxygen—High concentrations of oxygen may enhance the pulmonary toxicity of bleomycin. FIO$_2$ should be maintained at no higher than 25% when possible.

DRUG INTERACTION 2
Cisplatin—Cisplatin decreases renal clearance of bleomycin and, in so doing, may lead to higher drug levels, resulting in greater toxicity.

DRUG INTERACTION 3
Radiation therapy—Radiation therapy enhances the pulmonary toxicity of bleomycin.

DRUG INTERACTION 4
Brentuximab—Co-administration of bleomycin and brentuximab may increase the risk of pulmonary toxicity. As such, the concomitant use of these two agents is contraindicated.

SPECIAL CONSIDERATIONS

1. PFTs with special focus on DLCO and vital capacity should be obtained at baseline and before each cycle of therapy. A decrease of >15% in PFTs should mandate the immediate discontinuation of bleomycin, even in the absence of clinical symptoms. Increased risk of pulmonary toxicity when cumulative dose >400 units.
2. Chest X-ray should be obtained at baseline and before each cycle of therapy to monitor for evidence of infiltrates and/or interstitial lung findings.
3. Monitor for clinical signs of pulmonary dysfunction, including shortness of breath, dyspnea, decreased O_2 saturation, and decreased lung expansion.
4. Use with caution in patients with impaired renal function because drug clearance may be reduced. Doses should be reduced in the presence of renal dysfunction. Baseline CrCl should be obtained, and renal status should be monitored before each cycle.
5. Patients with lymphoma may be at increased risk for developing an anaphylactic reaction. This complication can be immediate or delayed. An anaphylaxis kit that includes epinephrine, antihistamines, and corticosteroids should be readily available at bedside during bleomycin administration.
6. Premedicate patients with acetaminophen 30 minutes before administration of drug and every 6 hours for 24 hours if fever and chills are noted.
7. Patients undergoing surgery must inform the surgeon and anesthesiologist of prior treatment with bleomycin. High concentrations of forced inspiratory oxygen (FIO_2) at the time of surgery may enhance the pulmonary toxicity of bleomycin.

TOXICITY 1

Skin reactions are the most common side effects and include erythema, hyperpigmentation of the skin, striae, and vesiculation. Skin peeling, thickening of the skin and nail beds, hyperkeratosis, and ulceration can also occur. These skin manifestations usually occur when the cumulative dose has reached 150–200 units.

TOXICITY 2

Pulmonary toxicity is dose-limiting in 10% of patients. Usually presents as pneumonitis with cough, dyspnea, dry inspiratory crackles, and infiltrates on chest X-ray. Increased incidence in patients >70 years of age and with cumulative doses >400 units. Rarely progresses to pulmonary fibrosis but can be fatal in about 1% of patients. PFTs are the most sensitive approach to follow, with specific focus on DLCO and vital capacity. A decrease of 15% or more in the PFTs should mandate immediate stoppage of the drug.

TOXICITY 3
Hypersensitivity reaction in the form of fever and chills observed in up to 25% of patients. True anaphylactoid reactions are rare but more common in patients with lymphoma.

TOXICITY 4
Vascular events, including myocardial infarction, stroke, and Raynaud's phenomenon, are rarely reported.

TOXICITY 5
Myelosuppression is relatively mild.

Blinatumomab

TRADE NAME	Blincyto	CLASSIFICATION	BiTE antibody
CATEGORY	Biologic response modifier agent, immunotherapy	DRUG MANUFACTURER	Amgen

MECHANISM OF ACTION
- Bispecific T-cell engaging (BiTE) antibody that binds to CD19 expressed on precursor B-cells and CD3 expressed on the surface of T cells. This antibody lacks the constant region of common monoclonal antibodies.
- This binding causes cytotoxic T cells to be physically linked to malignant CD19-positive B cells and triggers the signaling cascade, leading to the upregulation of cell adhesion molecules, production of cytolytic proteins, release of inflammatory cytokines, and the proliferation of T cells, ultimately resulting in lysis of CD19-positive B cells.
- CD19 is expressed in all stages of B-lineage acute lymphocytic leukemia (ALL), across all non-Hodgkin's lymphoma subtypes, and in CLL.
- Mechanism of action differs from that of conventional monoclonal antibodies, which use antibody-dependent cellular cytotoxicity and engage natural killer T cells, macrophages, and neutrophils to cause tumor cell death.

ABSORPTION
Administered only via the IV route.

DISTRIBUTION
Following continuous intravenous infusion, steady-state serum concentrations are achieved within 1 day and remain stable over time.

METABOLISM
Metabolism of blinatumomab has not been well characterized. As with other antibodies, it is assumed that blinatumomab is degraded to small peptides and amino acids via catabolic pathways. The mean elimination half-life is approximately 2 hours.

INDICATIONS
1. FDA-approved for the treatment of adult and pediatric patients with relapsed or refractory Philadelphia chromosome–negative, B-cell precursor ALL.
2. FDA-approved for the treatment of B-cell precursor ALL in first or second complete remission with minimal residual disease (MRD) greater than or equal to 0.1%.

DOSAGE RANGE
1. Treatment of MRD-positive, B-cell precursor ALL: A single cycle of therapy consists of 28 days of continuous IV infusion followed by a 14-day drug-free interval (total of 42 days).

   A treatment course consists of one cycle of blinatumomab for induction followed by up to three additional cycles for consolidation.
2. Treatment of relapsed or refractory B-cell precursor ALL: A single cycle of induction or consolidation therapy consists of 28 days of continuous IV infusion followed by a 14-day drug-free interval (total of 42 days).

   A single cycle of treatment of continued therapy consists of 28 days of continuous IV infusion followed by a 56-day treatment-free interval (total of 84 days).

   A treatment course consists of up to two cycles of blinatumomab for induction followed by three additional cycles for consolidation and up to four cycles of continued therapy.

   For patients >45 kg, the recommended dose for cycle 1 is 9 µg/day on days 1–7 and then 28 µg/day continuous IV infusion on days 8–28, followed by a 14-day treatment-free interval. For subsequent cycles, the dose is 28 µg/day on days 1–28 followed by a 14-day break.

   For patients <45 kg, the recommended dose for cycle 1 is 5 µg/m^2/day on days 1–7 and then 15 µg/m^2/day on days 8–28, followed by a 14-day treatment-free interval. For subsequent cycles, the dose is 15 µg/m^2/day on days 1–28, followed by a 14-day break.

DRUG INTERACTIONS
None well characterized to date.

SPECIAL CONSIDERATIONS
1. Hospitalization is recommended for the first 9 days of the first cycle of therapy and for the first 2 days of the second cycle.
2. Adult patients should be premedicated with 20 mg dexamethasone 1 hour prior to the first dose of therapy of each cycle, prior to a step dose (cycle 1, day 8), and when restarting an infusion after an interruption of

more than 4 hours. Pediatric patients should be premedicated with 5 mg/m^2 dexamethasone up to a maximum of 20 mg prior to the first dose of therapy in the first cycle, prior to a step dose (cycle 1, day 8), and when restarting an infusion after an interruption of more than 4 hours.

3. Monitor for infusion-related events, which may be clinically indistinguishable from the manifestations of cytokine release syndrome (CRS), with life-threatening or fatal consequences.

4. Monitor for CRS, which presents as fever, headache, nausea/vomiting, elevations in serum transaminases and increased serum bilirubin, and hypotension. In some cases, disseminated intravascular coagulation (DIC), capillary leak syndrome (CLS), and hemophagocytic lymphohistiocytosis/macrophage activation syndrome (HLH/MAS) have been reported as part of CRS. This is a black-box warning.

5. Monitor for neurologic toxicity, presenting as encephalopathy, convulsions, speech disorders, disturbances in consciousness, confusion and disorientation, and coordination and balance disorders. The median time to onset of any neurological toxicity is 7 days. This is a black-box warning.

6. Brain magnetic resonance imaging (MRI) changes showing leukoencephalopathy have been observed, especially in patients with prior treatment with cranial irradiation and chemotherapy (including systemic high-dose methotrexate or intrathecal cytarabine). The clinical significance of these imaging changes is unknown.

7. Monitor for signs and symptoms of infection, as blinatumomab therapy is associated with an increased risk of pneumonia, bacteremia, sepsis, opportunistic infection, and catheter-site infections.

8. Monitor CBCs while on therapy.

9. Monitor for tumor lysis syndrome, especially in patients with high numbers of circulating cells (>25,000/mm^3) or high tumor burden. Appropriate measures should be taken to prevent the development of tumor lysis syndrome while receiving blinatumomab therapy.

10. Patients should be advised against performing activities that require mental alertness, including operating heavy machinery and driving.

11. Closely monitor therapy in older patients (>65), as they experience a higher rate of neurological toxicities, including cognitive disorder, encephalopathy, confusion, and serious infections.

12. Monitor serum transaminases and serum bilirubin at baseline and periodically during therapy. Treatment should be stopped if the serum transaminases rise to >5 × ULN or if bilirubin rises to >3 × ULN. No dose modification is needed for patients with baseline CrCl >30 mL/min. There is currently no information available for patients with CrCL <30 mL/min or for patients on hemodialysis.

13. Pregnancy category C. Breastfeeding should be avoided.

TOXICITY 1
Infusion-related symptoms.

TOXICITY 2
Cytokine release syndrome (CRS).

TOXICITY 3
Tumor lysis syndrome characterized by hyperkalemia, hyperuricemia, hyperphosphatemia, hypocalcemia, and renal insufficiency. Usually occurs within the first 12–24 hours of treatment. Risk is increased in patients with high numbers of circulating malignant cells (>25,000/mm^3) and/or high tumor burden.

TOXICITY 4
Neurological toxicities with altered mental status, encephalopathy, seizures, speech disorders, confusion, balance disorders. Leukoencephalopathy with brain MRI changes can also be observed in rare cases.

TOXICITY 5
Myelosuppression with neutropenia, anemia, and thrombocytopenia.

TOXICITY 6
Increased risk of bacterial, fungal, viral, and opportunistic infections.

TOXICITY 7
GI toxicity in the form of nausea/vomiting, abdominal pain, diarrhea, constipation, and elevations in serum transaminases and serum bilirubin.

Bortezomib

TRADE NAME	Velcade	CLASSIFICATION	Proteasome inhibitor
CATEGORY	Chemotherapy drug	DRUG MANUFACTURER	Millennium: The Takeda Oncology Company

MECHANISM OF ACTION
- Reversible inhibitor of the 26S proteasome.
- The 26S proteasome is a large protein complex that degrades ubiquitinated proteins. This pathway plays an essential role in regulating the intracellular concentrations of various cellular proteins.
- Inhibition of the 26S proteasome prevents the targeted proteolysis of ubiquitinated proteins, and disruption of this normal pathway can affect multiple signaling pathways within the cell, leading to cell death.
- Results in downregulation of the NF-κB pathway. NF-κB is a transcription factor that stimulates the production of various growth factors, including IL-6, cell adhesion molecules, and anti-apoptotic proteins, all of which contribute to cell growth and chemoresistance. Inhibition of the NF-κB pathway by bortezomib leads to inhibition of cell growth and restores chemosensitivity.

MECHANISM OF RESISTANCE
- Activation of NF-κB pathway via proteasome-independent mechanisms.
- Mutations in the proteasome β5 subunit (PSMB5) gene, leading to overexpression of PSMB5 protein.
- Increased expression of the multidrug-resistant gene with elevated P170 protein levels, which leads to increased drug efflux and decreased intracellular drug accumulation.

ABSORPTION
Administered via the intravenous (IV) and subcutaneous (SC) routes. Total systemic exposure is equivalent for IV and SC administration.

DISTRIBUTION
Volume of distribution not well characterized. About 80% of drug bound to plasma proteins.

METABOLISM
Metabolized by the liver cytochrome P450 system. The major metabolic pathway is deboronation, forming two deboronated metabolites. The deboronated metabolites are inactive as 26S proteasome inhibitors. The elimination pathways for bortezomib have not been well characterized. Bortezomib has a mean elimination half-life of 76–108 hours upon multiple dosing with the 1.3 mg/m^2 dose.

INDICATIONS
1. FDA-approved for the treatment of multiple myeloma.
2. FDA-approved for the treatment of mantle cell lymphoma after at least one prior therapy.

DOSAGE RANGE

Recommended dose for relapsed multiple myeloma and mantle cell lymphoma is 1.3 mg/m^2 administered by IV or SC twice weekly for 2 weeks (on days 1, 4, 8, and 11) followed by a 10-day rest period (days 12–21).

DRUG INTERACTION 1

Ketoconazole and other CYP3A4 inhibitors—Co-administration of ketoconazole and other CYP3A4 inhibitors may decrease the metabolism of bortezomib, resulting in increased drug levels and potentially increased toxicity.

DRUG INTERACTION 2

CYP3A4 inducers—Co-administration of bortezomib with potent CYP3A4 inducers, such as rifampin, may increase the metabolism of bortezomib, resulting in decreased drug levels.

DRUG INTERACTION 3

St. John's Wort may alter the metabolism of bortezomib, resulting in decreased drug levels.

SPECIAL CONSIDERATIONS

1. Contraindicated in patients with hypersensitivity to boron, bortezomib, and/or mannitol.
2. Use with caution in patients with impaired liver function because drug metabolism and/or clearance may be reduced. Patients with mild hepatic impairment do not require dose modification. However, patients with moderate or severe hepatic impairment should be started at a reduced dose of 0.7 mg/m^2 in the first cycle. Depending on patient tolerability, the dose can be either increased to 1 mg/m^2 or further reduced to 0.5 mg/m^2 in subsequent cycles.
3. Dose adjustments of bortezomib are not necessary for patients with renal dysfunction. Since hemodialysis can reduce bortezomib concentrations, the drug should be administered after the dialysis procedure.
4. Use with caution in patients with a history of syncope, patients who are on antihypertensive medications, and patients who are dehydrated because bortezomib can cause orthostatic hypotension.
5. Bortezomib should be withheld at the onset of any grade 3 non-hematologic toxicity, excluding neuropathy, or any grade 4 hematologic toxicities. After symptoms have resolved, therapy can be restarted with a 25% dose reduction. With respect to neuropathy, the dose of bortezomib should be reduced to 1 mg/m^2 with grade 1 peripheral neuropathy with pain or grade 2 peripheral neuropathy. In the presence of grade 2 neurotoxicity, therapy should be withheld until symptoms have resolved and restarted at a dose of 0.7 mg/m^2 along with changing the treatment schedule to once per week. In the presence of grade 4 neurotoxicity, therapy should be discontinued.

6. The use of SC bortezomib may be considered in patients with pre-existing neuropathy or in those at high risk of developing peripheral neuropathy.
7. Patients should avoid taking green tea products and supplements, as they have been shown to bind to the boron moiety on bortezomib and, in so doing, inhibit clinical efficacy.
8. Patients should avoid taking St. John's Wort, as it has been shown to increase the metabolism of bortezomib, leading to lower effective drug levels.
9. Pregnancy category D. Breastfeeding should be avoided.

TOXICITY 1

Fatigue, malaise, and generalized weakness. Usually observed during the first and second cycles of therapy.

TOXICITY 2

GI toxicity in the form of nausea/vomiting and diarrhea.

TOXICITY 3

Myelosuppression with thrombocytopenia and neutropenia.

TOXICITY 4

Peripheral sensory neuropathy, although a mixed sensorimotor neuropathy has also been observed. Symptoms may improve and/or return to baseline upon discontinuation of bortezomib.

TOXICITY 5

Fever (>38°C) in up to 40% of patients.

TOXICITY 6

Orthostatic hypotension in up to 12% of patients.

TOXICITY 7

Congestive heart failure (CHF) and new onset of reduced LVEF. Rare cases of QT interval prolongation.

TOXICITY 8

Pulmonary toxicity in the form of pneumonitis, interstitial pneumonia, lung infiltrates, and acute respiratory distress syndrome (ARDS). Pulmonary hypertension has also been reported.

TOXICITY 9

Reversible posterior leukoencephalopathy syndrome (RPLS) is a rare event and presents with headache, seizure, lethargy, confusion, blindness, and other visual disturbances.

Bosutinib

TRADE NAME	Bosulif, SKI-606	CLASSIFICATION	Signal transduction inhibitor, Bcr-Abl inhibitor
CATEGORY	Targeted agent	DRUG MANUFACTURER	Pfizer

MECHANISM OF ACTION
- Potent inhibitor of the Bcr-Abl tyrosine kinase. Retains activity in 16 of 18 imatinib-resistant Bcr-Abl mutations.
- Does not have activity against T315I gatekeeper or V299L Bcr-Abl mutations.
- Potent inhibitor of the Src family (Src, Lyn, and Hck) kinases. Src family kinases (SFKs) are involved in cancer cell adhesion, migration, invasion, proliferation, differentiation, and survival.

MECHANISM OF RESISTANCE
Single-point mutations, either T315I or V299L, within the ATP-binding pocket of the Abl tyrosine kinase.

ABSORPTION
Well absorbed following oral administration, with peak plasma concentrations at 4–6 hours. Administration of a high-fat meal results in higher drug concentrations.

DISTRIBUTION
Exhibits extensive plasma protein binding (96%).

METABOLISM
Metabolized in the liver primarily by CYP3A4 microsomal enzymes, with all of the metabolites inactive. Approximately 91% and 3% of an administered dose of drug is eliminated in the feces and urine, respectively. The mean elimination half-life is 22.5 hours.

INDICATIONS

1. FDA-approved for the treatment of adult patients with chronic-, accelerated-, or blast-phase Philadelphia chromosome–positive (Ph+) CML with resistance or intolerance to prior therapy.
2. FDA-approved for newly diagnosed chronic phase Ph+ CML.

DOSAGE RANGE

1. Chronic, accelerated, or blast phase Ph+ CML with resistance or intolerance to prior therapy: 500 mg PO once daily with food.
2. Newly diagnosed chronic phase Ph+ CML: 400 mg PO once daily with food.
3. Consider dose escalation by increments of 100 mg once daily to a maximum of 600 mg PO once daily in patients who do not reach complete hematologic response (CHR) by week 8 or a complete cytogenetic response (CCyR) by week 12.

DRUG INTERACTIONS

1. Concomitant use of CYP3A inhibitors, such as ketoconazole, voriconazole, posaconazole, clarithromycin, fluconazole, erythromycin, diltiazem, aprepitant, verapamil, grapefruit juice, and ciprofloxacin, can decrease the metabolism of bosutinib, resulting in increased plasma drug levels and potentially increased toxicity.
2. Drugs that are moderate or strong CYP3A inducers, such as rifampin, phenytoin, carbamazepine, St. John's Wort, and phenobarbital, can increase the metabolism of bosutinib, resulting in decreased plasma drug levels and reduced clinical activity.
3. Proton pump inhibitors, such as lansoprazole, can decrease plasma concentrations of bosutinib.
4. Drugs that are P-glycoprotein substrates, such as digoxin, may have higher plasma concentrations when taken with bosutinib.

SPECIAL CONSIDERATIONS

1. Important to carefully review patient's list of medications, as bosutinib has several potential drug–drug interactions.
2. Monitor CBC weekly during the first month and then monthly thereafter.
3. Monitor liver function on a monthly basis for the first 3 months and periodically thereafter.
4. Dose of bosutinib should be reduced to 200 mg PO daily in the presence of pre-existing mild, moderate, and severe hepatic dysfunction.
5. Dose reduction is not required in the presence of mild or moderate renal impairment. The dose should be reduced to 300 mg PO daily in the presence of severe renal dysfunction (CrCl <30 mL/min).
6. Bosutinib should be taken with food, and drug tablets should not be crushed.
7. Avoid concomitant use of proton pump inhibitors (PPIs) while on bosutinib therapy. Consider using short-acting antacids or H2 blockers instead of PPIs.

8. Be aware of the potential for fluid retention that can manifest as pericardial effusion, pleural effusion, pulmonary edema, or peripheral edema.
9. Avoid Seville oranges, starfruit, pomelos, grapefruit juice, grapefruit products, and St. John's Wort while on therapy.
10. Pregnancy category D. Breastfeeding should be avoided.

TOXICITY 1
Gastrointestinal toxicity is common, presenting as diarrhea in more than 80%, nausea/vomiting, and abdominal pain.

TOXICITY 2
Myelosuppression with thrombocytopenia, anemia, and neutropenia.

TOXICITY 3
Skin rash occurs in about one-third of patients and is associated with pruritus.

TOXICITY 4
Elevation of serum transaminases (SGOT/SGPT), usually within the first 3 months of therapy.

TOXICITY 5
Fluid retention manifesting as peripheral edema, pericardial effusion, pleural effusion, or pulmonary edema.

TOXICITY 6
Fatigue and asthenia.

Brentuximab

TRADE NAME	Adcetris, SGN-35	CLASSIFICATION	Antibody drug conjugate
CATEGORY	Targeted agent, chemotherapy drug	DRUG MANUFACTURER	Seattle Genetics and Millennium: The Takeda Oncology Company

---

MECHANISM OF ACTION
- Brentuximab is a CD30-directed antibody–drug conjugate (ADC) that is made up of three components: (1) chimeric IgG1 antibody cAC10, specific for CD30; (2) microtubule-disrupting agent monomethyl auristatin E (MMAE); and (3) protease-cleavable linker that covalently attaches MMAE to cAC10. Approximately four molecules of MMAE are conjugated to each antibody molecule.

- Targets the CD30 antigen, a cell surface protein expressed on the surface of Hodgkin's Reed-Sternberg cells and on anaplastic large cell lymphomas (ALCLs), embryonal carcinomas, and select subtypes of B-cell–derived, non-Hodgkin's lymphomas and mature T-cell lymphomas. Normal expression of CD30 is highly restricted to a relatively small population of activated B cells and T cells and a small portion of eosinophils.
- Binding of the ADC to CD30-expressing cells is followed by internalization of the ADC–CD30 complex with subsequent release of MMAE via proteolytic cleavage.
- MMAE inhibits the microtubule network within the tumor cell, resulting in cell cycle arrest at the G2/M interphase and apoptotic death.
- Chimeric antibody mediates complement-dependent cell lysis (CDCC) in the presence of human complement and antibody-dependent cellular cytotoxicity (ADCC) with human effector cells.

MECHANISM OF RESISTANCE
None well characterized to date.

ABSORPTION
Administered only via the IV route.

DISTRIBUTION
Median time to peak drug concentration occurs immediately after infusion for the antibody-drug conjugate and approximately 2 to 3 days after infusion for MMAE. Steady-state blood levels for both the antibody-drug conjugate and MMAE are reached in 21 days.

METABOLISM
Only a small fraction of MMAE released from brentuximab is metabolized, which is mediated by CYP3A4 and CYP3A5. Approximately 25% of the total MMAE administered as part of the ADC infusion is recovered in feces and urine over a 1-week period, with 70% being recovered in feces. The terminal half-life estimates of the antibody–drug conjugate and MMAE are 4 to 6 days and 3 to 4 days, respectively.

INDICATIONS
1. FDA-approved for patients with previously untreated stage III or IV classical Hodgkin's lymphoma in combination with chemotherapy.
2. FDA-approved for patients with Hodgkin's lymphoma after failure of autologous stem cell transplant (ASCT) or after failure of at least two prior multiagent chemotherapy regimens in patients who are not ASCT candidates.
3. FDA-approved as post-autologous stem cell transplant consolidation for patients with Hodgkin's lymphoma at high risk for relapse or progression.
4. FDA-approved for patients with anaplastic large cell lymphoma after failure of at least one prior multiagent chemotherapy regimen.
5. FDA-approved for patients with primary cutaneous anaplastic large cell lymphoma or CD30-expressing mycosis fungoides who have received prior systemic therapy.

DOSAGE RANGE
1. Recommended dose as monotherapy is 1.8 mg/kg IV every 3 weeks.
2. Recommended dose in combination with chemotherapy is 1.2 mg/kg up to a maximum of 120 mg every 2 weeks for a maximum of 12 doses.

DRUG INTERACTIONS
Bleomycin—Co-administration of brentuximab with bleomycin may increase the risk of pulmonary toxicity. As such, the concomitant use of these two agents is contraindicated.

SPECIAL CONSIDERATIONS
1. Patients should be premedicated with acetaminophen and diphenhydramine to reduce the incidence of infusion-related reactions.
2. Monitor for infusion-related events, which usually occur 30–120 minutes after the start of the first infusion. Infusion should be immediately stopped if signs or symptoms of an allergic reaction are observed. Immediate institution of diphenhydramine, acetaminophen, corticosteroids, IV fluids, and/or vasopressors may be necessary. Resuscitation equipment should be readily available at bedside.
3. Monitor for tumor lysis syndrome, especially in patients with rapidly proliferating disease and/or high tumor burden.
4. Monitor CBCs at regular intervals during therapy.
5. Consider the diagnosis of progressive multifocal leukoencephalopathy (PML) in patients who present with new onset or changes in pre-existing neurological signs or symptoms. This represents a black-box warning.
6. Patients should not receive live, attenuated vaccines while on brentuximab therapy. In patients who have recently been vaccinated, brentuximab therapy should not be initiated for least 2 weeks.
7. Pregnancy category C. Breastfeeding should be avoided.

TOXICITY 1
Infusion-related symptoms, including fever, chills, urticaria, flushing, fatigue, headache, bronchospasm, rhinitis, dyspnea, angioedema, nausea, and/or hypotension.

TOXICITY 2
Tumor lysis syndrome characterized by hyperkalemia, hyperuricemia, hyperphosphatemia, hypocalcemia, and renal insufficiency. Usually occurs within the first 12–24 hours of treatment. Risk is increased in patients with rapidly proliferating tumor and/or high tumor burden.

TOXICITY 3
Myelosuppression with neutropenia and anemia.

TOXICITY 4
Peripheral sensory neuropathy is the most common neurologic side effect.

TOXICITY 5
Progressive multifocal leukoencephalopathy (PML).

TOXICITY 6
Skin reactions, including rash, pruritus, and Stevens-Johnson syndrome.

TOXICITY 7
Mild nausea/vomiting and diarrhea are the most common GI side effects.

Brexucabtagene autoleucel

TRADE NAME	Tecartus, KTE-X19, brexu-cel	**CLASSIFICATION**	CAR T-cell therapy
CATEGORY	Cellular therapy, immunotherapy	**DRUG MANUFACTURER**	Kite, Gilead

MECHANISM OF ACTION
- Brexucabtagene autoleucel is a CD19-directed genetically modified autologous T-cell immunotherapy that binds to CD19-expressing target cells and normal B cells.
- Prepared from the patient's own peripheral blood mononuclear cells, which are enriched for T cells, and then genetically modified ex vivo by retroviral transduction to express a chimeric antigen receptor (CAR) made up of a murine anti-CD19 single-chain variable fragment linked to CD28 and CD3-zeta co-stimulatory domains. The anti-CD19 CAR T cells are expanded ex vivo and infused back to the patient, where they target CR19-expressing cells.
- Lymphocyte depletion conditioning regimen with cyclophosphamide and fludarabine leads to increased systemic levels of IL-15 and other pro-inflammatory cytokines and chemokines that enhance CAR T-cell activity.
- The conditioning regimen may also decrease immunosuppressive regulatory T cells, activate antigen-presenting cells, and induce pro-inflammatory tumor cell damage.

MECHANISM OF RESISTANCE
- Selection of alternatively spliced CD19 isoforms that lack the CD19 epitope recognized by the CAR T cells.
- Antigen loss or modulation.
- Insufficient reactivity against tumors cells with low antigen density.
- Emergence of an antigen-negative clone.
- Lineage switching from lymphoid to myeloid leukemia phenotype.

ABSORPTION
Administered only via the IV route.

DISTRIBUTION
Peak levels of anti-CD19 CAR T cells are observed at 15 days after infusion.

METABOLISM
Metabolism has not been well characterized.

INDICATIONS
1. FDA-approved for relapsed or refractory mantle cell lymphoma. Approved under accelerated approval based on overall response rate and durability of response.
2. FDA-approved for relapsed or refractory B-cell ALL.

DOSAGE RANGE
1. Mantle cell lymphoma: target dose of 2×10^6 CAR-positive viable T cells per kilogram of body weight, with a maximum of 2×10^8 CAR-positive viable T cells
   A lymphodepleting chemotherapy regimen of cyclophosphamide 500 mg/m^2 IV and fludarabine 30 mg/m^2 IV on Days 3, 4, and 5 should be administered before infusion of brexucabtagene autoleucel.
2. B-cell ALL: target dose of 1×10^6 CAR-positive viable T cells per kilogram of body weight, with a maximum of 1×10^8 CAR-positive viable T cells
   A lymphodepleting chemotherapy regimen of fludarabine 25 mg/m^2 IV on Days 2, 3, and 4 and cyclophosphamide 900 mg/m^2 IV on the second day before should be administered before infusion of brexucabtagene autoleucel.
3. Patients should be pre-medicated with acetaminophen 650 mg PO and diphenhydramine 12.5 mg IV 1 hour before infusion of brexucabtagene autoleucel.

DRUG INTERACTIONS
None well characterized to date.

SPECIAL CONSIDERATIONS
1. Brexucabtagene autoleucel is available only through a restricted program under a Risk Evaluation and Mitigation Strategy (REMS).
2. Monitor for hypersensitivity infusion reactions. Patients should be pre-medicated with acetaminophen 650 mg PO and diphenhydramine 12.5 mg IV at 1 hour prior to CAR T-cell infusion. Prophylactic use of systemic corticosteroids should be avoided, as they may interfere with the clinical activity of brexucabtagene autoleucel.
3. Monitor patients at least daily for 7 days following infusion for signs and symptoms of cytokine release syndrome (CRS), which may be fatal or life-threatening in some cases. Please see package insert for complete guidelines regarding the appropriate management for CRS. This is a black-box warning.

4. Monitor for signs and symptoms of neurologic toxicities, which may be fatal or life-threatening in some cases. This is a black-box warning.
5. Monitor for signs and symptoms of infection.
6. Monitor CBCs periodically after infusion.
7. Immunoglobulin levels should be monitored after treatment with brexucabtagene autoleucel. Infection precautions, antibiotic prophylaxis, and immunoglobulin replacement may need to be instituted.
8. Patients should be advised not to drive and not to engage in operating heavy or potentially dangerous machinery for at least 8 weeks after receiving brexucabtagene autoleucel.
9. Patients will require lifelong monitoring for secondary malignancies.
10. No information is presently available regarding recommendations for breastfeeding during pregnancy. Insufficient data on the duration of contraception following treatment with brexucabtagene autoleucel.

TOXICITY 1
Hypersensitivity infusion reactions.

TOXICITY 2
CRS with fever, hypotension, tachycardia, chills, and hypoxia.

TOXICITY 3
Neurologic toxicity, which includes headache, confusional state, encephalopathy, tremors, dizziness, aphasia, imbalance and gait instability, and seizures.

TOXICITY 4
Myelosuppression with thrombocytopenia and neutropenia, which in some cases can be prolonged for several weeks after infusion.

TOXICITY 5
Infections with bacterial, viral, and fungal infections.

TOXICITY 6
Hypogammaglobulinemia.

TOXICITY 7
Hepatitis B reactivation.

TOXICITY 8
Hemophagocytic lymphohistiocytosis/macrophage activation syndrome (HLH/MAS).

TOXICITY 9
Secondary malignancies.

Brigatinib

TRADE NAME	Alunbrig	CLASSIFICATION	Signal transduction inhibitor, ALK inhibitor
CATEGORY	Targeted agent	DRUG MANUFACTURER	ARIAD, Takeda

MECHANISM OF ACTION
- Inhibits multiple receptor tyrosine kinases (RTKs), including anaplastic lymphoma kinase (ALK), insulin-like growth factor 1 receptor (IGF-1R), ROS1, FLT-3, and EGFR deletion and point mutations, which results in inhibition of tumor growth, tumor angiogenesis, and metastasis.
- Retains activity in NSCLC tumors resistant to crizotinib, including ALK mutations at L1196M, G1202R, C1156Y, F1174L, and R1275Q.

MECHANISM OF RESISTANCE
- Compound mutation at L1196M/G1202R of ALK protein.
- New fusion form of NTRK rearrangement.

ABSORPTION
The median time to peak drug levels ranges from 1 to 4 hours. Food with high fat content can reduce C_{max} by 13% with no effect on AUC. Brigatinib may be taken with or without food.

DISTRIBUTION
Approximately 66% of drug is bound to plasma proteins. Steady-state drug levels are achieved in approximately 15 days.

METABOLISM
Metabolized in the liver primarily by CYP3A4 and CYP2C8 microsomal enzymes, with N-demethylation and cysteine conjugation as the two main metabolic pathways. Elimination is mainly hepatic, with excretion in feces (65%), with nearly 40% as unchanged parent drug. Renal elimination accounts for about 25% of an administered dose. The terminal half-life of brigatinib is approximately 25 hours.

INDICATIONS
FDA-approved for the treatment of patients with ALK-positive metastatic NSCLC.

DOSAGE RANGE
Recommended dose is 90 mg PO daily for the first 7 days. If tolerated, the dose can be increased to 180 mg PO daily.

DRUG INTERACTION 1
Drugs such as ketoconazole, itraconazole, erythromycin, clarithromycin, atazanavir, indinavir, nefazodone, nelfinavir, ritonavir, saquinavir, telithromycin, and voriconazole may decrease the metabolism of brigatinib, resulting in increased drug levels and potentially increased toxicity.

DRUG INTERACTION 2
Drugs such as rifampin, phenytoin, phenobarbital, carbamazepine, and St. John's Wort may increase the metabolism of brigatinib, resulting in its inactivation and lower effective drug levels.

SPECIAL CONSIDERATIONS
1. Use with caution in patients with hepatic dysfunction, as brigatinib is eliminated mainly via the liver. No dose adjustment is needed for patients with mild hepatic dysfunction. The drug has not been evaluated in patients with moderate or severe hepatic dysfunction.
2. No dose adjustment is needed for patients with mild or moderate renal dysfunction. The drug has not been evaluated in the setting of severe renal dysfunction.
3. Patients receiving brigatinib along with oral warfarin anticoagulant therapy should have their coagulation parameters (PT and INR) monitored frequently, as elevations in INR and bleeding events may be observed.
4. Monitor patients for new or progressive pulmonary symptoms, including cough, dyspnea, and fever.
5. Monitor fasting blood sugar levels at baseline and periodically on treatment, especially in diabetic patients or in those on steroids.
6. Baseline and periodic evaluations of ECG and electrolyte status should be performed while on therapy. Use with caution in patients at risk of developing QT prolongation, including hypokalemia, hypomagnesemia, congenital long QT syndrome, and patients taking antiarrhythmic medications or any other drugs that may cause QT prolongation.
7. ALK testing using an FDA-approved test is required to confirm the presence of ALK-positive NSCLC for determining which patients should receive brigatinib therapy.
8. Closely monitor serum lipase and amylase levels during treatment.
9. Instruct patients to swallow tablets whole and to not crush or chew the tablets.
10. Avoid Seville oranges, starfruit, pomelos, grapefruit, and grapefruit products while on brigatinib therapy.
11. Pregnancy category D. Breastfeeding should be avoided.

TOXICITY 1
Hepatotoxicity with elevations in SGOT/SGPT.

TOXICITY 2
Nausea/vomiting, diarrhea, and abdominal pain are the most common GI side effects.

TOXICITY 3
Pulmonary toxicity with increased cough, dyspnea, fever, and pulmonary infiltrates. Severe, life-threatening interstitial lung disease (ILD)/pneumonitis can occur.

TOXICITY 4
Constitutional side effects with fatigue, asthenia, and anorexia.

TOXICITY 5
Cardiac toxicity with sinus bradycardia and hypertension.

TOXICITY 6
Hyperglycemia.

TOXICITY 7
Visual symptoms, including blurred vision, diplopia, and reduced visual acuity.

TOXICITY 8
Elevations in creatinine phosphokinase (CPK).

TOXICITY 9
Elevations in serum amylase and serum lipase.

TOXICITY 10
Peripheral edema.

Busulfan

$$CH_3-\overset{\overset{O}{\|}}{\underset{\underset{O}{\|}}{S}}-O-CH_2CH_2CH_2CH_2O-\overset{\overset{O}{\|}}{\underset{\underset{O}{\|}}{S}}-CH_3$$

TRADE NAME	Myleran, Busulfex	CLASSIFICATION	Alkylating agent
CATEGORY	Chemotherapy drug	DRUG MANUFACTURER	GlaxoSmithKline, Sagent

MECHANISM OF ACTION
- Methanesulfonate-type bifunctional alkylating agent.
- Interacts with cellular thiol groups and nucleic acids to form DNA–DNA and DNA–protein cross-links. Cross-linking of DNA results in inhibition of DNA synthesis and function.
- Cell cycle–nonspecific, active in all phases of the cell cycle.

MECHANISM OF RESISTANCE
- Decreased cellular uptake of drug.
- Increased intracellular thiol content due to glutathione or glutathione-related enzymes.
- Enhanced activity of DNA repair enzymes.

ABSORPTION
Excellent oral bioavailability, with peak levels in serum occurring within 2–4 hours after administration.

DISTRIBUTION
About 30% of drug is bound to plasma proteins. Has broad tissue distribution. Crosses the blood-brain barrier as well as the placental barrier.

METABOLISM
Metabolized primarily in the liver by the cytochrome P450 system. Metabolites, including sulfolane, 3-hydroxysulfolane, and methanesulfonic acid, are excreted in urine, with 50%–60% excreted within 48 hours. Metabolism may be influenced by circadian rhythm, with higher clearance rates observed in the evening, especially in younger patients. The terminal half-life is 2.5 hours.

INDICATIONS
1. Chronic myelogenous leukemia (CML) (standard dose).
2. Bone marrow/stem cell transplantation for refractory leukemia, lymphoma (high dose). Use in combination with cyclophosphamide as conditioning regimen prior to allogeneic stem cell transplantation for CML.

DOSAGE RANGE
1. CML—Usual dose for remission induction is 4–8 mg/day PO. Dosing on a weight basis is 1.8 mg/m^2/day. Maintenance dose is usually 1–3 mg/day PO.
2. Transplant setting—4 mg/kg/day IV for 4 days to a total dose of 16 mg/kg.

DRUG INTERACTION 1
Acetaminophen—Acetaminophen may decrease busulfan metabolism in the liver when given 72 hours before busulfan, resulting in enhanced toxicity.

DRUG INTERACTION 2
Itraconazole—Itraconazole reduces busulfan metabolism by up to 20%.

DRUG INTERACTION 3

Phenobarbital and phenytoin—Phenobarbital and phenytoin increase busulfan metabolism in the liver by inducing the activity of the liver microsomal system.

SPECIAL CONSIDERATIONS

1. Monitor CBC while on therapy. When the total WBC count has declined to approximately 15,000/mm^3, busulfan should be withheld until the nadir is reached and the counts begin to rise above this level. A decrease in the WBC count may not be seen during the first 10–15 days of therapy, and it may continue to fall for more than 1 month even after the drug has been stopped.
2. Monitor patients for pulmonary symptoms, as busulfan can cause interstitial pneumonitis.
3. Ingestion of busulfan on an empty stomach may decrease the risk of nausea and vomiting.
4. Therapeutic drug monitoring of busulfan is important in the setting of allogeneic stem cell transplantation, as a specific busulfan drug exposure has been associated with improved clinical outcomes.
5. Pregnancy category D. Breastfeeding should be avoided.

TOXICITY 1

Myelosuppression with pancytopenia is dose-limiting.

TOXICITY 2

Nausea/vomiting and diarrhea are common (>80% of patients) but generally mild with standard doses. Anorexia is also frequently observed.

TOXICITY 3

Mucositis is dose-related.

TOXICITY 4

Hyperpigmentation of skin, especially in hand creases and nail beds. Skin rash and pruritus also observed.

TOXICITY 5

Impotence, male sterility, amenorrhea, ovarian suppression, menopause, and infertility.

TOXICITY 6

Pulmonary symptoms, including cough, dyspnea, and fever, can be seen after long-term therapy. Interstitial pulmonary fibrosis, referred to as "busulfan lung," is a rare but severe side effect of therapy. May occur 1–10 years after discontinuation of therapy.

TOXICITY 7

Adrenal insufficiency is a rare event.

TOXICITY 8

Hepatotoxicity with elevations in LFTs. Hepatic veno-occlusive disease is observed with high doses of busulfan used in transplant setting.

TOXICITY 9

Insomnia, anxiety, dizziness, and depression are the most common neurologic side effects. Seizures can occur, usually with high-dose therapy.

TOXICITY 10

Increased risk of secondary malignancies, especially acute myelogenous leukemia, with long-term chronic use.

Cabazitaxel

TRADE NAME	Jevtana	CLASSIFICATION	Taxane, antimicrotubule agent
CATEGORY	Chemotherapy drug	DRUG MANUFACTURER	Sanofi-Aventis

MECHANISM OF ACTION
- Semisynthetic taxane prepared with a precursor extracted from yew needles.
- Binds to tubulin and promotes its assembly into microtubules while simultaneously inhibiting disassembly. This effect leads to stabilization of microtubules, which results in the inhibition of mitotic and interphase cellular functions.
- Cell cycle–specific agent with activity in the mitotic (M) phase.

MECHANISM OF RESISTANCE
- Alterations in tubulin with decreased affinity for drug.
- Unlike other taxanes, cabazitaxel is a poor substrate for the multidrug-resistance P-glycoprotein efflux pump and may be useful for treating multidrug-resistant tumors.

ABSORPTION
Administered only via the IV route.

DISTRIBUTION
Distributes widely to all body tissues and penetrates the blood-brain barrier. Extensive binding (89%–92%) to plasma proteins.

METABOLISM
Metabolized extensively in the liver (>95%), mainly by the CYP3A4 and CYP3A5 isoenzymes (80%–90%) and to a lesser extent by CYP2C8. Approximately 20 different metabolites are formed in the liver. Only about 24% is eliminated as the

parent form, with the majority (76%) of an administered dose being eliminated as metabolites. Renal clearance is minimal, with less than 4% of the drug cleared by the kidneys. Prolonged terminal half-life is about 77 hours. After a 1-hour infusion, approximately 80% of an administered dose is eliminated within 2 weeks.

INDICATIONS

FDA-approved in combination with prednisone for the treatment of patients with hormone-refractory, metastatic prostate cancer previously treated with a docetaxel-containing treatment regimen.

DOSAGE RANGE

Recommended dose is 20 mg/m^2 as a 1-hour infusion every 3 weeks in combination with oral prednisone 10 mg administered daily throughout cabazitaxel treatment. A higher dose of 25 mg/m^2 may be considered in certain select patients.

DRUG INTERACTION 1

Concomitant administration of CYP3A4 inhibitors such as ketoconazole, itraconazole, clarithromycin, atazanavir, indinavir, nefazodone, nelfinavir, ritonavir, saquinavir, telithromycin, and voriconazole may reduce cabazitaxel metabolism, resulting in increased plasma drug concentrations.

DRUG INTERACTION 2

Concomitant administration of CYP3A4 inducers such as phenytoin, carbamazepine, rifampin, phenobarbital, and St. John's Wort may enhance cabazitaxel metabolism, resulting in decreased plasma drug concentrations and potentially reduced clinical activity.

SPECIAL CONSIDERATIONS

1. Contraindicated in patients with history of severe hypersensitivity reactions to cabazitaxel or to other drugs formulated with polysorbate 80.
2. Monitor CBCs on a weekly basis during cycle 1 and before each treatment cycle thereafter. Contraindicated in patients with severe neutropenia (i.e., ANC <1,500 cells/mm^3). Prophylaxis with G-CSF should be considered in patients with high-risk clinical features (age >65, poor performance status, poor nutritional status, extensive prior radiation, other serious comorbid illnesses, or previous episodes of febrile neutropenia).
3. Patients should receive premedication with IV doses of an antihistamine, corticosteroid, and an H2-antagonist to prevent the incidence of hypersensitivity reactions.
4. Patients with a history of severe hypersensitivity reactions should **NOT** be rechallenged with cabazitaxel.
5. Dose reduction is not required in patients with mild hepatic dysfunction. The dose should be reduced to 15 mg/m^2 in patients with moderate hepatic dysfunction. Is contraindicated and should not be given and in patients with severe hepatic dysfunction (t. bilirubin >3 × ULN).

6. Dose reduction is not required in patients with mild, moderate, or severe renal dysfunction. No data is available for patients with end-stage renal disease or in those on dialysis, and caution should be used in these settings.
7. Pregnancy category D. Male patients with female partners should be advised to use effective contraception during treatment and for 4 months after the last dose.

TOXICITY 1
Myelosuppression with dose-limiting neutropenia. Thrombocytopenia and anemia are also observed. This is a black-box warning.

TOXICITY 2
Hypersensitivity reaction characterized by generalized skin rash, flushing, erythema, hypotension, dyspnea, and/or bronchospasm. Usually occurs within the first few minutes of infusion and more frequently with the first and second infusions. This is a black-box warning.

TOXICITY 3
Diarrhea, nausea/vomiting, constipation, abdominal pain, dysgeusia, and loss of appetite are the main GI side effects.

TOXICITY 4
Fatigue and asthenia.

TOXICITY 5
Neurotoxicity, mainly in the form of peripheral neuropathy, dizziness, and headache.

TOXICITY 6
Myalgias and arthralgias.

TOXICITY 7
Cardiac toxicity in the form of arrhythmias, hypotension, and peripheral edema.

TOXICITY 8
Alopecia occurs in 10% of patients.

TOXICITY 9
Hematuria and dysuria. Renal failure is a rare event.

C

Cabozantinib

TRADE NAME	Cabometyx, Cometriq	CLASSIFICATION	Signal transduction inhibitor, TKI
CATEGORY	Targeted agent	DRUG MANUFACTURER	Exelixis

MECHANISM OF ACTION
- Small-molecule inhibitor of tyrosine kinases associated with RET, MET, VEGFR-1, VEGFR-2, VEGFR-3, KIT, FLT-3, AXL, and TIE-2.
- Inhibition of the various receptor tyrosine kinases results in inhibition of critical signaling pathways involved in proliferation, growth, invasion/metastasis, angiogenesis, and maintenance of the tumor microenvironment.

MECHANISM OF RESISTANCE
None well characterized to date.

ABSORPTION
Oral absorption results in peak plasma concentrations at 2–6 hours and is increased by food with a high fat content.

DISTRIBUTION
Extensive binding to plasma proteins (>99.7%). With daily dosing, steady-state blood levels are achieved in about 15 days.

METABOLISM
Cabozantinib is metabolized in the liver, primarily by CYP3A4 enzymes. Approximately 80% of an administered dose is recovered, with 54% in feces and 27% in urine. The terminal half-life is on the order of 80–90 hours.

INDICATIONS
1. FDA-approved for adult and pediatric patients 12 years of age or older with locally advanced or metastatic differentiated thyroid cancer that has progressed on prior VEGFR-targeted therapy and who are radioactive iodine-refractory or ineligible.
2. FDA-approved for advanced renal cell cancer (RCC) as monotherapy.

3. FDA-approved for advanced renal cell cancer as first-line treatment in combination with nivolumab.
4. FDA-approved for hepatocellular cancer (HCC) following prior treatment with sorafenib.

DOSAGE RANGE
1. Medullary thyroid cancer—140 mg PO daily.
2. RCC—60 mg PO daily.
3. RCC—40 mg PO daily in combination with nivolumab 240 mg IV every 2 weeks or 480 mg IV every 4 weeks.
4. HCC—60 mg PO daily.

DRUG INTERACTIONS
- Drugs that stimulate liver microsomal CYP3A4 enzymes, including phenytoin, carbamazepine, rifampin, phenobarbital, and St. John's Wort, may increase the metabolism of cabozantinib, resulting in its inactivation and lower effective drug levels.
- Drugs that inhibit liver microsomal CYP3A4 enzymes, including ketoconazole, itraconazole, erythromycin, and clarithromycin, may reduce the metabolism of cabozantinib, resulting in increased drug levels and potentially increased toxicity.

SPECIAL CONSIDERATIONS
1. Patients should be instructed not to eat for at least 2 hours before and at least 1 hour after taking cabozantinib.
2. Dose adjustment of cabozantinib (Cabometyx) is not recommended for patients with mild hepatic dysfunction. The dose should be reduced in patients with moderate hepatic dysfunction (Child-Pugh B). For Cabometyx, the dose should be reduced to 40 mg once daily. Has not been studied in the setting of severe hepatic impairment (Child-Pugh C). The dose of cabozantinib (Cometriq) should be reduced to 80 mg daily for patients with mild or moderate hepatic dysfunction. Has not been studied in the setting of severe hepatic impairment.
3. Dose adjustment of cabozantinib (Cabometyx and Cometriq) is not recommended for patients with mild or moderate renal dysfunction. Has not been studied in the setting of severe renal impairment or end-stage renal disease.
4. Monitor for new GI signs and symptoms, as GI perforations and fistulas can occur.
5. Monitor blood pressure closely while on therapy. Use with caution in patients with uncontrolled hypertension.
6. Monitor patients for signs and symptoms of bleeding, as severe, sometimes fatal hemorrhage can occur. Do not use in patients with a recent history of hemorrhage or hemoptysis. This is a black-box warning.
7. Cabozantinib therapy should be discontinued in patients who develop arterial thromboembolic events, including myocardial infarction (MI) and cerebrovascular accident (CVA).

8. Routinely monitor urinary protein levels by urine dipstick analysis. Therapy should be discontinued for patients who develop nephrotic syndrome.
9. An oral examination should be performed prior to initiation of therapy and periodically while on therapy. Patients should be advised to practice good oral hygiene. Cabozantinib should be held for at least 3 weeks prior to any invasive dental procedure.
10. Dose modification is recommended in patients who experience the hand-foot syndrome.
11. Cabozantinib therapy should be discontinued in patients who develop the neurologic RPLS syndrome.
12. Cabozantinib tablets can **NOT** be substituted with cabozantinib capsules.
13. Embryo-fetal toxicity. Breastfeeding should be avoided.

TOXICITY 1
Mild-to-moderate skin reactions with rash, dry skin, alopecia, erythema, changes in hair color, and hyperkeratosis. Hand-foot syndrome occurs in up to 50% of patients, with grade 3/4 severity in 15% of patients.

TOXICITY 2
Diarrhea, nausea/vomiting, and mucositis are the most common GI side effects.

TOXICITY 3
Fatigue and asthenia.

TOXICITY 4
Hypertension.

TOXICITY 5
Bleeding complications, which in some cases, can be fatal.

TOXICITY 6
Osteonecrosis of the jaw, presenting as jaw pain, osteomyelitis, osteitis, bone erosion, and toothache.

TOXICITY 7
Proteinuria.

TOXICITY 8
RPLS with seizures, headache, visual disturbances, confusion, or altered mental function.

TOXICITY 9
Hepatotoxicity with elevations in SGOT, SGPT, and alkaline phosphatase.

Calaspargase pegol-mknl

TRADE NAME	Asparlas	CLASSIFICATION	Enzyme
CATEGORY	Chemotherapy drug	DRUG MANUFACTURER	Servier

MECHANISM OF ACTION
- Calaspargase pegol-mknl contains an asparagine-specific enzyme derived from *Escherichia coli*, as a conjugate of L-asparaginase and monomethoxy polyethylene glycol (mPEG) with a succinimidyl carbonase linker. The linker is a chemically stable bond between the mPEG moiety and the lysine groups of L-asparaginase.
- Tumor cells lack asparagine synthetase and thus require exogenous sources of L-asparagine.
- L-asparaginase hydrolyzes circulating L-asparagine to aspartic acid and ammonia.
- Depletion of the essential amino acid L-asparagine results in rapid inhibition of protein synthesis.

MECHANISM OF RESISTANCE
- Increased expression of the L-asparagine synthetase gene, which facilitates the cellular production of L-asparagine from endogenous sources.
- Formation of antibodies against L-asparaginase, resulting in inhibition of function.

ABSORPTION
Administered only via the IV route.

DISTRIBUTION
Apparent volume of distribution is 2.96 L and about 84.3% of the plasma volume.

METABOLISM
Metabolism is not well characterized. Minimal urinary and/or biliary excretion occurs. Plasma half-life is on the order of 16 days.

INDICATIONS
FDA-approved in combination with combination chemotherapy for acute lymphocytic leukemia in pediatric and young adults of age 1 month to 21 years.

DOSAGE RANGE
Recommended dose is 2,500 U/m^2 IV no more frequently than every 21 days.

DRUG INTERACTION 1
Methotrexate—L-asparaginase can inhibit the cytotoxic effects of methotrexate and thus rescue from methotrexate antitumor activity and toxicity. If given in combination, these two drugs should be administered 24 hours apart.

DRUG INTERACTION 2

Vincristine—L-asparaginase inhibits the clearance of vincristine, resulting in increased toxicity, especially neurotoxicity. Vincristine should be administered 12–24 hours before L-asparaginase.

SPECIAL CONSIDERATIONS

1. Monitor patients for allergic reactions and/or anaphylaxis. Resuscitation equipment and medications to treat anaphylaxis, including oxygen, epinephrine, IV steroids, and antihistamines, must be available. Patients should be observed for at least 1 hour after drug administration.
2. Monitor patient for allergic reactions and/or anaphylaxis. Contraindicated in patients with a prior history of anaphylactic reaction.
3. Monitor coagulation parameters, PT, PTT, INR, and serum fibrinogen levels.
4. Monitor LFTs and serum bilirubin levels at least weekly during the cycles of treatment that include calaspargase pegol-mknl through 6 weeks after the last dose of drug.
5. Contraindicated in patients with either active pancreatitis or a history of pancreatitis. If pancreatitis develops while on therapy, calaspargase pegol-mknl should be stopped immediately.
6. L-asparaginase can interfere with thyroid function tests. This effect is probably due to a marked reduction in serum concentration of thyroxine-binding globulin, which is observed within 2 days after the first dose. Levels of thyroxine-binding globulin return to normal within 4 weeks of the last dose.
7. Embryo-fetal toxicity with potential risk to fetus. Female patients should use effective contraception while on treatment and for at least 3 months after the final dose. The concomitant use of calaspargase pegol-mknl and oral contraceptives is not recommended because there is a potential for a drug-drug interaction between the two drugs.

TOXICITY 1

Hypersensitivity infusion reaction. Anaphylactic reaction may be life-threatening and presents as bronchospasm, respiratory distress, and hypotension.

TOXICITY 2

Mild elevation in LFTs, including serum bilirubin, alkaline phosphatase, and SGOT.

TOXICITY 3

Increased risk of both bleeding and clotting. Alterations in clotting with decreased levels of several clotting factors, including fibrinogen, factors IX and XI, antithrombin III, proteins C and S, plasminogen, and α-2-antiplasmin.

TOXICITY 4

Hepatotoxicity with elevations in LFTs and serum bilirubin.

TOXICITY 5

Pancreatitis usually manifested as transient increase in serum amylase or serum lipase levels.

Capecitabine

TRADE NAME	Xeloda	**CLASSIFICATION**	Antimetabolite, fluoropyrimidine
CATEGORY	Chemotherapy drug	**DRUG MANUFACTURER**	Roche

MECHANISM OF ACTION

- Fluoropyrimidine carbamate prodrug form of 5-FU. Capecitabine itself is inactive.
- Activation to cytotoxic forms is a complex process that involves three successive enzymatic steps. Metabolized in liver to 5'-deoxy-5-fluorocytidine (5'-DFCR) by the carboxylesterase enzyme and then to 5'-DFUR by cytidine deaminase (found in liver and in tumor tissues). Subsequently converted to 5-FU by the enzyme thymidine phosphorylase, which is expressed in higher levels in tumor versus normal tissue.
- Inhibition of the target enzyme thymidylate synthase (TS) by the 5-FU metabolite FdUMP.
- Incorporation of 5-FU metabolite FUTP into RNA, resulting in alterations in RNA processing and/or mRNA translation.
- Incorporation of 5-FU metabolite FdUTP into DNA, resulting in inhibition of DNA synthesis and function.
- Inhibition of TS leads to accumulation of dUMP and subsequent misincorporation of dUTP into DNA, resulting in inhibition of DNA synthesis and function.

MECHANISM OF RESISTANCE
- Increased expression of thymidylate synthase.
- Decreased levels of reduced folate substrate 5,10-methylenetetrahydrofolate.
- Decreased incorporation of 5-FU into RNA.
- Decreased incorporation of 5-FU into DNA.
- Increased activity of DNA repair enzymes, uracil glycosylase and dUTPase.
- Decreased expression of mismatch repair enzymes (hMLH1, hMSH2).
- Increased salvage of physiologic nucleosides, including thymidine.
- Increased expression of dihydropyrimidine dehydrogenase (DPD) .
- Alterations in TS with decreased binding affinity of enzyme for FdUMP.

ABSORPTION
Readily absorbed by the GI tract. Peak plasma levels are reached in 1.5 hours, while peak 5-FU levels are achieved at 2 hours after oral administration. The rate and extent of absorption are reduced by food.

DISTRIBUTION
Plasma protein binding of capecitabine and its metabolites is less than 60%. Primarily bound to albumin (35%).

METABOLISM
Capecitabine undergoes extensive enzymatic metabolism to 5-FU. After being absorbed as an intact molecule from the GI tract, it undergoes an initial hydrolysis reaction in the liver catalyzed by a carboxylesterase enzyme to 5'-DFCR. In the next step, 5'-DFCR is converted in the liver and other tissues to 5'-DFUR by the enzyme cytidine deaminase. Finally, 5'-DFUR is converted to 5-FU by the enzyme thymidine phosphorylase in tumor tissue as well as in normal tissues expressing this enzyme. Selective accumulation of 5-FU within tumor tissue (colorectal) versus normal tissue (colon) (3.2×) and plasma (21×) has been demonstrated in a population of colorectal cancer patients requiring definitive surgical resection who received capecitabine preoperatively.

Catabolism accounts for >85% of drug metabolism. Dihydropyrimidine dehydrogenase (DPD) is the main enzyme responsible for the catabolism of 5-FU, and it is present in liver and extrahepatic tissues such as GI mucosa, WBCs, and the kidneys. Greater than 90% of an administered dose of drug and its metabolites is cleared in the urine. The major metabolite excreted in urine is α-fluoro-β-alanine (FBAL). About 3% of the administered dose is excreted in urine as unchanged drug. The elimination half-life of capecitabine and capecitabine metabolites is on the order of 45–60 minutes.

INDICATIONS
1. Metastatic breast cancer—FDA-approved when used in combination with docetaxel for the treatment of patients with metastatic breast cancer after failure of prior anthracycline-containing chemotherapy.

2. Metastatic breast cancer—FDA-approved as monotherapy in patients refractory to both paclitaxel- and anthracycline-based chemotherapy or when anthracycline therapy is contraindicated.
3. Metastatic colorectal cancer—FDA-approved as first-line therapy when fluoropyrimidine therapy alone is preferred.
4. Stage III colon cancer—FDA-approved as adjuvant therapy when fluoropyrimidine therapy alone is preferred.
5. Clinical activity in gastric cancer, gastroesophageal cancer, and other GI cancers.

DOSAGE RANGE

1. Recommended dose is 1,250 mg/m^2 PO bid (morning and evening) for 2 weeks with 1 week rest. For combination therapy (capecitabine in combination with docetaxel) with docetaxel being dosed at 75 mg/m^2 day 1 of a 21-day cycle.
2. May decrease dose of capecitabine to 850–1,000 mg/m^2 bid on days 1–14 to reduce risk of toxicity without compromising efficacy (see Special Considerations, number 8).
3. An alternative dosing schedule for capecitabine monotherapy is 1,250–1,500 mg/m^2 PO bid for 1 week on and 1 week off. This schedule appears to be well tolerated, with no compromise in clinical efficacy.
4. Capecitabine should be used at lower doses (850–1,000 mg/m^2 bid on days 1–14) when used in combination with other cytotoxic agents, such as oxaliplatin.

DRUG INTERACTION 1

Capecitabine-warfarin interaction—Patients receiving concomitant capecitabine and oral coumarin-derivative anticoagulant therapy should have their coagulation parameters (PT and INR) monitored frequently in order to adjust the anticoagulant dose accordingly. A clinically important capecitabine–warfarin drug interaction has been documented. Altered coagulation parameters and/ or bleeding, including death, have been reported in patients taking capecitabine concomitantly with coumarin-derivative anticoagulants such as warfarin. Post-marketing reports have shown clinically significant increases in PT and INR in patients who were stabilized on anticoagulants at the time capecitabine was introduced. These events occurred within several days and up to several months after initiating capecitabine therapy and, in a few cases, within 1 month after stopping capecitabine. These events occurred in patients with and without liver metastases. Age >60 and a diagnosis of cancer independently predispose patients to an increased risk of coagulopathy.

DRUG INTERACTION 2

Aluminum hydroxide, magnesium hydroxide—Concomitant use of aluminum hydroxide– or magnesium hydroxide–containing antacids may increase the bioavailability of capecitabine by 16%–35%.

DRUG INTERACTION 3
Phenytoin—Capecitabine may increase phenytoin blood levels and subsequent phenytoin toxicity. Dose adjustment of phenytoin may be necessary.

DRUG INTERACTION 4
Leucovorin—Leucovorin enhances the toxicity of capecitabine.

SPECIAL CONSIDERATIONS
1. Capecitabine should be taken with a glass of water within 30 minutes after a meal.
2. Contraindicated in patients with known hypersensitivity to 5-FU.
3. Contraindicated in patients with known dihydropyrimidine dehydrogenase (DPD) deficiency.
4. No dose adjustments are necessary in patients with mild or moderate liver dysfunction. However, patients should be closely monitored.
5. In the setting of moderate renal dysfunction (baseline CrCl, 30–50 mL/min), a 25% dose reduction is recommended. Patients should be closely monitored because they may be at greater risk for increased toxicity. Contraindicated in patients with severe renal impairment (CrCl <30 mL/min).
6. Patients should be monitored for diarrhea and its associated sequelae, including dehydration, fluid imbalance, and infection. Elderly patients (>80 years of age) are especially vulnerable to the GI toxicity of capecitabine. Moderate to severe diarrhea (>grade 2) is an indication to interrupt therapy immediately. Subsequent doses should be reduced accordingly.
7. Drug therapy should be stopped immediately in the presence of grades 2 to 4 hyperbilirubinemia until complete resolution or a decrease in intensity to grade 1.
8. Drug therapy should be stopped immediately in the presence of grade 2 or higher adverse events until complete resolution or a decrease in intensity to grade 1. Treatment should continue at 75% of the initial starting dose for grade 2 or 3 toxicity. For grade 4 toxicity, if the physician chooses to continue treatment, treatment should continue at 50% of the initial starting dose.
9. Patients who experience unexpected, severe grade 3 or 4 myelosuppression, GI toxicity, and/or neurologic toxicity upon initiation of therapy may have an underlying deficiency in dihydropyrimidine dehydrogenase (DPD). Therapy must be discontinued immediately, and further testing to identify the presence of this pharmacogenetic syndrome should be considered.
10. Vitamin B6 (pyridoxine, 50 mg PO bid) may be used to prevent and/or reduce the incidence and severity of hand-foot syndrome. Dose may be increased to 100 mg PO bid if symptoms do not resolve within 3–4 days.
11. Celecoxib at a dose of 200 mg PO bid may be effective in preventing and/or reducing the incidence and severity of hand-foot syndrome. A low-dose nicotine patch has also been found to be effective in this setting.

12. In patients with hand-foot syndrome, the affected skin should be well hydrated using a bland and mild moisturizer. Instruct patients to soak affected hands and feet in cool to tepid water for 10 minutes, then apply petroleum jelly onto the wet skin. The use of lanolin-containing salves or ointments such as Bag Balm emollient may help.
13. Diltiazem can prevent capecitabine-induced coronary vasospasm and chest pain and may allow patients to continue to receive capecitabine.
14. Pregnancy category D. Breastfeeding should be avoided.

TOXICITY 1
Diarrhea is dose-limiting and observed in up to 55% of patients. Similar to GI toxicity observed with continuous infusion 5-FU. Mucositis, loss of appetite, and dehydration also noted.

TOXICITY 2
Hand-foot syndrome (palmar-plantar erythrodysesthesia). Severe hand-foot syndrome is seen in 15%–20% of patients. Characterized by tingling, numbness, pain, erythema, dryness, rash, swelling, increased pigmentation, and/or pruritus of the hands and feet. Similar to dermatologic toxicity observed with continuous infusion 5-FU.

TOXICITY 3
Nausea and vomiting occur in up to 50% of patients.

TOXICITY 4
Hepatotoxicity with elevations in serum bilirubin (20%–40%), alkaline phosphatase, and liver transaminases (SGOT, SGPT). Usually transient and clinically asymptomatic.

TOXICITY 5
Myelosuppression is observed less frequently than with IV 5-FU. Neutropenia more common than thrombocytopenia.

TOXICITY 6
Neurologic toxicity manifested by confusion, cerebellar ataxia, and rarely encephalopathy.

TOXICITY 7
Cardiac symptoms of chest pain, ECG changes, and serum enzyme elevation. Rare event but increased risk in patients with prior history of ischemic heart disease.

TOXICITY 8
Tear-duct stenosis, acute and chronic conjunctivitis.

Capmatinib

TRADE NAME	Tabrecta	CLASSIFICATION	Signal transduction inhibitor, MET inhibitor
CATEGORY	Targeted agent	DRUG MANUFACTURER	Novartis and Incyte

MECHANISM OF ACTION
- Small molecule inhibitor of mesenchymal-epithelial transition (MET) tyrosine kinase, including the mutant variant produced by exon 14 skipping.
- Leads to downstream inhibition of key signaling pathways involved in proliferation, motility, migration, and invasion.
- Amplification of MET is a predictive biomarker of sensitivity.

MECHANISM OF RESISTANCE
- Activation of EGFR signaling.
- Gene amplification of PIK3CA resulting in increased expression of PIK3CA.

ABSORPTION
Rapidly absorbed with a median time to peak drug levels of 1–2 hours after oral ingestion. Absorption after an oral dose is estimated to be >70%.

DISTRIBUTION
Extensive binding (96%) to plasma proteins. Steady-state drug levels are achieved in 3 days.

METABOLISM
Metabolized in the liver primarily by CYP3A4 microsomal enzymes and aldehyde oxidase. After an administered dose of drug, 78% is eliminated in feces (42% as parent drug) and 22% is eliminated in urine with only a negligible amount of parent drug. The terminal half-life of the drug is 6.5 hours.

INDICATIONS
FDA-approved for adult patients with metastatic NSCLC with a MET exon 14 skipping, as detected by an FDA-approved test.

DOSAGE RANGE
Recommended dose is 400 mg PO bid and can be taken with or without food.

DRUG INTERACTION 1
Drugs such as ketoconazole, itraconazole, erythromycin, clarithromycin, atazanavir, indinavir, nefazodone, nelfinavir, ritonavir, saquinavir, telithromycin, and voriconazole may decrease the metabolism of capmatinib, resulting in increased drug levels and potentially increased toxicity.

DRUG INTERACTION 2
Phenytoin and other drugs that stimulate the liver microsomal CYP3A4 enzymes, including carbamazepine, rifampin, phenobarbital, and St. John's Wort—These drugs may increase the metabolism of capmatinib, resulting in lower effective drug levels and potentially reduced activity.

SPECIAL CONSIDERATIONS
1. Dose reduction is not required in the setting of mild, moderate, and severe hepatic impairment.
2. Dose reduction is not required in the setting of mild to moderate renal impairment. Has not been studied in patients with severe renal impairment or in those with end-stage renal disease.
3. Monitor patients for new pulmonary symptoms because capmatinib can cause interstitial lung disease and pneumonitis.
4. Monitor LFTs at baseline and every 2 weeks during the first 3 months of therapy, then once a month or as clinically indicated.
5. Patients should be advised to avoid sun exposure and use sunscreen and protective clothing while on capmatinib therapy.
6. Can cause fetal harm when administered to a pregnant woman. Females of reproductive potential should use effective contraception during drug therapy and for at least one week after the final dose. Breastfeeding should be avoided.

TOXICITY 1
Peripheral edema.

TOXICITY 2
Nausea/vomiting.

TOXICITY 3
Anorexia and fatigue.

TOXICITY 4
Interstitial lung disease/pneumonitis with dyspnea, cough, and fever.

TOXICITY 5
Hepatotoxicity with elevations in SGOT, SGPT, and serum bilirubin.

TOXICITY 6
Photosensitivity.

Carboplatin

TRADE NAME	Paraplatin, CBDCA	**CLASSIFICATION**	Platinum analog
CATEGORY	Chemotherapy drug	**DRUG MANUFACTURER**	Bristol-Myers Squibb

MECHANISM OF ACTION
- Covalently binds to DNA with preferential binding to the N-7 position of guanine and adenine.
- Reacts with two different sites on DNA to produce cross-links, either intrastrand (>90%) or interstrand (<5%). Formation of DNA adducts results in inhibition of DNA synthesis and function as well as inhibition of transcription.
- Binding to nuclear and cytoplasmic proteins may result in cytotoxic effects.
- Cell cycle–nonspecific agent.

MECHANISM OF RESISTANCE
- Reduced accumulation of carboplatin due to alterations in cellular transport.
- Increased inactivation by thiol-containing proteins such as glutathione and glutathione-related enzymes.
- Enhanced DNA repair enzyme activity (e.g., ERCC-1).
- Deficiency in mismatch repair (MMR) enzymes (e.g., hMLH1, hMSH2).

ABSORPTION
Administered only via the IV route.

DISTRIBUTION
Widely distributed in body tissues. Crosses the blood-brain barrier and enters the CSF. Does not bind to plasma proteins and has an apparent volume of distribution of 16 L.

METABOLISM
Carboplatin does not undergo significant metabolism. As observed with cisplatin, carboplatin undergoes aquation reaction in the presence of low concentrations of chloride. This reaction is 100-fold slower with carboplatin when compared to cisplatin. Carboplatin is extensively cleared by the kidneys, with about 60%–70% of the drug excreted in urine within 24 hours. The elimination of carboplatin is slower than that of cisplatin, with a terminal half-life of 2–6 hours.

INDICATIONS
1. Ovarian cancer.
2. Germ cell tumors.
3. Head and neck cancer.
4. Small cell lung cancer (SCLC) and NSCLC.
5. Bladder cancer.
6. Relapsed and refractory acute leukemia.
7. Endometrial cancer.

DOSAGE RANGE
1. Dose of carboplatin is usually calculated to a target area under the curve (AUC) based on the glomerular filtration rate (GFR).
2. Calvert formula is used to calculate dose—Total dose (mg) = (target AUC) × (GFR + 25). Note: Dose is in mg, **NOT** mg/m^2.
3. Target AUC is usually between 5 and 7 mg/mL/min for previously untreated patients. In previously treated patients, lower AUCs (between 4 and 6 mg/mL/min) are recommended. AUCs >7 are not associated with improved response rates.
4. Bone marrow/stem cell transplant setting—Doses up to 1,600 mg/m^2 divided over several days.

DRUG INTERACTION
Myelosuppressive agents—Increased risk of myelosuppression when carboplatin is combined with other myelosuppressive drugs.

SPECIAL CONSIDERATIONS
1. Use with caution in patients with abnormal renal function. Dose reduction is required in the setting of renal dysfunction. Baseline CrCl must be obtained. Renal status must be closely monitored during therapy.
2. Although carboplatin is not as emetogenic as cisplatin, pretreatment with antiemetic agents is strongly recommended.
3. Avoid needles or IV administration sets containing aluminum because precipitation of drug may occur.
4. Contraindicated in patients with a history of severe allergic reactions to cisplatin, other platinum compounds, and mannitol.
5. In contrast to cisplatin, IV hydration pretreatment and post-treatment are not necessary. Patients should still be instructed to maintain adequate oral hydration.
6. Hemodialysis clears carboplatin at 25% of the rate of renal clearance. Peritoneal dialysis is unable to remove carboplatin.
7. Risk of hypersensitivity reactions increases from 1% to 27% in patients receiving more than 7 cycles of carboplatin-based therapy. For such patients, a 0.02-mL intradermal injection of an undiluted aliquot of their planned carboplatin dose can be administered 1 hour before each cycle of carboplatin. This skin test identifies patients in whom carboplatin may be safely administered.
8. Pregnancy category D. Breastfeeding should be avoided.

TOXICITY 1

Myelosuppression is significant and dose-limiting. Dose-dependent, cumulative toxicity is more severe in elderly patients. Thrombocytopenia is most commonly observed, with nadir by day 21.

TOXICITY 2

Nausea and vomiting. Delayed nausea and vomiting can also occur, albeit rarely. Significantly less emetogenic than cisplatin.

TOXICITY 3

Renal toxicity is significantly less common than with cisplatin.

TOXICITY 4

Peripheral neuropathy is observed in less than 10% of patients. Patients older than 65 years and/or previously treated with cisplatin may be at higher risk for developing neurologic toxicity.

TOXICITY 5

Mild and reversible elevation of liver enzymes, particularly alkaline phosphatase and SGOT.

TOXICITY 6

Allergic reaction. Can occur within a few minutes of starting therapy. Presents mainly as skin rash, urticaria, and pruritus. Bronchospasm and hypotension are uncommon.

TOXICITY 7

Alopecia is uncommon.

Carfilzomib

TRADE NAME	Kyprolis	CLASSIFICATION	Proteasome inhibitor
CATEGORY	Chemotherapy drug	DRUG MANUFACTURER	Onyx/Amgen

MECHANISM OF ACTION
- Tetrapeptide epoxyketone proteasome inhibitor of the 26S proteasome.
- Binds to the N-terminal threonine-containing active sites of the 20S proteasome, the proteolytic core within the 26S proteasome.
- The 26S proteasome is a large protein complex that degrades ubiquitinated proteins. This pathway plays an essential role in regulating the intracellular concentrations of various cellular proteins.
- Inhibition of the 26S proteasome prevents the targeted proteolysis of ubiquitinated proteins, and disruption of this normal pathway can affect multiple signaling pathways within the cell, leading to cell death.
- Results in downregulation of the NF-κB pathway. NF-κB is a transcription factor that stimulates the production of various growth factors, including IL-6, cell adhesion molecules, and anti-apoptotic proteins, all of which contribute to cell growth and chemoresistance.
- Can overcome resistance to bortezomib.
- Displays in vitro growth inhibitory activity in both solid tumors and hematologic malignancy cancer cells.

MECHANISM OF RESISTANCE
Increased expression of the multidrug-resistant gene with elevated P170 protein, leading to increased drug efflux and decreased intracellular accumulation.

ABSORPTION
Administered only via the IV route.

DISTRIBUTION
Extensive binding (97%) of drug bound to plasma proteins.

METABOLISM
Rapidly and extensively metabolized by peptidase cleavage and epoxide hydrolysis. The metabolites have no documented antitumor activity. Liver P450-mediated mechanisms play only a relatively minor role in drug metabolism. Rapidly cleared with a half-life of about 1 hour on day 1 of cycle 1.

INDICATIONS
1. FDA-approved for the treatment of patients with multiple myeloma who have received at least two prior therapies, including bortezomib and an immunomodulatory therapy.
2. FDA-approved in combination with lenalidomide and dexamethasone as second-line treatment for patients with multiple myeloma.

DOSAGE RANGE
Recommended dose for cycle 1 is 20 mg/m^2/day, and if tolerated, the dose can be increased to 27 mg/m^2/day for cycle 2 and all subsequent cycles. Carfilzomib is administered by IV on 2 consecutive days each week for 3 weeks (days 1, 2, 8, 9, 15, and 16) followed by a 12-day rest period (days 17–28).

DRUG INTERACTIONS
None well characterized to date.

SPECIAL CONSIDERATIONS

1. Monitor for cardiac complications. Patients with prior history of MI in the preceding 6 months, congestive heart failure (CHF), and conduction system abnormalities not controlled by medication may be at increased risk for cardiac complications.
2. Monitor pulmonary status given the risk of pulmonary arterial hypertension and pulmonary complications.
3. Monitor for infusion-related events, which can occur immediately following or up to 24 hours after drug administration. Premedication with dexamethasone 4 mg PO or IV prior to all doses of carfilzomib during cycle 1 and prior to all doses during the first cycle of dose escalation has been shown to reduce the incidence and severity of infusion reactions.
4. Patients should be well hydrated prior to drug administration to reduce the risk of renal toxicity.
5. Patients with high tumor burden are at increased risk for developing tumor lysis syndrome.
6. Monitor CBCs routinely because carfilzomib therapy is associated with thrombocytopenia, with nadirs occurring at around day 8 of each 28-day cycle.
7. Monitor LFTs on a routine basis because hepatotoxicity and rare cases of hepatic failure have been reported with carfilzomib.
8. In contrast to bortezomib and ixazomib, which each contain a boron moiety, the clinical activity of carfilzomib is not impaired by green tea and green tea supplements.
9. May cause fetal harm. Advise females of reproductive potential to use effective contraception during treatment and for 6 months following the last dose. Breastfeeding should be avoided while on therapy and for 2 weeks after the last dose.

TOXICITY 1
Fatigue and generalized weakness.

TOXICITY 2
Cardiac toxicity with CHF, MI, and rare cases of cardiac arrest.

TOXICITY 3
Myelosuppression with thrombocytopenia, neutropenia, and anemia.

TOXICITY 4
Hepatotoxicity with elevations in serum transaminases (SGOT, SGPT). Drug-induced hepatotoxicity with fatal outcomes has been reported.

TOXICITY 5
Pulmonary toxicity presenting as dyspnea in up to 35% of patients.

TOXICITY 6
Thrombotic microangiopathy syndromes with TTP and HUS.

TOXICITY 7
Neurologic toxicity with posterior reversible encephalopathy syndrome (PRES) and presents with headache, lethargy, confusion, blindness, seizure, and other visual and neurologic symptoms.

TOXICITY 8
Pulmonary arterial hypertension. Rare event observed in 2% of patients.

Carmustine

$$Cl-CH_2-CH_2-N-\overset{\overset{O}{||}}{C}-NH-CH_2-CH_2-Cl$$
$$|$$
$$NO$$

TRADE NAME	BCNU, Bischloro-ethylnitrosourea	CLASSIFICATION	Alkylating agent, nitrosourea
CATEGORY	Chemotherapy drug	DRUG MANUFACTURER	Bristol-Myers Squibb

MECHANISM OF ACTION
- Nitrosourea analog.
- Cell cycle–nonspecific.
- Chloroethyl metabolites interfere with the synthesis of DNA, RNA, and protein.

MECHANISM OF RESISTANCE
- Decreased cellular uptake of drug.
- Increased intracellular thiol content due to glutathione or glutathione-related enzymes.
- Enhanced activity of DNA repair enzymes.

ABSORPTION
Administered only via the IV route.

DISTRIBUTION
Lipid-soluble drug with broad tissue distribution. Crosses the blood-brain barrier, reaching concentrations >50% of those in plasma.

METABOLISM

After IV infusion, carmustine is rapidly taken up into tissues and degraded. Extensively metabolized in the liver. Approximately 60%–70% of drug is excreted in urine in its metabolite form, while 10% is excreted as respiratory CO_2. Short serum half-life of only 15–20 minutes.

INDICATIONS

1. Brain tumors—Glioblastoma multiforme, brain stem glioma, medulloblastoma, astrocytoma, and ependymoma.
2. Hodgkin's lymphoma.
3. Non-Hodgkin's lymphoma.
4. Multiple myeloma.
5. Glioblastoma multiforme—Implantable BCNU-impregnated wafer (Gliadel).

DOSAGE RANGE

1. Usual dose is 200 mg/m^2 IV every 6 weeks. Dose can sometimes be divided over 2 days.
2. Higher doses (450–600 mg/m^2) are used with stem cell rescue.
3. Implantable BCNU-impregnated wafers—Up to eight wafers are placed into the surgical resection site after excision of the primary brain tumor.

DRUG INTERACTION 1

Cimetidine—Cimetidine enhances the toxicity of carmustine.

DRUG INTERACTION 2

Amphotericin B—Amphotericin B enhances the cellular uptake of carmustine, thus resulting in increased toxicity, including renal toxicity.

DRUG INTERACTION 3

Digoxin—Carmustine may decrease the plasma levels of digoxin.

DRUG INTERACTION 4

Phenytoin—Carmustine may decrease the plasma levels of phenytoin.

SPECIAL CONSIDERATIONS

1. Administer carmustine slowly over a period of 1–2 hours to avoid intense pain and/or burning at the site of injection. Strategies to decrease pain and/or burning include diluting the drug, slowing the rate of administration, or placing ice above the IV injection site.
2. Monitor CBC while on therapy. Repeated cycles should not be given before 6 weeks, given the delayed and potentially cumulative myelosuppressive effects of carmustine.
3. PFTs should be obtained at baseline and monitored periodically during therapy. There is an increased risk of pulmonary toxicity in patients with a baseline forced vital capacity (FVC) or DLCO below 70% of predicted.
4. Pregnancy category D. Breastfeeding should be avoided.

TOXICITY 1
Myelosuppression is dose-limiting. Nadir typically occurs at 4–6 weeks.

TOXICITY 2
Nausea and vomiting may occur within 2 hours after a dose of drug and can last for up to 4–6 hours.

TOXICITY 3
Facial flushing and a burning sensation at the IV injection site. Skin contact with drug may cause brownish discoloration and pain.

TOXICITY 4
Hepatotoxicity with transient elevations in serum transaminases develops in up to 90% of patients within 1 week of therapy. With high-dose therapy, hepatic veno-occlusive disease may be observed in 5%–20% of patients.

TOXICITY 5
Impotence, male sterility, amenorrhea, ovarian suppression, menopause, and infertility. Gynecomastia is occasionally observed.

TOXICITY 6
Pulmonary toxicity is uncommon at low doses. At cumulative doses >1,400 mg/m^2, ILD and pulmonary fibrosis in the form of an insidious cough, dyspnea, pulmonary infiltrates, and/or respiratory failure may develop.

TOXICITY 7
Renal toxicity is uncommon at total cumulative doses <1,000 mg/m^2.

TOXICITY 8
Increased risk of secondary malignancies, especially acute myelogenous leukemia and myelodysplasia.

Cemiplimab-rwlc

TRADE NAME	Libtayo	CLASSIFICATION	Anti-PD1 monoclonal antibody
CATEGORY	Immunotherapy, immune checkpoint inhibitor	DRUG MANUFACTURER	Regeneron and Sanofi Genzyme

MECHANISM OF ACTION

- Fully human IgG4 monoclonal antibody that binds to the programmed death (PD)-1 receptor, which is expressed on T cells, and inhibits the interaction between the PD-L1 and PD-L2 ligands and the PD-1 receptor.
- Blockade of the PD-1 pathway-mediated immune checkpoint enhances T-cell immune response, leading to T-cell activation and proliferation.

MECHANISM OF RESISTANCE

- Increased expression and/or activity of other immune checkpoint pathways (e.g., TIGIT, TIM3, and LAG3).
- Increased expression of other immune escape mechanisms.
- Increased infiltration of immune suppressive populations within the tumor microenvironment, which include Tregs, myeloid-derived suppressor cells (MDSCs), and M2 macrophages.
- Release of various cytokines, chemokines, and metabolites within the tumor microenvironment, including CSF-1, tryptophan metabolites, TGF-β, and adenosine.

DISTRIBUTION

Steady-state concentrations are achieved by 4 months.

METABOLISM

Metabolism of cemiplimab has not been extensively characterized. The mean elimination half-life is on the order of 19 days.

INDICATIONS

1. FDA-approved for patients with metastatic cutaneous squamous cell cancer (CSCC) or locally advanced CSCC who are not candidates for curative surgery or curative radiation.
2. FDA-approved for patients with locally advanced basal cell cancer (BCC) previously treated with a hedgehog pathway inhibitor or for whom a hedgehog pathway inhibitor is not appropriate.
3. FDA-approved for patients with metastatic basal cell cancer (BCC) previously treated with a hedgehog pathway inhibitor or for whom a hedgehog pathway inhibitor is not appropriate. This indication is approved under accelerated approval based on response rate and duration of response.
4. FDA-approved in combination with platinum-based chemotherapy for first-line treatment of locally advanced NSCLC who are not candidates for curative surgery or curative radiation or metastatic NSCLC with no EGFR, ALK, or ROS1 alterations.
5. FDA-approved as monotherapy for first-line treatment of locally advanced NSCLC who are not candidates for curative surgery or curative radiation or metastatic NSCLC with no EGFR, ALK, or ROS1 alterations and whose tumors express high PD-L1 (TPS>50%) levels.

DOSAGE RANGE

Recommended dose is 350 mg IV every 3 weeks.

DRUG INTERACTIONS
None well characterized to date.

SPECIAL CONSIDERATIONS
1. Monitor patients for signs and symptoms of infusion reactions.
2. Associated with significant immune-mediated adverse reactions due to T-cell activation and proliferation. These immune-mediated reactions may involve any organ system, with the most common reactions being pneumonitis, enterocolitis, hepatitis, dermatitis, hypophysitis, nephritis, and thyroid dysfunction.
3. Should be withheld for any of the following:
   - Grade 2 pneumonitis
   - Grade 2 or 3 colitis
   - SGOT/SGPT >3 × ULN and up to 10 × ULN or total bilirubin increases up to 3 × ULN
   - Any other severe or grade 3 treatment-related toxicity
4. Should be permanently discontinued for any of the following:
   - Any life-threatening or grade 4 toxicity
   - Grade 3 or 4 pneumonitis
   - Grade 4 colitis
   - SGOT/SGPT >5 × ULN or total bilirubin >3 × ULN
   - Any severe or grade 3 toxicity that recurs
   - Inability to reduce steroid dose to 10 mg or less of prednisone or equivalent per day within 12 weeks
   - Persistent grade 2 or 3 toxicity that does not recover to grade 1 or resolve within 12 weeks after the last dose of drug
5. Monitor thyroid function prior to and during therapy.
6. Immune-mediated reactions may occur even after discontinuation of therapy.
7. Can cause fetal harm when given to a pregnant women. Female patients should use effective contraception while on treatment and for at least 4 months after the final dose. Breast feeding should be avoided during therapy and for 4 months after the final dose.

TOXICITY 1
Colitis with diarrhea and abdominal pain.

TOXICITY 2
Pneumonitis with dyspnea and cough.

TOXICITY 3
GI side effects with nausea/vomiting, dry mouth, and pancreatitis.

TOXICITY 4
Hepatotoxicity with elevations in SGOT/SGPT, alkaline phosphatase, and serum bilirubin.

TOXICITY 5
Neurologic toxicity with neuropathy, myositis, myasthenia gravis, and autoimmune neuropathy.

TOXICITY 6
Nephritis with renal dysfunction.

TOXICITY 7
Arthralgias and myalgias.

TOXICITY 8
Maculopapular skin rash, erythema, dermatitis, and pruritus.

TOXICITY 9
Immune-mediated endocrinopathies, with hypothyroidism, adrenal insufficiency, hypophysitis, and diabetes.

TOXICITY 10
Infusion reactions.

Ceritinib

TRADE NAME	Zykadia	CLASSIFICATION	Signal transduction inhibitor, TKI
CATEGORY	Targeted agent	DRUG MANUFACTURER	Novartis

MECHANISM OF ACTION
- Inhibits multiple receptor tyrosine kinases (RTKs), including anaplastic lymphoma kinase (ALK), insulin-like growth factor-1 receptor (IGF-1R), insulin receptor, and ROS1, which results in inhibition of tumor growth, tumor angiogenesis, and metastasis.
- Retains activity in NSCLC tumors resistant to crizotinib, including ALK mutations at L1196M, G1269A, I1171T, and S1206Y. Does not overcome resistance to G1202R or F1174C mutations.

MECHANISM OF RESISTANCE

- Development of ALK mutations, including G1202R, F1174C, F1174L, C1156Y, and L1152R.
- Epithelial to mesenchymal transition (EMT), with loss of E-cadherin expression.
- Activation of MEK and SRC signaling pathways.
- Multidrug-resistant phenotype, with increased expression of P170 glycoprotein.

ABSORPTION

Rapidly absorbed after an oral dose, with peak plasma levels achieved within 4–6 hours. Absolute oral bioavailability has not yet been determined. Food with a high fat content can significantly increase drug concentrations by up to 50%–73%.

DISTRIBUTION

Extensive binding (97%) to plasma proteins. Steady-state drug levels are achieved in approximately 15 days.

METABOLISM

Metabolized in the liver, primarily by CYP3A4 microsomal enzymes. Elimination is mainly hepatic, with excretion in feces (92%), and nearly 70% as unchanged parent drug. Renal elimination is relatively minor, with only 1.3% of an administered dose being recovered in the urine. The terminal half-life of ceritinib is approximately 40 hours.

INDICATIONS

FDA-approved for the treatment of patients with ALK-positive metastatic NSCLC who have progressed on or are intolerant to crizotinib.

DOSAGE RANGE

Recommended dose is 750 mg PO daily.

DRUG INTERACTION 1

Drugs such as ketoconazole, itraconazole, erythromycin, clarithromycin, atazanavir, indinavir, nefazodone, nelfinavir, ritonavir, saquinavir, telithromycin, and voriconazole may decrease the metabolism of ceritinib, resulting in increased drug levels and potentially increased toxicity.

DRUG INTERACTION 2

Drugs such as rifampin, phenytoin, phenobarbital, carbamazepine, and St. John's Wort may increase the metabolism of ceritinib, resulting in its inactivation and lower effective drug levels.

SPECIAL CONSIDERATIONS

1. Dose reduction is not required for patients with mild or moderate hepatic dysfunction. Dose should be reduced to 150 mg PO daily in the setting of severe hepatic dysfunction.

2. Dose reduction is not required for patients with mild or moderate renal dysfunction. Has not been studied in the setting of severe renal dysfunction or in end-stage renal disease.
3. Patients receiving ceritinib along with oral warfarin anticoagulant therapy should have their coagulation parameters (PT and INR) monitored frequently because elevations in INR and bleeding events have been observed.
4. Monitor LFTs and serum bilirubin on a monthly basis and as clinically indicated because ceritinib may cause hepatotoxicity. May need to suspend, dose-reduce, or permanently stop ceritinib with the development of drug-induced hepatotoxicity.
5. Monitor patients for new or progressive pulmonary symptoms, including cough, dyspnea, and fever.
6. Monitor blood sugar levels, especially in diabetic patients or in those on steroids.
7. Baseline and periodic evaluations of ECG and electrolyte status should be performed while on therapy. Use with caution in patients at risk of developing QT prolongation, including hypokalemia, hypomagnesemia, and congenital long QT syndrome, and in patients taking antiarrhythmic medications or any other drugs that may cause QT prolongation.
8. ALK testing using an FDA-approved test is required to confirm the presence of ALK-positive NSCLC for determining which patients should receive ceritinib therapy.
9. Ceritinib should be taken on an empty stomach and should not be taken within 2 hours of a meal.
10. Avoid the concomitant use of proton pump inhibitors, H2-receptor inhibitors, and antacids because these drugs may alter the pH of the upper GI tract, which could change ceritinib solubility, leading to reduced drug bioavailability and decreased systemic drug exposure.
11. Avoid Seville oranges, starfruit, pomelos, grapefruit, and grapefruit products while on ceritinib therapy.
12. May cause fetal harm. Breastfeeding should be avoided during treatment and for 2 weeks following the final dose.

TOXICITY 1

Hepatotoxicity with elevations in serum transaminases (SGOT, SGPT).

TOXICITY 2

Nausea/vomiting, diarrhea, and abdominal pain are the most common GI side effects. Pancreatitis can occur with elevations of serum amylase and lipase.

TOXICITY 3

Pulmonary toxicity with increased cough, dyspnea, fever, and pulmonary infiltrates.

TOXICITY 4

Constitutional side effects with fatigue, asthenia, and anorexia.

TOXICITY 5

Cardiac toxicity with QTc prolongation and sinus bradycardia.

TOXICITY 6

Hyperglycemia.

TOXICITY 7

Skin rash.

Cetuximab

TRADE NAME	Erbitux, IMC-C225	CLASSIFICATION	Anti-EGFR monoclonal antibody
CATEGORY	Biologic response modifier agent, targeted agent	DRUG MANUFACTURER	Bristol-Myers Squibb and ImClone/Eli Lilly

MECHANISM OF ACTION

- Recombinant chimeric IgG1 monoclonal antibody directed against the epidermal growth factor receptor (EGFR). EGFR is overexpressed in a broad range of human solid tumors, including colorectal cancer, head and neck cancer, NSCLC, pancreatic cancer, and breast cancer.
- Binds with nearly 10-fold higher affinity to EGFR than normal ligands EGF and TGF-α, which then results in inhibition of EGFR. Prevents both homodimerization and heterodimerization of the EGFR, which leads to inhibition of autophosphorylation and inhibition of EGFR signaling.
- Inhibition of the EGFR signaling pathway results in inhibition of critical mitogenic and anti-apoptotic signals involved in proliferation, growth, invasion/metastasis, and angiogenesis.
- Inhibition of the EGFR pathway enhances the response to chemotherapy and/or radiation therapy.
- Immunologic mechanisms may also be involved in antitumor activity, and they include recruitment of ADCC and/or complement-mediated cell lysis.

MECHANISM OF RESISTANCE

- Mutations in EGFR, leading to decreased binding affinity to cetuximab.
- Decreased expression of EGFR.
- Increased expression of TGF-α ligand.
- Presence of KRAS mutations, which mainly occur in codons 12 and 13.
- Presence of BRAF mutations.
- Presence of NRAS mutations.

- Increased expression of HER2 through gene amplification.
- Increased HER3 expression.
- Activation/induction of alternative cellular signaling pathways, such as PI3K/Akt and IGF-1R.
- Increased expression of lncRNA MIR100HG and two embedded miRNAs, miR-100 and miR-125, which then leads to activation of Wnt signaling.

DISTRIBUTION
Distribution in the body is not well characterized.

METABOLISM
Metabolism of cetuximab has not been extensively characterized. Half-life is on the order of 5–7 days.

INDICATIONS
1. FDA-approved for the treatment of RAS wild-type mCRC in combination with irinotecan in irinotecan-refractory disease or as monotherapy in patients who are deemed to be irinotecan-intolerant. The use of cetuximab is not recommended for the treatment of mCRC with RAS mutations.
2. FDA-approved in combination with FOLFIRI in the front-line treatment of wild-type RAS mCRC.
3. Head and neck cancer—FDA-approved for use in combination with radiation therapy for the initial treatment of locally or regionally advanced squamous cell cancer of the head and neck.
4. Head and neck cancer—FDA-approved for use in combination with platinum-based therapy with 5-FU for the first-line treatment of recurrent locoregional disease or metastatic squamous cell cancer of the head and neck.
5. Head and neck cancer—FDA-approved as monotherapy for the treatment of recurrent or metastatic squamous cell cancer of the head and neck progressing after platinum-based therapy.

DOSAGE RANGE
1. Loading dose of 400 mg/m^2 IV administered over 120 minutes, followed by maintenance dose of 250 mg/m^2 IV given on a weekly basis.
2. An alternative dosing schedule is 500 mg/m^2 IV every 2 weeks, with no need for a loading dose.

DRUG INTERACTIONS
None well characterized to date.

SPECIAL CONSIDERATIONS
1. Should be used with caution in patients with known hypersensitivity to murine proteins and/or any individual components.
2. The level of EGFR expression does not accurately predict cetuximab clinical activity. As such, EGFR testing is not required for the clinical use of cetuximab.

3. Extended KRAS and NRAS testing should be performed in all mCRC patients being considered for cetuximab therapy. Only patients with wild-type KRAS and NRAS should be treated with cetuximab, either as monotherapy or in combination with cytotoxic chemotherapy.
4. Development of skin toxicity is a surrogate marker for cetuximab clinical activity.
5. Use with caution in patients with underlying ILD because these patients are at increased risk for worsening of their ILD.
6. In patients who develop a skin rash, topical antibiotics such as clindamycin gel or erythromycin cream or either oral clindamycin, oral doxycycline, or oral minocycline may help. Patients should be warned to avoid sunlight exposure.
7. About 90% of patients experience infusion reactions with the first infusion despite the use of prophylactic antihistamine therapy. However, some patients may experience infusion reactions with later infusions.
8. Electrolyte status should be closely monitored, especially serum magnesium levels, because hypomagnesemia has been observed with cetuximab treatment.
9. Pregnancy category C. Breastfeeding should be avoided.

TOXICITY 1
Infusion-related symptoms with fever, chills, urticaria, flushing, fatigue, headache, bronchospasm, dyspnea, angioedema, and hypotension. Occurs in 40%–50% of patients, although severe reactions occur in less than 1%. Usually mild-to-moderate severity and observed most commonly with administration of the first infusion.

TOXICITY 2
Skin toxicity with pruritus, dry skin, and a pustular, acneiform skin rash. Presents mainly on the face, neck region, and upper trunk. Improves with continued treatment and resolves upon cessation of therapy.

TOXICITY 3
Pulmonary toxicity in the form of ILD manifested by increased cough, dyspnea, and pulmonary infiltrates. Observed in less than 1% of patients and more frequent in patients with underlying pulmonary disease.

TOXICITY 4
Hypomagnesemia.

TOXICITY 5
Asthenia and generalized malaise observed in nearly 50% of patients.

TOXICITY 6
Paronychial inflammation with swelling of the lateral nail folds of the toes and fingers. Occurs with prolonged use.

C

Chlorambucil

$$Cl-N-\langle\text{benzene ring}\rangle-CH_2CH_2CH_2CO_2H$$
$$Cl$$

TRADE NAME	Leukeran	**CLASSIFICATION**	Alkylating agent
CATEGORY	Chemotherapy drug	**DRUG MANUFACTURER**	GlaxoSmithKline

MECHANISM OF ACTION
- Aromatic analog of nitrogen mustard.
- Functions as a bifunctional alkylating agent.
- Forms cross-links with DNA, resulting in inhibition of DNA synthesis and function.
- Cell cycle–nonspecific. Active in all phases of the cell cycle.

MECHANISM OF RESISTANCE
- Decreased cellular uptake of drug.
- Increased activity of DNA repair enzymes.
- Increased expression of sulfhydryl proteins, including glutathione and glutathione-related enzymes.

ABSORPTION
Oral bioavailability is approximately 75% when taken with food. Maximum plasma levels are achieved within 1–2 hours after oral administration. Extensively bound to plasma proteins.

DISTRIBUTION
Distribution of chlorambucil has not been well studied.

METABOLISM
Metabolized extensively by the liver cytochrome P450 system to both active and inactive forms. Parent drug and its metabolites are eliminated by the kidneys, and 60% of drug metabolites are excreted in urine within 24 hours. The terminal elimination half-life is 1.5–2.5 hours for the parent drug and about 2.5–4 hours for drug metabolites.

INDICATIONS
1. Chronic lymphocytic leukemia (CLL).
2. Non-Hodgkin's lymphoma.
3. Hodgkin's lymphoma.
4. Waldenstrom's macroglobulinemia.

DOSAGE RANGE

CLL—0.1–0.2 mg/kg PO daily for 3–6 weeks, as required. This dose is for initiation of therapy. For maintenance therapy, a dose of 2–4 mg PO daily is recommended.

DRUG INTERACTIONS

Phenobarbital, phenytoin, and other drugs that stimulate the liver P450 system—Concurrent use of chlorambucil with these drugs may increase its metabolic activation, leading to increased formation of toxic metabolites.

SPECIAL CONSIDERATIONS

1. Careful review of patient's medication list is required.
2. Contraindicated within 1 month of radiation and/or cytotoxic therapy, recent smallpox vaccine, and seizure history.
3. Use with caution when combined with allopurinol or colchicine because drug-induced hyperuricemia may be exacerbated.
4. Monitor CBCs periodically while on therapy. Discontinuation of chlorambucil is not necessary at the first sign of a reduction in the WBCs. However, fall may continue for 10 days or more after the last dose.
5. Therapy should be discontinued promptly if generalized skin rash develops, because this side effect may rapidly progress to erythema multiforme, toxic epidermal necrolysis, or Stevens-Johnson syndrome.
6. Pregnancy category D. Breastfeeding should be avoided.

TOXICITY 1

Myelosuppression is dose-limiting. Neutropenia and thrombocytopenia observed equally, with delayed and prolonged nadir occurring 25–30 days and recovery by 40–45 days. Usually reversible, but irreversible bone marrow failure can occur.

TOXICITY 2

Mild nausea and vomiting are common.

TOXICITY 3

Hyperuricemia.

TOXICITY 4

Pulmonary fibrosis and pneumonitis are dose-related and potentially life-threatening. Relatively rare event.

TOXICITY 5

Seizures with increased risk in children with nephrotic syndrome and patients receiving large cumulative doses. Patients with a history of seizure disorder may be especially prone to seizures.

TOXICITY 6

Skin rash, urticaria on face, scalp, and trunk with spread to legs seen in the early stages of therapy. Stevens-Johnson syndrome and toxic epidermal neurolysis are rare events.

TOXICITY 7
Amenorrhea, oligospermia/azoospermia, and sterility.

TOXICITY 8
Increased risk of secondary malignancies, including acute myelogenous leukemia.

Cisplatin

TRADE NAME	CDDP, Platinol	CLASSIFICATION	Platinum analog
CATEGORY	Chemotherapy drug	DRUG MANUFACTURER	Bristol-Myers Squibb

MECHANISM OF ACTION
- Covalently binds to DNA, with preferential binding to the N-7 position of guanine and adenine.
- Reacts with two different sites on DNA to produce cross-links, either intrastrand (>90%) or interstrand (<5%). Formation of DNA adducts results in inhibition of DNA synthesis and function as well as inhibition of transcription.
- Binding to nuclear and cytoplasmic proteins may result in cytotoxic effects.

MECHANISM OF RESISTANCE
- Increased inactivation by thiol-containing proteins such as glutathione and glutathione-related enzymes.
- Increased DNA repair enzyme activity (e.g., ERCC-1).
- Deficiency in mismatch repair enzymes (e.g., hMHL1, hMSH2).
- Decreased drug accumulation due to alterations in cellular transport.

ABSORPTION
Administered via the IV or intraperitoneal (IP) routes. Systemic absorption is rapid and complete after IP administration.

DISTRIBUTION
Widely distributed to all tissues, with highest concentrations in the liver and kidneys. Less than 10% remaining in the plasma 1 hour after infusion.

METABOLISM

Plasma concentrations of cisplatin decay rapidly, with a half-life of approximately 20–30 minutes following bolus administration. Within the cytoplasm of the cell, low concentrations of chloride (4 mM) favor the aquation reaction whereby the chloride atom is replaced by a water molecule, resulting in a highly reactive species. Platinum clearance from plasma proceeds slowly after the first 2 hours due to covalent binding with serum proteins, such as albumin, transferrin, and γ-globulin. Approximately 10%–40% of a given dose of cisplatin is excreted in the urine in 24 hours, with 35%–50% being excreted in the urine after 5 days of administration. Approximately 15% of the drug is excreted unchanged.

INDICATIONS

1. Testicular cancer.
2. Ovarian cancer.
3. Bladder cancer.
4. Head and neck cancer.
5. Esophageal cancer.
6. SCLC and NSCLC.
7. Non-Hodgkin's lymphoma.
8. Trophoblastic neoplasms.

DOSAGE RANGE

1. Ovarian cancer—75 mg/m^2 IV on day 1 every 21 days as part of the cisplatin/paclitaxel regimen, and 100 mg/m^2 on day 1 every 21 days as part of the cisplatin/cyclophosphamide regimen.
2. Testicular cancer—20 mg/m^2 IV on days 1–5 every 21 days as part of the PEB regimen.
3. NSCLC—60–100 mg/m^2 IV on day 1 every 21 days as part of the cisplatin/etoposide or cisplatin/gemcitabine regimens.
4. Head and neck cancer—20 mg/m^2/day IV continuous infusion for 4 days.

DRUG INTERACTION 1

Phenytoin—Cisplatin decreases pharmacologic effect of phenytoin. For this reason, phenytoin dose may need to be increased with concurrent use with cisplatin.

DRUG INTERACTION 2

Amifostine, mesna—The nephrotoxic effect of cisplatin is inactivated by amifostine and mesna.

DRUG INTERACTION 3

Aminoglycosides, amphotericin B, other nephrotoxic agents—Increased renal toxicity with concurrent use of cisplatin and aminoglycosides, amphotericin B, and/or other nephrotoxic agents.

DRUG INTERACTION 4
Etoposide, methotrexate, ifosfamide, bleomycin—Cisplatin reduces the renal clearance of etoposide, methotrexate, ifosfamide, and bleomycin, resulting in the increased accumulation of each of these drugs.

DRUG INTERACTION 5
Etoposide—Cisplatin may enhance the antitumor activity of etoposide.

DRUG INTERACTION 6
Radiation therapy—Cisplatin acts as a radiosensitizing agent.

DRUG INTERACTION 7
Paclitaxel—Cisplatin should be administered after paclitaxel when cisplatin and paclitaxel are used in combination. This sequence prevents delayed paclitaxel excretion and increased toxicity.

DRUG INTERACTION 8
Aminoglycosides, furosemide—Risk of ototoxicity is increased when cisplatin is combined with aminoglycosides and loop diuretics such as furosemide.

SPECIAL CONSIDERATIONS
1. Contraindicated in patients with known hypersensitivity to cisplatin or other platinum analogs.
2. Use with caution in patients with abnormal renal function. Dose of drug must be reduced in the setting of renal dysfunction. Creatinine clearance should be obtained at baseline and before each cycle of therapy. Carefully monitor renal function (BUN and creatinine) as well as serum electrolytes (Na, Mg, Ca, K) during treatment.
3. Fluid status of patient is critical. Patients must be hydrated before, during, and after drug administration. Usual approach is to give at least 1 liter before and 1 liter post-drug treatment of 0.9% sodium chloride with 20 mEq of KCl. With higher doses of drug, more aggressive hydration should be considered, with at least 2 liters of fluid administered before drug. In this setting, urine output should be greater than 100 mL/hr. Furosemide diuresis may be used after every 2 liters of fluid.
4. Use with caution in patients with hearing impairment or pre-existing peripheral neuropathy. Baseline audiology exam and periodic evaluation during therapy are recommended to monitor the effects of drug on hearing. Contraindicated in patients with pre-existing hearing deficit.
5. Cisplatin is a potent emetogenic agent that can cause acute and/or delayed nausea/vomiting. Give antiemetic premedication to prevent cisplatin-induced nausea and vomiting. Prophylaxis against delayed emesis (>24 hours after the drug administration) is also recommended. A combination of a 5-HT3 antagonist (e.g., ondansetron or granisetron) and dexamethasone is standard therapy for prevention of nausea and vomiting.
6. Avoid aluminum needles when administering the drug because precipitate may form, resulting in decreased potency.
7. Cisplatin is inactivated in the presence of alkaline solutions containing sodium bicarbonate.

TOXICITY 1
Nephrotoxicity is dose-limiting toxicity in up to 35%–40% of patients. Effects on renal function are dose-related and usually observed at 10–20 days after therapy. Generally reversible. Electrolyte abnormalities, mainly hypomagnesemia, hypocalcemia, and hypokalemia, are common. Hyperuricemia rarely occurs.

TOXICITY 2
Nausea and vomiting. Two forms are observed: acute (within the first 24 hours) and delayed (>24 hours). Early form begins within 1 hour of starting cisplatin therapy, may last for 8–12 hours, and does not predict who will develop the delayed form. The delayed form can present 3–5 days after drug administration.

TOXICITY 3
Myelosuppression in 25%–30% of patients, with WBCs, platelets, and RBCs equally affected. Neutropenia and thrombocytopenia are more pronounced at higher doses. Coombs-positive hemolytic anemia rarely observed.

TOXICITY 4
Neurotoxicity usually in the form of peripheral sensory neuropathy. Paresthesias and numbness in a classic stocking-glove pattern. Tends to occur after several cycles of therapy, and risk increases with cumulative doses. Loss of motor function, focal encephalopathy, and seizures also observed. Neurologic effects may be irreversible.

TOXICITY 5
Ototoxicity with high-frequency hearing loss and tinnitus.

TOXICITY 6
Hypersensitivity reactions consisting of facial edema, wheezing, bronchospasm, and hypotension. Usually occur within a few minutes of drug administration.

TOXICITY 7
Ocular toxicity manifested as optic neuritis, papilledema, and cerebral blindness. Altered color perception may be observed in rare cases.

TOXICITY 8
Hepatotoxicity with elevation in LFTs, mainly SGOT and serum bilirubin.

TOXICITY 9
Metallic taste of foods and loss of appetite.

TOXICITY 10
Vascular events, including myocardial infarction, arteritis, cerebrovascular accidents, and thrombotic microangiopathy. Raynaud's phenomenon has been reported.

TOXICITY 11

Alopecia.

TOXICITY 12

Syndrome of inappropriate antidiuretic hormone (SIADH) secretion.

TOXICITY 13

Azoospermia, impotence, and sterility.

Cladribine

TRADE NAME	2-Chlorodeoxyadenosine, 2-CdA, Leustatin	CLASSIFICATION	Antimetabolite, purine analog
CATEGORY	Chemotherapy drug	DRUG MANUFACTURER	Ortho Biotech

MECHANISM OF ACTION

- Purine deoxyadenosine analog with high specificity for lymphoid cells.
- Presence of the 2-chloro group on adenine ring renders cladribine resistant to breakdown by adenosine deaminase.
- Antitumor activity against both dividing and resting cells.
- Metabolized intracellularly to 5'-triphosphate form (Cld-ATP), which is the presumed active species.
- Triphosphate metabolite incorporates into DNA resulting in inhibition of DNA chain extension and inhibition of DNA synthesis and function.
- Inhibition of ribonucleotide reductase.
- Depletes nicotine adenine dinucleotide (NAD) concentration, resulting in depletion of ATP.
- Induction of apoptosis (programmed cell death).

MECHANISM OF RESISTANCE

- Decreased expression of the activating enzyme deoxycylidine kinase, resulting in decreased formation of cytotoxic cladribine metabolites.
- Increased expression of 5'-nucleotidase, which dephosphorylates cladribine nucleotide metabolites Cld-AMP and Cld-ATP.

ABSORPTION
Oral absorption is variable with about 50% oral bioavailability. Nearly 100% of drug is bioavailable after SC injection.

DISTRIBUTION
Widely distributed throughout the body. About 20% of drug is bound to plasma proteins. Crosses the blood-brain barrier, but CSF concentrations reach only 25% of those in plasma.

METABOLISM
Extensively metabolized intracellularly to nucleotide metabolite forms. Intracellular concentrations of phosphorylated metabolites exceed those in plasma by several hundred-fold. Terminal half-life is on the order of 5–7 hours. Cleared by the kidneys via a cation organic carrier system. Renal clearance is approximately 50%, with 20%–35% of drug eliminated unchanged.

INDICATIONS
1. Hairy cell leukemia.
2. Chronic lymphocytic leukemia.
3. Non-Hodgkin's lymphoma (low-grade).

DOSAGE RANGE
Recommended dose is 0.09 mg/kg/day IV via continuous infusion for 7 days. One course is usually administered. If the patient does not respond to one course, it is unlikely that a response will be seen with a second course of therapy.

DRUG INTERACTIONS
None well characterized to date.

SPECIAL CONSIDERATIONS
1. Use with caution in patients with abnormal renal function.
2. Monitor for signs of infection. Patients are at increased risk for opportunistic infections, including herpes, fungus, and Pneumocystis jiroveci (PJP).
3. Monitor for signs of tumor lysis syndrome. Increased risk in patients with a high tumor cell burden.
4. Allopurinol should be given before initiation of therapy to prevent hyperuricemia.
5. Pregnancy category D. Breastfeeding should be avoided.

TOXICITY 1
Myelosuppression is dose-limiting toxicity. Neutropenia more commonly observed than anemia or thrombocytopenia, and neutrophil nadir occurs at 7–14 days, with recovery in 3–4 weeks.

TOXICITY 2
Immunosuppression with decrease in CD4 and CD8 cells. Increased risk of opportunistic infections, including fungus, herpes, and PJP. Complete recovery of CD4 counts to normal may take up to 40 months.

TOXICITY 3
Fever occurs in 40%–50% of patients. Most likely due to release of pyrogens and/or cytokines from tumor cells. Associated with fatigue, malaise, myalgias, arthralgias, and chills. Incidence decreases with continued therapy.

TOXICITY 4
Mild nausea and vomiting observed in less than 30% of patients.

TOXICITY 5
Tumor lysis syndrome. Rare event most often in the setting of high tumor cell burden.

TOXICITY 6
Skin reaction at the site of injection.

Clofarabine

TRADE NAME	Clolar	CLASSIFICATION	Antimetabolite, purine analog
CATEGORY	Chemotherapy drug	DRUG MANUFACTURER	Sanofi-Aventis

MECHANISM OF ACTION
- Purine deoxyadenosine nucleoside analog.
- Presence of the 2-fluoro group on the sugar ring renders clofarabine resistant to breakdown by adenosine deaminase.
- Cell cycle–specific with activity in the S-phase.

- Requires transport into the cell via a nucleoside transport protein. Once inside the cell, the drug undergoes activation eventually to the cytotoxic triphosphate nucleotide metabolite.
- Incorporation of clofarabine triphosphate into DNA, resulting in chain termination and inhibition of DNA synthesis and function.
- Clofarabine triphosphate inhibits DNA polymerases α, β, and γ, which, in turn, interferes with DNA synthesis, DNA repair, and DNA chain elongation.
- Clofarabine triphosphate disrupts the mitochondrial membrane, leading to release of cytochrome C and the induction of apoptosis.
- Inhibits the enzyme ribonucleotide reductase, resulting in decreased levels of essential deoxyribonucleotides for DNA synthesis and function.

MECHANISM OF RESISTANCE
- Decreased activation of drug through decreased expression of the activating enzyme deoxycytidine kinase.
- Decreased nucleoside transport of drug into cells.
- Increased expression of cytidine triphosphate (CTP) synthetase activity, resulting in increased concentrations of competing physiologic nucleotide substrate dCTP.

ABSORPTION
Administered only via the IV route.

DISTRIBUTION
Approximately 50% bound to plasma proteins, primarily to albumin.

METABOLISM
Extensively metabolized intracellularly to nucleotide metabolite forms. Clofarabine has high affinity for the activating enzyme deoxycytidine kinase and is a more efficient substrate for this enzyme than the normal substrate deoxyadenosine. Renal clearance is approximately 50%–60%. The pathways of non-renal elimination remain unknown. The terminal elimination half-life is on the order of 5 hours.

INDICATIONS
FDA-approved for the treatment of pediatric patients 1–21 years of age with relapsed or refractory acute lymphoblastic leukemia after at least two prior regimens.

DOSAGE RANGE
Recommended dose is 52 mg/m^2 IV over 2 hours daily for 5 days every 2–6 weeks.

DRUG INTERACTIONS
None well characterized to date.

SPECIAL CONSIDERATIONS

1. Use with caution in patients with abnormal renal function. The dose of clofarabine should be reduced by 50% in patients with CrCl of 30–60 mL/min. Use with caution in patients with CrCl < 30 mL/min or in those on dialysis because the drug has not been studied in these settings.
2. Because clofarabine is excreted mainly by the kidneys, drugs with known renal toxicity should be avoided during the 5 days of drug treatment.
3. Concomitant use of medications known to cause liver toxicity should be avoided.
4. Patients should be closely monitored for evidence of tumor lysis syndrome and systemic inflammatory response syndrome (SIRS)/capillary leak syndrome, which result from rapid reduction in peripheral leukemic cells following drug treatment. The use of hydrocortisone 100 mg/m^2 IV on days 1–3 may prevent the development of SIRS or capillary leak.
5. Embryo-fetal toxicity. Breastfeeding should be avoided while on treatment and for at least 2 weeks after the last dose.

TOXICITY 1
Myelosuppression is dose-limiting with neutropenia, anemia, and thrombocytopenia.

TOXICITY 2
Capillary leak syndrome/SIRS with tachypnea, tachycardia, pulmonary edema, and hypotension. Pericardial effusion observed in up to 35% of patients, but usually minimal to small and not hemodynamically significant.

TOXICITY 3
Nausea/vomiting and diarrhea are most common GI side effects.

TOXICITY 4
Hepatotoxicity with elevation of serum transaminases and bilirubin. Usually occurs within 1 week and reversible, with resolution in 14 days.

TOXICITY 5
Increased risk of opportunistic infections, including fungal, viral, and bacterial infections.

TOXICITY 6
Renal toxicity with elevation in serum creatinine observed in up to 10% of patients.

TOXICITY 7
Cardiac toxicity with left ventricular dysfunction and tachycardia.

Cobimetinib

TRADE NAME	Cotellic	CLASSIFICATION	Signal transduction inhibitor, MEK inhibitor
CATEGORY	Targeted agent	DRUG MANUFACTURER	Genentech/Roche

MECHANISM OF ACTION
- Reversible inhibitor of mitogen-activated extracellular signal-regulated kinase 1 (MEK1) and kinase 2 (MEK2).
- Results in inhibition of downstream regulators of the extracellular signal-regulated kinase (ERK) pathway, leading to inhibition of cellular proliferation.
- Inhibits growth of BRAF-V600 mutation-positive melanoma, such as V600E and V600K.

MECHANISM OF RESISTANCE
- Increased expression and/or activation of the PI3K/AKT pathway.
- Reactivation of the MAPK signaling pathway.
- Emergence of MEK2 mutations.
- Presence of NRAS mutations.
- Increased expression and/or activation of the HER2-neu pathway.

ABSORPTION
Oral bioavailability is on the order of 46%. Peak plasma drug concentrations are achieved in 2.4 hours after oral ingestion. Food with a high fat content does not affect C_{max} and AUC.

DISTRIBUTION
Extensive binding (95%) of cobimetinib to plasma proteins. Steady-state blood levels are achieved in 9 days.

METABOLISM

Metabolized mainly via CYP3A oxidation and UGT2B7 glucuronidation in the liver. Elimination is hepatic, with 76% of an administered dose excreted in feces (6.6% as parent drug), with renal elimination accounting for only about 18% of an administered dose (1.6% as parent drug). The median terminal half-life of cobimetinib is 44 hours.

INDICATIONS

1. FDA-approved for unresectable or metastatic melanoma with a BRAF-V600E or V600K mutation in combination with vemurafenib.
2. FDA-approved as a single agent for histiocytic neoplasms.

DOSAGE RANGE

Recommended dose is 60 mg PO daily for 21 days on a 28-day cycle. Can be taken with or without food.

DRUG INTERACTION 1

Phenytoin and other drugs that stimulate the liver microsomal CYP3A4 enzymes, including carbamazepine, rifampin, phenobarbital, and St. John's Wort—These drugs may increase the metabolism of cobimetinib, resulting in its inactivation and lower effective drug levels.

DRUG INTERACTION 2

Drugs that inhibit the liver microsomal CYP3A4 enzymes, including ketoconazole, itraconazole, erythromycin, and clarithromycin—These drugs may decrease the metabolism of cobimetinib, resulting in increased drug levels and potentially increased toxicity.

DRUG INTERACTION 3

Warfarin—Patients receiving warfarin should be closely monitored for alterations in their clotting parameters (PT and INR) and/or bleeding because cobimetinib may inhibit the metabolism of warfarin by the liver P450 system. Dose of warfarin may require careful adjustment in the presence of cobimetinib therapy.

SPECIAL CONSIDERATIONS

1. Baseline and periodic evaluations of LVEF, at 1 month after treatment initiation and every 3 months thereafter, should be performed while on therapy. The median time to first onset of LVEF reduction is 4 months. Treatment should be held if the absolute LVEF drops by 10% from pretreatment baseline. Therapy should be permanently stopped for symptomatic cardiomyopathy or persistent, asymptomatic LVEF dysfunction that does not resolve within 4 weeks.
2. Patients should be warned about the possibility of visual disturbances.
3. Eye exams should be done at baseline and with any new visual changes to rule out the possibility of serous retinopathy or retinal vein occlusion.
4. Monitor patients for symptoms and signs of bleeding.

5. Monitor patients for an increased risk of new primary cancers, both cutaneous and non-cutaneous, while on therapy and for up to 6 months following the last dose of cobimetinib.
6. Monitor patients for skin reactions.
7. Monitor liver function tests periodically during therapy.
8. Monitor patients for skin reactions. The median time to grade 3 or 4 skin toxicity is 11 days.
9. Patients should be educated to avoid sun exposure.
10. Baseline and periodic CPK levels while on therapy because rhabdomyolysis has been observed with cobimetinib therapy.
11. BRAF testing using an FDA-approved diagnostic test to confirm the presence of the BRAF-V600E or V600K mutations is required for determining which patients should receive cobimetinib therapy.
12. No dose adjustment is needed for patients with mild hepatic dysfunction. Caution should be used in patients with moderate or severe hepatic dysfunction.
13. No dose adjustment is needed for patients with mild or moderate renal dysfunction. Use with caution in patients with severe renal dysfunction.
14. Pregnancy category D. Breastfeeding should be avoided.

TOXICITY 1
Cardiac toxicity in the form of cardiomyopathy.

TOXICITY 2
Ocular side effects, including impaired vision, serous retinopathy, retinal detachment, and retinal vein occlusion.

TOXICITY 3
GI toxicity with diarrhea, nausea/vomiting, and mucositis.

TOXICITY 4
Skin toxicity with rash, dermatitis, acneiform rash, hand-foot syndrome, erythema, pruritus, and paronychia. Severe skin toxicity observed in 12% of patients.

TOXICITY 5
Hepatotoxicity.

TOXICITY 6
Increased risk of bleeding, with GI hemorrhage, reproductive hemorrhage, and hematuria being most commonly observed.

TOXICITY 7
Increased risk of cutaneous squamous cell cancer, keratoacanthoma, and basal cell cancer.

TOXICITY 8
Rhabdomyolysis occurs in 14% of patients.

TOXICITY 9
Photosensitivity.

TOXICITY 10
Hypertension.

Copanlisib

TRADE NAME	Aliqopa	CLASSIFICATION	Signal transduction inhibitor, PI3K inhibitor
CATEGORY	Targeted agent	DRUG MANUFACTURER	Bayer

MECHANISM OF ACTION
- Pan–class I phosphatidylinositol-3-kinase (PI3K) inhibitor with specific activity against the α and δ isoforms expressed in malignant B cells.
- Inhibits several key signaling pathways, including BCR, CXCR12-mediated chemotaxis of malignant B cells, and NF-κB.

MECHANISM OF RESISTANCE
None well characterized to date.

ABSORPTION
Administered only via the IV route.

DISTRIBUTION
Extensive binding (84.2%) to plasma proteins, with albumin being the main binding protein. Steady-state drug levels are reached in approximately 8 days.

METABOLISM
Metabolism in the liver primarily by CYP3A4 (>90%) and to a minor extent (<10%) by CYP1A1. Elimination is mainly hepatic (64%), with excretion in the feces. Renal elimination accounts for 22% of an administered dose. Approximately 50% of an administered dose is eliminated as unchanged, and 50% is eliminated in metabolite form. The terminal half-life of the parent drug is 38–39 hours.

INDICATIONS
FDA-approved for patients with relapsed follicular lymphoma who have received at least two prior systemic therapies. Accelerated approval was given based on overall response rate.

DOSAGE RANGE
Recommended dose is 60 mg IV on days 1, 8, and 15 of a 28-day schedule.

DRUG INTERACTION 1
Phenytoin and other drugs that stimulate the liver microsomal CYP3A4 enzymes, including carbamazepine, rifampin, phenobarbital, and St. John's Wort—These drugs may increase the metabolism of copanlisib, resulting in its inactivation and lower effective drug levels.

DRUG INTERACTION 2
Drugs that inhibit the liver microsomal CYP3A4 enzymes, including ketoconazole, itraconazole, erythromycin, and clarithromycin—These drugs may decrease the metabolism of copanlisib, resulting in increased drug levels and potentially increased toxicity.

DRUG INTERACTION 3
Warfarin—Patients receiving warfarin should be closely monitored for alterations in their clotting parameters (PT and INR) and/or bleeding because copanlisib may inhibit warfarin metabolism by the liver P450 system. Dose of warfarin may require careful adjustment in the presence of copanlisib therapy.

SPECIAL CONSIDERATIONS
1. Dose reduction is not required in the setting of mild hepatic impairment (Child-Pugh Class A). Has not been studied in the setting of moderate or severe hepatic impairment (total bilirubin $>1.5 \times$ ULN, any AST).
2. Dose reduction is not required in the setting of mild or moderate renal impairment. Has not been studied in the setting of severe renal impairment, in end-stage renal disease, or in patients on dialysis.
3. Monitor for signs and symptoms of infection. PJP prophylaxis should be considered for patients at increased risk.
4. Monitor blood glucose levels as copanlisib may cause infusion-related hyperglycemia. Patients with diabetes mellitus should have their blood glucose levels under control before starting therapy.
5. Monitor blood pressure as copanlisib may result in infusion-related hypertension. Blood pressure may remain elevated for up to 6–8 hours after drug infusion.
6. Monitor CBCs on a weekly basis.
7. Dose should be reduced to 45 mg when co-administered with a strong CYP3A4 inhibitor.
8. May cause fetal harm when administered to a pregnant woman. Breastfeeding should be avoided.

TOXICITY 1

Hyperglycemia.

TOXICITY 2

Hypertension.

TOXICITY 3

Myelosuppression with neutropenia and thrombocytopenia.

TOXICITY 4

Infections with pneumonia being most common. PJP is a rare event.

TOXICITY 5

Diarrhea and nausea/vomiting.

TOXICITY 6

Fatigue, asthenia, and anorexia.

TOXICITY 7

Non-infectious pneumonitis.

TOXICITY 8

Skin reactions, including maculopapular rash, pruritus, and exfoliative rash.

Crizotinib

TRADE NAME	Xalkori	CLASSIFICATION	Signal transduction inhibitor, ALK/RON inhibitor
CATEGORY	Targeted agent	DRUG MANUFACTURER	Pfizer

MECHANISM OF ACTION
- Inhibits multiple receptor tyrosine kinases (RTKs), including ALK, hepatocyte growth factor receptor (c-Met), ROS1, and recepteur d'origine nantais (RON), which results in inhibition of tumor growth, tumor angiogenesis, and metastasis.

MECHANISM OF RESISTANCE
- Mutations in the ALK kinase domain, with the most frequent ones being L1196M and G1269A.
- Mutations in EGFR.
- Mutations in ROS1 tyrosine kinase domain.
- Activation of non-ALK oncogenic pathways, including EGFR, MEK, ERK, SRC, and IGF-1R.
- EMT transition with downregulated expression of E-cadherin and increased expression of vimentin.
- Increased expression of miR-100-5p.
- Multidrug-resistant phenotype with increased expression of P170 glycoprotein.

ABSORPTION
Rapidly absorbed after an oral dose, with peak plasma levels achieved within 4–6 hours. Oral bioavailability on the order of 40%–60%. Food with a high fat content reduces oral bioavailability by up to 15%.

DISTRIBUTION
Extensive binding (90%) to plasma proteins. Steady-state drug concentrations are reached in 15 days.

METABOLISM
Metabolized in the liver primarily by CYP3A4 and CYP3A5 microsomal enzymes. Elimination is hepatic, with excretion in feces (~60%), with renal elimination accounting for 20% of an administered dose. Unchanged crizotinib represents approximately 50% of an administered dose in feces and about 2% in urine. The terminal half-life is approximately 40 hours.

INDICATIONS
1. FDA-approved for patients with locally advanced or metastatic NSCLC that is ALK- or ROS1-positive as detected by an FDA-approved test.
2. FDA-approved for pediatric patients 1 year of age and older and young adults with relapsed or refractory systemic anaplastic large cell lymphoma (ALCL) that is ALK-positive.
3. FDA-approved for adult and pediatric patients 1 year of age and older with unresectable, recurrent, or refractory inflammatory myofibroblastic tumor (IMT) that is ALK-positive.

DOSAGE RANGE

1. NSCLC: recommended dose is 250 mg PO bid.
2. ALCL: recommended dose is 280 mg/m² PO bid.
3. IMT: recommended dose for adult patients is 250 mg PO bid and for pediatric patients is 280 mg/m² PO bid.

DRUG INTERACTION 1

Drugs such as ketoconazole, itraconazole, erythromycin, clarithromycin, atazanavir, indinavir, nefazodone, nelfinavir, ritonavir, saquinavir, telithromycin, and voriconazole may decrease the metabolism of crizotinib, resulting in increased drug levels and potentially increased toxicity.

DRUG INTERACTION 2

Drugs such as rifampin, phenytoin, phenobarbital, carbamazepine, and St. John's Wort may increase the metabolism of crizotinib, resulting in its inactivation and lower effective drug levels.

DRUG INTERACTION 3

Proton pump inhibitors, H2-receptor inhibitors, and antacids—Drugs that alter the pH of the upper GI tract may alter crizotinib solubility, thereby reducing drug bioavailability and decreasing systemic drug exposure.

SPECIAL CONSIDERATIONS

1. Dose reduction is not required in NSCLC patients with mild hepatic dysfunction. Dose should be reduced to 200 mg PO bid in patients with moderate hepatic dysfunction, and reduced to 250 mg PO daily in patients with severe hepatic dysfunction.
2. Dose reduction is not required in patients with mild or moderate renal dysfunction. Dose reduction to 250 mg PO once daily is recommended in patients with severe renal dysfunction (CrCl <30 mL/min) not requiring dialysis.
3. Patients should be advised against performing activities that require mental alertness, including operating machinery and driving.
4. Patients receiving crizotinib along with oral warfarin anticoagulant therapy should have their coagulation parameters (PT and INR) monitored frequently because elevations in INR and bleeding events have been observed.
5. Monitor LFTs and serum bilirubin on a monthly basis and as clinically indicated because crizotinib may cause life-threatening and/or fatal hepatotoxicity. More frequent testing is required in patients who develop LFT elevations. May need to suspend, dose-reduce, or permanently stop crizotinib with the development of drug-induced hepatotoxicity.
6. Monitor patients for new or progressive pulmonary symptoms, including cough, dyspnea, and fever.
7. Patients should be aware of potential visual changes, including blurry vision, photosensitivity, and flashes/floaters. Careful eye exam should be performed in the setting of new or worsening floaters and/or photopsia to rule out the presence of retinal detachment.

8. Baseline and periodic evaluations of ECG and electrolyte status should be performed while on therapy. Use with caution in patients at risk of developing QT prolongation, including hypokalemia, hypomagnesemia, and congenital long QT syndrome, and patients taking antiarrhythmic medications or any other drugs that may cause QT prolongation.
9. ALK testing using an FDA-approved test is required to confirm the presence of ALK-positive NSCLC for determining which patients should receive crizotinib therapy.
10. Avoid Seville oranges, starfruit, pomelos, grapefruit, and grapefruit juice while on crizotinib therapy.
11. Male patients may experience symptoms of androgen deficiency with reduction in free testosterone levels while on crizotinib therapy.
12. May cause fetal harm. Breastfeeding should be avoided while on therapy and for 45 days after the last dose.

TOXICITY 1
Hepatotoxicity with elevations in serum transaminases (SGOT, SGPT). Rare cases of liver failure and death have been reported.

TOXICITY 2
Nausea/vomiting and diarrhea are the most common GI side effects.

TOXICITY 3
Pulmonary toxicity with increased cough, dyspnea, fever, and pulmonary infiltrates.

TOXICITY 4
Constitutional side effects with fatigue, asthenia, and anorexia.

TOXICITY 5
Cardiac toxicity with QTc prolongation and sinus bradycardia.

TOXICITY 6
Visual side effects, including diplopia, blurry vision, visual field defects, floaters/flashes, visual brightness, and reduced visual acuity.

TOXICITY 7
Peripheral sensory and/or motor neuropathy have been reported in up to 10% of patients.

TOXICITY 8
Symptoms associated with androgen deficiency and reduced testosterone levels.

Cyclophosphamide

TRADE NAME	Cytoxan, CTX	**CLASSIFICATION**	Alkylating agent
CATEGORY	Chemotherapy drug	**DRUG MANUFACTURER**	Bristol-Myers Squibb

MECHANISM OF ACTION
- Inactive in its parent form.
- Activated by the liver cytochrome P450 microsomal system to the cytotoxic metabolites phosphoramide mustard and acrolein.
- Cyclophosphamide metabolites form cross-links with DNA, resulting in inhibition of DNA synthesis and function.
- Cell cycle–nonspecific agent, active in all phases of the cell cycle.
- Potent immune modulator at low doses that targets suppressive regulatory immune cells within the tumor microenvironment while enhancing effector T cells.

MECHANISM OF RESISTANCE
- Decreased cellular uptake of drug.
- Decreased expression of drug-activating enzymes of the liver P450 system.
- Increased expression of sulfhydryl proteins, including glutathione and glutathione-associated enzymes.
- Increased expression of aldehyde dehydrogenase resulting in enhanced enzymatic detoxification of drug.
- Enhanced activity of DNA repair enzymes.

ABSORPTION
Well absorbed by the GI tract with oral bioavailability of nearly 90%.

DISTRIBUTION
Distributed throughout the body, including brain and CSF. Also distributed in milk and saliva. Minimal binding of parent drug to plasma proteins; however, about 60% of the phosphoramide mustard metabolite is bound to plasma proteins.

METABOLISM
Extensively metabolized in the liver by the cytochrome P450 system to both active and inactive forms. The active forms are 4-hydroxycyclophosphamide, phosphoramide mustard, and acrolein. Parent drug and metabolites are eliminated mainly in urine. Only about 10%-20% of drug is excreted in parent form in urine while only 4% of unchanged drug is excreted in stool via the hepatobiliary route. The elimination half-life ranges from 4–6 hours.

INDICATIONS
1. Breast cancer.
2. Non-Hodgkin's lymphoma.
3. Chronic lymphocytic leukemia.
4. Ovarian cancer.
5. Bone and soft tissue sarcoma.
6. Rhabdomyosarcoma.
7. Neuroblastoma and Wilms' tumor.

DOSAGE RANGE
1. Breast cancer—When given orally, the usual dose is 100 mg/m^2 PO on days 1–14 given every 28 days. When administered by IV, the usual dose is 600 mg/m^2 given every 21 days as part of the AC or CMF regimens.
2. Non-Hodgkin's lymphoma—Usual dose is 400–600 mg/m^2 IV on day 1 every 21 days, as part of the CVP regimen, and 750 mg/m^2 on day 1 every 21 days, as part of the CHOP regimen.
3. High-dose bone marrow transplantation—Usual dose in the setting of bone marrow transplantation is 60 mg/kg IV for 2 days.

DRUG INTERACTION 1
Phenobarbital, phenytoin, and other drugs that stimulate the liver P450 system—Increase the metabolic activation of cyclophosphamide to its cytotoxic metabolites.

DRUG INTERACTION 2
Anticoagulants—Cyclophosphamide increases the effect of anticoagulants, and thus the dose of anticoagulants may need to be decreased depending on the coagulation parameters, PT/INR.

DRUG INTERACTION 3
Digoxin—Cyclophosphamide decreases the plasma levels of digoxin by activating its metabolism in the liver.

DRUG INTERACTION 4
Doxorubicin—Cyclophosphamide may increase the risk of doxorubicin-induced cardiac toxicity.

SPECIAL CONSIDERATIONS
1. Use with caution in patients with abnormal renal function especially in those with severe renal dysfunction. Dose should be reduced in the setting of renal dysfunction. CrCl should be obtained at baseline and before each cycle of therapy.
2. Administer oral form of drug during the daytime.
3. Encourage fluid intake of at least 2–3 L/day to reduce the risk of hemorrhagic cystitis. High-dose therapy requires administration of IV fluids for hydration.
4. Encourage patients to empty bladder several times daily (on average, every 2 hours) to reduce the risk of bladder toxicity.
5. Pregnancy category D. Breastfeeding should be avoided.

TOXICITY 1
Myelosuppression is dose-limiting. Mainly neutropenia, with nadir occurring at 7–14 days, and with recovery by day 21. Thrombocytopenia may occur, usually with high-dose therapy.

TOXICITY 2
Bladder toxicity in the form of hemorrhagic cystitis, dysuria, and increased urinary frequency occurs in 5%–10% of patients. Time of onset is variable and may begin within 24 hours of therapy or may be delayed for up to several weeks. Usually reversible upon discontinuation of drug. Uroprotection with mesna and hydration must be used with high-dose therapy to prevent bladder toxicity.

TOXICITY 3
Nausea and vomiting. Usually dose-related, occurs within 2–4 hours of therapy and may last up to 24 hours. Anorexia is fairly common.

TOXICITY 4
Alopecia generally starting 2–3 weeks after starting therapy. Skin and nails may become hyperpigmented.

TOXICITY 5
Amenorrhea with ovarian failure. Sterility may be permanent.

TOXICITY 6
Cardiac toxicity is observed with high-dose therapy.

TOXICITY 7
Increased risk of secondary malignancies, including acute myelogenous leukemia and bladder cancer, especially in patients with chronic hemorrhagic cystitis.

TOXICITY 8
Immunosuppression with an increased risk of infections.

TOXICITY 9
SIADH.

TOXICITY 10
Hypersensitivity reaction with rhinitis and irritation of the nose and throat. Usually self-resolving in 1–3 days, but steroids and/or diphenhydramine may be required.

Cytarabine

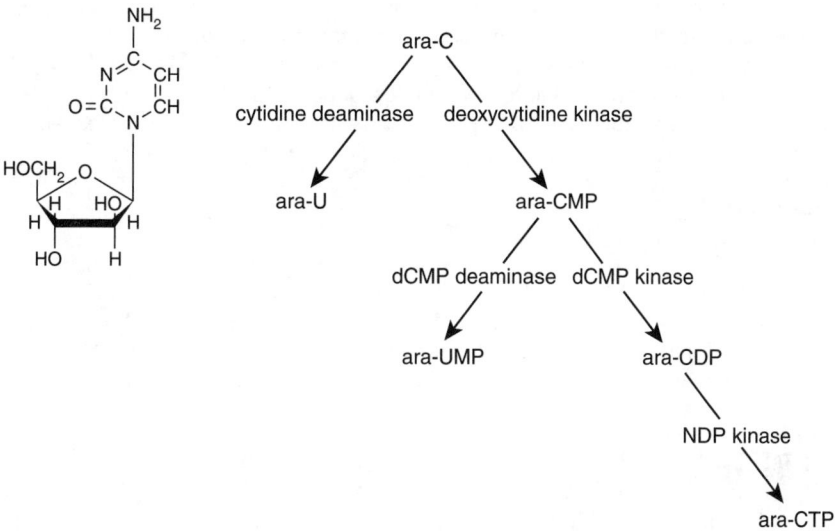

TRADE NAME	Cytosine arabinoside, Ara-C	CLASSIFICATION	Antimetabolite, deoxycytidine analog
CATEGORY	Chemotherapy drug	DRUG MANUFACTURER	Bedford Laboratories

MECHANISM OF ACTION

- Deoxycytidine analog originally isolated from the sponge Cryptotethya crypta.
- Cell cycle–specific with activity in the S-phase.
- Transported into the cell via a nucleoside transport protein and then undergoes intracellular activation first to the monophosphate metabolite with eventual formation of the ara-CTP triphosphate metabolite. Antitumor activity of cytarabine is determined by a balance between intracellular activation and degradation and the subsequent formation of cytotoxic ara-CTP metabolites.
- Incorporation of ara-CTP into DNA, resulting in chain termination and inhibition of DNA synthesis and function.
- Ara-CTP inhibits several DNA polymerases α, β, and γ, which then interferes with DNA synthesis, DNA repair, and DNA chain elongation.
- Ara-CTP inhibits ribonucleotide reductase, resulting in decreased levels of essential deoxyribonucleotides required for DNA synthesis and function.

MECHANISM OF RESISTANCE

- Decreased activation of drug through decreased expression of the anabolic enzyme deoxycytidine kinase.
- Increased breakdown of drug by the catabolic enzymes, cytidine deaminase and deoxycytidylate (dCMP) deaminase.
- Decreased nucleoside transport of drug into cells.
- Increased expression of CTP synthetase activity, resulting in increased concentrations of competing physiologic nucleotide substrate dCTP.

ABSORPTION

Administered only via the IV route.

DISTRIBUTION

Rapidly cleared from the bloodstream after IV administration. Distributes rapidly into tissues and total body water. Crosses the blood-brain barrier, with CSF levels reaching 20%–40% of those in plasma. Binding to plasma proteins has not been well characterized.

METABOLISM

Undergoes extensive metabolism with approximately 70%–80% of drug being recovered in the urine as the ara-U metabolite within 24 hours. Deamination occurs in liver, plasma, and peripheral tissues. The principal enzyme involved in drug catabolism is cytidine deaminase, which converts ara-C into the inactive metabolite ara-U. dCMP deaminase converts ara-CMP into ara-UMP, and this represents an additional catabolic pathway of the drug. The terminal elimination half-life is 2–6 hours. The half-life of ara-C in CSF is somewhat longer, ranging from 2–11 hours, due to the relatively low activity of cytidine deaminase present in CSF.

INDICATIONS

1. Acute myelogenous leukemia.
2. Acute lymphocytic leukemia.
3. Chronic myelogenous leukemia.
4. Leptomeningeal carcinomatosis.
5. Non-Hodgkin's lymphoma.

DOSAGE RANGE

Several different doses and schedules have been used:

1. Standard dose—100 mg/m^2/day IV on days 1–7 as a continuous IV infusion, in combination with an anthracycline as induction chemotherapy for AML.
2. High-dose—1.5–3.0 g/m^2 IV q 12 hours for 3 days as a high-dose, intensification regimen for AML.
3. SC—20 mg/m^2 SC for 10 days per month for 6 months, associated with IFN-α for treatment of CML.
4. Intrathecal—10–30 mg intrathecal (IT) up to three times weekly in the treatment of leptomeningeal carcinomatosis secondary to leukemia or lymphoma.

DRUG INTERACTION 1

Gentamicin—Cytarabine antagonizes the efficacy of gentamicin.

DRUG INTERACTION 2
5-Fluorocytosine—Cytarabine inhibits the efficacy of 5-fluorocytosine by preventing its cellular uptake.

DRUG INTERACTION 3
Digoxin—Cytarabine decreases the oral bioavailability of digoxin, thereby decreasing its efficacy. Digoxin levels should be monitored closely while on therapy.

DRUG INTERACTION 4
Alkylating agents, cisplatin, and ionizing radiation—Cytarabine enhances the cytotoxicity of various alkylating agents (cyclophosphamide, carmustine), cisplatin, and ionizing radiation by inhibiting DNA repair mechanisms. Concurrent use of high-dose cytarabine and cisplatin may increase risk of ototoxicity.

DRUG INTERACTION 5
Methotrexate—Pretreatment with methotrexate enhances the formation of ara-CTP metabolites, resulting in enhanced cytotoxicity.

DRUG INTERACTION 6
Fludarabine, hydroxyurea—Pretreatment with fludarabine and/or hydroxyurea potentiates the cytotoxicity of cytarabine by enhancing the formation of cytotoxic ara-CTP metabolites.

DRUG INTERACTION 7
GM-CSF, interleukin-3—Cytokines, including GM-CSF and interleukin-3, enhance cytarabine-mediated apoptosis mechanisms.

DRUG INTERACTION 8
L-asparaginase—Increased risk of pancreatitis when L-asparaginase is given before cytarabine.

SPECIAL CONSIDERATIONS
1. Monitor CBCs on a regular basis during therapy.
2. Use with caution in patients with abnormal liver and/or renal function. Dose modification should be considered in this setting because patients are at increased risk for toxicity. Monitor hepatic and renal function during therapy.
3. Alkalinization of the urine (pH >7), allopurinol, and vigorous IV hydration are recommended to prevent tumor lysis syndrome in patients with acute myelogenous leukemia.
4. High-dose therapy should be administered over a 1- to 2-hour period.
5. Conjunctivitis is observed with high-dose therapy because the drug is excreted in tears. Patients should be treated with hydrocortisone eye drops (2 drops OU qid for 10 days) on the night before the start of therapy.
6. Pregnancy category D. Breastfeeding should be avoided.

TOXICITY 1
Myelosuppression is dose-limiting. Neutropenia and thrombocytopenia are common. Nadir usually occurs by days 7–10, with recovery by days 14–21. Megaloblastic anemia has also been observed.

TOXICITY 2
Nausea and vomiting. Mild-to-moderate emetogenic agent, with increased severity observed with high-dose therapy. Anorexia, diarrhea, and mucositis usually occur 7–10 days after therapy.

TOXICITY 3
Cerebellar ataxia, lethargy, and confusion. Neurotoxicity develops in up to 10% of patients. Onset usually 5 days after drug treatment and lasts up to 1 week. In most cases, CNS toxicities are mild and reversible. Risk factors for neurotoxicity include high-dose therapy, age older than 40, and abnormal renal and/or liver function.

TOXICITY 4
Transient hepatic dysfunction with elevation of serum transaminases and bilirubin. Most often associated with high-dose therapy.

TOXICITY 5
Acute pancreatitis.

TOXICITY 6
Ara-C syndrome. Described in pediatric patients and represents an allergic reaction to cytarabine. Characterized by fever, myalgia, malaise, bone pain, maculopapular skin rash, conjunctivitis, and occasional chest pain. Usually occurs within 12 hours of drug infusion. Steroids appear to be effective in treating and/or preventing the onset of this syndrome.

TOXICITY 7
Pulmonary complications include non-cardiogenic pulmonary edema, acute respiratory distress, and *Streptococcus viridans* pneumonia. Usually observed with high-dose therapy.

TOXICITY 8
Erythema of skin, alopecia, and hidradenitis are usually mild and self-limited. Hand-foot syndrome observed rarely with high-dose therapy.

TOXICITY 9
Conjunctivitis and keratitis. Usually associated with high-dose regimens.

TOXICITY 10
Seizures, alterations in mental status, and fever may be observed within the first 24 hours after IT administration.

Dabrafenib

TRADE NAME	Tafinlar	**CLASSIFICATION**	Signal transduction inhibitor, BRAF inhibitor
CATEGORY	Targeted agent	**DRUG MANUFACTURER**	GlaxoSmithKline

MECHANISM OF ACTION
- Inhibits mutant forms of BRAF serine-threonine kinase, including BRAF-V600E, which results in inhibition of mitogen-activated protein kinase (MAPK) signaling.
- Inhibits wild-type BRAF and CRAF kinases. This inhibitory activity against wild-type BRAF is in sharp contrast to vemurafenib.

MECHANISM OF RESISTANCE
- Increased expression of MAPK signaling.
- Mutations in MAP2K1, which encodes MEK1 kinase, and MAP2K2 gene, which encodes MEK2 kinase. These mutations lead to activation of MAPK signaling downstream of RAF.
- BRAF amplification.
- NRAS mutations.
- Activation/induction of alternative cellular signaling pathways, such as FGFR, EGFR, and PI3K/Akt.
- Reactivation of Ras/Raf signaling.

ABSORPTION
High oral bioavailability on the order of 95%. Time to peak drug concentrations is 2 hours. Food with a high fat content reduces both C_{max} and AUC.

DISTRIBUTION
Extensive binding (>99%) of dabrafenib to plasma proteins.

METABOLISM
Metabolized in the liver primarily by CYP2C8 and CYP3A4 microsomal enzymes to produce the hydroxy-dabrafenib metabolite, which is further metabolized by CYP3A4 to the carboxy-dabrafenib metabolite. The hydroxy metabolite as well as

other metabolites may have clinical activity. Elimination is primarily hepatic with excretion in feces (~70%), with renal elimination accounting for about 25% of the administered dose. The median terminal half-life of dabrafenib is approximately 8 hours.

INDICATIONS

1. FDA-approved as a single agent for unresectable or metastatic melanoma with BRAF-V600E mutation as determined by an FDA-approved diagnostic test.
2. FDA-approved in combination with trametinib for unresectable or metastatic melanoma with BRAF-V600E mutation as determined by an FDA-approved diagnostic test.
3. FDA-approved in combination with trametinib for the adjuvant treatment of melanoma with BRAF-V600E or V600K mutations as determined by an FDA-approved diagnostic test, following complete surgical resection.
4. FDA-approved in combination with trametinib for metastatic NSCLC with BRAF-V600E mutation as determined by an FDA-approved diagnostic test.
5. FDA-approved in combination with trametinib for locally advanced or metastatic anaplastic thyroid cancer (ATC) with BRAF-V600E mutation as determined by an FDA-approved diagnostic test, and with no appropriate locoregional treatment options.
6. FDA-approved in combination with trametinib for adult and pediatric patients 6 years of age and older with unresectable or metastatic solid tumors with BRAF-V600E mutation who have progressed following prior treatment and have no satisfactory alternative treatment options. This indication is approved under accelerated approval based on overall response rate and duration of response.
7. FDA-approved for pediatric patients 1 year of age and older with low-grade glioma with a BRAF-V600E mutation who require systemic therapy.

DOSAGE RANGE

1. Recommended dose as a single agent and in combination for adult patients is 150 mg PO bid. Should be taken at least 1 hour before or at least 2 hours after a meal.
2. Recommended dose for capsules or tablets for oral suspension in pediatric patients is based on body weight as outlined in the package insert.

DRUG INTERACTION 1

Drugs such as ketoconazole, itraconazole, erythromycin, clarithromycin, atazanavir, indinavir, nefazodone, nelfinavir, ritonavir, saquinavir, telithromycin, and voriconazole may decrease the metabolism of dabrafenib, resulting in increased drug levels and potentially increased toxicity.

DRUG INTERACTION 2

Drugs such as rifampin, phenytoin, phenobarbital, carbamazepine, and St. John's Wort may increase the metabolism of dabrafenib, resulting in lower effective drug levels.

DRUG INTERACTION 3

Warfarin—Dabrafenib may alter the anticoagulant effect of warfarin by prolonging the PT and INR. Coagulation parameters (PT and INR) need to be closely monitored, and dose of warfarin may require adjustment.

SPECIAL CONSIDERATIONS

1. Careful skin exams should be done at baseline, every 2 months while on therapy, and for up to 6 months following discontinuation of therapy given the increased incidence of cutaneous squamous cell cancers and keratoacanthomas.
2. Monitor body temperature, as dabrafenib can cause febrile drug reactions. Should be withheld for fevers >101.3°F, and patients should be carefully evaluated for infection.
3. Monitor serum glucose levels in patients with diabetes or hyperglycemia.
4. Monitor patients for eye reactions, including uveitis and iritis.
5. BRAF testing using an FDA-approved diagnostic test to confirm the presence of the BRAF-V600E mutation is required.
6. No dose adjustment is needed for patients with mild hepatic dysfunction. Caution should be used in patients with moderate or severe hepatic dysfunction
7. No dose adjustment is needed for patients with mild or moderate renal dysfunction. Caution should be used in patients with severe renal dysfunction.
8. Avoid Seville oranges, pomelos, starfruit, grapefruit, and grapefruit products while on dabrafenib therapy.
9. May cause fetal harm. Females of reproductive potential should use non-hormonal methods of contraception during treatment and for at least 2 weeks after the last dose or at least 4 months after the last dose taken in combination with trametinib. Breastfeeding should be avoided.

TOXICITY 1

Cutaneous squamous cell cancers and keratoacanthomas occur in up to 10% of patients. Usually occur within 6–8 weeks of starting therapy.

TOXICITY 2

Skin reactions, including hyperkeratosis, hand-foot syndrome, and rash.

TOXICITY 3

Fever.

TOXICITY 4

Hyperglycemia.

TOXICITY 5

Arthralgias and myalgias.

TOXICITY 6

Ophthalmologic side effects, including uveitis, iritis, and photophobia.

TOXICITY 7
Constipation is the most common GI side effect.

TOXICITY 8
Fatigue.

Dacarbazine

TRADE NAME	DIC, DTIC-dome, Imidazole carboxamide	CLASSIFICATION	Nonclassic alkylating agent
CATEGORY	Chemotherapy drug	DRUG MANUFACTURER	Ben Venue Laboratories, Bayer

MECHANISM OF ACTION
- Cell cycle–nonspecific drug.
- Initially developed as a purine antimetabolite, but antitumor activity is not mediated via inhibition of purine biosynthesis.
- Metabolic activation is required for antitumor activity.
- While the precise mechanism of cytotoxicity is unclear, dacarbazine methylates nucleic acids, and in so doing, inhibits DNA, RNA, and protein synthesis.

MECHANISM OF RESISTANCE
Increased activity of DNA repair enzymes such as O6-alkylguanine-DNA alkyltransferase (AGAT).

ABSORPTION
IV administration is preferred, as there is slow and variable oral absorption.

DISTRIBUTION
Widely distributed in body tissues. About 20% of drug is loosely bound to plasma proteins.

METABOLISM

Metabolized in the liver by the microsomal P450 system to active metabolites (MTIC, AIC). About 40%–50% of the parent drug is excreted unchanged in urine within 6 hours, and tubular secretion appears to predominate. The elimination half-life of the drug is 5–6 hours.

INDICATIONS

1. Metastatic malignant melanoma.
2. Hodgkin's lymphoma.
3. Soft tissue sarcomas.
4. Neuroblastoma.

DOSAGE RANGE

1. Hodgkin's lymphoma—375 mg/m^2 IV on days 1 and 15 every 28 days, as part of the ABVD regimen.
2. Soft tissue sarcoma—250 mg/m^2/day IV continuous infusion on days 1–4 as part of the AD regimen and 750 mg/m^2 IV on day 1 every 21 days as part of the CYVADIC regimen.
3. Melanoma—As a single agent, 250 mg/m^2 IV for 5 days or 800–1,000 mg/m^2 IV every 3 weeks.

DRUG INTERACTION 1

Heparin, lidocaine, and hydrocortisone—Incompatible with dacarbazine.

DRUG INTERACTION 2

Phenytoin, phenobarbital—Decreased efficacy of dacarbazine when administered with phenytoin and phenobarbital, as these drugs induce dacarbazine metabolism by the liver P450 system.

SPECIAL CONSIDERATIONS

1. Dacarbazine is a potent vesicant, and should be carefully administered to avoid the risk of extravasation.
2. Dacarbazine is a highly emetogenic agent. Use aggressive antiemetics before drug administration to decrease risk of nausea and vomiting.
3. No specific guidelines for dacarbazine dosing in the setting of hepatic and/or renal dysfunction. However, dose modification should be considered in patients with moderate to severe hepatic and/or renal dysfunction
4. Patients should avoid sun exposure for several days after dacarbazine therapy.
5. Pregnancy category C. Breastfeeding should be avoided.

TOXICITY 1

Myelosuppression is dose-limiting toxicity. Leukopenia and thrombocytopenia are equally likely, with nadir occurring at 21–25 days.

TOXICITY 2

Nausea and vomiting can be significant, usually occurring within 1–3 hours and lasting for up to 12 hours. Aggressive antiemetic therapy strongly recommended. Anorexia is common, but diarrhea occurs rarely.

TOXICITY 3

Flu-like syndrome in the form of fever, chills, malaise, myalgias, and arthralgias. May last for several days after therapy.

TOXICITY 4

Pain and/or burning at the site of injection.

TOXICITY 5

Hepatotoxicity with elevation in LFTs. Associated with an acute sinusoidal obstruction syndrome and hepatic necrosis that can lead to death.

TOXICITY 6

CNS toxicity in the form of paresthesias, neuropathies, ataxia, lethargy, headache, confusion, and seizures.

TOXICITY 7

Increased risk of photosensitivity.

TOXICITY 8

Teratogenic, mutagenic, and carcinogenic.

Dacomitinib

TRADE NAME	Izimpro	CLASSIFICATION	Signal transduction inhibitor, EGFR inhibitor
CATEGORY	Targeted agent	DRUG MANUFACTURER	Pfizer

MECHANISM OF ACTION

- Potent and selective small-molecule inhibitor of EGFR, which binds irreversibly to specific mutant forms of EGFR, including T790M, L858R, and exon 19 deletion.
- Potent inhibitor of HER2 and HER4.
- Inhibition of mutant EGFR and HER2 and HER4 results in inhibition of critical mitogenic and antiapoptotic signals involved in proliferation, growth, invasion/metastasis, angiogenesis, and response to chemotherapy and/or radiation therapy.

MECHANISM OF RESISTANCE

- Amplification of the c-Met gene, with increased gene copy number.
- Presence of BRAF mutations.
- Activation/induction of alternative cellular signaling pathways such as PI3K/Akt.

ABSORPTION

Oral bioavailability is on the order of 80%, and there is no food effect on absorption. Peak plasma drug levels are achieved in 6 hours after ingestion.

DISTRIBUTION

Extensive binding (98%) to plasma proteins. Steady-state drug levels are reached in approximately 14 days.

METABOLISM

Metabolism in the liver primarily by CYP3A4 microsomal enzymes, via oxidation and glutathione conjugation pathways. Formation of the active O-desmethyl dacomitinib metabolite, which involves CYP2D6. Elimination is mainly hepatic (nearly 80%), with excretion in feces. Only 20% of drug eliminated in feces is unchanged parent drug, with the large majority in metabolite forms. Renal elimination of parent drug and its metabolites account for only 3% of an administered dose. The terminal half-life of the parent drug is about 70 hours.

INDICATIONS

FDA-approved for first-line treatment of metastatic NSCLC with EGFR exon 19 deletions or exon 21 L858R substitution mutations as detected by an FDA-approved test.

DOSAGE RANGE

Recommended dose is 45 mg/day PO.

DRUG INTERACTION 1

Proton pump inhibitors—These drugs may reduce the oral bioavailability of dacomitinib, leading to reduced drug levels.

DRUG INTERACTION 2

CYP2D6 substrates—Patients should be warned of the concomitant use of dacomitinib with CYP2D6 substrates as there can be increased concentration of these drugs, which may then lead to increased risk of toxicities.

SPECIAL CONSIDERATIONS

1. Dose reduction is not recommended in patients with mild or moderate hepatic dysfunction. Has not been studied in patients with severe hepatic dysfunction, and caution should be used in this setting.
2. Dose reduction is not recommended in patients with mild or moderate renal dysfunction. Has not been studied in patients with severe renal dysfunction or in those on hemodialysis, and caution should be used in these settings.
3. Monitor patients for new or progressive pulmonary symptoms, including cough, dyspnea, and fever.
4. Patients should be warned about the increased risk of diarrhea. Anti-diarrheal treatment with loperamide should be initiated with new onset diarrhea.
5. If acid reduction is necessary, treatment with antacids and H2-receptor antagonists should be used. Patients should be educated to take dacomitinib at least 6 hours before or 10 hours after the H2-receptor antagonist.
6. May cause fetal harm, and effective contraception should be practiced while on therapy and for at least 17 days after the last dose of drug. Breastfeeding should be avoided.

TOXICITY 1

Skin toxicity with rash, dry skin, pruritus, and nail bed changes.

TOXICITY 2

Diarrhea is most common GI toxicity. Mild nausea/vomiting, mucositis, and constipation are also observed.

TOXICITY 3

Pulmonary toxicity in the form of ILD manifested by increased cough, dyspnea, fever, and pulmonary infiltrates. Observed in only about 3% of patients.

TOXICITY 4

Fatigue, anorexia, and reduced appetite.

Dactinomycin-D

TRADE NAME	Actinomycin-D, Cosmegen	CLASSIFICATION	Antitumor antibiotic
CATEGORY	Chemotherapy drug	DRUG MANUFACTURER	Bedford Laboratories

MECHANISM OF ACTION
- Product of the *Streptomyces* species.
- Consists of a tricyclic phenoxazine chromophore, which is linked to two short, identical cyclic polypeptides.
- Chromophore moiety preferentially binds to guanine-cytidine base pairs. Binding to single- and double-stranded DNA results in inhibition of DNA synthesis and function.
- Formation of oxygen free radicals results in single- and double-stranded DNA breaks and subsequent inhibition of DNA synthesis and function.
- Inhibition of RNA and protein synthesis may also contribute to the cytotoxic effects.

MECHANISM OF RESISTANCE
- Reduced cellular uptake of drug, resulting in decreased intracellular drug accumulation.
- Increased expression of the multidrug-resistant gene with elevated P170 protein levels leads to increased drug efflux and decreased intracellular drug accumulation.

ABSORPTION
Administered only via the IV route.

DISTRIBUTION
After an IV bolus injection, dactinomycin rapidly disappears from the circulation in about 2 minutes. Concentrates in nucleated blood cells. Does not cross the blood-brain barrier. Appears to be highly bound to plasma proteins.

METABOLISM

Clinical pharmacology is not well characterized. Metabolized only to small extent. Most of drug is eliminated in unchanged form by hepatobiliary (50%) and renal (20%) excretion. Terminal elimination half-life ranges from 30 to 40 hours.

INDICATIONS

1. Wilms' tumor.
2. Rhabdomyosarcoma.
3. Germ cell tumors.
4. Gestational trophoblastic disease.
5. Ewing's sarcoma.

DOSAGE RANGE

1. Adults—0.4–0.45 mg/m^2 IV on days 1–5 every 2–3 weeks.
2. Children—0.015 mg/kg/day (up to a maximum dose of 0.5 mg/day) IV on days 1–5 over a period of 16–45 weeks, depending on the specific regimen.

DRUG INTERACTIONS

None well characterized to date.

SPECIAL CONSIDERATIONS

1. Administer drug slowly by IV push to avoid extravasation.
2. Contraindicated in patients actively infected with chickenpox or herpes zoster, as generalized infection may result in death.
3. Use with caution in patients either previously treated with radiation therapy or currently receiving radiation therapy. Increased risk of radiation-recall skin reaction.
4. Patients should be cautioned against sun exposure while on therapy.
5. Pregnancy category C. May be excreted in breast milk. Breastfeeding should be avoided.

TOXICITY 1

Myelosuppression is dose-limiting and can be severe. Neutropenia and thrombocytopenia equally observed. Nadir occurs at days 8–14 after administration.

TOXICITY 2

Nausea and vomiting and onset usually within the first 2 hours of therapy, lasts for up to 24 hours, and in some cases, may be severe.

TOXICITY 3

Mucositis and/or diarrhea. Usually occurs within 5–7 days and can be severe.

TOXICITY 4

Alopecia is common.

TOXICITY 5
Hyperpigmentation of skin, erythema, and increased sensitivity to sunlight. Radiation-recall reaction with erythema and desquamation of skin observed with prior or concurrent radiation therapy.

TOXICITY 6
Potent vesicant. Tissue damage occurs with extravasation of drug.

TOXICITY 7
Elevation of serum transaminases in less than 15% of patients. Dose- and schedule-dependent. Hepatic veno-occlusive disease observed rarely with higher doses and daily schedule.

Daratumumab

TRADE NAME	Darzalex	CLASSIFICATION	Anti-CD38 monoclonal antibody
CATEGORY	Biologic response modifier agent, targeted agent	DRUG MANUFACTURER	Janssen Pharmaceuticals, Johnson & Johnson

MECHANISM OF ACTION
- Daratumumab is an IgG1κ human monoclonal antibody directed against CD38, which is a cell surface glycoprotein that is highly expressed on multiple myeloma cells. CD38 is expressed at low levels on normal lymphoid and myeloid cells.
- Inhibits the growth of CD38-expressing tumor cells by inducing apoptosis directly through Fc-mediated cross-linking as well as by immune-mediated tumor cell lysis through complement-dependent cytotoxicity (CDCC), antibody-dependent cell-mediated cytotoxicity (ADCC), and antibody-dependent cellular phagocytosis.
- Myeloid-derived suppressor cells (MDSCs) and regulatory T cells are sensitive to daratumumab-mediated cell lysis.

MECHANISM OF RESISTANCE
None well characterized to date.

ABSORPTION
Administered via the IV and SC routes.

DISTRIBUTION
Steady-state drug levels are achieved by 5 months with the every-4-week dosing schedule.

METABOLISM
Metabolism has not been well characterized. Mean terminal half-life is approximately 18 days.

INDICATIONS
1. FDA-approved as monotherapy for patients with multiple myeloma who have received at least 3 prior lines of therapy, including a proteasome inhibitor and an immunomodulatory agent, or who are double-refractory to a proteasome inhibitor and an immunomodulatory agent.
2. FDA-approved in combination with pomalidomide and dexamethasone for patients with multiple myeloma who have received at least 2 prior therapies, including lenalidomide and a proteasome inhibitor.
3. FDA-approved in combination with bortezomib and dexamethasone in patients with multiple myeloma who have received at least 1 prior therapy.
4. FDA-approved in combination with bortezomib, melphalan, and prednisone in newly diagnosed patients with multiple myeloma who are ineligible for autologous stem cell transplant (ASCT).
5. FDA-approved in combination with lenalidomide and dexamethasone in newly diagnosed patients with multiple myeloma who are ineligible for ASCT and in patients with relapsed or refractory multiple myeloma who have received at least 1 prior therapy.
6. FDA-approved in combination with bortezomib, thalidomide, and dexamethasone in newly diagnosed patients who are eligible for ASCT.
7. FDA-approved in combination with bortezomib, cyclophosphamide, and dexamethasone in newly diagnosed patients with light chain amyloidosis (AL). Approved under accelerated approval based on response rate.
8. FDA-approved in combination with carfilzomib and dexamethasone in patients with relapsed or refractory multiple myeloma who have received 1–3 prior lines of therapy.

DOSAGE RANGE
Recommended dose is 16 mg/kg on a weekly basis for weeks 1–8, then every 2 weeks for weeks 9–24, and finally every 4 weeks from week 25 onward until disease progression.

DRUG INTERACTION
No known significant interactions have been characterized to date.

SPECIAL CONSIDERATIONS

1. Daratumumab should be administered by IV infusion at the appropriate infusion rate. Consider increasing infusion rate only in the absence of infusion reactions. Please see package insert for specific details on the appropriate infusion rate.

2. Approximately 50% of infusion reactions occur with the first infusion, and nearly all reactions occur during the infusion or within 4 hours of completing the infusion.

3. Premedication with antihistamines (diphenhydramine 25–50 mg PO or IV), antipyretics (acetaminophen 650–1,000 mg), and corticosteroids (methylprednisolone 100 mg or equivalent dose of an intermediate-acting or long-acting steroid) is required to reduce the risk of infusion reactions. Interrupt the infusion for any reaction and manage as appropriate. Administer daratumumab in a clinical facility with immediate access to resuscitative measures (e.g., glucocorticoids, epinephrine, bronchodilators, and/or oxygen).

4. Administer oral corticosteroids (20 mg methylprednisolone) on the first and second days after all infusions to reduce the risk of delayed infusion reactions. For patients with chronic obstructive pulmonary disease, consider short- and long-acting bronchodilators and inhaled corticosteroids.

5. Blood transfusion centers should be informed that a patient has received daratumumab, as this drug can bind to CD38 on red blood cells. This binding may result in a positive indirect antiglobulin test (Coombs test), and this effect may persist for up to 6 months after the last infusion.

6. Patients should be typed and screened for red blood cell transfusions prior to starting daratumumab therapy.

7. Daratumumab may interfere with an accurate assessment of the myeloma response, as the drug may be detected on serum protein electrophoresis and immunofixation assays that are used to monitor for endogenous M-protein levels.

8. No dose adjustments are recommended for patients with renal dysfunction.

9. No dose adjustments are recommended for patients with mild hepatic dysfunction. Has not been studied in the setting of moderate or severe hepatic dysfunction.

10. Monitor CBCs on a periodic basis.

11. Prophylaxis for herpes zoster virus reactivation is recommended.

12. May cause fetal harm. Women of reproductive potential should be advised to use effective contraception during treatment and for 3 months after the last dose. Breast feeding should be avoided while on treatment.

TOXICITY 1

Myelosuppression with neutropenia, thrombocytopenia, and anemia.

TOXICITY 2
Infusion reactions with bronchospasm, cough, wheezing, dyspnea, laryngeal edema, and hypertension.

TOXICITY 3
Nasal congestion and allergic rhinitis.

TOXICITY 4
Fatigue, reduced appetite, and headache.

TOXICITY 5
Arthralgias, musculoskeletal chest pain, and back pain.

TOXICITY 6
Increased risk of infections, including upper respiratory infection, nasopharyngitis, and pneumonia. Reactivation of herpes zoster virus has been reported in 3% of patients.

TOXICITY 7
GI side effects with mild nausea/vomiting, diarrhea, and constipation.

Daratumumab and Hyaluronidase-fihj

TRADE NAME	Darzalex faspro	**CLASSIFICATION**	Anti-CD38 monoclonal antibody
CATEGORY	Biologic response modifier agent, targeted agent	**DRUG MANUFACTURER**	Janssen, Johnson & Johnson

MECHANISM OF ACTION
- Daratumumab is an IgG1κ human monoclonal antibody directed against CD38, which is a cell surface glycoprotein that is highly expressed on multiple myeloma cells. CD38 is expressed at low levels on normal lymphoid and myeloid cells.
- Inhibits the growth of CD38-expressing tumor cells by inducing apoptosis directly through Fc-mediated cross-linking as well as by immune-mediated tumor cell lysis through complement-dependent cytotoxicity (CDCC), antibody-dependent cell-mediated cytotoxicity (ADCC), and antibody-dependent cellular phagocytosis.

- Myeloid-derived suppressor cells (MDSCs) and regulatory T cells are sensitive to daratumumab-mediated cell lysis.
- Hyaluronidase increases the permeability of the subcutaneous tissue by depolymerizing hyaluronan, which is a key polysaccharide present in the extracellular matrix of the subcutaneous tissue.

MECHANISM OF RESISTANCE
None well characterized to date.

ABSORPTION
Administered only via the SC route. Absolute bioavailability is nearly 70%, and peak drug levels are achieved in 3–4 days.

DISTRIBUTION
Estimated mean volume of distribution is 5.2 L.

METABOLISM
Metabolism has not been well characterized. Mean terminal half-life is on the order of 20–28 days.

INDICATIONS
1. FDA-approved as monotherapy for patients with multiple myeloma who have received at least 3 prior lines of therapy, including a proteasome inhibitor and an immunomodulatory agent, or who are double-refractory to a proteasome inhibitor and an immunomodulatory agent.
2. FDA-approved in combination with pomalidomide and dexamethasone for patients with multiple myeloma who have received at least 1 prior therapy, including lenalidomide and a proteasome inhibitor.
3. FDA-approved in combination with bortezomib and dexamethasone in patients with multiple myeloma who have received at least 1 prior therapy.
4. FDA-approved in combination with bortezomib, melphalan, and prednisone in newly diagnosed patients with multiple myeloma who are ineligible for autologous stem cell transplant (ASCT).
5. FDA-approved in combination with lenalidomide and dexamethasone in newly diagnosed patients with multiple myeloma who are ineligible for ASCT and in patients with relapsed or refractory multiple myeloma who have received at least 1 prior therapy.
6. FDA-approved in combination with bortezomib, thalidomide, and dexamethasone in newly diagnosed patients with multiple myeloma who are eligible for ASCT.
7. FDA-approved in combination with bortezomib, cyclophosphamide, and dexamethasone in newly diagnosed patients with light chain amyloidosis. Approved under accelerated approval based on response rate.
8. FDA-approved in combination with carfilzomib and dexamethasone in patients with relapsed or refractory multiple myeloma who have received 1–3 prior lines of therapy.

DOSAGE RANGE

Recommended dose is 1,800 mg daratumumab and 30,000 units of hyaluronidase SC into the abdomen according to the recommended schedule as monotherapy or as part of a combination regimen.

DRUG INTERACTION

No significant interactions have been characterized to date.

SPECIAL CONSIDERATIONS

1. Contraindicated in patients with a history of severe hypersensitivity to daratumumab, hyaluronidase, or any of the components of the formulation.
2. Monitor for hypersensitivity and local injection site reactions.
3. Premedication with antihistamines (diphenhydramine 25–50 mg PO or IV), antipyretics (acetaminophen 650–1,000 mg), and corticosteroids (methylprednisolone 100 mg or equivalent dose of an intermediate-acting or long-acting steroid) is recommended to reduce the risk of hypersensitivity reactions.
4. Monitor CBCs on a periodic basis.
5. Monitor patients with cardiac involvement of light chain amyloidosis on a frequent basis for signs and symptoms of cardiac toxicity.
6. Blood transfusion centers should be informed that a patient has received daratumumab, as this drug can bind to CD38 on red blood cells. This binding may result in a positive indirect antiglobulin test (Coombs test), and this effect may persist for up to 6 months after the last infusion.
7. Patients should be typed and screened for red blood cell transfusions prior to starting daratumumab therapy.
8. Daratumumab may interfere with an accurate assessment of the myeloma response, as the drug may be detected on serum protein electrophoresis and immunofixation assays that are used to monitor for endogenous M-protein levels.
9. No dose adjustments are recommended for patients with renal dysfunction.
10. No dose adjustments are recommended for patients with mild hepatic dysfunction. Has not been studied in the setting of moderate or severe hepatic dysfunction.
11. May cause fetal harm when administered to a pregnant woman. Women of reproductive potential need to use effective contraception while on treatment and for 3 months after the last dose. Breastfeeding should be avoided.

TOXICITY 1

Myelosuppression with neutropenia, thrombocytopenia, and anemia.

TOXICITY 2

Hypersensitivity reactions and local injection site reactions.

TOXICITY 3
Infections with URIs and pneumonia.

TOXICITY 4
Fatigue and anorexia.

TOXICITY 5
GI side effects with mild nausea/vomiting, diarrhea, and constipation.

TOXICITY 6
Arthralgias, musculoskeletal chest pain, and back pain.

Dasatinib

TRADE NAME	Sprycel, BMS-354825	CLASSIFICATION	Signal transduction inhibitor, Bcr-Abl and Src inhibitor
CATEGORY	Targeted agent	DRUG MANUFACTURER	Bristol-Meyers Squibb

MECHANISM OF ACTION
- Potent inhibitor of the Bcr-Abl kinase and Src family of kinases (Src, Lck, Yes, Fyn), c-Kit, and PDGFR-β.
- Differs from imatinib in that it binds to the active and inactive conformations of the Abl kinase domain and overcomes imatinib resistance resulting from Bcr-Abl mutations.

MECHANISM OF RESISTANCE
- Gatekeeper mutation T315I within the ATP-binding pocket of the Abl tyrosine kinase.
- Increased expression/activation of MOS, TPL2, and ERK1/2.
- BCR:ABL1 overexpression due to Ph chromosome duplication, BCR:ABL1 gene amplification, or increased transcription of the BCR:ABL1 gene.

ABSORPTION
Rapidly absorbed following oral administration with good oral bioavailability. Peak plasma concentrations are observed between 30 minutes and 6 hours of oral ingestion.

DISTRIBUTION
Extensive distribution in the extravascular space. Binding of parent drug and its active metabolite to plasma proteins in the range of 90%–95%.

METABOLISM
Metabolized in the liver primarily by CYP3A4 liver microsomal enzymes. Other liver P450 enzymes, such as UGT, play a relatively minor role in metabolism. Approximately 85% of an administered dose is eliminated in feces within 10 days. The terminal half-life of the parent drug is on the order of 4–6 hours.

INDICATIONS
1. FDA-approved for the treatment of adults with chronic phase (CP), accelerated phase (AP), or myeloid blast (MB) or lymphoid blast (LB) phase Ph+ CML with resistance or intolerance to prior therapy including imatinib.
2. FDA-approved for the treatment of adults with Ph+ ALL with resistance or intolerance to prior therapy.
3. FDA-approved in newly diagnosed adult patients with Ph+ chronic phase CML.
4. FDA-approved in pediatric patients 1 year of age and older with Ph+ CML in chronic phase.
5. FDA-approved in combination with chemotherapy in pediatric patients 1 year of age and older with newly diagnosed Ph+ ALL.

DOSAGE RANGE
1. Chronic phase CML, adults: 100 mg PO once daily. A lower dose of 50 mg PO once daily can be used, as it is well tolerated and active.
2. Accelerated phase CML, myeloid or lymphoid blast phase CML, or Ph+ ALL, adults: 140 mg PO once daily.
3. Chronic phase CML, pediatrics: starting dose based on body weight.

DRUG INTERACTION 1
Dasatinib is an inhibitor of CYP3A4 and may decrease the metabolic clearance of drugs that are metabolized by CYP3A4.

DRUG INTERACTION 2
Drugs such as ketoconazole, itraconazole, erythromycin, and clarithromycin decrease the metabolism of dasatinib, resulting in increased drug levels and potentially increased toxicity.

DRUG INTERACTION 3
Drugs such as rifampin, phenytoin, phenobarbital, carbamazepine, and St. John's Wort increase the metabolism of dasatinib, resulting in its inactivation and potentially lower effective drug levels.

DRUG INTERACTION 4
Solubility of dasatinib is pH-dependent. In the presence of famotidine, PPIs, and/or antacids, dasatinib drug concentrations are reduced.

SPECIAL CONSIDERATIONS
1. Oral dasatinib tablets can be taken with or without food but must not be crushed or cut.
2. Important to review patient's list of medications, as dasatinib has several potential drug–drug interactions.
3. Patients should be warned about not taking the herbal medicine St. John's Wort while on dasatinib therapy.
4. Monitor CBC on a weekly basis for the first 2 months and periodically thereafter.
5. Use with caution when patients are on aspirin, NSAIDs, or anticoagulation, as there is an increased risk of bleeding.
6. Monitor electrolyte status, especially calcium and phosphate levels, as oral calcium supplementation may be required.
7. Sexually active patients on dasatinib therapy should use adequate contraception.
8. Avoid Seville oranges, starfruit, pomelos, grapefruit, and grapefruit juice while on dasatinib therapy.
9. Patients should be closely monitored for depressive symptoms and suicide ideation while on therapy.
10. Pregnancy category D. Breastfeeding should be avoided.

TOXICITY 1
Myelosuppression with thrombocytopenia, neutropenia, and anemia.

TOXICITY 2
Bleeding complications in up to 40% of patients resulting from platelet dysfunction.

TOXICITY 3
Fluid retention occurs in 50% of patients, with peripheral edema and pleural effusions. Usually mild to moderate severity.

TOXICITY 4
GI toxicity in the form of diarrhea, nausea/vomiting, and abdominal pain.

TOXICITY 5
Fatigue, asthenia, and anorexia.

TOXICITY 6
Elevations in serum transaminases and/or bilirubin.

TOXICITY 7
Hypocalcemia and hypophosphatemia.

TOXICITY 8
Cardiac toxicity in the form of heart failure and QTc prolongation. Occurs rarely (3%–4%). Pulmonary hypertension can also occur (5%).

TOXICITY 9
Insomnia, depression, and suicidal ideation.

Daunorubicin

TRADE NAME	Daunomycin, Cerubidine, Rubidomycin	CLASSIFICATION	Antitumor antibiotic, anthracycline
CATEGORY	Chemotherapy drug	DRUG MANUFACTURER	Ben Venue, Bedford Laboratories

MECHANISM OF ACTION
- Cell cycle–nonspecific agent.
- Intercalates into DNA, resulting in inhibition of DNA synthesis and function.
- Inhibits transcription through inhibition of DNA-dependent RNA polymerase.
- Inhibits topoisomerase II by forming a cleavable complex with DNA and topoisomerase II to create uncompensated DNA helix torsional tension, leading to eventual DNA breaks.
- Formation of cytotoxic oxygen free radicals results in single- and double-stranded DNA breaks, with inhibition of DNA synthesis and function.

MECHANISM OF RESISTANCE
- Increased expression of the multidrug-resistant gene with elevated P170 levels, which leads to increased drug efflux and decreased intracellular drug accumulation.
- Decreased expression of topoisomerase II.

- Mutation in topoisomerase II, with decreased binding affinity to drug.
- Increased expression of sulfhydryl proteins, including glutathione and glutathione-dependent enzymes.

ABSORPTION
Administered only via the IV route.

DISTRIBUTION
Significantly more lipid soluble than doxorubicin. Widely distributed to tissues, with high concentrations in heart, liver, lungs, kidneys, and spleen. Does not cross the blood-brain barrier. Moderate binding to plasma proteins (60%–70%).

METABOLISM
Metabolism in the liver, with formation of one of its primary metabolites, daunorubicinol, which has antitumor activity. Parent compound and its metabolites are excreted mainly through the hepatobiliary system into feces. Renal clearance accounts for only 10%–20% of drug elimination. The half-life of the parent drug is 20 hours, while the half-life of the daunorubicinol metabolite is 30–40 hours.

INDICATIONS
1. Acute myelogenous leukemia—Remission induction and relapse.
2. Acute lymphoblastic leukemia—Remission induction and relapse.

DOSAGE RANGE
1. AML—45 mg/m^2 IV on days 1–3 of the first course of induction therapy and on days 1 and 2 on subsequent courses. Used in combination with continuous infusion ara-C.
2. ALL—45 mg/m^2 IV on days 1–3 in combination with vincristine, prednisone, and L-asparaginase.
3. Single agent—40 mg/m^2 IV every 2 weeks.

DRUG INTERACTION 1
Dexamethasone, heparin—Daunorubicin is incompatible with dexamethasone and heparin, as a precipitate will form.

DRUG INTERACTION 2
Dexrazoxane—Cardiotoxic effects of daunorubicin are inhibited by the iron chelating agent dexrazoxane (ICRF-187, Zinecard).

SPECIAL CONSIDERATIONS
1. Use with caution in patients with abnormal liver function. Dose reduction is recommended in the setting of liver dysfunction.
2. Because daunorubicin is a vesicant, administer slowly over 60 minutes with a rapidly flowing IV. Careful administration of the drug, usually through a central venous catheter, is necessary as the drug is a potent vesicant. Close monitoring is necessary to avoid extravasation.

If extravasation is suspected, immediately stop infusion, withdraw fluid, elevate extremity, and apply ice to involved site. In severe cases, consult a plastic surgeon.

3. Monitor cardiac function before (baseline) and periodically during therapy with either multigated acquisition (MUGA) radionuclide scan or echocardiogram to assess left ventricular ejection fraction (LVEF). Risk of cardiac toxicity is higher in patients >70 years of age, in patients with prior history of hypertension or pre-existing heart disease, and in patients previously treated with anthracyclines or prior radiation therapy to the chest. Cumulative doses of >550 mg/m^2 are associated with increased risk for cardiac toxicity.

4. Use with caution in patients previously treated with radiation therapy, as daunorubicin can cause a radiation-recall skin reaction.

5. Patients should be cautioned to avoid sun exposure and to wear sun protection when outside.

6. Patients should be warned about the potential for red-orange discoloration of urine that may occur for 1–2 days after drug administration.

7. Pregnancy category D. Breastfeeding should be avoided.

TOXICITY 1

Myelosuppression is dose-limiting, with neutropenia being more common than thrombocytopenia. Nadir occurs at 10–14 days, with recovery by day 21.

TOXICITY 2

Nausea and vomiting. Usually mild, occurring in 50% of patients within 1–2 hours of treatment.

TOXICITY 3

Mucositis and diarrhea are common within the first week of treatment but not dose-limiting.

TOXICITY 4

Cardiac toxicity. Acute form presents within the first 2–3 days as arrhythmias and/or conduction abnormalities, ECG changes, pericarditis, and/or myocarditis. Usually transient and mostly asymptomatic.

Chronic form associated with a dose-dependent, dilated cardiomyopathy and congestive heart failure. Incidence increases with cumulative doses >550 mg/m^2.

TOXICITY 5

Potent vesicant. Extravasation can lead to tissue necrosis and chemical thrombophlebitis at the injection site.

TOXICITY 6

Hyperpigmentation of nails, rarely skin rash, and urticaria. Radiation-recall skin reaction can occur at prior sites of irradiation. Increased hypersensitivity to sunlight.

TOXICITY 7

Alopecia is universal. Usually reversible within 5–7 weeks after termination of treatment.

TOXICITY 8

Red-orange discoloration of urine. Lasts 1–2 days after drug administration.

Daunorubicin Liposome

TRADE NAME	DaunoXome	**CLASSIFICATION**	Antitumor antibiotic, anthracycline
CATEGORY	Chemotherapy drug	**DRUG MANUFACTURER**	Diatos

MECHANISM OF ACTION

- Liposomal encapsulation of daunorubicin.
- Protected from chemical and enzymatic degradation; displays reduced plasma protein binding; and shows decreased uptake in normal tissues when compared to parent compound, daunorubicin.
- Penetrates tumor tissue into which daunorubicin is released, possibly through increased permeability of tumor neovasculature to liposome particles.
- Cell cycle–nonspecific agent.
- Intercalates into DNA, resulting in inhibition of DNA synthesis and function.
- Inhibits transcription through inhibition of DNA-dependent RNA polymerase.
- Inhibits topoisomerase II by forming a cleavable complex with DNA and topoisomerase II to create uncompensated DNA helix torsional tension, leading to eventual DNA breaks.
- Formation of oxygen free radicals results in single- and double-stranded DNA breaks, with subsequent inhibition of DNA synthesis and function.

MECHANISM OF RESISTANCE

- Increased expression of the multidrug-resistant gene with elevated P170 levels. This leads to increased drug efflux and decreased intracellular drug accumulation.
- Decreased expression of topoisomerase II.
- Mutation in topoisomerase II, with decreased binding affinity to drug.
- Increased expression of sulfhydryl proteins, including glutathione and glutathione-dependent enzymes.

ABSORPTION
Administered only via the IV route.

DISTRIBUTION
Small, steady-state volume of distribution (6 L) in contrast to the parent drug, daunorubicin. Distribution is limited mainly to the intravascular compartment. Does not cross the blood-brain barrier. Minimal binding to plasma proteins.

METABOLISM
Metabolism in the liver, but the primary metabolite, daunorubicinol, is present only in low concentrations. Cleared from plasma at 17 mL/min in contrast to daunorubicin, which is cleared at 240 mL/min. Elimination half-life is about 4–5 hours, far shorter than that of daunorubicin.

INDICATIONS
HIV-associated, advanced Kaposi's sarcoma—First-line therapy.

DOSAGE RANGE
Recommended dose is 40 mg/m^2 IV every 2 weeks.

DRUG INTERACTIONS
None well characterized to date.

SPECIAL CONSIDERATIONS
1. Use with caution in patients with abnormal liver function. Dose reduction is required in the setting of liver dysfunction.
2. Because the parent drug, daunorubicin, is a vesicant, administer slowly over 60 minutes with a rapidly flowing IV. Careful monitoring is necessary to avoid extravasation. If extravasation is suspected, immediately stop infusion, withdraw fluid, elevate extremity, and apply ice to involved site. May administer local steroids. In severe cases, consult a plastic surgeon.
3. Monitor cardiac function before (baseline) and periodically during therapy with either MUGA radionuclide scan or echocardiogram to assess LVEF. Risk of cardiac toxicity is higher in patients >70 years of age, in patients with prior history of hypertension or pre-existing heart disease, and in patients previously treated with anthracyclines or prior radiation therapy to the chest. Cumulative doses of >320 mg/m^2 are associated with increased risk for cardiac toxicity.
4. Patients may develop back pain, flushing, and chest tightness during the first 5 minutes of infusion. These symptoms are probably related to the liposomal component of the drug. Infusion should be discontinued until symptoms resolve and then resumed at a slower rate.
5. Pregnancy category D. Breastfeeding should be avoided.

TOXICITY 1
Myelosuppression is dose-limiting with neutropenia being moderate to severe.

TOXICITY 2
Nausea and vomiting occur in 50% of patients and usually mild.

TOXICITY 3
Mucositis and diarrhea are common but not dose-limiting.

TOXICITY 4
Cardiac toxicity. Acute form presents within the first 2–3 days as arrhythmias and/or conduction abnormalities, ECG changes, pericarditis, and/or myocarditis. Usually transient and mostly asymptomatic.

Chronic form associated with a dose-dependent, dilated cardiomyopathy associated with congestive heart failure. Incidence increases when cumulative doses are >320 mg/m^2.

TOXICITY 5
Infusion-related reaction. Occurs within the first 5 minutes of infusion and manifested by back pain, flushing, and tightness in chest and throat. Observed in about 15% of patients and usually with the first infusion. Improves upon termination of infusion and typically does not recur upon reinstitution at a slower infusion rate.

TOXICITY 6
Potent vesicant. Extravasation can lead to tissue necrosis and chemical thrombophlebitis at the site of injection.

TOXICITY 7
Hyperpigmentation of nails, rarely skin rash, and urticaria. Radiation-recall skin reaction can occur at prior sites of irradiation. Increased hypersensitivity to sunlight.

TOXICITY 8
Alopecia. Lower incidence than its parent compound, daunorubicin.

Daunorubicin and Cytarabine Liposome

TRADE NAME	Vyxeos, CPX-351	CLASSIFICATION	Anthracycline and antimetabolite
CATEGORY	Chemotherapy drug	DRUG MANUFACTURER	Jazz Pharmaceuticals

MECHANISM OF ACTION

- Daunorubicin and cytarabine liposome is a combination of daunorubicin and cytarabine in a fixed 1:5 molar ratio encapsulated for IV administration. The 1:5 molar ratio has been shown in pre-clinical studies to provide maximal cell kill of leukemic cells.
- Daunorubicin is not cell cycle-specific and works in all phases of the cell cycle.
- Daunorubicin directly intercalates into DNA, resulting in inhibition of DNA synthesis and function.
- Daunorubicin inhibits transcription through inhibition of DNA-dependent RNA polymerase.
- Daunorubicin inhibits topoisomerase II by forming a cleavable complex with DNA and topoisomerase II to create uncompensated DNA helix torsional tension, leading to eventual DNA breaks.
- Daunorubicin can form iron-dependent cytotoxic oxygen free radicals, resulting in single- and double-stranded DNA breaks, with inhibition of DNA synthesis and function.
- Cytarabine is a cell cycle–specific agent with activity in the S-phase.
- Cytarabine is a nucleoside analog that requires intracellular activation to the nucleotide metabolite ara-cytidine triphosphate (ara-CTP). Antitumor activity of cytarabine is determined by a balance between intracellular activation and degradation and the subsequent formation of cytotoxic ara-CTP metabolites.

- Incorporation of ara-CTP into DNA, resulting in chain termination and inhibition of DNA synthesis and function.
- Ara-CTP inhibits several DNA polymerases α, β, and γ, which then interfere with DNA synthesis, DNA repair, and DNA chain elongation.
- Ara-CTP inhibits ribonucleotide reductase, resulting in decreased levels of essential deoxyribonucleotides required for DNA synthesis and function.

MECHANISM OF RESISTANCE
Daunorubicin
- Increased expression of the multidrug-resistant gene with elevated P170 levels, which leads to increased drug efflux of daunorubicin and decreased intracellular drug accumulation.
- Decreased expression of topoisomerase II.
- Mutation in topoisomerase II, with decreased binding affinity to drug.
- Increased expression of sulfhydryl proteins, including glutathione and glutathione-dependent enzymes.

Cytarabine
- Decreased activation of drug through decreased expression of the anabolic enzyme deoxycytidine kinase.
- Increased breakdown of drug by the catabolic enzymes cytidine deaminase and deoxycytidylate (dCMP) deaminase.
- Decreased nucleoside transport of drug into cells.
- Increased expression of CTP synthetase activity, resulting in increased concentrations of competing physiologic nucleotide substrate dCTP.

ABSORPTION
Administered only via the IV route.

DISTRIBUTION
Binding to plasma proteins has not been evaluated.

METABOLISM
Daunorubicin is metabolized in the liver, with formation of one of its primary metabolites, daunorubicinol, which has antitumor activity. Parent daunorubicin and its metabolites are excreted mainly through the hepatobiliary system into feces. Renal clearance of daunorubicin accounts for only 9% of drug elimination. The half-life of daunorubicin in the liposome form is 31.5 hours.

Cytarabine undergoes extensive metabolism, with approximately 70% of the drug being recovered in the urine as the uracil arabinoside (ara-U) metabolite. Deamination occurs in liver, plasma, and peripheral tissues. The principal enzyme involved in drug catabolism is cytidine deaminase, which converts ara-C into the inactive metabolite ara-U. dCMP deaminase converts ara-CMP into ara-uridine monophosphate (ara-UMP), and this represents an additional catabolic pathway of the drug. The half-life of cytarabine in the liposome form is 40.4 hours.

INDICATIONS
FDA-approved for newly diagnosed therapy-related AML (t-AML) or AML with myelodysplasia-related changes (AML-MRC).

DOSAGE RANGE
1. Induction: Administer liposome (daunorubicin 44 mg/m^2 and cytarabine 100 mg/m^2) IV on days 1, 3, and 5 for cycle 1, and on days 1 and 3 for subsequent cycles if needed.
2. Consolidation: Administer liposome (daunorubicin 29 mg/m^2 and cytarabine 65 mg/m^2) IV on days 1 and 3.

DRUG INTERACTION 1
Cardiotoxic agents—Concomitant use with other cardiotoxic agents may increase the risk of cardiac toxicity.

DRUG INTERACTION 2
Hepatotoxic agents—Concomitant use with other hepatotoxic agents may increase the risk of hepatotoxicity.

SPECIAL CONSIDERATIONS
1. Dose reduction is not required in patients with serum bilirubin levels <3 mg/dL. Has not been studied in patients with serum bilirubin levels >3 mg/dL, and caution should be used in this setting.
2. Dose reduction is not required for patients with mild or moderate renal dysfunction. Has not been studied in patients with severe renal dysfunction or end-stage renal disease, and caution should be used in these settings.
3. Should be administered via an infusion pump through a central venous catheter.
4. Monitor patients for infusion reactions. In the presence of mild or moderate infusion reactions, the rate of infusion should be interrupted or slowed, and symptoms should be treated appropriately. If severe or life-threatening reactions occur, the drug should be discontinued permanently, the symptoms should be treated, and the patient closely monitored until all symptoms resolve.
5. Monitor CBCs on a regular basis while on therapy.
6. Monitor cardiac function before (baseline) and periodically during therapy with either multigated acquisition (MUGA) radionuclide scan or echocardiogram to assess left ventricular ejection fraction (LVEF). Risk of cardiac toxicity is higher in patients >70 years of age, in patients with prior history of hypertension or pre-existing heart disease, and in patients

previously treated with anthracyclines or prior radiation therapy to the chest. Cumulative doses of >550 mg/m^2 are associated with increased risk for cardiac toxicity.
7. Use with caution in patients previously treated with radiation therapy, as daunorubicin can cause a radiation-recall skin reaction.
8. Patients should be cautioned to avoid sun exposure and to wear sun protection when outside.
9. Monitor patients for signs and symptoms of acute copper toxicity.
10. The drug can cause fetal harm when administered to a pregnant woman. Breastfeeding should be avoided.

TOXICITY 1
Myelosuppression is dose-limiting with neutropenia and thrombocytopenia.

TOXICITY 2
Mild nausea and vomiting, mucositis, and diarrhea.

TOXICITY 3
Infusion-related hypersensitivity reactions.

TOXICITY 4
Cardiac toxicity. Acute form presents within the first 2–3 days as arrhythmias and/or conduction abnormalities, ECG changes, pericarditis, and/or myocarditis. Usually transient and mostly asymptomatic.

Chronic form associated with a dose-dependent, dilated cardiomyopathy and congestive heart failure. Incidence increases with cumulative doses >550 mg/m^2.

TOXICITY 5
Strong vesicant. Extravasation can lead to tissue necrosis and chemical thrombophlebitis at the injection site.

TOXICITY 6
Hemorrhagic events with epistaxis most common. Serious bleeding events, including CNS hemorrhages, have been reported rarely.

TOXICITY 7
Maculopapular skin rash and pruritus.

Decitabine

Decitabine

TRADE NAME	5-Aza-2'-deoxycytidine, Dacogen	**CLASSIFICATION**	Antimetabolite, deoxycytidine analog
CATEGORY	Chemotherapy drug, hypomethylating agent	**DRUG MANUFACTURER**	Eisai

MECHANISM OF ACTION
- Deoxycytidine analog.
- Cell cycle–specific with activity in the S-phase.
- Requires activation to the nucleotide metabolite decitabine triphosphate.
- Incorporation of decitabine triphosphate into DNA results in inhibition of DNA methyltransferases, which then leads to loss of DNA methylation. Aberrantly silenced genes, such as tumor suppressor genes, are then reactivated and expressed.

MECHANISM OF RESISTANCE
None well characterized to date.

ABSORPTION
Administered only via the IV route.

DISTRIBUTION
Distribution in humans has not been fully characterized. Drug crosses blood-brain barrier. Plasma protein binding of decitabine is negligible.

METABOLISM
Precise route of elimination and metabolic fate of decitabine is not known in humans. One of the elimination pathways is via deamination by cytidine deaminase, found principally in the liver but also in plasma, granulocytes, intestinal epithelium, and peripheral tissues.

INDICATIONS

FDA-approved for treatment of patients with myelodysplastic syndromes (MDS), including previously treated and untreated, de novo, and secondary MDS of all French-American-British subtypes (refractory anemia, refractory anemia with ringed sideroblasts, refractory anemia with excess blasts, refractory anemia with excess blasts in transformation, and chronic myelomonocytic leukemia), and intermediate-1, intermediate-2, and high-risk International Prognostic Scoring System groups.

DOSAGE RANGE

1. Recommended dose is 15 mg/m^2 continuous infusion IV over 3 hours repeated every 8 hours for 3 days. Cycles should be repeated every 6 weeks.
2. An alternative schedule is 20 mg/m^2 IV over 1 hour daily for 5 days given every 28 days.

DRUG INTERACTIONS

None well characterized to date.

SPECIAL CONSIDERATIONS

1. Patients should be treated for a minimum of 4 cycles. In some cases, a complete or partial response may take longer than 4 cycles.
2. Monitor CBCs on a regular basis during therapy. See prescribing information for recommendations regarding dose adjustments.
3. Decitabine therapy should not be resumed if serum creatinine $\geq$2 mg/dL, SGPT and/or total bilirubin 2 $\times$ ULN, and in the presence of active or uncontrolled infection.
4. Use with caution in patients with underlying liver and/or kidney dysfunction.
5. Pregnancy category D. Breastfeeding should be avoided.

TOXICITY 1

Myelosuppression with pancytopenia is dose-limiting.

TOXICITY 2

Fatigue and anorexia.

TOXICITY 3

GI toxicity with nausea/vomiting, constipation, and abdominal pain.

TOXICITY 4

Hyperbilirubinemia.

TOXICITY 5

Peripheral edema.

Decitabine-Cedazuridine

Decitabine

Cedazuridine

TRADE NAME	Inqovi	CLASSIFICATION	Antimetabolite
CATEGORY	Chemotherapy drug, hypomethylating agent	DRUG MANUFACTURER	Taiho

MECHANISM OF ACTION
- Decitabine is a deoxycytidine analog, while cedazuridine is a uridine nucleoside inhibitor of cytidine deaminase. Concomitant administration of cedazuridine with decitabine inhibits the degradation of decitabine, allowing for increased systemic decitabine exposure.
- Cell cycle–specific with activity in the S-phase.
- Decitabine is transported inside the cell via a nucleoside transport protein and then activated intracellularly eventually to the nucleotide metabolite decitabine triphosphate.
- Incorporation of decitabine triphosphate into DNA results in inhibition of DNA methyltransferases, which then leads to loss of DNA methylation. Aberrantly silenced genes, such as tumor suppressor genes, are then reactivated and expressed.

MECHANISM OF RESISTANCE
None well characterized to date.

ABSORPTION
Oral bioavailability of cedazuridine is modest at 20%. The presence of cedazuridine results in increased oral bioavailablity of decitabine. The median time to decitabine C_{max} is 1 hour after ingestion, while the median time to cedazuridine C_{max} is 3 hours after ingestion. Food does not appear to affect oral absorption.

DISTRIBUTION
Distribution in humans has not been fully characterized. The drug crosses the blood-brain barrier. Plasma protein binding of decitabine is negligible.

METABOLISM
One of the elimination pathways of decitabine is via deamination by cytidine deaminase, found principally in the liver but also in plasma, granulocytes, intestinal epithelium, and peripheral tissues.

INDICATIONS
FDA-approved for treatment of patients with MDS, including previously treated and untreated, de novo, and secondary MDS of all French-American-British subtypes (refractory anemia, refractory anemia with ringed sideroblasts, refractory anemia with excess blasts, refractory anemia with excess blasts in transformation, and chronic myelomonocytic leukemia), and intermediate-1, intermediate-2, and high-risk International Prognostic Scoring System groups.

DOSAGE RANGE
Recommended dose is 1 tablet (35 mg decitabine and 100 mg cedazuridine) PO once daily on days 1–5 of a 28-day cycle.

DRUG INTERACTION
Concomitant administration of decitabine/cedazuridine with drugs that are metabolized by cytidine deaminase may result in increased systemic exposure with the potential for increased toxicity.

SPECIAL CONSIDERATIONS
1. Decitabine/cedazuridine should **NOT** be substituted for IV decitabine within a given cycle.
2. Patients should be treated for a minimum of 4 cycles. In some cases, a complete or partial response may take longer than 4 cycles.
3. Monitor CBC on a regular basis during therapy. See prescribing information for specific recommendations regarding dose adjustments.
4. Decitabine/cedazuridine therapy should not be resumed if serum creatinine ≥2 mg/dL, SGPT and/or total bilirubin 2 × ULN, and in the presence of active or uncontrolled infection.
5. Dose reduction is not recommended in patients with mild hepatic impairment. The decitabine/cedazuridine combination has not been studied in patients with moderate or severe hepatic impairment.
6. Dose reduction is not recommended in patients with mild or moderate renal impairment. The decitabine/cedazuridine combination has not been studied in patients with severe renal impairment or in those with end-stage renal disease.
7. Can cause fetal harm when given to a pregnant woman. Females of reproductive potential should use effective contraception during treatment and for at least 6 months after the last dose. Breastfeeding should be avoided.
8. Male patients should be educated about the possibility of impairment of male fertility, the reversibility of which is unknown.

TOXICITY 1
Myelosuppression with pancytopenia is dose-limiting.

TOXICITY 2
Fatigue and anorexia.

TOXICITY 3
GI toxicity in the form of nausea/vomiting, constipation, and abdominal pain.

TOXICITY 4
Hepatotoxicity with elevations in SGOT/SGPT, alkaline phosphatase, and serum bilirubin.

TOXICITY 5
Peripheral edema.

Degarelix

TRADE NAME	Firmagon	CLASSIFICATION	GnRH antagonist
CATEGORY	Hormonal agent	DRUG MANUFACTURER	Ferring

MECHANISM OF ACTION
Binds immediately and reversibly to GnRH receptors of the pituitary gland, which leads to inhibition of luteinizing hormone (LH) and follicle-stimulating hormone (FSH) production. Causes a rapid and sustained suppression of testosterone without the initial surge that is observed with LHRH agonist therapy.

ABSORPTION

Not orally absorbed because of extensive proteolysis in the hepatobiliary system. Forms a depot upon subcutaneous administration from which degarelix is released into the circulation.

DISTRIBUTION

Approximately 90% of degarelix is bound to plasma proteins. Distribution throughout total body water.

METABOLISM

Metabolism occurs mainly via hydrolysis, with excretion of peptide fragments in feces. Approximately 70%–80% is eliminated in feces, while the remaining 20%–30% is eliminated in urine. The elimination half-life is approximately 53 days.

INDICATIONS

Advanced prostate cancer.

DOSAGE RANGE

Administer 240 mg SC as a starting dose and then 80 mg SC every 28 days.

DRUG INTERACTIONS

None well characterized to date.

SPECIAL CONSIDERATIONS

1. Initiation of treatment with degarelix does not induce a transient tumor flare in contrast to LHRH agonists, such as goserelin and leuprolide.
2. Serum testosterone levels decrease to castrate levels within 3 days of initiation of therapy.
3. Use with caution in patients with congenital long QT syndrome, electrolyte abnormalities, and CHF, and in patients on antiarrhythmic medications, such as quinidine, procainamide, amiodarone, or sotalol, as long-term androgen deprivation therapy prolongs the QT interval.
4. Pregnancy category X. Breastfeeding should be avoided.

TOXICITY 1

Hot flashes with decreased libido and impotence.

TOXICITY 2

Local discomfort at the site of injection with erythema, swelling, and/or induration.

TOXICITY 3

Weight gain.

D

TOXICITY 4
Mild elevations in serum transaminases.

TOXICITY 5
Fatigue.

Denileukin diftitox

TRADE NAME	Ontak, DAB389	**CLASSIFICATION**	Cytokine, diptheria toxin
CATEGORY	Biologic response modifier agent, immunotherapy	**DRUG MANUFACTURER**	Eisai

MECHANISM OF ACTION
- Recombinant fusion protein composed of amino acid sequences of human interleukin-2 (IL-2) and the enzymatic and translocation domains of diphtheria toxin.
- Specifically binds to the CD25 component of the IL-2 receptor and then internalized via endocytosis.
- Upon release of diphtheria toxin into cytosol, cellular protein synthesis is inhibited, and cell death via apoptosis occurs.

ABSORPTION
Administered only via the IV route.

DISTRIBUTION
Volume of distribution is similar to that of circulating blood, and the initial distribution half-life is approximately 2–5 minutes.

METABOLISM
Metabolized primarily via catabolism by proteolytic degradation pathways. The elimination half-life is 70–80 minutes.

INDICATIONS
Persistent or recurrent cutaneous T-cell lymphoma in which the malignant cells express the CD25 component of the IL-2 receptor.

DOSAGE RANGE
Recommended dose is 9 or 18 mg/kg/day IV on days 1–5 every 21 days.

DRUG INTERACTIONS
None well characterized to date.

SPECIAL CONSIDERATIONS
1. Expression of CD25 on tumor skin biopsy must be confirmed before administration of denileukin diftitox. A testing service is available and can be reached by calling 1-800-964-5836.
2. Contraindicated in patients with a known hypersensitivity to denileukin diftitox or any of its components, including IL-2 and diphtheria toxin.
3. Use with caution in patients with pre-existing cardiac and pulmonary disease, as they are at increased risk for developing serious and sometimes fatal reactions.
4. Resuscitative equipment and medications, including IV antihistamines, corticosteroids, and epinephrine, should be readily available at bedside prior to treatment.
5. Monitor serum albumin at baseline and during therapy. Low serum albumin levels place patient at increased risk for vascular leak syndrome. Delay administration of denileukin until the serum albumin is 3 g/dL.
6. Patients should be monitored closely throughout the entire treatment, including vital signs, pre- and post-infusion weights, and evidence of peripheral edema.
7. Premedication with acetaminophen, NSAIDs, and antihistamines can help to reduce the incidence and severity of hypersensitivity reactions.
8. Pregnancy category C. Breastfeeding should be avoided.

TOXICITY 1
Flu-like symptoms with fever, chills, asthenia, myalgias, arthralgias, and headache. Usually mild, transient, and easily manageable.

TOXICITY 2
Hypersensitivity reaction manifested by hypotension, back pain, dyspnea, skin rash, chest pain or tightness, tachycardia, dysphagia, and rarely anaphylaxis. Observed in nearly 70% of patients during or within the first 24 hours of drug infusion.

TOXICITY 3
Vascular leak syndrome characterized by hypotension, edema, and/or hypoalbuminemia. Usually self-limited process. Pre-existing low serum albumin (<3 g/dL) predisposes patients to this syndrome.

TOXICITY 4
Diarrhea may be delayed with prolonged duration. Anorexia along with nausea and vomiting also observed.

TOXICITY 5

Myelosuppression is uncommon, with anemia occurring more frequently than neutropenia.

TOXICITY 6

Hepatotoxicity with elevations in serum transaminases and hypoalbuminemia (albumin <2.3 g/dL) in 15%–20% of patients. Usually occurs during the first course and resolves within 2 weeks of stopping therapy.

Docetaxel

TRADE NAME	Taxotere	CLASSIFICATION	Taxane, antimicrotubule agent
CATEGORY	Chemotherapy drug	DRUG MANUFACTURER	Sanofi-Aventis

MECHANISM OF ACTION

- Semisynthetic taxane. Derived from the needles of the European yew tree.
- High-affinity binding to microtubules enhances tubulin polymerization. Normal dynamic process of microtubule network is inhibited, leading to inhibition of mitosis and cell division.
- Cell cycle–specific agent with activity in the mitotic (M) phase.

MECHANISM OF RESISTANCE

- Alterations in tubulin, with decreased affinity for drug.
- Multidrug-resistant (MDR-1) phenotype with increased expression of P170 glycoprotein. Results in enhanced drug efflux with decreased intracellular accumulation of drug. Cross-resistant to other natural products, including vinca alkaloids, anthracyclines, taxanes, and etoposide.

ABSORPTION
Administered only via the IV route.

DISTRIBUTION
Distributes widely to all body tissues. Extensive binding (>90%) to plasma and cellular proteins.

METABOLISM
Extensively metabolized by the hepatic P450 microsomal system. About 75% of drug is excreted via fecal elimination. Less than 10% is eliminated as the parent compound, with the majority being eliminated as metabolites. Renal clearance is relatively minor, with less than 10% of drug clearance via the kidneys. Plasma elimination is tri-exponential with a terminal half-life of 11 hours.

INDICATIONS
1. Breast cancer—FDA-approved for the treatment of locally advanced or metastatic breast cancer after failure of prior chemotherapy.
2. Breast cancer—FDA-approved in combination with doxorubicin and cyclophosphamide for adjuvant treatment of patients with node-positive breast cancer.
3. NSCLC—FDA-approved for locally advanced or metastatic disease after failure of prior platinum-based chemotherapy.
4. NSCLC—FDA-approved in combination with cisplatin for treatment of patients with locally advanced or metastatic disease who have not previously received chemotherapy.
5. Prostate cancer—FDA-approved in combination with prednisone for androgen-independent (hormone-refractory) metastatic prostate cancer.
6. Gastric cancer—FDA-approved in combination with cisplatin and 5-fluorouracil (5-FU) for advanced gastric cancer, including adenocarcinoma of the gastroesophageal junction, in patients who have not received prior chemotherapy.
7. Head and neck cancer—FDA-approved for use in combination with cisplatin and 5-FU for induction treatment of patients with inoperable, locally advanced disease.
8. SCLC.
9. Refractory ovarian cancer.
10. Bladder cancer.

DOSAGE RANGE
1. Metastatic breast cancer—60, 75, and 100 mg/m^2 IV every 3 weeks or 35–40 mg/m^2 IV weekly for 3 weeks with 1-week rest.
2. Breast cancer—75 mg/m^2 IV every 3 weeks in combination with cyclophosphamide and doxorubicin for adjuvant therapy.
3. NSCLC—75 mg/m^2 IV every 3 weeks or 35–40 mg/m^2 IV weekly for 3 weeks with 1-week rest after platinum-based chemotherapy.
4. NSCLC—75 mg/m^2 IV every 3 weeks in combination with cisplatin in patients who have not received prior chemotherapy.

5. Metastatic prostate cancer—75 mg/m^2 IV every 3 weeks in combination with prednisone.
6. Advanced gastric cancer—75 mg/m^2 IV every 3 weeks in combination with cisplatin and 5-FU.
7. Head and neck cancer—75 mg/m^2 IV every 3 weeks in combination with cisplatin and 5-FU for induction therapy of locally advanced disease.

DRUG INTERACTION 1
Radiation therapy—Docetaxel acts as a radiosensitizing agent.

DRUG INTERACTION 2
Inhibitors and/or activators of the liver cytochrome P450 CYP3A4 enzyme system—Concurrent use with drugs such as cyclosporine, ketoconazole, and erythromycin may affect docetaxel metabolism and its subsequent antitumor and toxic effects.

SPECIAL CONSIDERATIONS
1. Use with caution in patients with abnormal liver function. Patients with abnormal liver function are at higher risk for toxicity, including treatment-related mortality.
2. Monitor CBCs on a periodic basis. Docetaxel therapy should not be given to patients with neutrophil counts of <1,500 cells/mm^3.
3. Patients should receive steroid premedication to reduce the incidence and severity of fluid retention and hypersensitivity reactions. Give dexamethasone 8 mg PO bid for 3 days beginning 1 day before drug administration.
4. Monitor patients for allergic and/or hypersensitivity reactions, which are related to the polysorbate 80 vehicle in which the drug is formulated. Usually occur with the first and second treatments. Emergency equipment, including Ambu bag, ECG machine, fluids, pressors, and other drugs for resuscitation, must be at bedside before initiation of treatment.
5. Contraindicated in patients with known hypersensitivity reactions to docetaxel and/or polysorbate 80.
6. Use only glass, polypropylene bottles, or polypropylene or polyolefin plastic bags for drug infusion. Administer only through polyethylene-lined administration sets.
7. Monitor patient's weight, measure daily input and output, and evaluate for peripheral edema.
8. Pregnancy category D. Breastfeeding should be avoided.

TOXICITY 1
Myelosuppression with neutropenia is dose-limiting. Nadir is usually observed at days 7–10, with recovery by day 14. Thrombocytopenia and anemia are also observed.

TOXICITY 2

Hypersensitivity reactions with generalized skin rash, erythema, hypotension, dyspnea, and/or bronchospasm. Usually occur within the first 2–3 minutes of an infusion and almost always within the first 10 minutes. Most frequently observed with first or second treatments. Usually prevented by premedication with steroid; overall incidence decreased to less than 3%. When it occurs during drug infusion, treat with hydrocortisone IV, diphenhydramine 50 mg IV, and/or cimetidine 300 mg IV.

TOXICITY 3

Fluid retention syndrome. Presents as weight gain, peripheral and/or generalized edema, pleural effusion, and ascites. Incidence increases with total doses >400 mg/m^2. Occurs in about 50% of patients.

TOXICITY 4

Maculopapular skin rash and dry, itchy skin. Most commonly affects forearms and hands. Brown discoloration of fingernails may occur. Observed in up to 50% of patients usually within 1 week after therapy.

TOXICITY 5

Alopecia occurs in up to 80% of patients.

TOXICITY 6

Mucositis and/or diarrhea seen in 40% of patients. Mild to moderate nausea and vomiting, usually of brief duration.

TOXICITY 7

Peripheral neuropathy is less commonly observed with docetaxel than with paclitaxel.

TOXICITY 8

Generalized fatigue and asthenia are common, occurring in 60%–70% of patients. Arthralgias and myalgias also observed.

TOXICITY 9

Reversible elevations in serum transaminases, alkaline phosphatase, and bilirubin.

TOXICITY 10

Phlebitis and/or swelling at the injection site.

Dostarlimab-gxly

TRADE NAME	Jemperli, MK-3475	**CLASSIFICATION**	Anti-PD-1 mononclonal antibody
CATEGORY	Immunotherapy, immune checkpoint inhibitor	**DRUG MANUFACTURER**	GlaxoSmithKline

MECHANISM OF ACTION
- Humanized IgG4 antibody that binds to the PD-1 receptor, which is expressed on T cells, and inhibits the interaction between the PD-L1 and PD-L2 ligands and the PD-1 receptor.
- Blockade of the PD-1 pathway-mediated immune checkpoint enhances T-cell immune response, leading to T-cell activation and proliferation.

MECHANISM OF RESISTANCE
- Increased expression and/or activity of other immune checkpoint pathways (e.g., TIGIT, TIM3, and LAG3).
- Increased expression of other immune escape mechanisms.
- Increased infiltration of immune suppressive cells within the tumor microenvironment, which include Tregs, myeloid-derived suppressor cells (MDSCs), and M2 macrophages.
- Release of various cytokines, chemokines, and metabolites within the tumor microenvironment, including CSF-1, tryptophan metabolites, TGF-β, and adenosine.

DISTRIBUTION
Distribution in body has not been well characterized.

METABOLISM
Metabolism has not been extensively characterized. As with other antibodies, it is expected to be broken down into small peptide and amino acids via catabolic pathways. The terminal half-life is on the order of 25 days.

INDICATIONS
1. FDA-approved for adult patients as monotherapy for mismatch repair deficient (dMMR) recurrent or advanced endometrial cancer that has progressed on or following prior therapy with a platinum-based regimen.
2. FDA-approved for adult patients in combination with carboplatin and paclitaxel followed by dostarlimab monotherapy for mismatch repair deficient (dMMR) primary advanced or recurrent endometrial cancer.
3. FDA-approved for adult patients with dMMR recurrent or advanced solid tumors that have progressed on or following prior treatment and who have no other alternative treatment options.

DOSAGE RANGE

1. dMMR recurrent or advanced endometrial cancer monotherapy: 500 mg IV every 3 weeks for 6 doses followed by 1,000 mg IV every 6 weeks.
2. dMMR recurrent or advanced endometrial cancer in combination with carboplatin and paclitaxel: 500 mg IV every 3 weeks for 6 doses followed by 1,000 mg IV as monotherapy every 6 weeks.
3. dMMR recurrent or advanced solid tumors: Dose 1–4: 500 mg IV every 3 weeks. Starting 3 weeks after Dose 4 (Dose 5 onward): 1,000 mg IV every 6 weeks.

DRUG INTERACTIONS

None well characterized to date.

SPECIAL CONSIDERATIONS

1. Dostarlimab can result in significant immune-mediated adverse reactions due to T-cell activation and proliferation. These immune-mediated reactions may involve any organ system, with the most common reactions being pneumonitis, colitis, hepatitis, hypophysitis, nephritis, and thyroid dysfunction.
2. Monitor for symptoms and signs of immune-mediated adverse reactions.
3. Monitor liver function tests, serum creatinine, and thyroid function at baseline and periodically during therapy.
4. Monitor patients for infusion-related reactions. The infusion rate may need to be interrupted, slowed, or permanently discontinued depending on the severity of the reaction.
5. Dose modification is not needed for patients with hepatic or renal dysfunction.
6. Embryo-fetal toxicity. Females of reproductive potential need to use effective contraception while on treatment and for 4 months after the last dose.

TOXICITY 1

Infusion reactions.

TOXICITY 2

Fatigue, anorexia, and asthenia.

TOXICITY 3

Colitis with diarrhea and abdominal pain.

TOXICITY 4

Pneumonitis with dyspnea and cough.

TOXICITY 5

Hepatitis with elevations in SGOT/SGPT, alkaline phosphatase, and serum bilirubin.

TOXICITY 6
Neurologic toxicity with neuropathy, myositis, and myasthenia gravis.

TOXICITY 7
Renal toxicity with nephritis.

TOXICITY 8
Musculoskeletal symptoms with arthralgias, oligoarthritis or polyarthritis, tenosynovitis, polymyalgia rheumatica, and myalgias.

TOXICITY 9
Endocrinopathies, including hypophysitis, hypothyroidism, adrenal insufficiency, and diabetes.

TOXICITY 10
Maculopapular skin rash, erythema, dermatitis, and pruritus.

Doxorubicin

TRADE NAME	Adriamycin, Hydroxydaunorubicin	CLASSIFICATION	Antitumor antibiotic, anthracycline
CATEGORY	Chemotherapy drug	DRUG MANUFACTURER	Bedford Laboratories

MECHANISM OF ACTION
- Anthracycline antibiotic isolated from *Streptomyces* species.
- Intercalates into DNA, resulting in inhibition of DNA synthesis and function.
- Inhibits transcription through inhibition of DNA-dependent RNA polymerase.
- Inhibits topoisomerase II by forming a cleavable complex with DNA and topoisomerase II to create uncompensated DNA helix torsional tension, leading to eventual DNA breaks.

- Formation of cytotoxic oxygen free radicals results in single- and double-stranded DNA breaks, with subsequent inhibition of DNA synthesis and function.

MECHANISM OF RESISTANCE
- Increased expression of the multidrug-resistant gene with elevated P170 levels, which leads to increased drug efflux and decreased intracellular drug accumulation.
- Decreased expression of topoisomerase II.
- Mutations in topoisomerase II, with decreased binding affinity to doxorubicin.
- Increased expression of sulfhydryl proteins, including glutathione and glutathione-dependent proteins.

ABSORPTION
Administered only via the IV route.

DISTRIBUTION
Widely distributed to tissues. Does not cross the blood-brain barrier. About 75% of doxorubicin and its metabolites is bound to plasma proteins.

METABOLISM
Metabolized extensively in the liver to the active hydroxylated metabolite, doxorubicinol, as well as to inactive metabolites. About 40%–50% of drug is eliminated via biliary excretion in feces. Less than 10% of drug is cleared by the kidneys. Prolonged terminal half-life of 20–48 hours.

INDICATIONS
1. Breast cancer.
2. Hodgkin's and non-Hodgkin's lymphoma.
3. Soft tissue sarcoma.
4. Ovarian cancer.
5. SCLC and NSCLC.
6. Bladder cancer.
7. Thyroid cancer.
8. Hepatoma.
9. Gastric cancer.
10. Wilms' tumor.
11. Neuroblastoma.
12. Acute lymphoblastic leukemia.

DOSAGE RANGE
1. Single agent—60–75 mg/m^2 IV every 3 weeks.
2. Single agent—15–20 mg/m^2 IV weekly.
3. Combination therapy—45–60 mg/m^2 every 3 weeks.
4. Continuous infusion—60–90 mg/m^2 IV over 96 hours.

DRUG INTERACTION 1
Dexamethasone, 5-FU, heparin—Doxorubicin is incompatible with dexamethasone, 5-FU, and heparin, as concurrent use will lead to precipitate formation.

DRUG INTERACTION 2
Dexrazoxane—The cardiotoxic effects of doxorubicin are inhibited by the iron-chelating agent dexrazoxane.

DRUG INTERACTION 3
Cyclophosphamide—Increased risk of hemorrhagic cystitis and cardiac toxicity when doxorubicin is given with cyclophosphamide. Important to be able to distinguish between hemorrhagic cystitis and the normal red-orange urine observed with doxorubicin therapy.

DRUG INTERACTION 4
Phenobarbital, phenytoin—Increased plasma clearance of doxorubicin when given concurrently with barbiturates and/or phenytoin.

DRUG INTERACTION 5
Trastuzumab, mitomycin-C—Increased risk of cardiac toxicity when doxorubicin is given with trastuzumab or mitomycin-C.

DRUG INTERACTION 6
6-Mercaptopurine—Increased risk of hepatotoxicity when doxorubicin is given with 6-mercaptopurine.

SPECIAL CONSIDERATIONS
1. Use with caution in patients with abnormal liver function. Dose reduction is recommended in the setting of liver dysfunction.
2. Because doxorubicin is a potent vesicant, administer slowly with a rapidly flowing IV. Avoid using veins over joints or in extremities with compromised venous and/or lymphatic drainage. Use of a central venous catheter is recommended for patients with difficult venous access and mandatory for prolonged infusions. Careful monitoring is necessary to avoid extravasation. If extravasation is suspected, immediately stop infusion, withdraw fluid, elevate extremity, and apply ice to involved site. May administer local steroids. In severe cases, consult a plastic surgeon.
3. Monitor cardiac function before (baseline) and periodically during therapy with either MUGA radionuclide scan or echocardiogram to assess LVEF. Risk of cardiac toxicity is higher in patients >70 years of age, in patients with prior history of hypertension or pre-existing heart disease, in patients previously treated with anthracyclines, or in patients with prior radiation therapy to the chest. Cumulative doses of >450 mg/m^2 are associated with increased risk for cardiac toxicity.
4. Risk of cardiac toxicity is decreased with weekly or continuous infusion schedules. Use of the iron chelating agent dexrazoxane (ICRF-187) is effective at reducing the development of cardiac toxicity.

5. Use with caution in patients previously treated with radiation therapy, as doxorubicin can cause radiation-recall skin reaction. Increased risk of skin toxicity when doxorubicin is given concurrently with radiation therapy.
6. Patients should be cautioned to avoid sun exposure and to wear sun protection when outside.
7. Patients should be warned about the potential for red-orange discoloration of urine for 1–2 days after drug administration.
8. Pregnancy category D. Breastfeeding should be avoided.

TOXICITY 1
Myelosuppression is dose-limiting, with neutropenia more common than thrombocytopenia or anemia. Nadir usually occurs at days 10–14, with full recovery by day 21.

TOXICITY 2
Nausea and vomiting. Usually mild, occurring in 50% of patients within the first 1–2 hours of treatment.

TOXICITY 3
GI toxicity with mucositis and diarrhea.

TOXICITY 4
Cardiac toxicity. Acute form presents within the first 2–3 days as arrhythmias and/or conduction abnormalities, ECG changes, pericarditis, and/or myocarditis. Usually transient and mostly asymptomatic and not dose-related.

Chronic form results in a dose-dependent, dilated cardiomyopathy associated with congestive heart failure. Risk increases when cumulative doses are >450 mg/m^2.

TOXICITY 5
Potent vesicant. Extravasation can lead to tissue necrosis and chemical thrombophlebitis at the site of injection.

TOXICITY 6
Hyperpigmentation of nails, rarely skin rash, and urticaria. Radiation-recall skin reaction can occur at prior sites of irradiation. Increased hypersensitivity to sunlight.

TOXICITY 7
Alopecia is universal but usually reversible within 3 months after termination of treatment.

TOXICITY 8
Red-orange discoloration of urine. Usually occurs within 1–2 days after drug administration.

TOXICITY 9
Allergic, hypersensitivity reactions are rare.

Doxorubicin liposome

TRADE NAME	Doxil	**CLASSIFICATION**	Antitumor antibiotic, anthracycline
CATEGORY	Chemotherapy drug	**DRUG MANUFACTURER**	Janssen, Sun Pharma

MECHANISM OF ACTION
- Liposomal encapsulation of doxorubicin.
- Protected from chemical and enzymatic degradation, reduced plasma protein binding, and decreased uptake in normal tissues.
- Penetrates tumor tissue into which doxorubicin is released.
- Intercalates into DNA, resulting in inhibition of DNA synthesis and function.
- Inhibits transcription through inhibition of DNA-dependent RNA polymerase.
- Inhibits topoisomerase II by forming a cleavable complex with DNA and topoisomerase II. This creates uncompensated DNA helix torsional tension, leading to eventual DNA breaks.
- Formation of cytotoxic oxygen free radicals results in single- and double-stranded DNA breaks and subsequent inhibition of DNA synthesis and function.

MECHANISM OF RESISTANCE
- Increased expression of the multidrug-resistant gene with elevated P170 protein levels, which leads to increased drug efflux and decreased intracellular drug accumulation.
- Decreased expression of topoisomerase II.
- Mutations in topoisomerase II, with decreased binding affinity to drug.
- Increased expression of sulfhydryl proteins, including glutathione and glutathione-dependent proteins.

ABSORPTION
Administered only via the IV route.

DISTRIBUTION
Mainly confined to the intravascular compartment. In contrast to parent drug, doxorubicin, liposomal doxorubicin has a small volume of distribution. Does not cross the blood-brain barrier. Binding to plasma proteins has not been well characterized.

METABOLISM
Plasma clearance of liposomal doxorubicin is slower than that of doxorubicin, resulting in AUCs that are significantly greater than an equivalent dose of doxorubicin. Prolonged terminal half-life of about 55 hours.

INDICATIONS

1. AIDS-related Kaposi's sarcoma—Used in patients with disease that has progressed on prior combination chemotherapy and/or in patients who are intolerant to such therapy.
2. Ovarian cancer—Metastatic disease refractory to both paclitaxel and platinum-based chemotherapy regimens.
3. Multiple myeloma—FDA-approved in combination with bortezomib in patients who have not previously received bortezomib and who have received at least one prior therapy.

DOSAGE RANGE

1. Kaposi's sarcoma—20 mg/m^2 IV every 21 days.
2. Ovarian cancer—50 mg/m^2 IV every 28 days.
3. Multiple myeloma—30 mg/m^2 IV on day 4 after bortezomib, which is administered at 1.3 mg/m^2 IV on days 1, 4, 8, and 11 every 21 days.

DRUG INTERACTIONS

None well characterized to date.

SPECIAL CONSIDERATIONS

1. Liposomal doxorubicin should **NOT** be substituted for doxorubicin and should be used only where indicated.
2. Use with caution in patients with abnormal liver function. Dose reduction is required in the setting of liver dysfunction.
3. Infusions of liposomal doxorubicin should be given at an initial rate of 1 mg/min over a period of at least 30 minutes to avoid the risk of infusion-associated reactions, which is a black-box warning. This reaction is thought to be related to the lipid component of liposomal doxorubicin. In the event of such a reaction, with flushing, dyspnea, or facial swelling, the infusion should be stopped immediately. If symptoms are minor, can restart infusion at 50% the initial rate. Patients should not be rechallenged in the face of a severe hypersensitivity reaction.
4. Careful monitoring is necessary to avoid extravasation. If extravasation is suspected, immediately stop infusion, withdraw fluid, elevate extremity, and apply ice to involved site. May administer local steroids. In severe cases, consult a plastic surgeon.
5. Monitor cardiac function before (baseline) and periodically during therapy with either MUGA radionuclide scan or echocardiogram to assess LVEF. Risk of cardiac toxicity is increased at total cumulative doses of doxorubicin approaching 450 mg/m^2. It is also higher in patients >70 years of age, in patients with prior history of hypertension or pre-existing heart disease, in patients previously treated with anthracyclines, or in patients with prior radiation therapy to the chest. This is a black-box warning.
6. Monitor CBC weekly while on therapy.

7. Patients should be cautioned about the risk of hand-foot syndrome.
8. Patients should be warned about the potential for red-orange discoloration of urine for 1–2 days after drug administration.
9. Pregnancy category D. Breastfeeding should be avoided.

TOXICITY 1

Myelosuppression is dose-limiting with neutropenia more common than thrombocytopenia or anemia. Nadir usually occurs at days 10–14, with full recovery by day 21.

TOXICITY 2

Mild nausea and vomiting occurs in 20% of patients.

TOXICITY 3

GI toxicity with mucositis and diarrhea.

TOXICITY 4

Cardiac toxicity. Acute form presents within the first 2–3 days as arrhythmias and/or conduction abnormalities, ECG changes, pericarditis, and/or myocarditis. Usually transient and mostly asymptomatic, and not dose-related.

Chronic form results in a dose-dependent dilated cardiomyopathy associated with congestive heart failure.

TOXICITY 5

Skin toxicity manifested as the hand-foot syndrome with skin rash, swelling, erythema, pain, and/or desquamation. Usually mild with onset at 5–6 weeks after the start of treatment. May require subsequent dose reduction. More commonly observed in ovarian cancer patients (37%) than in those with Kaposi's sarcoma (5%).

TOXICITY 6

Hyperpigmentation of nails, skin rash, and urticaria. Radiation-recall skin reaction can occur at prior sites of irradiation.

TOXICITY 7

Alopecia is common but generally reversible within 3 months after termination of treatment.

TOXICITY 8

Infusion reaction with flushing, dyspnea, facial swelling, headache, back pain, tightness in the chest and throat, and/or hypotension. Occurs in about 5%–10% of patients, usually with the first treatment. Upon stopping the infusion, resolves within several hours to a day.

TOXICITY 9

Red-orange discoloration of urine. Usually occurs within 1–2 days after drug administration.

Durvalumab

TRADE NAME	Imfinzi, MEDI4736	CLASSIFICATION	Anti PD-L1 monoclonal antibody
CATEGORY	Immune checkpoint inhibitor, immunotherapy	DRUG MANUFACTURER	MedImmune/ AstraZeneca

MECHANISM OF ACTION
- Human IgG1 κ antibody that binds to the PD-L1 ligand expressed on tumor cells and/or tumor infiltrating cells, which then blocks the interaction between the PD-L1 ligand and the PD-1 and B7.1 receptors found on T cells and antigen-presenting cells.
- Blockade of the PD-1 pathway-mediated immune checkpoint overcomes immune escape mechanisms and enhances T-cell immune response, leading to T-cell activation and proliferation.

MECHANISM OF RESISTANCE
- Increased expression and/or activity of other immune checkpoint pathways (e.g., TIGIT, TIM3, and LAG3).
- Increased expression of other immune escape mechanisms.
- Increased infiltration of immune suppressive populations within the tumor microenvironment, which include Tregs, myeloid-derived suppressor cells (MDSCs), and M2 macrophages.
- Release of various cytokines, chemokines, and metabolites within the tumor microenvironment, including CSF-1, tryptophan metabolites, TGF-β, and adenosine.

DISTRIBUTION
Mean volume of distribution is 5.6 L. Steady-state concentrations are achieved at 16 weeks.

METABOLISM
Metabolism of durvalumab has not been extensively characterized. The mean elimination half-life is on the order of 17 days.

INDICATIONS
1. FDA-approved for unresectable stage III NSCLC in which disease has not progressed following concurrent platinum-based chemotherapy and radiation therapy.
2. FDA-approved in combination with tremelimumab and platinum-based chemotherapy for metastatic NSCLC with no sensitizing EGFR mutations or ALK alterations.
3. FDA-approved in combination with etoposide and either carboplatin or cisplatin as first-line treatment of extensive stage SCLC.

4. FDA-approved in combination with gemcitabine and cisplatin for locally advanced or metastatic biliary tract cancer.
5. FDA-approved in combination with tremelimumab for unresectable hepatocellular cancer (HCC).

DOSAGE RANGE

1. Stage III NSCLC: Weight >30 kg–10 mg/kg IV every 2 weeks or 1,500 mg every 4 weeks.
   Weight <30 kg–20 mg/kg IV every 2 weeks
2. Metastatic NSCLC: Weight >30 kg–1,500 mg IV every 3 weeks in combination with tremelimumab and platinum-based chemotherapy for 4 cycles and then 1,500 mg IV every 4 weeks as monotherapy for 4 doses and a fifth dose of tremelimumab 75 mg in combination with durvalumab dose 6 at week 16.
   Weight <30 kg–20 mg/kg IV every 3 weeks in combination with tremelimumab and platinum-based chemotherapy and then 20 mg/kg IV every 4 weeks as monotherapy and a fifth dose of tremelimumab 1 mg/kg in combination with durvalumab dose 6 at week 16.
3. SCLC: Weight >30 kg–1,500 mg IV every 3 weeks in combination with chemotherapy and then 1,500 mg IV every 4 weeks as monotherapy.
   Weight <30 kg–20 mg/kg IV every 3 weeks in combination with chemotherapy and then 10 mg/kg IV every 2 week as monotherapy.
4. Biliary tract cancer: Weight >30 kg–1,500 mg IV every 3 weeks in combination with chemotherapy and then 1,500 mg IV every 4 weeks as monotherapy.
   Weight <30 kg–20 mg/kg IV every 3 weeks in combination with chemotherapy and then 20 mg/kg IV every 2 weeks as monotherapy.
5. HCC: Weight >30 kg–1,500 mg IV in combination with tremelimumab 300 mg as a single dose on Cycle 1 Day 1 followed by durvalumab 1,500 mg IV every 4 weeks as monotherapy.
   Weight <30 kg–20 mg/kg IV in combination with tremelimumab 4 mg/kg as a single dose on Cycle 1 Day 1 followed by durvalumab 20 mg/kg IV every 4 weeks as monotherapy.

DRUG INTERACTIONS

None well characterized to date.

SPECIAL CONSIDERATIONS

1. Associated with significant immune-mediated adverse reactions due to T-cell activation and proliferation. These immune-mediated reactions may involve any organ system, with the most common reactions being pneumonitis, enterocolitis, hepatitis, dermatitis, hypophysitis, nephritis, and thyroid dysfunction.
2. Mild hepatic impairment does not affect durvalumab pharmacokinetics. However, the effect of moderate or severe hepatic impairment on drug metabolism has not been well characterized.
3. Mild to moderate renal impairment does not affect durvalumab pharmacokinetics. However, the effect of severe renal impairment on drug metabolism has not been well characterized.

4. Durvalumab should be withheld for any of the following:
   - Grade 2 pneumonitis
   - Grade 2 colitis
   - SGOT/SGPT >3–5 × ULN or total bilirubin >1.5–3 × ULN
   - Serum creatinine >1.5–3 × ULN
   - Any other severe or grade 3 treatment-related toxicity
5. Durvalumab should be permanently discontinued for any of the following:
   - Any life-threatening or grade 4 toxicity
   - Grades 3 or 4 pneumonitis
   - Grades 3 or 4 colitis
   - SGOT/SGPT >8 × ULN or total bilirubin >5 × ULN
   - Serum creatinine >3–6 × ULN
6. Monitor thyroid and adrenal function prior to and during therapy.
7. Immune-mediated reactions may occur even after discontinuation of therapy.
8. Durvalumab can cause fetal harm, and women should use effective contraception while on therapy and for at least 3 months following the last dose of therapy.
9. Breastfeeding is not recommended during therapy and for at least 3 months after the last dose of therapy.

TOXICITY 1
Fatigue, anorexia, and asthenia.

TOXICITY 2
Pneumonitis with dyspnea and cough.

TOXICITY 3
Hepatotoxicity with elevations in SGOT/SGPT and serum bilirubin.

TOXICITY 4
Colitis with diarrhea and abdominal pain.

TOXICITY 5
Endocrinopathies, which include hypothyroidism, hyperthyroidism, adrenal insufficiency, diabetes mellitus, and hypophysitis/hypopituitarism.

TOXICITY 6
Neurologic toxicity with neuropathy, myositis, myasthenia gravis, and Guillain-Barré syndrome.

TOXICITY 7
Renal toxicity with nephritis.

TOXICITY 8
Maculopapular skin rash, erythema, dermatitis, and pruritus.

TOXICITY 9
Infusion-related reactions.

TOXICITY 10
Musculoskeletal symptoms, which may present with arthralgias, oligoarthritis, polyarthritis, tenosynovitis, polymyalgia rheumatica, and myalgias.

Duvelisib

TRADE NAME	Copiktra	CLASSIFICATION	Signal transduction inhibitor, PI3K inhibitor
CATEGORY	Targeted agent	DRUG MANUFACTURER	Verastem Oncology

MECHANISM OF ACTION
- Phosphatidylinositol-3-kinase (PI3K) inhibitor with specific activity against PI3K-δ and PI3K-γ isoforms expressed in normal and malignant B cells.
- Inhibits several key signaling pathways, including B cell receptor signaling and CXCR12-mediated chemotaxis of malignant B cells.
- Inhibits CXCL12-induced T-cell migration and M-CSF and IL-4 driven M2 polarization of macrophages, which leads to a more prominent immunostimulatory tumor environment that activates effector T cells.

MECHANISM OF RESISTANCE
- Increased expression of IL-6.
- Activation of STAT3 and NF-κB signaling.

ABSORPTION
Absolute oral bioavailability is approximately 42%. Peak plasma drug levels are achieved in 1–2 hours after ingestion, and food does not appear to alter bioavailability.

DISTRIBUTION
Extensive binding (98%) to plasma proteins. Steady-state drug levels are reached in approximately 3 days.

METABOLISM
Metabolism occurs primarily by CYP3A4 liver microsomal enzymes. Elimination is mainly hepatic (79%), with excretion in feces. Renal elimination accounts for 14% of an administered dose. Approximately 11% of an administered dose is eliminated in feces as unchanged parent drug. The terminal half-life of the parent drug is 4.7 hours.

INDICATIONS
FDA-approved for relapsed or refractory CLL or small lymphocytic lymphoma (SLL) after at least 2 prior therapies.

DOSAGE RANGE
Recommended dose is 25 mg PO bid.

DRUG INTERACTION 1
Phenytoin and other drugs that stimulate the liver microsomal CYP3A4 enzymes, including carbamazepine, rifampin, phenobarbital, and St. John's Wort—These drugs may increase the metabolism of duvelisib, resulting in lower effective drug levels.

DRUG INTERACTION 2
Drugs that inhibit the liver microsomal CYP3A4 enzymes, including ketoconazole, itraconazole, erythromycin, and clarithromycin—These drugs may decrease the metabolism of duvelisib, resulting in increased drug levels and potentially increased toxicity.

SPECIAL CONSIDERATIONS
1. Dose reduction is not required in the setting of mild, moderate, and severe hepatic impairment (Child-Pugh Class A, B, and C).
2. Dose reduction is not required in the setting of mild or moderate renal impairment. Has not been studied in the setting of severe renal impairment, end-stage renal disease, or in patients on dialysis.
3. Monitor for signs and symptoms of severe hypersensitivity reactions.
4. Monitor blood glucose levels at least once per week for the first 8 weeks of treatment, followed by once every 2 weeks, and then as clinically indicated. Patients with diabetes mellitus should have their blood glucose levels under control before starting therapy.
5. Monitor for signs and symptoms of infection as fatal and/or serious infections can occur in up to 30% of patients. There is an increased risk for opportunistic infections, including Pneumocystis jiroveci (PJP). Patients should be empirically placed on PJP prophylaxis. This is a black-box warning.

6. Patients should be educated on the signs and symptoms of serious skin reactions. Patients with a prior history of Stevens-Johnson syndrome, erythema multiforme, or toxic epidermal necrolysis should not be treated. This is a black-box warning.
7. Monitor patients for severe diarrhea or colitis as fatal and/or serious diarrhea or colitis occur in nearly 20% of patients. Patients should start on anti-diarrheal medication, increase oral fluid intake, and notify their physician if diarrhea occurs while on therapy. This is a black-box warning.
8. Monitor patients for new onset pulmonary symptoms. This is a black-box warning.
9. May cause fetal harm when administered to a pregnant woman. Breastfeeding should be avoided.

TOXICITY 1
Myelosuppression with neutropenia.

TOXICITY 2
Hepatotoxicity with elevations in SGOT/SGPT and serum bilirubin.

TOXICITY 3
Skin toxicity with maculopapular skin rash and more serious reactions, including Stevens-Johnson syndrome, erythema multiforme, and toxic epidermal necrolysis.

TOXICITY 4
Infections with pneumonia, sepsis, and lower respiratory infections. There is an increased risk of PJP and CMV reactivation/infections.

TOXICITY 5
GI toxicity with diarrhea or colitis, nausea/vomiting, and mucositis.

TOXICITY 6
Pulmonary toxicity with cough, dyspnea, hypoxia and interstitial infiltrates..

TOXICITY 7
Fatigue, asthenia, and anorexia.

Elacestrant

TRADE NAME	Orserdu	CLASSIFICATION	Estrogen receptor degrader
CATEGORY	Hormonal agent	DRUG MANUFACTURER	Stemline Therapeutics

MECHANISM OF ACTION
- First orally available non-steroidal selective estrogen receptor degrader (SERD).
- Binds to ER-α resulting in degradation of ER-α protein mediated by the proteasomal pathway.
- Maintains activity in ER+, HER2-breast tumors resistant to fulvestrant and CDK 4/6 inhibitors and in those harboring *ESR1* mutations.
- *ESR1* mutations present in 30%–40% of metastatic ER+ breast cancer.

MECHANISM OF RESISTANCE
None well-characterized to date.

ABSORPTION
Median time to reach peak plasma levels is 1–4 hours.

DISTRIBUTION
Extensive binding with approximately 99% of drug bound to plasma proteins. Steady-state drug levels are reached by day 6.

METABOLISM
Extensively metabolized in liver by microsomal CYP3A4 enzymes and to lesser extent by CYP2C9 and CYP2A6. Major route of elimination is in feces (approximately 82%), with renal excretion accounting for <10% of drug clearance. Long terminal half-life on the order of 30–50 hours.

INDICATIONS
FDA-approved for post-menopausal women or adult men with ER+, HER2-negative, *ESR1*-mutated advanced or metastatic breast cancer with disease progression following at least one line of endocrine therapy.

DOSAGE RANGE
Recommended dose is 345 mg PO daily with food.

DRUG INTERACTION 1
Drugs such as ketoconazole, itraconazole, erythromycin, clarithromycin, atazanavir, indinavir, nefazodone, nelfinavir, ritonavir, saquinavir, telithromycin, and voriconazole may decrease the metabolism of elacestrant, resulting in increased drug levels and potentially increased toxicity.

DRUG INTERACTION 2
Phenytoin and other drugs that stimulate the liver microsomal CYP3A4 enzymes, including carbamazepine, rifampin, phenobarbital, and St. John's Wort—These drugs may increase the metabolism of elacestrant, resulting in lower effective drug levels and potentially reduced activity.

DRUG INTERACTION 3
Certain P-gp substrates–Avoid concomitant use of elacestrant with certain P-gp substrates, such as digoxin, verapamil, and diltiazem, or BCRP substrates, as elacestrant is a P-gp and BCRP inhibitor.

SPECIAL CONSIDERATIONS
1. No dose adjustments are required for patients with mild or moderate renal dysfunction. Has not been studied in patients with severe renal dysfunction or end-stage renal disease.
2. No dose adjustments are required for patients with mild liver dysfunction. Dose should be reduced to 258 mg in patients with moderate hepatic dysfunction. Has not been studied in patients with severe hepatic dysfunction.
3. Monitor lipid profile at baseline and periodically while on therapy.
4. Tablets should be swallowed whole and should be taken with food to reduce nausea/vomiting.
5. May cause fetal harm when administered to a pregnant woman. Females should use effective contraception during treatment and for 1 week after the last dose. Breastfeeding should be avoided while on treatment and for 1 week after the last dose.

TOXICITY 1
Fatigue, anorexia, and asthenia.

TOXICITY 2
Mild nausea/vomiting and dyspepsia.

TOXICITY 3
Dyslipidemia with hypercholesterolemia and hypertriglyceridemia.

TOXICITY 4
Musculoskeletal pain and arthralgias.

TOXICITY 5
Hot flashes.

Elotuzumab

TRADE NAME	Empliciti	**CLASSIFICATION**	Anti-SLAMF7 monoclonal antibody
CATEGORY	Biologic response modifier agent, immunotherapy	**DRUG MANUFACTURER**	Bristol-Myers Squibb

MECHANISM OF ACTION
- Elotuzumab is an IgG1-κ humanized monoclonal antibody directed against the extracellular domain of human signaling lymphocyte activation molecule family 7 (SLAMF7).
- SLAMF7 is a glycoprotein with a limited expression pattern. It is expressed on more than 95% of myeloma cells and on natural killer (NK) cells, on plasma cells, and on specific immune cell subsets within the hematopoietic lineage, albeit at lower levels.
- Does not interact with other members of the SLAM family.
- Directly activates NK cells through SLAMF7 signaling pathway and Fc receptors and mediates NK cell–mediated antibody-dependent cellular cytotoxicity (ADCC).
- Activation of NK cells by elotuzumab may result in the release of inflammatory cytokines that then leads to the recruitment of other immune cells to enhance the anti-myeloma effect.
- Does not bind to $CD34^+$ hematopoietic stem cells.

MECHANISM OF RESISTANCE
None well characterized to date.

ABSORPTION
Administered only via the IV route.

DISTRIBUTION
Steady state is achieved by approximately 6 weeks.

METABOLISM
Metabolism occurs by proteolytic catabolism with breakdown to small peptides and individual amino acids. The elimination of elotuzumab increases with increasing body weight, which supports the use of weight-based dosing. The mean terminal half-life is approximately 18 days.

INDICATIONS
1. FDA-approved in combination with lenalidomide and dexamethasone for patients with multiple myeloma who have received at least 1–3 prior lines of therapy.
2. FDA-approved in combination with pomalidomide and dexamethasone for patients with multiple myeloma who have received at least 2 prior lines of therapy, including lenalidomide and a proteasome inhibitor.

DOSAGE RANGE
1. Recommended dose in combination with lenalidomide and dexamethasone is 10 mg/kg IV on a weekly basis for the first 2 cycles, then every 2 weeks thereafter.
2. Recommended dose in combination with pomalidomide and dexamethasone is 10 mg/kg IV on a weekly basis for the first 2 cycles and then 20 mg/kg every 4 weeks thereafter.

DRUG INTERACTION
None well characterized to date.

SPECIAL CONSIDERATIONS
1. Monitor patients for infusion reactions, which generally occur during the first infusion.
2. Premedication with antihistamines (diphenhydramine 25–50 mg PO or IV), antipyretics (acetaminophen 650–1,000 mg), and corticosteroids (methylprednisolone 100 mg or equivalent dose of an intermediate- or long-acting steroid) is required to reduce the risk of infusion reactions, and should be given 30–60 minutes prior to infusion. Interrupt the infusion for any reaction and manage as appropriate. Administer elotuzumab in a clinical facility with immediate access to resuscitative measures (e.g., glucocorticoids, epinephrine, bronchodilators, and/or oxygen). For patients who experience a severe infusion reaction, therapy should be permanently discontinued.
3. Monitor for signs and symptoms of infection.
4. Monitor liver function tests (LFTs) at baseline and periodically while on therapy. Elotuzumab should be held for > grade 3 elevation of LFTs, and restarting the drug may occur after LFTs return to baseline values.
5. Elotuzumab may interfere with an accurate assessment of the myeloma response, as the drug may be detected on serum protein electrophoresis and immunofixation assays that are used to monitor for endogenous M-protein levels.
6. No dose adjustments are recommended for patients with renal dysfunction.

7. No dose adjustments are recommended for patients with mild hepatic dysfunction. Has not been studied in the setting of moderate or severe hepatic dysfunction, and caution should be used in these settings.
8. No studies with elotuzumab have been done in pregnant women, nor is information available on the potential risk of breastfeeding.

TOXICITY 1
Infusion reactions with chills, fever, bronchospasm, cough, wheezing, dyspnea, laryngeal edema, and hypotension.

TOXICITY 2
Increased risk of infections, including upper respiratory infection (URI), nasopharyngitis, and pneumonia. Opportunistic infections, including fungal infections and herpes zoster, have been observed.

TOXICITY 3
Fatigue and anorexia.

TOXICITY 4
Hepatotoxicity with elevations in SGOT/SGPT and alkaline phosphatase.

TOXICITY 5
Increased risk of second primary cancers.

TOXICITY 6
GI side effects with mild nausea/vomiting, diarrhea, and constipation.

Enasidenib

TRADE NAME	Idhifa, AG-221/CC-90007	CLASSIFICATION	Signal transduction inhibitor, IDH2 inhibitor
CATEGORY	Targeted agent	DRUG MANUFACTURER	Agios and Celgene

MECHANISM OF ACTION

- Small-molecule inhibitor of isocitrate dehydrogenase 2 (IDH2). Specifically targets the mutant IDH2 variants R140Q, R172S, and R172K at significantly lower concentrations than the wild-type IDH enzyme.
- IDH2 mutations occur in up to 20% of AML patients, and they are associated with an increased level of an oncometabolite 2-hydroxyglutarate (2-HG), which induces a block in cell differentiation.
- Treatment with enasidenib leads to reduced 2-HG levels, induces myeloid differentiation, and reduces abnormal histone hypermethylation.

MECHANISM OF RESISTANCE

- IDH2 mutations through trans or cis dimer-interface mutations.
- Second-site IDH1 mutations.
- Mutations in NRAS and MAPK genes leading to activation of NRAS and MAPK signaling.
- Mutations in other receptor tyrosine kinase (RTK) pathway genes, such as KRAS, PTPN11, KIT, and FLT3.

ABSORPTION

Oral bioavailability is approximately 57%. Peak plasma drug levels are achieved in 4 hours after ingestion.

DISTRIBUTION

Extensive binding (98.5%) to plasma proteins. Steady-state drug levels are reached in approximately 29 days.

METABOLISM

Metabolism in the liver by multiple CYP enzymes, including CYP1A2, CYP2B6, CYP2C8, CYP2C9, CYP2D6, and CYP3A4. Metabolized also by multiple UGT enzymes, including UGT1A1, UGT1A3, UGT1A4, UGT1A89, UGT2B7, and UGT2B15. Following an administered dose, 89% of an administered dose is eliminated in feces and 11% is eliminated in urine. The terminal half-life is approximately 137 hours.

INDICATIONS

FDA-approved for relapsed or refractory AML with an IDH2 mutation as detected by an FDA-approved diagnostic test.

DOSAGE RANGE

Recommended dose is 100 mg PO daily for a minimum of 6 months.

DRUG INTERACTION 1

Drugs such as ketoconazole, itraconazole, erythromycin, clarithromycin, atazanavir, indinavir, nefazodone, nelfinavir, ritonavir, saquinavir, telithromycin, and voriconazole may decrease the metabolism of enasidenib, resulting in increased drug levels and potentially increased toxicity.

DRUG INTERACTION 2
Drugs such as rifampin, phenytoin, phenobarbital, carbamazepine, and St. John's Wort may increase the metabolism of enasidenib, resulting in lower effective drug levels.

SPECIAL CONSIDERATIONS
1. Dose reduction is not required in the setting of mild hepatic impairment (Child-Pugh Class A). Has not been studied in the setting of moderate and severe hepatic impairment, and dose reduction may be necessary.
2. Dose reduction is not required if CrCl >30 mL/min.
3. Monitor for the development of the differentiation syndrome, which may be fatal if not appropriately treated. Can present as early as 10 days and up to 5 months after start of therapy. Steroids (dexamethasone 10 mg IV every 12 hours) should be initiated if differentiation syndrome is suspected with hemodynamic monitoring. In the presence of non-infectious leukocytosis, treatment with hydroxyurea or leukapheresis should be instituted. This is a black-box warning.
4. Monitor CBCs and blood chemistries at baseline and at least every 2 weeks for the first 3 months of therapy.
5. Monitor for tumor lysis syndrome, as the induction of myeloid proliferation from enasidenib can cause a rapid reduction in AML cells.
6. Patients should be selected based on the presence of IDH2 mutations in the blood or bone marrow.
7. May cause fetal harm when administered to a pregnant woman. Females of reproductive potential should use effective contraception during drug therapy and for at least 30 days after the final dose. Breastfeeding should be avoided.

TOXICITY 1
Hepatotoxicity with elevations in indirect serum bilirubin levels and no associated increase in LFTs.

TOXICITY 2
Differentiation syndrome with dyspnea, hypoxia, pulmonary infiltrates, pleural effusion, fever, pericardial effusion, and peripheral edema. Hepatic, renal, and multi-organ dysfunction have also been observed.

TOXICITY 3
Nausea/vomiting and diarrhea.

TOXICITY 4
Fatigue and anorexia.

TOXICITY 5
Non-infectious leukocytosis.

TOXICITY 6
Tumor lysis syndrome is a rare event.

Encorafenib

TRADE NAME	Braftovi	**CLASSIFICATION**	Signal transduction inhibitor, BRAF inhibitor
CATEGORY	Targeted agent	**DRUG MANUFACTURER**	Array BioPharma

MECHANISM OF ACTION
- Inhibits mutant forms of BRAF serine-threonine kinase, including BRAF-V600E, which results in inhibition of mitogen-activated protein kinase (MAPK) signaling.
- Inhibits wild-type BRAF and CRAF kinases. This inhibitory activity against wild-type BRAF is similar to dabrafenib but in sharp contrast to vemurafenib.
- May inhibit other kinases, including JNK1, JNK2, JNK3, LIMK1, LIMK2, MEK4, and STK36.

MECHANISM OF RESISTANCE
- Increased expression of MAPK signaling.
- Activation/induction of alternative cellular signaling pathways, such as FGFR, EGFR, and PI3K/Akt.
- Reactivation of Ras/Raf signaling.

ABSORPTION
High oral bioavailability on the order of 86%. Time to peak drug concentrations is 2 hours. Food with a high fat content reduces C_{max} but not AUC.

DISTRIBUTION
Significant binding (86%) of encorafenib to plasma proteins. Steady-state drug levels are reached in 15 days.

METABOLISM

Metabolized in the liver through N-dealklyation by CYP3A4, CYP2C19, and CYP2D6 microsomal enzymes. Elimination occurs in equal proportion in feces and urine, with each accounting for approximately 47% of an administered dose. The mean terminal half-life of encorafenib is approximately 3.5 hours.

INDICATIONS

1. FDA-approved in combination with binimetinib for unresectable or metastatic melanoma with BRAF-V600E or V600K mutation as determined by an FDA-approved diagnostic test.
2. FDA-approved in combination with cetuximab for metastatic colorectal cancer with a BRAF-V600E mutation.
3. Clinical activity in combination with binimetinib and cetuximab for metastatic colorectal cancer with a BRAF-V600E mutation.

DOSAGE RANGE

1. Melanoma: Recommended dose is 450 mg PO once daily in combination with binimetinib.
2. Colorectal cancer: Recommended dose is 300 mg PO once daily in combination with cetuximab.

DRUG INTERACTION 1

Drugs such as ketoconazole, itraconazole, erythromycin, clarithromycin, atazanavir, indinavir, nefazodone, nelfinavir, ritonavir, saquinavir, telithromycin, and voriconazole may decrease the metabolism of encorafenib, resulting in increased drug levels and potentially increased toxicity.

DRUG INTERACTION 2

Drugs such as rifampin, phenytoin, phenobarbital, carbamazepine, and St. John's Wort may increase the metabolism of encorafenib, resulting in lower effective drug levels.

DRUG INTERACTION 3

CYP3A4 substrates—Co-administration of encorafenib with CYP3A4 substrates, such as hormonal contraceptives, may result in reduced efficacy of these agents and/or increased toxicity.

SPECIAL CONSIDERATIONS

1. Careful skin exams should be done at baseline, every 2 months while on therapy, and for up to 6 months following discontinuation of therapy given the increased incidence of cutaneous squamous cell cancers and keratoacanthomas.
2. Patients should be closely monitored for signs and symptoms of non-cutaneous malignancies.
3. Monitor serum glucose levels in patients with diabetes or hyperglycemia.
4. Monitor patients for eye reactions, including uveitis and iritis.
5. BRAF testing using an FDA-approved diagnostic test to confirm the presence of the BRAF-V600E mutation is required.

6. No dose adjustment is needed for patients with mild hepatic dysfunction and in those with mild or moderate renal dysfunction. Caution should be used in patients with moderate or severe hepatic dysfunction and in those with severe renal dysfunction. Guidelines for dosing in these settings of hepatic and renal impairment have not been established.
7. Dosing guidelines are in place in the setting of co-administration of moderate or strong CYP3A4 inhibitors. Please see package insert for details on dosing.
8. Pregnancy category D. Breastfeeding should be avoided.

TOXICITY 1
Cutaneous squamous cell cancers and keratoacanthomas occur in up to 3% of patients. The median time to first occurrence is about 6 months. A new primary melanoma can also be observed.

TOXICITY 2
Skin reactions, including hyperkeratosis, rash, dry skin, alopecia, and pruritus.

TOXICITY 3
Fatigue.

TOXICITY 4
Hemorrhage with GI bleeding complications. Intracranial bleeding in the setting of metastatic brain disease can occur.

TOXICITY 5
Arthralgias and myalgias.

TOXICITY 6
Ophthalmologic side effects, including uveitis, iritis, and photophobia.

TOXICITY 7
Nausea/vomiting, abdominal pain, and constipation are the most common GI side effects.

TOXICITY 8
QTc prolongation.

TOXICITY 9
Hyperglycemia.

Enfortumab vedotin-ejfv

TRADE NAME	Padcev, AGS-22M6E, AGS-22CE	CLASSIFICATION	Antibody-drug conjugate
CATEGORY	Biologic response modifier agent, chemotherapy drug	DRUG MANUFACTURER	Astellas

MECHANISM OF ACTION
- Antibody-drug conjugate made up of a fully human monoclonal antibody directed against Nectin-4 conjugated to the microtubule-disrupting anti-mitotic agent monomethyl auristatin E (MMAE). Approximately 4 molecules of MMAE are conjugated to each antibody molecule.
- Upon binding to Nectin-4, enfortumab vedotin is rapidly internalized into lysosomes, and MMAE is then released in the cell to bind to microtubules, which inhibits mitosis and cell division, resulting in cell death. MMAE biological activity is similar to that of other anti-microtubule inhibitors and works in the M-phase of the cell cycle.
- Nectin-4 is a transmembrane protein that is a family member of related immunoglobulin-like adhesion molecules involved in cell-cell adhesion and processes involved in oncogenesis.
- Nectin-4 is highly expressed in several solid tumors, including urothelial, breast, gastric, and lung cancers.

MECHANISM OF RESISTANCE
None well characterized to date.

ABSORPTION
Administered only via the IV route.

DISTRIBUTION
Moderate binding (77%) of drug to plasma proteins. Steady-state levels of MMAE are achieved within 21 days.

METABOLISM

Enfortumab vedotin is metabolized via catabolism to small peptides, amino acids, unconjugated MMAE, and unconjugated MMAE-related catabolites. MMAE serves as a substrate for CYP3A4 liver microsomal enzymes. The median terminal half-life of the antibody-conjugated MMAE is about 12 days, while the unconjugated MMAE terminal half-life is about 4 days after the first dose of the antibody-drug conjugate.

INDICATIONS

1. FDA-approved as monotherapy for patients with metastatic urothelial cancer following treatment with a PD-1 or PD-L1 inhibitor and platinum-based chemotherapy in the neoadjuvant/adjuvant, locally advanced, or metastatic setting.
2. FDA-approved in combination with pembrolizumab for patients with locally advanced or metastatic urothelial cancer who are not eligible for cisplatin-containing chemotherapy.

DOSAGE RANGE

1. Monotherapy: 1.25 mg/kg (up to a maximum of 125 mg) IV on days 1, 8, and 15 on a 28-day schedule.
2. Combination therapy: 1.25 mg/kg (up to a maximum of 125 mg) IV on days 1 and 8 on a 21-day schedule.

DRUG INTERACTION 1

Drugs such as ketoconazole, itraconazole, erythromycin, clarithromycin, atazanavir, indinavir, nefazodone, nelfinavir, ritonavir, saquinavir, telithromycin, and voriconazole may decrease the metabolism of MMAE, resulting in increased drug levels and potentially increased toxicity.

DRUG INTERACTION 2

Phenytoin and other drugs that stimulate the liver microsomal CYP3A4 enzymes, including carbamazepine, rifampin, phenobarbital, and St. John's Wort—These drugs may increase the metabolism of MMAE, resulting in lower effective drug levels.

SPECIAL CONSIDERATIONS

1. Monitor for infusion site extravasation. If extravasation occurs, the infusion should be stopped, and the patient monitored for infusion reactions.
2. Serum glucose levels need to be closely monitored while on therapy, especially in patients with pre-existing diabetes. Therapy should be held when blood glucose levels >250 mg/dL.

3. Monitor for ocular disorders, which include dry eye, blurred vision, and keratitis. The median time to develop eye disorders is on the order of 2 months. The use of artificial tears should be considered for prophylaxis of dry eyes.
4. Dose reduction is not required for patients with mild hepatic dysfunction. There is limited safety information for patients with moderate or severe hepatic dysfunction, and use should be avoided in these settings.
5. Dose reduction is not required for patients with mild, moderate, or severe renal dysfunction. Has not been studied in patients with end-stage renal disease and/or in those on hemodialysis.
6. Can cause fetal harm when given to a pregnant woman. Females of reproductive potential should use effective contraception during treatment and for at least 2 months after the last dose. Males with female partners of reproductive potential should use effective contraception while on treatment and for at least 4 months after the last dose. Breastfeeding should be avoided.

TOXICITY 1
Fatigue and anorexia.

TOXICITY 2
Nausea/vomiting, loss of taste.

TOXICITY 3
Peripheral neuropathy.

TOXICITY 4
Hyperglycemia.

TOXICITY 5
Skin toxicity with maculopapular skin rash, pruritus, and dry skin.

TOXICITY 6
Ocular toxicity with dry eye, blurred vision, keratitis, and limbal stem cell deficiency.

TOXICITY 7
Infusion site extravasations.

Entrectinib

TRADE NAME	Rozlytrek, RXDX-101	**CLASSIFICATION**		Signal transduction inhibitor, TRK inhibitor
CATEGORY	Targeted agent	**DRUG MANUFACTURER**		Roche

MECHANISM OF ACTION

- Potent inhibitor of tropomyosin receptor kinases (TRK), TRKA, TRKB, and TRKC, which are encoded by NTRK1, NTRK2, and NTRK3, respectively.
- NTRK gene fusions involve chromosomal rearrangements between an expressed 5' partner and a 3' partner encoding a tyrosine kinase. These oncogenic fusions represent a novel oncogenic driver and have been identified in up to 1% of all solid cancers.
- Inhibits ROS1 and ALK as well as JAK2 and TNK2. The active metabolite of entrectinib, M5, has similar inhibitory activity against TRK, ROS1, and ALK.
- Rationally designed to cross the blood-brain barrier to treat brain metastases with NTRK1-, NTRK2-, NTRK3-, ROS1-, and ALK-rearranged cancers.

MECHANISM OF RESISTANCE

- Mutations in the TRK kinase domain, including TRKA-G595R, TRKA-G667C, and TRKC-G623R.
- Activation of RAS and ERK signaling. Mutations in KRAS G12C have been identified.
- Mutations in IGF1R, which leads to activation of the IGF1R signaling pathway.

ABSORPTION

Oral bioavailability is modest at 34%. The median time to C_{max} is 4–6 hours after ingestion. Food does not appear to affect oral absorption.

DISTRIBUTION
Extensive binding (>99%) of entrectinib and its active metabolite M5 to plasma proteins. Steady-state drug levels are achieved in approximately 2 weeks.

METABOLISM
Metabolized in the liver primarily by CYP3A4 microsomal enzymes. M5 is the active metabolite, and it is the only major active metabolite identified in the peripheral blood. Elimination is primarily in feces (83%) with 36% of an administered dose in the parent form and 22% in the M5 metabolite form, with only minimal excretion of drug in urine (3%). The terminal half-lives of entrectinib and M5 are approximately 20–22 and 40 hours, respectively.

INDICATIONS
1. FDA-approved for adult and pediatric patients 12 years and older with metastatic solid tumors that have an NTRK gene fusion without a known acquired resistance mutation, are metastatic or where surgical resection is likely to result in severe morbidity, and have progressed following treatment or have no satisfactory alternative treatments.
2. FDA-approved for adult patients with metastatic NSCLC whose tumors are ROS1-positive.

DOSAGE RANGE
1. ROS1-positive NSCLC: recommended dose is 600 mg PO once daily.
2. NTRK gene fusion-positive solid tumors: recommended dose is 600 mg PO once daily.

DRUG INTERACTION 1
Drugs such as ketoconazole, itraconazole, erythromycin, clarithromycin, atazanavir, indinavir, nefazodone, nelfinavir, ritonavir, saquinavir, telithromycin, and voriconazole may decrease the metabolism of entrectinib, resulting in increased drug levels and potentially increased toxicity.

DRUG INTERACTION 2
Drugs such as rifampin, phenytoin, phenobarbital, carbamazepine, and St. John's Wort may increase the metabolism of entrectinib, resulting in its inactivation and lower effective drug levels.

SPECIAL CONSIDERATIONS
1. No dose adjustment is needed for patients with mild hepatic dysfunction. Has not been studied in patients with moderate or severe hepatic dysfunction.
2. No dose adjustment is needed for patients with mild or moderate renal dysfunction. Has not been studied in patients with severe renal impairment or those with end-stage renal disease.
3. Should be avoided in patients taking moderate and strong CYP3A4 inducers.
4. Should be avoided in patients taking moderate and strong CYP3A4 inhibitors. If strong CYP3A4 inhibitors are required, the dose of entrectinib should be reduced.

5. Baseline and periodic evaluations of left ventricular ejection fraction (LVEF) should be performed while on therapy. Monitor patients for signs and symptoms of CHF.
6. Patients should be warned not to drive or operate hazardous machinery if experiencing any type of CNS effects.
7. Monitor LFTs every 2 weeks during the first month of therapy, then monthly thereafter and as clinically indicated.
8. Baseline and periodic evaluations of ECG, with focus on QT interval. Electrolyte status should be monitored while on therapy. Use with caution in patients at risk of developing QT prolongation, including hypokalemia, hypomagnesemia, and congenital long QT syndrome, and patients taking antiarrhythmic medications or any other drugs that may cause QT prolongation.
9. NTRK testing using an FDA-approved test is required to confirm the presence of NTRK gene fusions.
10. Can cause fetal harm when administered to a pregnant woman. Females of reproductive potential should use effective contraception during drug therapy and for at least 5 weeks after the final dose. Breastfeeding should be avoided.

TOXICITY 1
Neurotoxicity with cognitive impairment, confusion, attention deficits, mood disorders, dizziness, and sleep impairment.

TOXICITY 2
Hepatotoxicity with elevations in SGOT and SGPT.

TOXICITY 3
Nausea/vomiting, constipation, diarrhea, and abdominal pain.

TOXICITY 4
Fatigue and anorexia.

TOXICITY 5
CHF.

TOXICITY 6
Vision disorders with blurred vision, photophobia, diplopia, photopsia, cataracts, and vitreous floaters.

TOXICITY 7
QT prolongation.

TOXICITY 8
Increased risk of skeletal fractures.

TOXICITY 9
Hyperuricemia.

Enzalutamide

TRADE NAME	Xtandi	CLASSIFICATION	Antiandrogen
CATEGORY	Hormonal agent	DRUG MANUFACTURER	Astellas/Medivation

MECHANISM OF ACTION
- Pure androgen receptor (AR) antagonist that acts on different steps in the androgen receptor signaling pathway.
- Competitively inhibits androgen binding to ARs and by inhibiting AR nuclear translocation and co-activator recruitment of the ligand-receptor complex.
- Inhibits the androgen-AR pathway at the receptor and post-receptor ligand binding level.
- N-desmethyl enzalutamide metabolite exhibits similar antitumor activity to enzalutamide.

MECHANISM OF RESISTANCE
- Androgen receptor gene rearrangement, promoting synthesis of constitutively active truncated androgen receptor splice variants that lack the androgen receptor ligand-binding domain.
- Resistance may also be mediated by NF-κB2/p52 via activation of androgen receptor and splice variants.
- Decreased expression of androgen receptor.
- Mutation in androgen receptor leading to decreased binding affinity to enzalutamide.

ABSORPTION
Rapidly absorbed following oral administration. Peak plasma levels observed 0.5–3 hours after oral ingestion. Steady-state drug levels achieved by day 28 following daily dosing. Co-administration with food does not alter the extent of absorption.

DISTRIBUTION
Mean apparent volume of distribution after a single oral dose is 110 L (29% CV). Extensive binding (97%–98%) to plasma proteins, primarily albumin. N-desmethyl enzalutamide metabolite also exhibits extensive binding to plasma proteins (95%).

METABOLISM

Following oral administration, the major metabolites are enzalutamide, N-desmethyl enzalutamide, and an inactive carboxylic acid metabolite. CYP2C8 and CYP3A4 are the main liver microsomal enzymes responsible for drug metabolism. CYP2C8 is primarily responsible for the formation of the active metabolite N-dimethyl enzalutamide. Primarily eliminated by hepatic metabolism. Mean terminal half-life for enzalutamide is 5.8 days, and the mean terminal half-life for N-desmethyl enzalutamide is 7.8 to 8.6 days.

INDICATIONS

1. FDA-approved for metastatic castration-resistant prostate cancer in patients who have received prior chemotherapy containing docetaxel.
2. FDA-approved for first-line treatment of metastatic castration-resistant prostate cancer.

DOSAGE RANGE

Recommended dose is 160 mg PO once daily. Patients should also receive a GnRH analog at the same time or should have had bilateral orchiectomy.

DRUG INTERACTIONS

1. Co-administration with strong CYP2C8 inhibitors, such as gemfibrozil, increases the plasma drug concentrations of both enzalutamide and N-desmethyl enzalutamide.
2. Co-administration with strong or moderate CYP2C8 inducers (e.g., rifampin) may alter the plasma exposure of enzalutamide.
3. Co-administration with strong CYP3A4 inhibitors (e.g., itraconazole) may increase the plasma drug concentration of enzalutamide and N-desmethyl enzalutamide.
4. Co-administration with strong CYP3A4 inducers (e.g., carbamazepine, phenobarbital, phenytoin, rifabutin, rifampin, rifapentine) and moderate CYP3A4 inducers (e.g., bosentan, efavirenz, etravirine, modafinil, nafcillin) and St. John's Wort) may decrease the plasma drug concentration of enzalutamide.
5. Avoid co-administration with certain CYP2C9 or CYP2C19 substrates.

SPECIAL CONSIDERATIONS

1. No initial dosage adjustment is necessary for patients with mild or moderate renal impairment. Has not been studied in patients with severe renal impairment (CrCL <30 mL/min) or end-stage renal disease.
2. No initial dosage adjustment is necessary for patients with mild or moderate hepatic impairment. Patients with severe hepatic impairment (Child-Pugh Class C) have not been evaluated.
3. Closely monitor patients for seizure activity. It is unclear which patients are at increased risk for developing seizures.
4. Male patients with female partners of reproductive potential should use effective contraception during treatment and for 3 months after the last dose of drug.

TOXICITY 1
Asthenia and fatigue occur in 50% of patients.

TOXICITY 2
Musculoskeletal adverse events occur, including back pain, arthralgia, musculoskeletal pain, muscle weakness, musculoskeletal stiffness, and non-pathologic bone fractures.

TOXICITY 3
Diarrhea occurs in about 20% of patients and is usually mild.

TOXICITY 4
Hot flashes occur in 20% of patients.

TOXICITY 5
Peripheral edema.

TOXICITY 6
Seizures occur rarely in <1% of patients, which usually resolve upon discontinuation of therapy.

Epcoritamab

TRADE NAME	Epkinly	**CLASSIFICATION**	BiTE antibody targeting CD20 and CD3
CATEGORY	Biologic response modifier agent, immunotherapy	**DRUG MANUFACTURER**	Genmab and AbbVie

MECHANISM OF ACTION
- Bispecific T-cell engaging (BiTE) humanized IgG1 antibody that binds to the CD20 antigen expressed on malignant B cells and CD3 expressed on the surface of T cells.
- Binding of this bispecific antibody causes cytotoxic T cells to be physically linked to malignant CD20-positive lymphoma cells and triggers the signaling cascade, leading to upregulation of cell adhesion molecules, production of cytolytic proteins, release of inflammatory cytokines, and proliferation of T cells, ultimately resulting in lysis of CD20-positive malignant B cells.
- CD20 is expressed on more than 90% of all B-cell non-Hodgkin's lymphomas and leukemias.

- CD20 is not expressed on early pre–B cells, plasma cells, normal bone marrow stem cells, antigen-presenting dendritic reticulum cells, or other normal tissues.
- Mechanism of action differs from classic anti-CD20 monoclonal antibodies that induce direct cell death by inhibition of CD20 intracellular signaling and by antibody-dependent cellular cytotoxicity and complement-mediated cellular cytotoxicity.

ABSORPTION
Administered via the SC route. Mean bioavailability is approximately 70% when administered SC. Time to reach maximal concentrations occurs at days 3–8 after SC injection. Maximal drug levels are achieved at the end of the IV infusion in cycle 2.

DISTRIBUTION
Following SC administration, steady-state levels are achieved after 12 weekly treatments.

METABOLISM
Metabolism has not been well characterized. As with other antibodies, it is assumed that epcoritamab is degraded to small peptides and amino acids via catabolic pathways. The terminal half-life is approximately 22 days.

INDICATIONS
FDA-approved for the treatment of adult patients with relapsed or refractory diffuse large B-cell lymphoma, including DLBCL arising from indolent lymphoma and high-grade B-cell lymphoma after 2 or more lines of systemic therapy. Approved under accelerated approval based on response rate and duration of response.

DOSAGE RANGE
1. Administered only as SC injection according to the step-up dosing schedule as outlined.
2. Cycle 1, Day 1 – 0.16 mg; Cycle 1, Day 8 – 0.8 mg; Cycle 1, Day 15 – 48 mg; Cycle 1, Day 22 – 48 mg.
3. Cycles 2 and 3, Days 1, 8, 15, and 22 – 48 mg.
4. Cycles 4–9, Days 1 and 15 – 48 mg.
5. Cycles 10 and beyond, Day 1 – 48 mg

DRUG INTERACTION
Epcoritamab treatment results in release of cytokines that may suppress the activity of CYP3A4 enzymes. This may then lead to increased exposure of drugs that are CYP3A4 substrates.

SPECIAL CONSIDERATIONS

1. Patients should be premedicated one to three hours prior to each step-up dose and first treatment dose to reduce the risk of CRS with 16 mg dexamethasone (oral or IV), H1 receptor antagonist (oral or IV diphenhydramine), and an antipyretic (oral or IV acetaminophen).
2. Monitor for CRS, which occurs most frequently with the first two cycles of therapy. This is a black-box warning.
3. Monitor for neurologic toxicity, especially for the immune effector cell-associated neurotoxicity syndrome (ICANS). This is a black-box warning.
4. Monitor for signs and symptoms of infection. Patients should be given PJP prophylaxis prior to starting on therapy. Prophylaxis against herpes virus prior to starting on therapy should also be considered.
5. Monitor CBCs while on therapy.
6. Dose reduction is not required in patients with mild hepatic dysfunction. Has not been studied in setting of moderate or severe hepatic dysfunction.
7. Dose reduction is not required in patients with mild or moderate renal dysfunction. Has not been studied in setting of severe renal dysfunction or end-stage renal disease.
8. May cause fetal harm. Women should be advised to use effective contraception during treatment and for 4 months after the last dose of treatment. Breastfeeding should be avoided while on therapy and for 4 months after the last dose.

TOXICITY 1

Cytokine release syndrome (CRS) with fever, chills, hypotension, tachycardia, hypoxia, and headache.

TOXICITY 2

Myelosuppression with neutropenia, anemia, and thrombocytopenia.

TOXICITY 3

Neurological toxicities with headache, motor dysfunction, sensory neuropathy, and encephalopathy. ICANS can present with confusional state and dysgraphia.

TOXICITY 5

Injection site reactions.

TOXICITY 6

Increased risk of viral, bacterial, fungal, and opportunistic infections.

TOXICITY 7

Tumor lysis syndrome.

Epirubicin

TRADE NAME	4 Epi-doxorubicin, Ellence	CLASSIFICATION	Antitumor antibiotic, anthracycline
CATEGORY	Chemotherapy drug	DRUG MANUFACTURER	Pfizer

MECHANISM OF ACTION
- Anthracycline derivative of doxorubicin.
- Intercalates into DNA, which results in inhibition of DNA synthesis and function.
- Inhibits topoisomerase II by forming a cleavable complex with topoisomerase II and DNA.
- Formation of cytotoxic oxygen free radicals, which can cause single- and double-stranded DNA breaks.

MECHANISM OF RESISTANCE
- Increased expression of the multidrug-resistant gene with enhanced drug efflux. This results in decreased intracellular drug accumulation.
- Decreased expression of topoisomerase II.
- Mutation in topoisomerase II, with decreased binding affinity to drug.
- Increased expression of glutathione and glutathione-associated enzymes.

ABSORPTION
Administered only via the IV route.

DISTRIBUTION
Rapid and extensive distribution to formed blood elements and to body tissues. Does not cross the blood-brain barrier. Extensively bound (about 80%) to plasma proteins. Peak plasma levels are achieved immediately.

METABOLISM
Extensive metabolism by the liver microsomal P450 system. Both active (epirubicinol) and inactive metabolites are formed in the liver, and elimination is mainly through the hepatobiliary route. Renal clearance accounts for only 20% of drug elimination. The half-life is approximately 30–38 hours for the parent compound and 20–31 hours for the epirubicinol metabolite.

INDICATIONS

1. Breast cancer—FDA-approved as part of adjuvant therapy in women with axillary node involvement following resection of primary breast cancer.
2. Metastatic breast cancer.
3. Gastric cancer—Active in the treatment of metastatic disease as well as early-stage disease.

DOSAGE RANGE

1. Recommended dose is 100–120 mg/m^2 IV every 3 weeks.
2. In heavily pretreated patients, consider starting at lower dose of 75–90 mg/m^2 IV every 3 weeks.
3. Alternative schedule is 12–25 mg/m^2 IV on a weekly basis.

DRUG INTERACTION 1

Heparin—Epirubicin is incompatible with heparin as a precipitate will form.

DRUG INTERACTION 2

5-FU, cyclophosphamide—Increased risk of myelosuppression when epirubicin is used in combination with 5-FU and cyclophosphamide.

DRUG INTERACTION 3

Cimetidine—Cimetidine decreases the AUC of epirubicin by 50% and should be discontinued upon initiation of epirubicin therapy.

SPECIAL CONSIDERATIONS

1. Use with caution in patients with abnormal liver function. Dose modification should be considered in patients with liver dysfunction.
2. Use with caution in patients with severe renal impairment. Dose should be reduced by at least 50% when serum creatinine >5 mg/dL.
3. Use with caution in elderly patients, as they are at increased risk for developing toxicity.
4. Careful monitoring of drug administration is necessary to avoid extravasation. If extravasation is suspected, stop infusion immediately, withdraw fluid, elevate arm, and apply ice to site. In severe cases, consult plastic surgeon.
5. Monitor cardiac function before (baseline) and periodically during therapy with either MUGA radionuclide scan or echocardiogram to assess LVEF. Risk of cardiac toxicity is higher in elderly patients >70 years of age, in patients with prior history of hypertension or pre-existing heart disease, in patients previously treated with anthracyclines, or in patients with prior radiation therapy to the chest. In patients with no prior history of anthracycline therapy, cumulative doses of 900 mg/m^2 are associated with increased risk for cardiac toxicity.
6. Continuous infusion and weekly schedules are associated with decreased risk of cardiac toxicity. Dexrazoxane may be helpful in preventing epirubicin-mediated cardiac toxicity.
7. Monitor weekly CBC while on therapy.

8. Use with caution in patients previously treated with radiation therapy, as epirubicin may induce a radiation-recall reaction.
9. Patients may experience red-orange discoloration of urine for 24 hours after drug administration.
10. Pregnancy category D. Breastfeeding should be avoided.

TOXICITY 1

Myelosuppression is dose-limiting toxicity with neutropenia more common than thrombocytopenia. Nadir typically occurs 8–14 days after treatment, with recovery of blood counts by day 21. Risk of myelosuppression greater in elderly patients and in those previously treated with chemotherapy and/or radiation therapy.

TOXICITY 2

Mild nausea and vomiting. Occur less frequently than with doxorubicin.

TOXICITY 3

Mucositis and diarrhea. Dose-dependent, common, and generally mild.

TOXICITY 4

Cardiac toxicity. Cardiac effects are similar to but less severe than those of doxorubicin. Acute toxicity presents as rhythm or conduction disturbances, chest pain, and myopericarditis syndrome that typically occurs within the first 24–48 hours of drug administration. Transient and mostly asymptomatic, not dose-related.

Chronic form of cardiac toxicity presents as a dilated cardiomyopathy with congestive heart failure. Risk of congestive heart failure increases significantly with cumulative doses >900 mg/m^2.

TOXICITY 5

Alopecia occurs within 10 days of initiation of therapy and regrowth of hair upon termination of treatment. Less commonly observed than with doxorubicin and occurs in only 25%–50% of patients.

TOXICITY 6

Potent vesicant. Extravasation can lead to tissue injury, inflammation, and chemical thrombophlebitis at the site of injection.

TOXICITY 7

Skin rash, flushing, hyperpigmentation of skin and nails, and photosensitivity. Radiation-recall skin reaction can occur at previous sites of irradiation.

TOXICITY 8

Red-orange discoloration of urine for 24 hours after drug administration.

Erdafitinib

TRADE NAME	Balversa	**CLASSIFICATION**	Signal transduction inhibitor, FGFR inhibitor
CATEGORY	Targeted agent	**DRUG MANUFACTURER**	Astex and Janssen

MECHANISM OF ACTION
- Pan-fibroblast growth factor receptor (FGFR) inhibitor that targets FGFR1, FGFR2, FGFR3, and FGFR4. Leads to inhibition of FGFR-mediated signaling, which involves tumor cell growth, proliferation, migration, angiogenesis, and survival.
- Broad-spectrum activity against a wide range of solid tumors, including cholangiocarcinoma, hepatocellular cancer, non–small cell lung cancer, prostate cancer, and esophageal cancer.

MECHANISM OF RESISTANCE
- Mutations in gatekeeper residues in FGFR, such as FGFR1 V561M and FGFR2 V565I.
- Mutations in the FGFR4 kinase domain including V550L, V550M, and V550E.
- Upregulation of ERB-B2, MET and ERK/MAPK signaling pathways.
- Activation of P4HA2 expression mediated by HIF-1α.

ABSORPTION
Oral bioavailability is modest at 34%. The median time to peak drug levels is 2.5 hours after ingestion.

DISTRIBUTION
Extensive binding (99.8%) of drug is bound to plasma proteins, mainly α-1-acid glycoprotein. Steady-state drug levels are achieved in approximately 2 weeks.

METABOLISM
Metabolized in the liver primarily by CYP2C9 and CYP3A4 microsomal enzymes. The relative contribution of CYP2C9 and CYP3A4 in the total clearance of erdafinitib is 39% and 20%, respectively. Approximately 69% of an administered dose is eliminated in feces, with 19% in the unchanged parent form, and 19% is eliminated in urine, with 13% as unchanged parent drug. Terminal half-life of erdafitinib is approximately 59 hours.

INDICATIONS

FDA-approved for patients with locally advanced or metastatic urothelial carcinoma that has an FGFR2 or FGFR3 genetic alteration and following progression from at least one line of prior platinum-containing chemotherapy, including within 12 months of neoadjuvant or adjuvant platinum-based chemotherapy.

DOSAGE RANGE

Recommended dose is 8 mg PO once daily with a dose increase to 9 mg PO daily if appropriate criteria are met.

DRUG INTERACTION 1

Drugs such as ketoconazole, itraconazole, erythromycin, clarithromycin, atazanavir, indinavir, nefazodone, nelfinavir, ritonavir, saquinavir, telithromycin, and voriconazole may decrease the metabolism of erdafitinib, resulting in increased drug levels and potentially increased toxicity.

DRUG INTERACTION 2

Phenytoin and other drugs that stimulate the liver microsomal CYP3A4 enzymes, including carbamazepine, rifampin, phenobarbital, and St. John's Wort—These drugs may increase the metabolism of erdafitinib, resulting in lower effective drug levels.

DRUG INTERACTION 3

Avoid concomitant use of agents that alter serum phosphate levels as erdafitinib increases serum phosphate levels. Such drugs include potassium phosphate supplements, vitamin D supplements, antacids, phosphate-containing enemas or laxatives, and drugs known to have phosphate as an excipient.

SPECIAL CONSIDERATIONS

1. Patients should be seen by a dietician and must have a restricted phosphate diet to 600–800 mg daily.
2. Closely monitor serum phosphate levels at 14–21 days after starting on therapy. The dose of erdafinitib can be increased to 9 mg once daily if the serum phosphate level is <5.5 mg/dL. Serum phosphate levels should then be monitored on a monthly basis. If the serum phosphate level is >7.0 mg/dL, an oral phosphate binder should be used until the serum phosphate levels returns to <5.5 mg/dL.
3. Monthly eye exams should be performed during the first 4 months of therapy and every 3 months thereafter. The eye exam should include visual acuity, slit lamp examination, fundoscopy, and optical coherence tomography.
4. Erdafitinib plasma concentrations are predicted to be 50% higher in patients with the CYP2C9*3/*3 genotype. Patients who are known or suspected to have the CYP2C9*3/*3 genotype should be closely monitored for increased toxicity. This pharmacogenetic syndrome is present in 0.4% to 3% of the population.

5. Erdafitinib should be withheld in the presence of central serious retinopathy (CSR) and retinal pigment epithelial detachment (RPED) and permanently discontinued if these ocular disorders do not resolve within 4 weeks or if grade 4 in severity.
6. Can cause fetal harm when administered to a pregnant woman. Females of reproductive potential should use effective contraception during drug therapy and for 1 month after the final dose. Breastfeeding should be avoided.

TOXICITY 1
Hyperphosphatemia.

TOXICITY 2
Ocular disorders with central serious retinopathy (CSR) and retinal pigment epithelial detachment (RPED) leading to visual field defects. Dry eye symptoms occur in nearly 30% of patients.

TOXICITY 3
Mucositis, diarrhea, dry mouth, nausea/vomiting, and abdominal pain.

TOXICITY 4
Fatigue and anorexia.

TOXICITY 5
Onycholysis, dry skin, palmar-plantar erythrodysesthesia, alopecia, nail dystrophy, and nail discoloration.

Eribulin

TRADE NAME	Halaven	CLASSIFICATION	Nontaxane, antimicrotubule agent
CATEGORY	Chemotherapy drug	DRUG MANUFACTURER	Eisai

MECHANISM OF ACTION

- Synthetic analog of halichondrin B, a product isolated from the marine sponge *Halichondria okadai*.
- Potent anti-microtubule agent, with a novel mechanism that is distinct from other known anti-microtubule agents.
- Cell cycle–specific, as it leads to a block in the G2-M phase of the cell cycle.
- Inhibits microtubule growth by sequestering tubulin in non-productive aggregates, with no effect on microtubule shortening.
- Maintains activity in various taxane-resistant tumor cell lines.

MECHANISM OF RESISTANCE

- Increased expression of ATP-binding cassette subfamily B member (ABCB1) and subfamily 11 (ABCC11).
- Activation of NF-κB signaling.
- Activation of PI3K signaling.

ABSORPTION

Administered only via the IV route.

DISTRIBUTION

Rapidly and extensively distributed with a mean volume of distribution of 43–114 L/m^2. Variable binding to plasma proteins that ranges from 49% to 65%.

METABOLISM

No major eribulin metabolites have been identified. Elimination occurs primarily via the hepatobiliary route as parent drug in feces (82%), with only a small amount of drug excreted in the urine (9%). The mean elimination half-life is approximately 40 hours.

INDICATIONS

1. FDA-approved for patients with metastatic breast cancer who have previously received at least two chemotherapeutic regimens for the treatment of metastatic disease. Prior therapy should have included an anthracycline and a taxane in either the adjuvant or metastatic setting.
2. FDA-approved for patients with unresectable or metastatic liposarcoma who have received a prior anthracycline-containing regimen.

DOSAGE RANGE

Recommended dose is 1.4 mg/m^2 IV on days 1 and 8 of a 21-day cycle.

DRUG INTERACTION

Drugs that are associated with QT prolongation—arsenic trioxide, astemizole, bepridil, certain phenothiazines (chlorpromazine, mesoridazine, and thioridazine), chloroquine, clarithromycin, Class IA antiarrhythmics (disopyramide, procainamide, quinidine), Class III antiarrhythmics (amiodarone, bretylium, dofetilide, ibutilide, sotalol), dextromethorphan, droperidol, erythromycin, grepafloxacin, halofantrine, haloperidol, methadone, pentamidine, posaconazole, saquinavir, sparfloxacin, terfenadine, and troleandomycin.

SPECIAL CONSIDERATIONS

1. Use with caution in patients with moderate renal impairment (CrCl 30–50 mL/min). In this setting, a lower starting dose of 1.1 mg/m^2 is recommended. The safety of this drug is not known in patients with severe renal impairment (CrCl <30 mL/min).
2. Use with caution in patients with mild hepatic impairment (Child-Pugh Class A). In this setting, a lower starting dose of 1.1 mg/m^2 is recommended. In patients with moderate hepatic impairment (Child-Pugh Class B), a dose of 0.7 mg/m^2 is recommended. Has not been studied in patients with severe hepatic impairment (Child-Pugh Class C).
3. Closely monitor CBCs on a periodic basis.
4. Monitor ECG with QTc measurement at baseline and periodically during therapy, as QTc prolongation has been observed. Use with caution in patients with a history of CHF, bradyarrhythmias, concomitant use of drugs that prolong QT interval, congenital QT syndrome, and electrolyte abnormalities (hypokalemia and hypomagnesemia).
5. Pregnancy category D. Breastfeeding should be avoided.

TOXICITY 1

Myelosuppression with dose-limiting neutropenia. Thrombocytopenia and anemia are observed at a much lower extent.

TOXICITY 2

Fatigue, asthenia, and anorexia.

TOXICITY 3

GI side effects in the form of nausea/vomiting, mucositis, diarrhea, dyspepsia, and dry mouth.

TOXICITY 4

Peripheral neuropathy.

TOXICITY 5

QTc prolongation occurs rarely.

Erlotinib

H₃C–SO₃H (methanesulfonic acid salt, as depicted: •H$_3$C–SO$_3$H)

TRADE NAME	Tarceva, OSI-774	CLASSIFICATION	Signal transduction inhibitor, EGFR inhibitor
CATEGORY	Targeted agent	DRUG MANUFACTURER	OSI, Genentech/ Roche

MECHANISM OF ACTION

- Potent and selective small-molecule inhibitor of the kinase activity of wild-type and certain activating mutations of epidermal growth factor receptor (EGFR), resulting in inhibition of EGFR autophosphorylation and inhibition of EGFR signaling.
- Inhibition of the EGFR tyrosine kinase results in inhibition of critical mitogenic and antiapoptotic signals involved in proliferation, growth, metastasis, angiogenesis, and response to chemotherapy and/or radiation therapy.
- Active in the absence or presence of EGFR-activating mutations, although activity appears to be higher in tumors that express EGFR-activating mutations.

MECHANISM OF RESISTANCE

- Mutations in the EGFR tyrosine kinase leading to decreased binding affinity to erlotinib.
- Presence of KRAS mutations.
- Presence of BRAF mutations.
- Activation/induction of alternative cellular signaling pathways such as PI3K/Akt and IGF-1R.
- Increased expression of HER2 through gene amplification.
- Increased expression of c-Met through gene amplification.
- Increased expression of NF-κB signaling pathway.

ABSORPTION
Oral bioavailability is approximately 60% and increased by food to almost 100%.

DISTRIBUTION
Extensive binding (90%) to plasma proteins, including albumin and a1-acid glycoprotein, and extensive tissue distribution. Peak plasma levels are achieved 4 hours after ingestion. Steady-state drug concentrations are reached in 7–8 days.

METABOLISM
Metabolism in the liver primarily by the CYP3A4 microsomal enzyme and by CYP1A2 to a lesser extent. Elimination is mainly hepatic, with excretion in the feces. Renal elimination of parent drug and its metabolites accounts for only about 8% of an administered dose. Following a 100-mg oral dose, 91% of the dose is recovered: 83% in feces (1% of the dose as intact parent) and 8% in urine (0.3% of the dose as intact parent). The terminal half-life of the parent drug is 36 hours.

INDICATIONS
1. FDA-approved as first-line treatment of metastatic NSCLC with EGFR exon 19 deletion or exon 21 (L858R) mutations.
2. FDA-approved in combination with ramucirumab for first-line treatment of metastatic NSCLC with EGFR exon 19 deletions or exon 21 (L858R) mutations.
3. FDA-approved as monotherapy for treatment of locally advanced or metastatic NSCLC after failure of at least one prior chemotherapy regimen.
4. FDA-approved as maintenance treatment of patients with locally advanced or metastatic NSCLC whose disease has not progressed after four cycles of platinum-based first-line chemotherapy.
5. FDA-approved in combination with gemcitabine for the first-line treatment of locally advanced unresectable or metastatic pancreatic cancer.

DOSAGE RANGE
1. NSCLC—Recommended dose is 150 mg/day PO. For elderly or frail patients, low-dose erlotinib at 50 mg/day may be considered.
2. Pancreatic cancer—Recommended dose is 100 mg/day PO in combination with gemcitabine.

DRUG INTERACTION 1
Phenytoin and other drugs that stimulate the liver microsomal CYP3A4 enzymes, including carbamazepine, rifampin, phenobarbital, and St. John's Wort—These drugs may increase the metabolism of erlotinib, resulting in its inactivation and lower effective drug levels.

DRUG INTERACTION 2
Drugs that inhibit the liver microsomal CYP3A4 enzymes, including ketoconazole, itraconazole, erythromycin, and clarithromycin—These drugs may decrease the metabolism of erlotinib, resulting in increased drug levels and potentially increased toxicity.

DRUG INTERACTION 3
Warfarin—Patients receiving warfarin should be closely monitored for alterations in their clotting parameters (PT and INR) and/or bleeding, as erlotinib may inhibit the metabolism of warfarin by the liver P450 system. Dose of warfarin may require careful adjustment in the presence of erlotinib therapy.

SPECIAL CONSIDERATIONS
1. Use with caution in patients with hepatic impairment. Dose reduction and/or interruption should be considered.
2. Has not been studied in the setting of renal impairment.
3. Nonsmokers and patients with EGFR-positive tumors are more sensitive to erlotinib therapy.
4. Erlotinib should not be used in combination with platinum-based chemotherapy, as there is no evidence of clinical benefit.
5. Closely monitor patients for new or progressive pulmonary symptoms, including cough, dyspnea, and fever. Erlotinib therapy should be interrupted pending further diagnostic evaluation.
6. Consider increasing the dose of erlotinib to 300 mg in patients with NSCLC who are actively smoking, as the metabolism of erlotinib by CYP1A1/1A2 in the liver is induced.
7. In patients who develop a skin rash, topical antibiotics such as clindamycin gel or erythromycin cream/gel or oral clindamycin, oral doxycycline, or oral minocycline may help.
8. Avoid Seville oranges, starfruit, pomelos, grapefruit products, and grapefruit juice while on erlotinib therapy.
9. Avoid the concomitant use of PPIs and H2-blockers, as they can reduce the oral bioavailability of erlotinib. If an H2-blocker must be used, erlotinib should be taken 10 hours after the H2-blocker and at least 2 hours before the next H2-blocker.
10. Pregnancy category D. Breastfeeding should be avoided.

TOXICITY 1
Pruritus, dry skin with mainly a pustular, acneiform skin rash occurring most often on face and upper trunk. Nail changes, paronychia, painful fissures or cracking of the skin on hands and feet, and hair growth abnormalities, including alopecia, thinning hair with increased fragility (trichorrhexis), darkening and increased thickness of eyelashes and eyebrows (trichomegaly), and hirsutism.

TOXICITY 2
Diarrhea is most common GI toxicity. Mild nausea/vomiting and mucositis.

TOXICITY 3
Pulmonary toxicity in the form of ILD manifested by increased cough, dyspnea, fever, and pulmonary infiltrates. Occurs rarely and observed in less than 1% of patients and more frequent in patients with underlying pulmonary disease.

TOXICITY 4
Mild-to-moderate elevations in serum transaminases. Usually transient and clinically asymptomatic.

TOXICITY 5
Anorexia.

TOXICITY 6
Conjunctivitis and keratitis. Rare cases of corneal perforation and ulceration.

TOXICITY 7
Rare episodes of GI hemorrhage.

TOXICITY 8
Radiation-recall skin reactions.

Estramustine

TRADE NAME	Estracyte, Emcyt	CLASSIFICATION	Antimicrotubule agent
CATEGORY	Chemotherapy drug	DRUG MANUFACTURER	Pfizer

MECHANISM OF ACTION
- Conjugate of nornitrogen mustard and estradiol phosphate.
- Cell cycle–specific agent with activity in the mitosis (M) phase.
- Initially designed to target cancer cells expressing estrogen receptors. However, active against estrogen receptor–negative tumor cells.
- This drug was initially designed as an alkylating agent, but it has no alkylating activity.
- Inhibits microtubule structure and function and the process of microtubule assembly by binding to microtubule-associated proteins (MAPs).

MECHANISM OF RESISTANCE
- Mechanisms of cellular resistance are different from those identified for other anti-microtubule agents.
- Estramustine-resistant cells do not express increased levels of P170 glycoprotein and are not cross-resistant to other anti-microtubule agents and/or natural products.
- Estramustine-resistant cells display increased efflux of drug with decreased drug accumulation. The underlying mechanism(s) remain(s) ill-defined.

ABSORPTION
Highly bioavailable via the oral route, with 70%–75% of an oral dose absorbed.

METABOLISM
Supplied as the estramustine phosphate form, which renders it more water-soluble. Rapidly dephosphorylated in the GI tract so that the dephosphorylated form predominates about 4 hours after ingestion. Metabolized primarily in the liver. About 15%–20% of the drug is excreted in urine. Only small amounts of unmetabolized drug are found. Biliary and fecal excretion of alkylating and estrogenic metabolites has also been demonstrated. Prolonged half-life of 20–24 hours.

INDICATIONS
Hormone-refractory, metastatic prostate cancer.

DOSAGE RANGE
1. Single agent: 14 mg/kg/day PO in 3–4 divided doses.
2. Combination: 600 mg/m^2/day PO days 1–42 every 8 weeks, as part of the estramustine/vinblastine regimen.

DRUG INTERACTIONS
None well characterized to date.

SPECIAL CONSIDERATIONS
1. Contraindicated in patients with active thrombophlebitis or thromboembolic disorders. Closely monitor patients with history of heart disease and/or stroke.
2. Contraindicated in patients with known hypersensitivity to estradiol or nitrogen mustard.
3. Contraindicated in patients with peptic ulcer disease, severe liver disease, or cardiac disease.
4. Instruct patients to take estramustine with water 1 hour before meals or 2 hours after meals to decrease the risk of GI upset.
5. Administer prophylactic antiemetics to avoid nausea and vomiting.
6. Instruct patients that milk, milk products, and calcium-rich foods may impair absorption of drug.

TOXICITY 1

Nausea and vomiting. Occur within 2 hours of ingestion. Usually mild and respond to antiemetic therapy. However, intractable vomiting may occur after prolonged therapy (6–8 weeks).

TOXICITY 2

Gynecomastia is reported in up to 50% of patients. Can be prevented by prophylactic breast irradiation.

TOXICITY 3

Diarrhea occurs in about 15%–25% of patients.

TOXICITY 4

Cardiovascular complications are rare and include congestive heart failure, cardiac ischemia, and thromboembolism.

TOXICITY 5

Myelosuppression is rare.

TOXICITY 6

Skin rash.

Etoposide

TRADE NAME	VePesid, VP-16	CLASSIFICATION	Epipodophyllotoxin, topoisomerase II inhibitor
CATEGORY	Chemotherapy drug	DRUG MANUFACTURER	Bristol-Myers Squibb

MECHANISM OF ACTION

- Plant alkaloid extracted from the *Podophyllum peltatum* mandrake plant.
- Cell cycle–specific agent with activity in the late S- and G2-phases.
- Inhibits topoisomerase II by stabilizing the topoisomerase II-DNA complex and preventing the unwinding of DNA.

MECHANISM OF RESISTANCE

- Multidrug-resistant phenotype with increased expression of P170 glycoprotein. Results in enhanced drug efflux and decreased intracellular accumulation of drug. Cross-resistant to vinca alkaloids, anthracyclines, taxanes, and other natural products.
- Decreased expression of topoisomerase II.
- Mutations in topoisomerase II with decreased binding affinity to drug.
- Enhanced activity of DNA repair enzymes.

ABSORPTION

Oral bioavailability is approximately 50%, requiring an oral dose to be twice that of an IV dose. However, oral bioavailability is non-linear and decreases with higher doses of drug (>200 mg). Food does not affect oral absorption.

DISTRIBUTION

Rapidly distributed into all body fluids and tissues. Large fraction of etoposide (90%–95%) is protein-bound, mainly to albumin. Decreased albumin levels result in a higher fraction of free drug and a potentially higher incidence of host toxicity.

METABOLISM

Metabolized primarily by the liver via glucuronidation to hydroxyacid metabolites, which are less active than the parent compound. About 30%–50% of etoposide is excreted in urine, and only 2%–6% is excreted in stool via hepatobiliary excretion. The elimination half-life ranges from 3 to 10 hours.

INDICATIONS

1. Germ cell tumors.
2. SCLC.
3. NSCLC.
4. Non-Hodgkin's lymphoma.
5. Hodgkin's lymphoma.
6. Gastric cancer.
7. High-dose therapy in transplant setting for various malignancies, including breast cancer, lymphoma, and ovarian cancer.

DOSAGE RANGE

1. Testicular cancer—As part of the PEB regimen, 100 mg/m^2 IV on days 1–5 with cycles repeated every 3 weeks.
2. SCLC—As part of cisplatin/VP-16 regimen, 100–120 mg/m^2 IV on days 1–3 with cycles repeated every 3 weeks.
3. SCLC—50 mg/m^2/day PO for 21 days.

DRUG INTERACTIONS

Warfarin—Etoposide may alter the anticoagulant effect of warfarin by prolonging the PT and INR. Coagulation parameters (PT and INR) need to be closely monitored, and dose of warfarin may require adjustment.

SPECIAL CONSIDERATIONS

1. Use with caution in patients with abnormal renal function. Dose reduction is recommended in patients with renal dysfunction. Baseline CrCl should be obtained, and renal status should be carefully monitored during therapy.
2. Use with caution in patients with abnormal liver function. Dose reduction is recommended in this setting.
3. Administer drug over a period of at least 30–60 minutes to avoid the risk of hypotension. Should the blood pressure drop, immediately discontinue the drug and administer IV fluids. Rate of administration must be reduced upon restarting therapy.
4. Carefully monitor for anaphylactic reactions. More commonly observed during the initial infusion of therapy and probably related to the polysorbate 80 vehicle in which the drug is formulated. In rare instances, such an allergic reaction can be fatal. The drug should be immediately stopped, and treatment with antihistamines, steroids, H2-blockers such as cimetidine, and pressor agents should be administered.
5. Closely monitor injection site for signs of phlebitis, and avoid extravasation.
6. Pregnancy category D. Breastfeeding should be avoided.

TOXICITY 1
Myelosuppression is dose-limiting, with neutropenia more common than thrombocytopenia. Nadir usually occurs 10–14 days after therapy, with recovery by day 21.

TOXICITY 2
Nausea and vomiting occur in about 30%–40% of patients and generally mild to moderate. More commonly observed with oral administration.

TOXICITY 3
Anorexia.

TOXICITY 4
Alopecia observed in nearly two-thirds of patients.

TOXICITY 5
Mucositis and diarrhea are unusual with standard doses but more often observed with high doses in transplant setting.

TOXICITY 6
Hypersensitivity reaction with chills, fever, bronchospasm, dyspnea, tachycardia, facial and tongue swelling, and hypotension. Occurs in less than 2% of patients.

TOXICITY 7
Metallic taste during infusion of drug.

TOXICITY 8
Local inflammatory reaction at injection site.

TOXICITY 9
Radiation-recall skin changes.

TOXICITY 10
Increased risk of secondary malignancies, especially acute myelogenous leukemia (M4, M5 subtype). Associated with 11:23 translocation. Usually develops within 2–3 years of treatment and in the absence of preceding myelodysplastic syndrome.

Etoposide phosphate

TRADE NAME	Etopophos	CLASSIFICATION	Epipodophyllotoxin, topoisomerase II inhibitor
CATEGORY	Chemotherapy drug	DRUG MANUFACTURER	Bristol-Myers Squibb

MECHANISM OF ACTION
- Water-soluble prodrug form of etoposide.
- Cell cycle–specific agent with activity in late S- and G2-phases.
- Must first be dephosphorylated for etoposide to be active.
- Once activated, it inhibits topoisomerase II by stabilizing the topoisomerase II–DNA complex and preventing the unwinding of DNA.

MECHANISM OF RESISTANCE
- Multidrug-resistant phenotype with increased expression of P170 glycoprotein. Results in enhanced drug efflux and decreased intracellular accumulation of drug.
- Decreased expression of topoisomerase II.
- Mutations in topoisomerase II with decreased binding affinity to drug.
- Enhanced activity of DNA repair enzymes.

ABSORPTION
Administered only via the IV route.

DISTRIBUTION
Rapidly distributed into all body fluids and tissues. Large fraction of drug (90%–95%) is protein-bound, mainly to albumin. Decreased albumin levels result in a higher fraction of free drug and a potentially higher incidence of toxicity.

METABOLISM
Rapidly and completely converted to etoposide in plasma, which is then metabolized primarily by the liver to hydroxyacid metabolites. These metabolites are less active than the parent compound. The elimination half-life of the drug ranges from 3 to 10 hours. About 15%–20% of the drug is excreted in urine and about 2%–6% is excreted in stool within 72 hours after IV administration.

INDICATIONS
1. Germ cell tumors.
2. SCLC.
3. NSCLC.

DOSAGE RANGE
1. Testicular cancer: 100 mg/m^2 IV on days 1–5 with cycles repeated every 3 weeks.
2. SCLC: 100 mg/m^2 IV on days 1–3 with cycles repeated every 3 weeks.

DRUG INTERACTIONS
Warfarin—Etoposide may alter the anticoagulant effect of warfarin by prolonging the PT and INR. Coagulation parameters need to be closely monitored, and dose of warfarin may require adjustment.

SPECIAL CONSIDERATIONS
1. Use with caution in patients with abnormal renal function. Dose reduction is recommended in this setting. Baseline CrCl should be obtained, and renal status should be closely monitored during therapy.
2. Use with caution in patients with abnormal liver function. Dose reduction is recommended in this setting.
3. Administer drug over a period of at least 30–60 minutes to avoid the risk of hypotension. Should the blood pressure drop, immediately discontinue the drug and administer IV fluids. The rate of administration must be reduced upon restarting therapy.

4. Carefully monitor for anaphylactic reactions. Occur more frequently during the initial infusion of therapy. In rare instances, such an allergic reaction can be fatal. The drug should be immediately stopped, and treatment with antihistamines, steroids, H2-blockers such as cimetidine, and pressor agents should be administered.
5. Closely monitor injection site for signs of phlebitis. Carefully avoid extravasation.
6. Pregnancy category D. Breastfeeding should be avoided.

TOXICITY 1
Myelosuppression is dose-limiting, with neutropenia more common than thrombocytopenia. Nadir usually occurs 10–14 days after therapy, with recovery by day 21.

TOXICITY 2
Nausea and vomiting occur in about 30%–40% of patients and generally mild to moderate.

TOXICITY 3
Anorexia.

TOXICITY 4
Alopecia.

TOXICITY 5
Mucositis and diarrhea are only occasionally seen.

TOXICITY 6
Hypersensitivity reaction with chills, fever, bronchospasm, dyspnea, tachycardia, facial and tongue swelling, and hypotension.

TOXICITY 7
Metallic taste during infusion of drug.

TOXICITY 8
Local inflammatory reaction at the injection site.

TOXICITY 9
Radiation-recall skin changes.

TOXICITY 10
Increased risk of secondary malignancies, especially acute myelogenous leukemia (M4, M5 subtype). Associated with 11:23 translocation. Typically develops within 2–3 years of treatment and in the absence of preceding myelodysplastic syndrome.

Everolimus

OCH$_2$
OO
OH
H$_3$C
O
OH
O
O
O
O
O
H$_3$CO
OCH$_3$
OPO$_3$H$_2$

TRADE NAME	Afinitor, RAD001	**CLASSIFICATION**	Signal transduction inhibitor, mTOR inhibitor
CATEGORY	Targeted agent	**DRUG MANUFACTURER**	Novartis

MECHANISM OF ACTION
- Potent inhibitor of the mammalian target of rapamycin (mTOR), a serine-threonine kinase that is a key component of cellular signaling pathways involved in the growth and proliferation of tumor cells.
- Inhibitor of hypoxia-inducible factor (HIF-1), which leads to reduced expression of VEGF.
- Inhibition of mTOR signaling results in cell cycle arrest, induction of apoptosis, and inhibition of angiogenesis.

MECHANISM OF RESISTANCE
- Increased expression of cell cycle–activating proteins cdk2 and cyclin A.
- Increased expression of cell cycle–activating proteins cdk1 and cyclin B.
- Activation of EIF4E by aurora kinase A.
- Increased expression/activation of mTORC2/Akt signaling.
- Increased expression/activation of ERK and STAT3 signaling.

ABSORPTION
Peak drug levels are achieved 1–2 hours after oral administration. Food with a high fat content reduces oral bioavailability by up to 20%.

DISTRIBUTION
Significant binding (up to 75%) to plasma proteins. Steady-state drug concentrations are reached within 2 weeks after once-daily dosing.

METABOLISM

Metabolism in the liver primarily by CYP3A4 microsomal enzymes. Six main metabolites have been identified, including 3 monohydroxylated metabolites, 2 hydrolytic ring-opened products, and a phosphatidylcholine conjugate of everolimus. These metabolites are significantly less active than the parent compound. Elimination is mainly via the hepatobiliary route, with excretion in feces, and renal elimination of parent drug and its metabolites accounts for only 5% of an administered dose. The terminal half-life of the parent drug is 30 hours.

INDICATIONS

1. FDA-approved for the treatment of advanced renal cell cancer after failure on sunitinib or sorafenib.
2. FDA-approved in combination with lenvatinib for the treatment of advanced renal cell cancer following one prior anti-angiogenic therapy.
3. FDA-approved for advanced pancreatic neuroendocrine tumors (PNETs) and for progressive, well-differentiated, non-functional neuroendocrine tumors (NETs) of GI or lung origin that are unresectable, locally advanced, or metastatic. This agent is not indicated for the treatment of functional carcinoid tumors.
4. FDA-approved for patients with renal angiomyolipoma and tuberous sclerosis complex (TSC) not requiring surgery.
5. FDA-approved for subependymal giant cell astrocytoma associated with TSC patients who require treatment but are not candidates for curative surgery.
6. FDA-approved for TSC-associated partial-onset seizure patients aged 2 years and older.
7. FDA-approved in combination with exemestane for postmenopausal women with advanced hormone receptor (HR)–positive, HER2-negative breast cancer with recurrent or progressive disease after failure of treatment with either letrozole or anastrozole.

DOSAGE RANGE

Recommended dose for advanced breast cancer, NET, and renal cell cancer is 10 mg PO once daily.

DRUG INTERACTION 1

Phenytoin and other drugs that induce liver microsomal CYP3A4 enzymes, including carbamazepine, rifampin, phenobarbital, dexamethasone, and St. John's Wort—These drugs may increase the metabolism of everolimus, resulting in its inactivation and lower effective drug levels.

DRUG INTERACTION 2

Drugs that inhibit liver microsomal CYP3A4 enzymes, including ketoconazole, itraconazole, fluconazole, verapamil or diltiazem, erythromycin, and clarithromycin—These drugs may decrease the metabolism of everolimus, resulting in increased drug levels and potentially increased toxicity.

SPECIAL CONSIDERATIONS

1. Everolimus should be taken once daily at the same time with or without food. The tablets should be swallowed whole with a glass of water and never chewed or crushed.
2. Use with caution in patients with moderate liver impairment (Child-Pugh Class B), and dose should be reduced to 5 mg daily. Should not be used in patients with severe liver impairment (Child-Pugh Class C).
3. Consider increasing dose in 5-mg increments up to a maximum of 20 mg once daily if used in combination with drugs that are strong inducers of CYP3A4.
4. Closely monitor patients for new or progressive pulmonary symptoms, including cough, dyspnea, and fever. Non-infectious pneumonitis is a class effect of rapamycin analogs, and everolimus therapy should be interrupted pending further diagnostic evaluation.
5. Patients are at increased risk for developing opportunistic infections, such as pneumonia, other bacterial infections, and invasive fungal infections.
6. Monitor serum glucose levels in all patients, especially those with diabetes mellitus.
7. Monitor serum triglyceride and cholesterol levels while on therapy.
8. Avoid alcohol or mouthwashes containing peroxide in the setting of oral ulcerations, as they may worsen the condition.
9. Avoid grapefruit products while on everolimus, as they can result in a significant increase in drug levels.
10. Avoid the use of live vaccines and/or close contact with those who have received live vaccines while on everolimus.
11. Pregnancy category D. Breastfeeding should be avoided.

TOXICITY 1
Asthenia and fatigue.

TOXICITY 2
Mucositis, oral ulcerations, and diarrhea.

TOXICITY 3
Nausea/vomiting and anorexia.

TOXICITY 4
Increased risk of opportunistic infections, such as pneumonia, other bacterial infections, and invasive fungal infections.

TOXICITY 5
Pulmonary toxicity in the form of increased cough, dyspnea, fever, and pulmonary infiltrates.

TOXICITY 6
Skin rash.

TOXICITY 7
Myelosuppression with anemia, thrombocytopenia, and neutropenia.

TOXICITY 8
Hyperlipidemia with increased serum triglycerides and/or cholesterol in up to 70%–75% of patients.

TOXICITY 9
Hyperglycemia in up to 50% of patients.

TOXICITY 10
Mild liver toxicity with elevation in serum transaminases and alkaline phosphatase.

Exemestane

TRADE NAME	Aromasin	CLASSIFICATION	Steroidal aromatase inhibitor
CATEGORY	Hormonal agent	DRUG MANUFACTURER	Pfizer

MECHANISM OF ACTION
- Permanently binds to and irreversibly inactivates aromatase.
- Inhibits the synthesis of estrogens by inhibiting the conversion of adrenal androgens (androstenedione and testosterone) to estrogens (estrone, estrone sulfate, and estradiol).
- No inhibitory effect on adrenal corticosteroid or aldosterone biosynthesis.

MECHANISM OF RESISTANCE

- Some degree of cross-resistance exists between exemestane and nonsteroidal aromatase inhibitors.
- Activation of growth factor signaling pathways, specifically HER2 and IGF1-R, with cross-talk with the ER signaling pathway, resulting in activation of PI3K/Akt and various MAPKs.
- Increased expression and activation of the NF-κB signaling pathway.
- Increased expression of Nrf2 as a result of lower ubiquitination/degradation.

ABSORPTION

Excellent bioavailability via the oral route, with 85% of a dose absorbed within 2 hours of ingestion. Absorption is not affected by food.

DISTRIBUTION

Widely distributed throughout the body. About 90% of drug is bound to plasma proteins. Steady-state levels of drug are achieved after 7 days of a once-daily administration.

METABOLISM

Extensively metabolized in the liver by CYP3A4 enzymes (up to 85%) to inactive forms. The major route of elimination is hepatobiliary, with excretion in feces, with renal excretion accounting for only 10% of drug clearance. The half-life of drug is about 24 hours.

INDICATIONS

Treatment of advanced breast cancer in postmenopausal women whose disease has progressed following tamoxifen therapy.

DOSAGE RANGE

Recommended dose is 25 mg PO once daily after a meal.

DRUG INTERACTION 1

Phenytoin and other drugs that stimulate the liver microsomal CYP3A4 enzymes, including carbamazepine, rifampin, phenobarbital, and St. John's Wort—These drugs may increase the metabolism of exemestane, resulting in its inactivation and lower effective drug levels.

DRUG INTERACTION 2

Drugs that inhibit the liver microsomal CYP3A4 enzymes, including ketoconazole, itraconazole, erythromycin, and clarithromycin—These drugs may decrease the metabolism of exemestane, resulting in increased drug levels and potentially increased toxicity.

SPECIAL CONSIDERATIONS

1. No dose adjustments are required for patients with either hepatic or renal dysfunction.
2. Should not be administered to premenopausal women.

3. Should not be administered with estrogen-containing agents, as they may interfere with antitumor activity.
4. Caution patients about the risk of hot flashes.
5. No need for glucocorticoid and/or mineralocorticoid replacement.
6. Pregnancy category D. Breastfeeding should be avoided.

TOXICITY 1
Hot flashes.

TOXICITY 2
Mild nausea.

TOXICITY 3
Fatigue.

TOXICITY 4
Headache.

TOXICITY 5
Musculoskeletal symptoms including carpal tunnel syndrome.

Floxuridine

TRADE NAME	5-Fluoro-2'-deoxyuridine, FUDR	CLASSIFICATION	Antimetabolite, fluropyrimidine
CATEGORY	Chemotherapy drug	DRUG MANUFACTURER	Roche, Mayne Pharma

MECHANISM OF ACTION
- Fluoropyrimidine deoxynucleoside analog.
- Cell cycle–specific with activity in the S-phase.
- Requires transport into the cell via a nucleoside transport protein.
- Requires activation to cytotoxic metabolite forms. Metabolized to 5-FU metabolite FdUMP, which inhibits thymidylate synthase (TS). This results in inhibition of DNA synthesis, function, and repair.
- Incorporation of 5-FU metabolite FUTP into RNA, resulting in alterations in RNA processing and/or mRNA translation.
- Incorporation of 5-FU metabolite FdUTP into DNA, resulting in inhibition of DNA synthesis and function.
- Inhibition of TS leads to accumulation of dUMP, which becomes misincorporated into DNA in the form of dUTP, resulting in inhibition of DNA synthesis and function.

MECHANISM OF RESISTANCE
- Increased expression of thymidylate synthase.
- Decreased levels of reduced folate substrate 5, 10-methylenetetrahydrofolate.
- Decreased incorporation of 5-FU into RNA.
- Decreased incorporation of 5-FU into DNA.
- Increased activity of DNA repair enzymes, uracil glycosylase and dUTPase.
- Increased salvage of physiologic nucleosides, including thymidine.
- Increased expression of dihydropyrimidine dehydrogenase.
- Decreased expression of mismatch repair enzymes (hMLH1, hMSH2).
- Alterations in TS, with decreased binding affinity of enzyme for FdUMP.

ABSORPTION
Administered only via the IV and intra-arterial (IA) routes.

DISTRIBUTION
After IV administration, floxuridine is rapidly extracted by the liver via first-pass metabolism. After hepatic IA administration, greater than 90% of drug is extracted by hepatocytes. Binding to plasma proteins has not been well characterized.

METABOLISM
Undergoes extensive enzymatic metabolism in the liver to 5-FU and 5-FU metabolites. Catabolism accounts for >85% of drug metabolism, which is mediated by dihydropyrimidine dehydrogenase (DPD). DPD is present in liver and extrahepatic tissues, including GI mucosa, WBCs, and the kidneys. About 30% of an administered dose of drug is cleared in urine, mainly as inactive metabolites. The terminal elimination half-life is 20 hours.

INDICATIONS
1. Metastatic colorectal cancer—Intrahepatic arterial treatment of colorectal cancer metastatic to the liver.
2. Metastatic GI adenocarcinoma—Patients with metastatic disease confined to the liver.

DOSAGE RANGE
Recommended dose is 0.1–0.6 mg/kg/day IA for 7–14 days via hepatic artery.

DRUG INTERACTION 1
Leucovorin—Leucovorin enhances the toxicity and antitumor activity of floxuridine. Stabilizes the TS-FdUMP-reduced folate ternary complex, resulting in maximal inhibition of TS.

DRUG INTERACTION 2
Thymidine—Rescues against the toxic effects of floxuridine.

DRUG INTERACTION 3
Vistonuridine (PN401)—Rescues against the toxic effects of floxuridine.

SPECIAL CONSIDERATIONS
1. Contraindicated in patients with poor nutritional status, depressed bone marrow function, or potentially serious infection.
2. No dose adjustments are necessary in patients with mild and moderate liver dysfunction or abnormal renal function. However, patients should be closely monitored, as they may be at increased risk of toxicity.

3. Patients should be placed on an H2-blocker, such as ranitidine 150 mg PO bid, to prevent the onset of peptic ulcer disease while on therapy. Onset of ulcer-like pain is an indication to stop therapy, as hemorrhage and/or perforation may occur.
4. Patients who experience unexpected, severe grades 3 or 4 toxicities with initiation of therapy may have an underlying deficiency in dihydropyrimidine dehydrogenase (DPD). Therapy must be discontinued immediately. Further testing to identify the presence of this pharmacogenetic syndrome should be considered.
5. Pregnancy category D. Breastfeeding should be avoided.

TOXICITY 1
Hepatotoxicity is dose-limiting. Presents as abdominal pain and elevated alkaline phosphatase, liver transaminases, and bilirubin. Sclerosing cholangitis is a rare event. Other GI toxicities include duodenitis, duodenal ulcer, and gastritis.

TOXICITY 2
Nausea and vomiting are mild. Mucositis and diarrhea also observed.

TOXICITY 3
Hand-foot syndrome (palmar-plantar erythrodysesthesia). Characterized by tingling, numbness, pain, erythema, dryness, rash, swelling, increased pigmentation, and/or pruritus of the hands and feet.

TOXICITY 4
Myelosuppression. Nadir occurs at 7–10 days, with full recovery by 14–17 days.

TOXICITY 5
Neurologic toxicity manifested by somnolence, confusion, seizures, cerebellar ataxia, and rarely encephalopathy.

TOXICITY 6
Cardiac symptoms of chest pain, ECG changes, and serum enzyme elevation. Rare event but increased risk in patients with prior history of ischemic heart disease.

TOXICITY 7
Blepharitis, tear-duct stenosis, acute and chronic conjunctivitis.

TOXICITY 8
Catheter-related complications include leakage, catheter occlusion, perforation, dislodgement, infection, bleeding at catheter site, and thrombosis and/or embolism of hepatic artery.

F

Fludarabine

TRADE NAME	2-Fluoro-ara-AMP, Fludara	CLASSIFICATION	Antimetabolite, fluoropyrimidine
CATEGORY	Chemotherapy drug	DRUG MANUFACTURER	Sagent Pharmaceuticals and Antisoma (oral form)

MECHANISM OF ACTION
- 5'-Monophosphate analog of arabinofuranosyladenosine (F-ara-A) with high specificity for lymphoid cells. Presence of the 2-fluoro group on adenine ring renders fludarabine resistant to breakdown by adenosine deaminase.
- Considered a prodrug and inactive in its parent form. Following administration, it is rapidly dephosphorylated to 2-fluoro-ara-adenosine (F-ara-A). F-ara-A enters cells via a nucleoside transport system and is then phosphorylated first to its monophosphate form and eventually to the active 5'-triphosphate metabolite (F-ara-ATP).
- Antitumor activity against both dividing and resting cells.
- Triphosphate metabolite incorporates into DNA, resulting in inhibition of DNA chain extension.
- Inhibition of ribonucleotide reductase by fludarabine triphosphate.
- Inhibition of DNA polymerase-α and DNA polymerase-β by the triphosphate metabolite, resulting in inhibition of DNA synthesis and DNA repair.
- Induction of apoptosis (programmed cell death).

MECHANISM OF RESISTANCE
- Decreased expression of the activating enzyme, deoxycytidine kinase.
- Decreased nucleoside transport of drug into cells.

ABSORPTION
Orally bioavailable, in the range of 50%–65%, and an oral tablet form is available. Absorption is not affected by food.

DISTRIBUTION
Widely distributed throughout the body. Concentrates in high levels in liver, kidney, and spleen. Binding to plasma proteins has not been well characterized.

METABOLISM
Rapidly converted to 2-fluoro-ara-A, which enters cells via the nucleoside transport system and is rephosphorylated by deoxycytidine kinase to fludarabine monophosphate. This metabolite undergoes two subsequent phosphorylation steps to yield fludarabine triphosphate, the active species. Major route of elimination is via the kidneys, and approximately 25% of 2-fluoro-ara-A is excreted unchanged in urine. The terminal half-life is on the order of 10–20 hours.

INDICATIONS
1. Chronic lymphocytic leukemia (CLL).
2. Non-Hodgkin's lymphoma (low-grade).
3. Cutaneous T-cell lymphoma.

DOSAGE RANGE
1. Recommended dose is 25 mg/m² IV on days 1–5 every 28 days.
2. For oral usage, the recommended dose is 40 mg/m² PO on days 1–5 every 28 days.

DRUG INTERACTION 1
Cytarabine—Fludarabine may enhance the antitumor activity of cytarabine by inducing the expression of deoxycytidine kinase.

DRUG INTERACTION 2
Cyclophosphamide, cisplatin, mitoxantrone—Fludarabine may enhance the antitumor activity of cyclophosphamide, cisplatin, and mitoxantrone by inhibiting nucleotide excision repair mechanisms.

SPECIAL CONSIDERATIONS
1. Use with caution in patients with abnormal renal function. Dose reduction is not required for CrCl >80 mL/min. For CrCl between 50 and 79 mL/min, the dose should be reduced to 20 mg/m², and for CrCl between 30 and 49 mL/min, the dose should be reduced to 15 mg/m². Fludarabine should not be administered to patients with CrCl <30 mL/min.
2. Use with caution in elderly patients and in those with bone marrow impairment, as they are at increased risk of toxicity.
3. Monitor for signs of infection. Patients are at increased risk for opportunistic infections, including herpes, fungi, and PJP. Patients should be empirically placed on trimethoprim/sulfamethoxazole prophylaxis, 1 DS tablet PO bid 3 times/week.
4. Monitor for signs of tumor lysis syndrome, especially in patients with a high tumor cell burden. May occur as early as within the first week of treatment.

5. Allopurinol may be given prior to initiation of fludarabine therapy to prevent hyperuricemia.
6. Use irradiated blood products in patients requiring transfusions, as transfusion-associated graft-versus-host disease can occur rarely after transfusion of non-irradiated products in patients treated with fludarabine.
7. Used as part of an immunosuppressive lymphodepletion conditioning regimen with cyclophosphamide in adoptive immunotherapy and chimeric antigen receptor (CAR) T-cell therapy.
8. Pregnancy category D. Breastfeeding should be avoided.

TOXICITY 1
Myelosuppression is dose-limiting. Neutrophil nadir occurs in 10–13 days, with recovery by day 14–21. Autoimmune hemolytic anemia and drug-induced aplastic anemia can also occur.

TOXICITY 2
Immunosuppression. Decrease in CD4 and CD8 T cells occurs in most patients. Increased risk of opportunistic infections, including fungus, herpes, and PJP. Recovery of CD4 count is slow and may take over a year to return to normal.

TOXICITY 3
Nausea and vomiting are usually mild.

TOXICITY 4
Fever occurs in 20%–30% of patients. Most likely due to release of pyrogens and/or cytokines from tumor cells. Associated with fatigue, malaise, myalgias, arthralgias, and chills.

TOXICITY 5
Hypersensitivity reaction with maculopapular skin rash, erythema, and pruritus.

TOXICITY 6
Tumor lysis syndrome. Rarely seen (in less than 1%–2% of patients) and most often in the setting of high tumor-cell burden.

TOXICITY 7
Transient elevation in serum transaminases. Clinically asymptomatic.

5-Fluorouracil

TRADE NAME	5-FU, Efudex	CLASSIFICATION	Antimetabolite, fluoropyrimidine
CATEGORY	Chemotherapy drug	DRUG MANUFACTURER	Roche

MECHANISM OF ACTION

- Fluoropyrimidine analog.
- Cell cycle–specific with activity in the S-phase.
- Inactive in its parent form and requires activation to cytotoxic metabolite forms.
- Inhibition of the target enzyme thymidylate synthase (TS) by the 5-FU metabolite, FdUMP.
- Incorporation of the 5-FU metabolite FUTP into RNA, resulting in alterations in RNA processing and/or mRNA translation.
- Incorporation of the 5-FU metabolite FdUTP into DNA, resulting in inhibition of DNA synthesis and function.
- Inhibition of TS leads to accumulation of dUMP, which then gets misincorporated into DNA in the form of dUTP, resulting in inhibition of DNA synthesis and function.

MECHANISM OF RESISTANCE

- Increased expression of thymidylate synthase (TS).
- Decreased levels of reduced folate substrate 5, 10-methylenetetrahydrofolate for TS reaction.
- Decreased incorporation of 5-FU into RNA.
- Decreased incorporation of 5-FU into DNA.
- Increased activity of DNA repair enzymes, uracil glycosylase and dUTPase.
- Increased salvage of physiologic nucleosides, including thymidine.
- Increased expression of dihydropyrimidine dehydrogenase (DPD).
- Decreased expression of mismatch repair enzymes (hMLH1, hMSH2).
- Alterations in TS, with decreased binding affinity of enzyme for FdUMP.

ABSORPTION

Administered only via the IV route.

DISTRIBUTION

After IV administration, 5-FU is widely distributed to tissues, with highest concentration in GI mucosa, bone marrow, and liver. Penetrates into third-space fluid collections such as ascites and pleural effusions. Crosses the blood-brain barrier and distributes into CSF and brain tissue. Binding to plasma proteins has not been well characterized.

METABOLISM

Undergoes extensive enzymatic metabolism intracellularly to cytotoxic metabolites. Catabolism accounts for >85% of drug metabolism. DPD is the main enzyme responsible for 5-FU catabolism, and it is highly expressed in liver and extrahepatic tissues such as GI mucosa, WBCs, and kidney. Greater than 90% of an administered dose of drug is cleared in urine and lungs. The terminal elimination half-life is short, ranging from 10 to 20 min.

INDICATIONS

1. Colorectal cancer—Adjuvant setting and advanced disease.
2. Breast cancer—Adjuvant setting and advanced disease.
3. GI malignancies, including anal, esophageal, gastric, and pancreatic cancer.
4. Head and neck cancer.
5. Hepatoma.
6. Ovarian cancer.
7. Topical use in basal cell cancer of skin and actinic keratoses.

DOSAGE RANGE

1. Bolus monthly schedule: 425–450 mg/m^2 IV on days 1–5 every 28 days.
2. Bolus weekly schedule: 500–600 mg/m^2 IV every week for 6 weeks every 8 weeks.
3. 24-hour infusion: 2,400–2,600 mg/m^2 IV every week.
4. 96-hour infusion: 800–1,000 mg/m^2/day IV.
5. 120-hour infusion: 1,000 mg/m^2/day IV on days 1–5 every 21–28 days.
6. Protracted continuous infusion: 200–400 mg/m^2/day IV.

DRUG INTERACTION 1

Leucovorin—Leucovorin enhances the antitumor activity and toxicity of 5-FU. Stabilizes the TS-FdUMP-reduced folate ternary complex, resulting in maximal inhibition of TS.

DRUG INTERACTION 2

Methotrexate, trimetrexate—Antifolate analogs increase the formation of 5-FU nucleotide metabolites when given 24 hours before 5-FU.

DRUG INTERACTION 3

Thymidine—Rescues against the TS- and DNA-mediated toxic effects of 5-FU.

DRUG INTERACTION 4

Vistonuridine (uridine triacetate)—Rescues against the toxic effects of 5-FU.

SPECIAL CONSIDERATIONS

1. No dose adjustments are necessary in patients with mild to moderate liver or renal dysfunction. However, patients should be closely monitored, as they may be at increased risk for toxicity.
2. Contraindicated in patients with bone marrow depression, poor nutritional status, infection, active ischemic heart disease, or history of myocardial infarction within previous 6 months.
3. Patients should be monitored closely for mucositis and/or diarrhea, as there is increased potential for dehydration, fluid imbalance, and infection. Elderly patients are at especially high risk for GI toxicity.
4. Patients who experience unexpected, severe grades 3 or 4 myelosuppression, GI toxicity, and/or neurologic toxicity with initiation of therapy may have an underlying deficiency in DPD. Therapy must be discontinued immediately. Further testing to identify the presence of this pharmacogenetic syndrome (autosomal recessive) should be considered.
5. Vistonuridine, at a dose of 10 g PO every 6 hours for 20 doses, may be used in patients who have been overdosed with 5-FU or in those who experience severe toxicity.
6. Vitamin B6 (pyridoxine 50 mg PO bid), celecoxib (200 mg PO bid), and nicotine patch may be used to prevent and/or reduce the incidence and severity of hand-foot syndrome.
7. Use of ice chips in mouth 10–15 minutes pre- and 10–15 minutes post-IV bolus injections of 5-FU may reduce the incidence and severity of mucositis.
8. Pregnancy category D. Breastfeeding should be avoided.

TOXICITY 1

Myelosuppression. Dose-limiting for the bolus schedules and less frequently observed with infusional therapy. Neutropenia and thrombocytopenia more common than anemia.

TOXICITY 2

Mucositis and/or diarrhea. May be severe and dose-limiting for infusional schedules. Nausea and vomiting are mild and rare.

TOXICITY 3

Hand-foot syndrome (palmar-plantar erythrodysesthesia). Characterized by tingling, numbness, pain, erythema, dryness, rash, swelling, increased pigmentation, nail changes, pruritus of the hands and feet, and/or desquamation. Most often observed with infusional therapy and can be dose-limiting.

TOXICITY 4

Neurologic toxicity manifested by somnolence, confusion, altered mental status, seizures, cerebellar ataxia, and rarely encephalopathy.

TOXICITY 5

Cardiac symptoms of chest pain, ECG changes, and serum enzyme elevation. Rare event but increased risk in patients with prior history of ischemic heart disease.

TOXICITY 6

Blepharitis, tear-duct stenosis, acute and chronic conjunctivitis.

TOXICITY 7

Dry skin, photosensitivity, and pigmentation of the infused vein are common.

TOXICITY 8

Metallic taste in mouth during IV bolus injection.

Flutamide

TRADE NAME	Eulexin	CLASSIFICATION	Antiandrogen
CATEGORY	Hormonal agent	DRUG MANUFACTURER	Schering, Taj Pharmaceuticals

MECHANISM OF ACTION

Nonsteroidal, antiandrogen agent binds to androgen receptor and inhibits androgen uptake as well as inhibiting androgen binding in nucleus in androgen-sensitive prostate cancer cells.

MECHANISM OF RESISTANCE

- Decreased expression of androgen receptor.
- Mutation in androgen receptor, leading to decreased binding affinity to flutamide.

ABSORPTION

Rapidly and completely absorbed by the GI tract. Peak plasma levels observed 1–2 hours after oral administration.

DISTRIBUTION

Distribution is not well characterized. Flutamide and its metabolites are extensively bound to plasma proteins (92%–96%).

METABOLISM

Extensive metabolism by the liver cytochrome P450 system to both active and inactive metabolites. The main metabolite, α-hydroxyflutamide, is biologically active. Flutamide and its metabolites are cleared primarily in urine, and only 4% of drug is eliminated in feces. The elimination half-life of flutamide is about 8 hours, whereas the half-life of the α-hydroxyflutamide metabolite is 8–10 hours.

INDICATIONS

1. Locally confined stage B2–C prostate cancer.
2. Stage D2 metastatic prostate cancer.

DOSAGE RANGE

Recommended dose is 250 mg PO tid at 8-hour intervals.

DRUG INTERACTIONS

Warfarin—Flutamide can inhibit metabolism of warfarin by the liver P450 system, leading to increased anticoagulant effect. Coagulation parameters (PT and INR) must be followed closely when warfarin and flutamide are taken concurrently, and dose adjustments may be needed.

SPECIAL CONSIDERATIONS

1. Monitor LFTs at baseline and during therapy. In the presence of elevated serum transaminases to 2–3 × ULN, therapy should be terminated.
2. Caution patients about the risk of diarrhea, and if severe, flutamide may need to be stopped.
3. Caution patients about the potential for hot flashes. Consider the use of clonidine 0.1–0.2 mg PO daily, megestrol acetate 20 mg PO bid, or soy tablets 1 tablet PO tid for prevention and/or treatment.
4. Instruct patients on the potential risk of altered sexual function and impotence.
5. Pregnancy category D. Breastfeeding should be avoided.

TOXICITY 1

Hot flashes occur in 60% of patients, decreased libido (35%), impotence (30%), gynecomastia (10%), nipple pain, and galactorrhea.

TOXICITY 2

GI toxicity with nausea/vomiting and diarrhea.

TOXICITY 3

Transient elevations in serum transaminases are rare but may necessitate discontinuation of therapy.

TOXICITY 4

Amber-green discoloration of urine secondary to flutamide and/or its metabolites.

Fulvestrant

OH

HO ''''(CH$_2$)$_9$SO(CH$_2$)$_3$CF$_2$CF$_3$

TRADE NAME	Faslodex	**CLASSIFICATION**	Estrogen receptor antagonist
CATEGORY	Hormonal agent	**DRUG MANUFACTURER**	AstraZeneca

MECHANISM OF ACTION
- Potent and selective antagonist of the estrogen receptor (ER) with no known agonist effects. Affinity to the ER is comparable to that of estradiol.
- Downregulates the expression of the ER, presumably through enhanced degradation.

MECHANISM OF RESISTANCE
- Decreased expression of ER.
- Decreased expression of G protein-coupled estrogen receptor 1 (GPER).
- Increased expression of cell division protein kinase 6 (CDK6).
- Increased expression of growth factor receptors, such as EGFR and HER2/neu.

ABSORPTION
Not absorbed orally. After IM injection, peak plasma levels are achieved in approximately 7 days and are maintained for at least 1 month.

DISTRIBUTION
Rapidly and widely distributed throughout the body. Approximately 99% of drug is bound to plasma proteins, and very high-density lipoprotein (VHDL), low-density lipoprotein (LDL), and high-density lipoprotein (HDL) are the main binding proteins.

METABOLISM
Extensively metabolized in the liver by microsomal CYP3A4 enzymes to both active and inactive forms. Steady-state levels of drug are achieved after 7 days of a once-monthly administration and are maintained for at least up to 1 month. The major route of elimination is via the hepatobiliary route in stool (approximately 90%), with renal excretion accounting for only 1% of drug clearance. The half-life of fulvestrant is on the order of 40 days.

INDICATIONS

1. Metastatic breast cancer—Treatment of hormone receptor (HR)–positive, HER2-negative advanced breast cancer in postmenopausal women not previously treated with endocrine therapy.
2. Metastatic breast cancer—Treatment of HR-positive metastatic breast cancer in postmenopausal women, with disease progression following endocrine therapy.
3. Metastatic breast cancer—Treatment of HR-positive, HER2-negative advanced or metastatic breast cancer in combination with palbociclib or abemaciclib in women with disease progression following endocrine therapy.
4. Metastatic breast cancer—Treatment of HR-positive, HER2-negative advanced or metastatic breast cancer in combination with ribociclib in postmenopausal women as initial endocrine-based therapy or following disease progression on endocrine therapy.

DOSAGE RANGE

Recommended dose as monotherapy and in combination with palbociclib, abemaciclib, or ribociclib is 500 mg IM on days 1, 15, 29, and once monthly thereafter.

DRUG INTERACTIONS

None well characterized to date.

SPECIAL CONSIDERATIONS

1. No dose adjustments are required for patients with renal dysfunction.
2. No dose adjustments are required for patients with mild liver dysfunction. In patients with moderate liver dysfunction (Child-Pugh Class B), a dose of 250 mg IM is recommended on days 1, 15, 29, and once monthly thereafter. The safety and efficacy of fulvestrant have not been studied in patients with severe hepatic impairment.
3. Use with caution in patients with bleeding diatheses, thrombocytopenia, and/or in those receiving anticoagulation therapy.
4. Fulvestrant can interfere with measurement of serum estradiol levels by immunoassay, which can result in falsely elevated estradiol levels.
5. Pregnancy category D. Breastfeeding should be avoided, as it is not known whether fulvestrant is excreted in human milk.

TOXICITY 1

Asthenia occurs in up to 25% of patients.

TOXICITY 2

Mild nausea and vomiting. Constipation and/or diarrhea can also occur.

TOXICITY 3

Hot flashes seen in 20% of patients.

TOXICITY 4

Mild headache.

TOXICITY 5

Injection site reactions with mild pain and inflammation that are usually transient in nature.

TOXICITY 6

Back pain and arthralgias. Flu-like syndrome in the form of fever, malaise, and myalgias. Occurs in 10% of patients.

TOXICITY 7

Dry, scaling skin rash.

Futibatinib

TRADE NAME	Lytgobi, TAS-120	CLASSIFICATION	Signal transduction inhibitor, FGFR inhibitor
CATEGORY	Targeted agent	DRUG MANUFACTURER	Taiho

MECHANISM OF ACTION

- Structurally novel, irreversible, highly selective pan-fibroblast growth factor receptor (FGFR) small molecule inhibitor.
- Leads to inhibition of FGFR-mediated signaling in tumors with activating FGFR amplification, mutations, fusions, and other rearrangements.
- FGFR signaling plays a critical role in tumor cell growth, proliferation, migration, angiogenesis, and survival.
- FGFR signaling pathway activated in 15%–20% of intrahepatic cholangiocarcinoma and in other tumor types, including bladder cancer, breast cancer, NSCLC, endometrial cancer, and head and neck cancer.

MECHANISM OF RESISTANCE

- Mutations in gatekeeper residues in FGFR, such as FGFR1 V561M and FGFR2 V565I.
- Mutations in the FGFR4 kinase domain including V550L, V550M, and V550E.
- Upregulation of ERB-B2, MET and ERK/MAPK signaling pathways.

ABSORPTION

Median time to peak drug levels is 2 hours after oral ingestion.

DISTRIBUTION

Extensive binding (95%) of drug mainly to plasma proteins.

METABOLISM

Metabolized in the liver primarily by CYP3A4 and to a lesser extent by CYP2C9 and CYP2D6. Approximately 91% of an administered dose is eliminated in feces mainly in parent form and only 9% eliminated in urine. The mean terminal half-life of futibatinib is approximately 3 hours.

INDICATIONS

FDA-approved for previously treated, unresectable locally advanced or metastatic intrahepatic cholangiocarcinoma with an FGFR2 fusion or other rearrangement as detected by an FDA-approved test. Accelerated approval based on overall response rate and duration of response.

DOSAGE RANGE

Recommended dose is 20 mg PO once daily.

DRUG INTERACTION 1

Drugs such as ketoconazole, itraconazole, erythromycin, clarithromycin, atazanavir, indinavir, nefazodone, nelfinavir, ritonavir, saquinavir, telithromycin, and voriconazole may decrease the metabolism of futibatinib, resulting in increased drug levels and potentially increased toxicity.

DRUG INTERACTION 2

Phenytoin and other drugs that stimulate the liver microsomal CYP3A4 enzymes, including carbamazepine, rifampin, phenobarbital, and St. John's Wort—These drugs may increase the metabolism of futibatinib, resulting in lower effective drug levels.

DRUG INTERACTION 3

Avoid concomitant use of P-gp or BCRP substrates as futibatinib may increase exposure of these drugs leading to potentially increased toxicity.

SPECIAL CONSIDERATIONS

1. Patients should be seen by a dietician and placed on a restricted phosphate diet to 600–800 mg daily.

2. Closely monitor serum phosphate levels while on therapy. The median time to onset of hyperphosphatemia is 5 days. Serum phosphate levels should be monitored on a monthly basis. If the serum phosphate level is >5.5 mg/dL, ensure that a restricted phosphate diet is being correctly followed. For serum phosphate levels >7.5 mg/dL, phosphate-lowering therapy, such as an oral phosphate binder, should be used, and the dose of drug should be held, reduced, or permanently discontinued based on duration and severity of the hyperphosphatemia.

3. Comprehensive eye exam, including optical coherence tomography (OCT), should be performed at baseline, every 2 months for the first 6 months, and then every 3 months thereafter while on treatment. With the onset of new visual symptoms, patients should have an immediate evaluation with OCT, with follow-up every 3 weeks until resolution of symptoms or discontinuation of treatment.

4. No need for dose reduction in setting of mild hepatic impairment. Has not been studied in the setting of moderate or severe hepatic impairment.

5. No need for dose reduction in setting of mild or moderate renal impairment. Has not been studied in the setting of severe renal impairment or end-stage renal disease.

6. Concomitant use of a dual P-gp and strong CYP3A inducer should be avoided.

7. Concomitant use of a dual P-gp and strong CYP3A inhibitor should be avoided.

8. Embryo-fetal toxicity. Can cause fetal harm when administered to a pregnant woman. Females of reproductive potential should use effective contraception during drug therapy and for 1 week after the final dose. Breastfeeding should be avoided.

TOXICITY 1

Hyperphosphatemia. Soft tissue mineralization, calcinosis, and vascular calcification may occur.

TOXICITY 2

Ocular disorders with retinal pigment epithelial detachment (RPED) leading to blurred vision, visual floaters, or photopsia. Dry eye symptoms are common.

TOXICITY 3

Dry skin, palmar-plantar erythrodysesthesia, paronychia, and nail disorder, discoloration, dystrophy, and onycholysis.

TOXICITY 4

Fatigue and anorexia.

TOXICITY 5

Diarrhea, mucositis, dry mouth, and nausea/vomiting.

TOXICITY 6

Myalgias and arthralgias.

Gefitinib

TRADE NAME	Iressa, ZD1839	**CLASSIFICATION**	Signal transduction inhibitor, EGFR inhibitor
CATEGORY	Targeted agent	**DRUG MANUFACTURER**	AstraZeneca

MECHANISM OF ACTION
- Potent and selective small molecule inhibitor of the kinase activity of wild-type and certain activating mutations of EGFR, exon 19 deletion or exon 21 (L858R) substitution mutations, resulting in inhibition of EGFR autophosphorylation and inhibition of EGFR signaling.
- Inhibition of the EGFR tyrosine kinase results in inhibition of critical mitogenic and antiapoptotic signals involved in proliferation, growth, metastasis, angiogenesis, and response to chemotherapy and/or radiation therapy.

MECHANISM OF RESISTANCE
- Mutations in the EGFR tyrosine kinase, leading to decreased binding affinity to gefitinib.
- Presence of KRAS mutations.
- Activation/induction of alternative cellular signaling pathways, such as PI3K/Akt and IGF-1R.

ABSORPTION
Oral absorption is relatively slow, and oral bioavailability is approximately 60%. Food does not affect drug absorption. Peak drug levels are reached in 3–7 hours.

DISTRIBUTION
Extensive binding (90%) to plasma proteins, including albumin and α1-acid glycoprotein, and extensive tissue distribution. Steady-state drug concentrations are reached in 7–10 days.

METABOLISM

Metabolism in the liver primarily by CYP3A4 and CYP2D6 microsomal enzymes. Other cytochrome P450 enzymes play a minor role in its metabolism. The main metabolite is the O-desmethyl piperazine derivative, and this metabolite is significantly less potent than the parent drug. Elimination is mainly via the hepatobiliary route, with excretion in feces, and renal elimination of parent drug and its metabolites accounts for less than 4% of an administered dose. The terminal half-life of the parent drug is 41 hours.

INDICATIONS

FDA-approved for first-line treatment of metastatic NSCLC with EGFR exon 19 deletion or exon 21 (L858R) substitution mutations as detected by an FDA-approved test.

DOSAGE RANGE

Recommended dose is 250 mg/day PO.

DRUG INTERACTION 1

Dilantin and other drugs that stimulate the liver microsomal CYP3A4 enzyme, including carbamazepine, rifampin, phenobarbital, and St. John's Wort—These drugs increase the metabolism of gefitinib, resulting in its inactivation and lower effective drug levels.

DRUG INTERACTION 2

Drugs that inhibit the liver microsomal CYP3A4 enzyme, including ketoconazole, itraconazole, erythromycin, and clarithromycin—These drugs decrease the metabolism of gefitinib, resulting in increased drug levels and potentially increased toxicity.

DRUG INTERACTION 3

Warfarin—Patients receiving warfarin should be closely monitored for alterations in their clotting parameters (PT and INR) and/or bleeding, as gefitinib inhibits the metabolism of warfarin by the liver P450 system. Dose of warfarin may require careful adjustment in the presence of gefitinib therapy.

DRUG INTERACTION 4

Acid-reducing agents—Drugs that elevate gastric pH, such as proton pump inhibitors, H2-receptor antagonists, and antacids, may reduce the plasma drug levels of gefitinib. Avoid concomitant use of gefitinib with these agents.

SPECIAL CONSIDERATIONS

1. Clinical responses may be observed quickly within the first week of initiation of therapy.
2. Patients with bronchoalveolar NSCLC may be more sensitive to gefitinib therapy than other histologic subtypes. Females and nonsmokers also show increased sensitivity to gefitinib therapy.

3. Closely monitor patients with central lesions, as they may be at increased risk for complications of hemoptysis.
4. Dose of gefitinib may need to be increased when used in patients with seizure disorders who are receiving phenytoin, as the metabolism of gefitinib by the liver P450 system is enhanced in the presence of phenytoin. The dose of gefitinib should be increased to 500 mg daily when patients are taking phenytoin and other strong CYP3A4 inducers.
5. Coagulation parameters (PT/INR) should be closely monitored when patients are receiving both gefitinib and warfarin, as gefitinib inhibits the metabolism of warfarin by the liver P450 system.
6. In patients who develop a skin rash, topical antibiotics such as clindamycin gel or either oral clindamycin and/or oral minocycline may help.
7. Avoid Seville oranges, starfruit, pomelos, grapefruit, and grapefruit juice while on gefitinib.
8. For patients who need to be on proton-pump inhibitors, gefinitib should be taken 12 hours after the last dose or 12 hours before the next dose of the proton-pump inhibitor. For H2-receptor antagonists or antacids, gefitinib should be taken 6 hours after or 6 hours before these acid-reducing agents.
9. Pregnancy category D. Breastfeeding should be avoided.

TOXICITY 1
Elevations in blood pressure, especially in those with underlying hypertension.

TOXICITY 2
Pruritus, dry skin with mainly a pustular, acneiform skin rash.

TOXICITY 3
Mild-to-moderate elevations in serum transaminases. Usually transient and clinically asymptomatic.

TOXICITY 4
Asthenia and anorexia.

TOXICITY 5
Mild nausea/vomiting and mucositis.

TOXICITY 6
Conjunctivitis, blepharitis, and corneal erosions. Abnormal eyelash growth may occur in some patients.

TOXICITY 7
Rare episodes of hemoptysis and GI hemorrhage.

G

Gemcitabine

TRADE NAME	Gemzar	CLASSIFICATION	Antimetabolite
CATEGORY	Chemotherapy drug	DRUG MANUFACTURER	Eli Lilly

MECHANISM OF ACTION

- Fluorine-substituted deoxycytidine analog.
- Cell cycle–specific with activity in the S-phase.
- Requires transport into the cell via a nucleoside transport protein. Once inside the cell, undergoes intracellular activation by deoxycytidine kinase to the monophosphate form, with eventual metabolism to the cytotoxic gemcitabine triphosphate metabolite. Antitumor activity of gemcitabine is determined by a balance between intracellular activation and degradation and the formation of cytotoxic triphosphate metabolites.
- Incorporation of gemcitabine triphosphate metabolite into DNA, resulting in chain termination and inhibition of DNA synthesis and function.
- Triphosphate metabolite inhibits DNA polymerases α, β, and γ, which, in turn, interferes with DNA synthesis, DNA repair, and DNA chain elongation.
- Inhibition of the enzyme ribonucleotide reductase by both gemcitabine triphosphate and gemcitabine diphosphate, resulting in decreased levels of essential deoxyribonucleotides for DNA synthesis and function.
- Incorporation of gemcitabine triphosphate into RNA, resulting in alterations in RNA processing and mRNA translation.

MECHANISM OF RESISTANCE

- Decreased activation of drug through decreased expression/activity of the anabolic enzyme deoxycytidine kinase.
- Increased breakdown of drug by the catabolic enzymes cytidine deaminase and dCMP deaminase.
- Decreased nucleoside transport of drug into cells.
- Increased concentration of the competing physiologic nucleotide dCTP, through increased expression of CTP synthetase.
- Increased expression of ribonucleotide reductase (RR).

ABSORPTION
Administered only via the IV route.

DISTRIBUTION
With infusions <70 min, gemcitabine is not extensively distributed. In contrast, with longer infusions, gemcitabine is slowly and widely distributed into body tissues. Does not cross the blood-brain barrier. Binding to plasma proteins is negligible.

METABOLISM
Undergoes extensive metabolism by deamination to the difluorouridine (dFdU) metabolite, with approximately >90% of drug being recovered in urine in this form. Deamination occurs in liver, plasma, and peripheral tissues. The principal enzyme involved in drug catabolism is cytidine deaminase. The terminal elimination half-life is dependent on the infusion time. With short infusions <70 minutes, the half-life ranges from 30 to 90 minutes, while for longer infusions >70 minutes, the half-life is increased to 4–10 hours. Plasma clearance is also dependent on gender and age. Clearance is 30% lower in women and in elderly patients.

INDICATIONS
1. Pancreatic cancer—FDA-approved as monotherapy or in combination with erlotinib for first-line treatment of locally advanced or metastatic disease.
2. Pancreatic cancer—FDA-approved in combination with Abraxane for first-line treatment of metastatic disease.
3. NSCLC—FDA-approved in combination with cisplatin for treatment of inoperable, locally advanced, or metastatic disease.
4. Breast cancer—FDA-approved in combination with paclitaxel for first-line treatment of metastatic breast cancer after failure of prior anthracycline-containing adjuvant chemotherapy.
5. Ovarian cancer—FDA-approved in combination with carboplatin for patients with advanced ovarian cancer that has relapsed at least 6 months after completion of platinum-based therapy.
6. Bladder cancer.
7. Soft tissue sarcoma.
8. Hodgkin's lymphoma.
9. Non-Hodgkin's lymphoma.

DOSAGE RANGE
1. Pancreatic cancer: 1,000 mg/m^2 IV every week for 7 weeks, with 1-week rest. Treatment then continues weekly for 3 weeks, followed by 1-week rest.
2. Pancreatic cancer: 1,000 mg/m^2 IV on days 1, 8, and 15 in combination with Abraxane 125 mg/m^2 IV on days 1, 8, and 15, with cycles repeated every 28 days.
3. Bladder cancer: 1,000 mg/m^2 IV on days 1, 8, and 15 every 28 days.
4. NSCLC: 1,200 mg/m^2 IV on days 1, 8, and 15 every 28 days.

DRUG INTERACTION 1

Cisplatin—Gemcitabine enhances cisplatin cytotoxicity by increasing the formation of cytotoxic platinum-DNA adducts.

DRUG INTERACTION 2

Radiation therapy—Gemcitabine is a potent radiosensitizer.

SPECIAL CONSIDERATIONS

1. Monitor CBCs on a regular basis during therapy. Dose reduction is recommended based on the degree of hematologic toxicity.
2. Use with caution in patients with abnormal liver and/or renal function as there may be an increased risk for toxicity.
3. Use with caution in women and in elderly patients, as gemcitabine clearance is decreased.
4. Pregnancy category D. Breastfeeding should be avoided.

TOXICITY 1

Myelosuppression is dose-limiting, with neutropenia more common than thrombocytopenia. Nadir typically occurs by days 10–14, with recovery by day 21.

TOXICITY 2

Nausea and vomiting. Usually mild to moderate, occur in 70% of patients. Diarrhea and/or mucositis observed in 15%–20% of patients.

TOXICITY 3

Flu-like syndrome manifested by fever, malaise, chills, headache, and myalgias. Seen in 20% of patients. Fever, in the absence of infection, develops in 40% of patients within the first 6–12 hours after treatment but generally is mild.

TOXICITY 4

Hepatotoxicity with elevation of serum transaminases and bilirubin.

TOXICITY 5

Pulmonary toxicity in the form of mild dyspnea and drug-induced pneumonitis. ARDS has been reported rarely.

TOXICITY 6

Infusion reaction presents as flushing, facial swelling, headache, dyspnea, and/ or hypotension. Usually related to the rate of infusion and resolves with slowing or discontinuation of infusion.

TOXICITY 7

Mild proteinuria and hematuria. In rare cases, thromboangiopathic syndromes, including hemolytic-uremic syndrome (HUS) and thrombotic thrombocytopenic purpura (TTP), have been reported.

TOXICITY 8

Maculopapular skin rash with pruritus generally involving the trunk and extremities. Radiation-recall dermatitis may occur. Alopecia is rarely observed.

Gemtuzumab ozogamicin

TRADE NAME	Mylotarg, CMC-544	**CLASSIFICATION**	Antibody-drug conjugate
CATEGORY	Biologic response modifier agent, chemotherapy drug	**DRUG MANUFACTURER**	Pfizer

MECHANISM OF ACTION
- CD33-directed antibody-drug conjugate that is made up of gemtuzumab, a humanized IgG4 κ antibody specific for the cell surface glycoprotein CD33, and N-acetyl-gamma-calicheamicin, a cytotoxic enediyne antibiotic derived from the soil microorganism *Micromonospora echinospora*.
- Upon binding to CD33, gemtuzumab ozogamicin is rapidly internalized into lysosomes, and calicheamicin is then released to interact with the minor groove of DNA, leading to site-specific double-strand DNA breaks. Calicheamicin causes cell cycle arrest in the G2-M phase, which is then followed by apoptosis.
- CD33 is expressed on the surface of myeloid leukemic blasts and immature normal cells of myelomonocytic lineage but not expressed on other normal tissues, including hematopoietic stem cells.

MECHANISM OF RESISTANCE
- Reduced binding of gemtuzumab ozogamicin to CD33.
- Altered internalization of the gemtuzumab ozogamicin-CD33 complex into cells.
- Activated PI3K/AKT signaling.

ABSORPTION
Administered only via the IV route.

DISTRIBUTION
Extensive binding (97%) of gemtuzumab ozogamicin to plasma proteins.

METABOLISM
Primarily metabolized by non-enzymatic reduction. The median terminal half-life is on the order of 62 days after the first dose and 90 hours after the second dose.

INDICATIONS
1. FDA-approved for adult and pediatric patients aged 1 month or older with newly diagnosed CD33-positive AML.
2. FDA-approved for adult and pediatric patients 2 years and older with relapsed or refractory CD33-positive AML.

DOSAGE RANGE

1. Newly diagnosed AML (combination therapy): Adult patients
   - Induction: 3 mg/m^2 on days 1, 4, and 7 in combination with daunorubicin and cytarabine.
   - Consolidation: 3 mg/m^2 on day 1 in combination with daunorubicin and cytarabine.
2. Newly diagnosed AML (combination therapy): Pediatric patients 1 month or older
   - Induction: 3 mg/m^2 for patients with BSA >0.6 m^2 on days 1, 4, and 7 in combination with daunorubicin and cytarabine.
   - Induction: 0.1 mg/kg for patient with BSA <0.6 m^2 on day 1 in combination with daunorubicin and cytarabine.
3. Newly diagnosed AML (monotherapy):
   - Induction: 6 mg/m^2 on day 1, and 3 mg/m^2 on day 8.
   - Continuation: 2 mg/m^2 on day 1, repeated every 4 weeks for up to 8 cycles.
   - Relapsed or refractory AML (monotherapy): 3 mg/m^2 IV on days 1, 4, and 7.

DRUG INTERACTIONS

None well characterized to date.

SPECIAL CONSIDERATIONS

1. Gemtuzumab ozogamicin should **NOT** be given by IV push or bolus and must be administered as a 2-hour infusion.
2. Monitor for infusion-related reactions. Patients should be premedicated with a corticosteroid, antihistamine, and acetaminophen prior to all infusions. Patients should be monitored during and for at least 1 hour after the completion of the infusion.
3. Monitor CBC prior to each treatment cycle. Gemtuzumab ozogamicin is myelosuppressive, and thrombocytopenia with serious or life-threatening hemorrhage has been observed. Please see package insert for details regarding dose modifications for hematologic toxicities. CBCs should be monitored at least 3 times per week until recovery from hematologic toxicity.
4. Monitor liver function tests (LFTs) and serum bilirubin levels closely, as hepatotoxicity, including hepatic veno-occlusive disease (VOD), has been observed. This is a black-box warning. Risk of VOD is greater in patients who receive higher doses of gemtuzumab ozogamicin as monotherapy, in patients with moderate or severe hepatic dysfunction prior to receiving gemtuzumab ozogamicin, in patients treated with gemtuzumab ozogamicin after hematopoietic stem cell transplantation (HSCT), and in those who undergo HSCT after gemtuzumab ozogamicin.

5. Cytoreduction is recommended in patients with WBC count >30,000 prior to the first dose of therapy to prevent and/or reduce the risk of tumor lysis syndrome.

6. ECGs should be obtained at baseline and periodically on treatment to assess QT interval. Monitoring should be more frequent when medications known to prolong the QT interval are used concomitantly with gemtuzumab ozogamicin.

7. Dose reduction is not required in patients with mild or moderate renal dysfunction. Has not been studied in setting of severe renal dysfunction or end-stage renal disease.

8. Dose reduction is not required in patients with mild hepatic dysfunction. Has not been studied in setting of moderate or severe hepatic dysfunction.

9. Can cause fetal harm when given to a pregnant woman. Females of reproductive potential should use effective contraception during treatment and for at least 6 months after the last dose. Males with female partners of reproductive potential should use effective contraception while on treatment and for at least 3 months after the last dose. Breastfeeding should be avoided.

TOXICITY 1
Myelosuppression with thrombocytopenia and neutropenia.

TOXICITY 2
Infusion-related reactions.

TOXICITY 3
Hepatotoxicity with elevation in LFTs. Severe and sometimes fatal hepatic veno-occlusive disease (VOD) observed in 5% of patients during or following HSCT after completion of treatment.

TOXICITY 4
QT interval prolongation.

TOXICITY 5
Asthenia, fatigue, and pyrexia.

TOXICITY 6
Hemorrhagic events with intracranial hematoma and subdural hematoma.

G

Gilteritinib

TRADE NAME	Xospata	CLASSIFICATION	Signal transduction inhibitor, FLT3 inhibitor
CATEGORY	Targeted agent	DRUG MANUFACTURER	Astellas

MECHANISM OF ACTION
- Inhibits multiple receptor tyrosine kinases, including FMS-like tyrosine kinase 3 (FLT3) and AXL.
- FLT3 is one of the most frequently mutated genes in AML, with mutations occurring in up to 30% of patients.
- Potent activity against FLT3 receptors with internal tandem duplications (ITD) and tyrosine kinase domain mutations.

MECHANISM OF RESISTANCE
- NRAS or KRAS mutations leading to activation of the RAS/MAPK signaling pathway.
- Tyrosine kinase domain (TKD) mutations in FLT3-ITD, including N676K, D835V, and Y842C and F691L gatekeeper mutation.
- BCR-ABL1 fusion.

ABSORPTION
Median time to peak drug levels is 4–6 hours after ingestion. Food with high fat content reduces C_{max} and AUC by 26% and <10%, respectively.

DISTRIBUTION
Extensive binding (94%) of drug to plasma proteins, mainly serum albumin. Steady-state drug levels are achieved in approximately 15 days.

METABOLISM
Metabolized in the liver primarily by CYP3A4 microsomal enzymes. The main metabolites are M17 (formed by N-dealklyation and oxidation), M16, and M10, the latter two of which are formed via N-dealklyation. Approximately 65% of an administered dose is eliminated in feces and 16% is eliminated in urine. The terminal half-life is approximately 113 hours.

INDICATIONS

FDA-approved for patients with relapsed or refractory AML with a FLT3 mutation as detected by an FDA-approved test.

DOSAGE RANGE

Recommended dose is 120 mg PO once daily with or without food.

DRUG INTERACTION 1

Drugs such as ketoconazole, itraconazole, erythromycin, clarithromycin, atazanavir, indinavir, nefazodone, nelfinavir, ritonavir, saquinavir, telithromycin, and voriconazole may decrease the metabolism of gilteritinib, resulting in increased drug levels and potentially increased toxicity.

DRUG INTERACTION 2

Drugs such as rifampin, phenytoin, phenobarbital, carbamazepine, and St. John's Wort may increase the metabolism of gilteritinib, resulting in lower effective drug levels.

SPECIAL CONSIDERATIONS

1. Dose adjustment is not required for patients with mild or moderate hepatic impairment. Has not been studied in patients with severe hepatic impairment, and there are no formal recommendations for dosing in this setting.
2. Dose adjustment is not required for patients with mild or moderate renal impairment (CrCl 30–80 mL/min). Has not been studied in patients with severe renal impairment or in those on hemodialysis, and there are no formal recommendations for dosing in these settings.
3. Response to therapy may be delayed, and for this reason, treatment should be given for at least 6 months to allow time for a clinical response.
4. Monitor for the development of the differentiation syndrome, which may be fatal if not appropriately treated. Can present as early as 2 days and up to 75 days after start of therapy, and has been observed with or without leukocytosis. Steroids (dexamethasone 10 mg IV every 12 hours) should be initiated if differentiation syndrome is suspected with hemodynamic monitoring. In the presence of non-infectious leukocytosis, treatment with hydroxyurea or leukapheresis should be instituted. This is a black-box warning.
5. Monitor CBCs and blood chemistries, including CPK, at baseline, at least once weekly for the first month, once every other week for the second month, and once monthly for the duration of therapy.
6. Monitor ECGs at baseline, on days 1 and 15 of cycle 1, and prior to the start of the next two subsequent cycles, as gilteritinib therapy can result in QT interval prolongation.
7. Gilteritinib therapy should be discontinued in patients who develop posterior reversible encephalopathy syndrome (PRES).
8. Can cause fetal harm. Females of reproductive potential should use effective contraception during drug therapy and for at least 6 months after the final dose. Breastfeeding should be avoided.

TOXICITY 1
Differentiation syndrome with fever, dyspnea, pleural effusion, pericardial effusions, pulmonary edema, hypotension, peripheral edema, skin rash, and renal dysfunction.

TOXICITY 2
Pancreatitis.

TOXICITY 3
Posterior reversible encephalopathy syndrome (PRES).

TOXICITY 4
QTc prolongation.

TOXICITY 5
Fatigue, malaise, anorexia.

TOXICITY 6
Myalgias and arthralgias.

Glasdegib

TRADE NAME	Daurismo	**CLASSIFICATION**	Signal transduction inhibitor, Hedgehog inhibitor
CATEGORY	Targeted agent	**DRUG MANUFACTURER**	Pfizer

MECHANISM OF ACTION
- Inhibits the Hedgehog (Hh) pathway by binding to and inhibiting the transmembrane protein Smoothened (SMO).
- Aberrant Hh signaling has been identified in human leukemias and, specifically, in leukemia stem cells.

MECHANISM OF RESISTANCE
None well characterized to date.

ABSORPTION
Oral bioavailability is 77%. The median time to peak drug levels is 1.3 to 1.8 hours after ingestion. Food with high-fat content reduces AUC and C_{max} by 16% and 31%, respectively.

DISTRIBUTION
Extensive binding (91%) of drug to plasma proteins. Steady-state drug levels are achieved in approximately 8 days.

METABOLISM
Metabolized in the liver primarily by CYP3A4 microsomal enzymes with minor contributions by CYP2C8 and UGT1A9. Following an administered dose, nearly 50% of the dose is eliminated in urine and 42% is eliminated in feces. The terminal half-life is approximately 17.4 hours.

INDICATIONS
FDA-approved in combination with low-dose cytarabine for newly diagnosed AML in patients who are >75 years of age or who have comorbidities that preclude the use of intensive induction chemotherapy.

DOSAGE RANGE
Recommended dose is 100 mg PO once daily on days 1–28 in combination with cytarabine 20 mg SC bid on days 1–10 of each 28-day cycle.

DRUG INTERACTION 1
Drugs such as ketoconazole, itraconazole, erythromycin, clarithromycin, atazanavir, indinavir, nefazodone, nelfinavir, ritonavir, saquinavir, telithromycin, and voriconazole may decrease the metabolism of glasdegib, resulting in increased drug levels and potentially increased toxicity.

DRUG INTERACTION 2
Drugs such as rifampin, phenytoin, phenobarbital, carbamazepine, and St. John's Wort may increase the metabolism of glasdegib, resulting in lower effective drug levels.

SPECIAL CONSIDERATIONS
1. Dose adjustment is not required for patients with mild hepatic impairment. Has not been studied in patients with moderate or severe hepatic impairment.
2. Dose adjustment is not required for patients with mild or moderate renal impairment (CrCl 30–80 mL/min). Has not been studied in patients with severe renal impairment or in those on hemodialysis.
3. Monitor CBCs and blood chemistries, including serum creatinine kinase levels at baseline, and at least once weekly for the first month. Monitor electrolytes and renal function once monthly for the duration of therapy.
4. Monitor ECGs at baseline, at 1 week after initiation, and then once monthly for the next 2 months, as glasdegib therapy can result in QTc interval prolongation.

5. Avoid concomitant use of other drugs that can prolong the QTc interval.
6. Patients should be advised not to donate blood or blood products during treatment with glasdegib and for at least 30 days after the last dose.
7. Can cause fetal death or severe birth defects when administered to a pregnant woman. Females of reproductive potential should use effective contraception during drug therapy and for at least 30 days after the final dose. Breastfeeding should be avoided. This represents a black-box warning.

TOXICITY 1
Myelosuppression with anemia, thrombocytopenia, and neutropenia.

TOXICITY 2
Fatigue and anorexia.

TOXICITY 3
Nausea/vomiting, abdominal pain, constipation, and diarrhea.

TOXICITY 4
QTc prolongation.

TOXICITY 5
Pneumonia.

TOXICITY 6
Renal insufficiency.

TOXICITY 7
Muscle spasms and musculoskeletal pain.

Glofitamab

TRADE NAME	Columvi	**CLASSIFICATION**	BiTE anti-CD20 monoclonal antibody
CATEGORY	Biologic response modifier agent, immunotherapy	**DRUG MANUFACTURER**	Genentech

MECHANISM OF ACTION
- Bispecific T-cell engaging (BiTE) humanized IgG1 antibody that binds to CD20 antigen expressed on malignant B cells and to CD3 receptor expressed on the surface of T cells.

- This binding causes cytotoxic T cells to be physically linked to malignant CD20-positive lymphoma cells and triggers the signaling cascade, leading to upregulation of cell adhesion molecules, production of cytolytic proteins, release of inflammatory cytokines, and proliferation of T cells, ultimately resulting in lysis of CD20-positive malignant B cells.
- CD20 is expressed on more than 90% of all B-cell non-Hodgkin's lymphomas and leukemias.
- CD20 is not expressed on early pre–B cells, plasma cells, normal bone marrow stem cells, antigen-presenting dendritic reticulum cells, or other normal tissues.
- Mechanism of action differs from classic anti-CD20 monoclonal antibodies that induce direct cell death by inhibition of CD20 intracellular signaling and by antibody-dependent cellular cytotoxicity and complement-mediated cellular cytotoxicity.

ABSORPTION
Administered only via the IV route.

DISTRIBUTION
Volume of distribution on the order of 5.6 L (24%).

METABOLISM
Metabolism has not been well characterized. As with other antibodies, it is assumed that glofitamab is degraded to small peptides and amino acids via catabolic pathways. The terminal half-life is on the order of 6-11 days.

INDICATIONS
FDA-approved for the treatment of adult patients with relapsed or refractory diffuse large B-cell lymphoma, including DLBCL arising from follicular lymphoma after 2 or more lines of systemic therapy. Approved under accelerated approval based on response rate and duration of response.

DOSAGE RANGE
1. Administered in combination with obinutuzumab and as an IV injection according to the step-up dosing schedule as outlined
2. Pretreat on Cycle 1, Day 1 with a single 1,000 mg dose of obinutuzumab before initiation of glofitamab
3. Cycle 1, Day 8 – 2.5 mg; Cycle 1, Day 15 – 10 mg
4. Cycles 2–12 – 30 mg
5. Cycles repeated every 21 days up to a maximum of 12 cycles, inclusive of Cycle 1 step-up dosing.

DRUG INTERACTION
Glofitamab treatment results in release of cytokines that may suppress the activity of CYP3A4 enzymes. This may then lead to increased exposure of drugs that are CYP3A4 substrates.

SPECIAL CONSIDERATIONS

1. Patients should be premedicated one to three hours prior to each step-up dose and first treatment dose to reduce the risk of CRS with 16 mg dexamethasone (oral or IV), H1 receptor antagonist (oral or IV diphenhydramine), and an antipyretic (oral or IV acetaminophen).
2. Monitor for CRS, which occurs most frequently with the first two cycles of therapy. This is a black-box warning.
3. Monitor for neurologic toxicity, especially for the immune effector cell-associated neurotoxicity syndrome (ICANS).
4. Monitor for signs and symptoms of infection. Should not be administered to patients with an active infection. Consider PJP prophylaxis prior to starting on therapy.
5. Monitor CBCs while on therapy.
6. Monitor for evidence of tumor flare, which can occur in setting of bulky tumors or disease located close to airways or a vital organ.
7. Dose reduction is not required in patients with mild hepatic dysfunction. Has not been studied in setting of moderate or severe hepatic dysfunction.
8. Dose reduction is not required in patients with mild or moderate renal dysfunction. Has not been studied in setting of severe renal dysfunction or end-stage renal disease.
9. May cause fetal harm. Women should be advised to use effective contraception during treatment and for 1 month after the last dose of treatment. Breastfeeding should be avoided while on therapy and for 1 month after the last dose.

TOXICITY 1
Cytokine release syndrome (CRS) with fever, chills, hypotension, tachycardia, hypoxia, and headache.

TOXICITY 2
Myelosuppression with neutropenia, anemia, and thrombocytopenia.

TOXICITY 3
Neurological toxicities with headache, motor dysfunction, sensory neuropathy, and encephalopathy. ICANS can present with confusional state and dysgraphia.

TOXICITY 5
Tumor flare.

TOXICITY 6
Increased risk of viral, bacterial, fungal, and opportunistic infections. Can cause severe or fatal infections.

TOXICITY 7
Tumor lysis syndrome.

Goserelin

TRADE NAME	Zoladex	**CLASSIFICATION**	LHRH agonist
CATEGORY	Hormonal agent	**DRUG MANUFACTURER**	AstraZeneca

MECHANISM OF ACTION

- Administration leads to initial release of follicle-stimulating hormone (FSH) and luteinizing hormone (LH), followed by suppression of gonadotropin secretion as a result of desensitization of the pituitary to gonadotropin-releasing hormone. This results in decreased secretion of LH and FSH from the pituitary.

ABSORPTION

Bioavailability of SC administered drug is 75%–90%.

DISTRIBUTION

Distribution is not well characterized. Slowly released over a 28-day period. Peak serum concentrations are achieved 10–15 days after drug administration. About 30% of goserelin is bound to plasma proteins.

METABOLISM

Metabolism occurs mainly via hydrolysis of the C-terminal amino acids. Goserelin is nearly completely eliminated in urine. The elimination half-life is normally 4–5 hours but is prolonged in patients with impaired renal function (12 hours).

INDICATIONS

Advanced prostate cancer.

DOSAGE RANGE

Administer 3.6 mg SC every 28 days or 10.8 mg SC every 90 days.

DRUG INTERACTIONS

None well characterized to date.

SPECIAL CONSIDERATIONS

1. Initiation of treatment with goserelin may induce a transient tumor flare. Goserelin should not be given in patients with impending ureteral obstruction and/or spinal cord compression or in those with painful bone metastases.
2. Serum testosterone levels decrease to castrate levels within 2–4 weeks after initiation of therapy.
3. Use with caution in patients with abnormal renal function.
4. Caution patients about the potential for hot flashes. Consider the use of soy tablets, 1 tablet PO tid, for prevention and/or treatment.

TOXICITY 1

Hot flashes, decreased libido, impotence, and gynecomastia.

TOXICITY 2

Tumor flare occurs in up to 20% of patients, usually within the first 2 weeks of starting therapy. Presents as increased bone pain, urinary retention, or back pain with spinal cord compression. Usually prevented by pretreating with an antiandrogen agent such as flutamide, bicalutamide, or nilutamide.

TOXICITY 3

Local discomfort at the site of injection.

TOXICITY 4

Elevated serum cholesterol levels.

TOXICITY 5

Hypersensitivity reaction.

TOXICITY 6

Nausea and vomiting are relatively uncommon.

Hydroxyurea

$$H_2N - \overset{\overset{\displaystyle O}{\|}}{C} - \overset{\overset{\displaystyle H}{|}}{N} - OH$$

TRADE NAME	Hydrea	CLASSIFICATION	Antimetabolite
CATEGORY	Chemotherapy drug	DRUG MANUFACTURER	MGI Pharma

MECHANISM OF ACTION
- Cell cycle–specific analog of urea with activity in the S-phase.
- Inhibits the enzyme ribonucleotide reductase (RR), a key enzyme that converts ribonucleotides to deoxyribonucleotides, which are critical precursors for de novo DNA synthesis and DNA repair.

MECHANISM OF RESISTANCE
Increased expression of ribonucleotide reductase due to gene amplification, increased transcription, and post-transcriptional mechanisms.

ABSORPTION
Oral absorption is rapid and nearly complete, with oral bioavailability ranging between 80% and 100%. Peak plasma concentrations are achieved in 1–4 hours. The effect of food on oral absorption is not known.

DISTRIBUTION
Widely distributed in all tissues. High concentrations are found in third-space collections, including pleural effusions and ascites. Crosses the blood-brain barrier and enters the CSF. Excreted in significant levels in human breast milk.

METABOLISM
Approximately 50% of drug is metabolized in the liver, and about 50% of drug is excreted unchanged in urine. The carbon dioxide that results from drug metabolism is released through the lungs. Plasma half-life is on the order of 3–4.5 hours.

INDICATIONS
1. Chronic myelogenous leukemia.
2. Essential thrombocytosis.
3. Polycythemia vera.
4. Acute myelogenous leukemia, blast crisis.
5. Head and neck cancer (in combination with radiation therapy).
6. Refractory ovarian cancer.
7. Sickle cell disease.

DOSAGE RANGE

1. Continuous therapy: 20–30 mg/kg PO daily.
2. Intermittent therapy: 80 mg/kg PO every third day.
3. Combination therapy with irradiation of head and neck cancer: 80 mg/kg PO every third day. In this setting, hydroxyurea is used as a radiation sensitizer and initiated at least 7 days before radiation therapy.

DRUG INTERACTION 1

5-FU—Hydroxyurea may enhance the risk of 5-FU toxicity.

DRUG INTERACTION 2

Antiretroviral agents—Hydroxyurea may enhance the activity of various anti-HIV agents, including azidothymidine (AZT), dideoxycytidine (ddC), and dideoxyinosine (ddI).

SPECIAL CONSIDERATIONS

1. Contraindicated in patients with bone marrow suppression presenting as WBC <2,500/mm^3 or platelet count <100,000/mm^3.
2. Monitor CBC on a weekly basis during therapy. Treatment should be held if the WBC count falls to less than 2,500/mm^3 or the platelet count drops to less than 100,000/mm^3. Once blood counts rise above these values, therapy can be resumed.
3. Use with caution in patients previously treated with chemotherapy and/or radiation therapy, as there is an increased risk of myelosuppression.
4. The need for dose adjustment in patients with hepatic impairment is not known.
5. Use with caution in patients with abnormal renal function. Dose should be reduced in patients with CrCl <60 mL/min and in patients with end-stage renal disease.
6. Pregnancy category D. Breastfeeding should be avoided, as the drug is excreted in human breast milk.

TOXICITY 1

Myelosuppression with neutropenia is dose-limiting. Median onset 7–10 days, with recovery of WBC counts 7–10 days after stopping the drug. Median onset of thrombocytopenia and anemia usually by day 10. Effect on bone marrow may be more severe in patients previously treated with chemotherapy and/or radiation therapy.

TOXICITY 2

Nausea and vomiting are generally mild. Incidence can be reduced by dividing the daily dose into two or three doses. Mucositis may also occur.

TOXICITY 3

Skin toxicity with maculopapular rash, facial and acral erythema, hyperpigmentation, dry skin with atrophy, and pruritus.

TOXICITY 4
Radiation-recall skin reaction.

TOXICITY 5
Headache, drowsiness, and confusion.

TOXICITY 6
Hepatotoxicity with transient elevations of serum transaminases and bilirubin.

TOXICITY 7
Teratogenic. Carcinogenic potential is not known.

Ibritumomab

TRADE NAME	Zevalin, IDEC-Y2B8	**CLASSIFICATION**	Immunoconjugate, anti-CD20 monoclonal antibody
CATEGORY	Biologic response modifier agent	**DRUG MANUFACTURER**	Spectrum

MECHANISM OF ACTION
- Immunoconjugate consisting of a stable thiourea covalent bond between the monoclonal antibody ibritumomab and the linker-chelator tiuxetan. This linker-chelator provides a high-affinity, conformationally restricted site for indium-111 and/or yttrium-90.
- The antibody moiety is ibritumomab, which targets the CD20 antigen, a 35-kDa cell surface non-glycosylated phosphoprotein expressed during early pre–B-cell development until the plasma cell stage. Binding of antibodies to CD20 induces a transmembrane signal that blocks cell activation and cell cycle progression.
- CD20 is expressed on more than 90% of all B-cell non-Hodgkin's lymphomas and leukemias. CD20 is not expressed on early pre–B cells, plasma cells, normal bone marrow stem cells, antigen-presenting dendritic reticulum cells, or other normal tissues.
- The beta emission from yttrium-90 induces cellular damage by the formation of free radicals in the target and neighboring cells.

ABSORPTION
Administered only via the IV route.

DISTRIBUTION
Peak and trough levels of rituximab correlate inversely with the number of circulating CD20-positive B cells. When In-111-ibritumomab is administered without unlabeled ibritumomab, only 18% of known sites of disease are imaged. In contrast, when In-111-ibritumomab administration is preceded by unlabeled ibritumomab, up to 90% of known sites of disease are imaged.

METABOLISM
Mean effective half-life of yttrium-90 in blood is 30 hours, and mean area under the fraction of injected activity (FIA) versus time curve in blood is 39 hours. Over a period of 7 days, a median of 7.2% of the injected activity is excreted in urine.

INDICATIONS
1. FDA-approved for relapsed and/or refractory low-grade, follicular, or transformed B-cell non-Hodgkin's lymphoma (NHL), including patients refractory to rituximab therapy.

2. FDA-approved for patients with previously untreated follicular NHL who achieve either a PR or CR to first-line chemotherapy.

DOSAGE RANGE

The regimen consists of the following: On day 1, an IV infusion of 250 mg/m^2 of rituximab; on day 7 and days 8 or 9, an IV infusion of 250 mg/m^2 of rituximab; and within 4 hours of each rituximab infusion, a therapeutic dose of 0.4 mCi/kg for patients with platelet counts greater than 150,000 or 0.3 mCi/kg for patients with platelet counts between 100,000 and 149,000. In either case, the maximum allowable dose of ibritumomab is 32 mCi, and patients should not be treated with a platelet count <100,000.

DRUG INTERACTIONS

None well characterized to date.

SPECIAL CONSIDERATIONS

1. Contraindicated in patients with known type I hypersensitivity, anaphylactic reactions to murine proteins, or sensitivity to any component of the product, including rituximab, yttrium chloride, and indium chloride.
2. Should not be administered to patients with an altered biodistribution of In-111 ibritumomab.
3. The prescribed and administered dose of yttrium-90 should **NOT** exceed the absolute maximum allowable dose of 32 mCi.
4. This therapy should be used only by physicians and healthcare professionals who are qualified and experienced in the safe use and handling of radioisotopes.
5. Patients should be premedicated with acetaminophen and diphenhydramine before each infusion of rituximab to reduce the incidence of infusion-related reactions.
6. Rituximab infusion should be started at an initial rate of 50 mg/hour. If no toxicity is observed during the first hour, the infusion rate can be escalated by increments of 50 mg/hour every 30 minutes to a maximum of 400 mg/hour. If the first treatment is well tolerated, the starting infusion rate for the second infusion can be administered at 100 mg/hour with 100-mg/hour increments at 30-minute intervals up to 400 mg/hour. Rituximab should **NOT** be given by IV push.
7. Monitor for infusion-related events resulting from rituximab infusion, which usually occur 30–120 minutes after the start of the first infusion. Infusion should be immediately stopped if signs or symptoms of an allergic reaction are observed. Immediate institution of diphenhydramine, acetaminophen, corticosteroids, IV fluids, and/or vasopressors may be necessary. In most instances, the infusion can be restarted at a reduced rate (50%) once symptoms have completely resolved. Resuscitation equipment should be readily available at bedside.
8. Infusion-related deaths within 24 hours of rituximab infusions have been reported.
9. Should not be given to patients with >25% involvement of the bone marrow by lymphoma and/or impaired bone marrow reserve.

10. Should not be given to patients with platelet counts below 100,000.
11. CBCs and platelet counts should be monitored weekly following ibritumomab therapy and should continue until levels recover.
12. Should be given only as a single-course treatment.
13. May have direct toxic effects on the male and female reproductive organs, and effective contraception should be used during therapy and for up to 12 months following the completion of therapy.
14. Pregnancy category D. Breastfeeding should be avoided, as it is not known whether ibritumomab is excreted in human milk.

TOXICITY 1

Infusion-related symptoms, including fever, chills, urticaria, flushing, fatigue, headache, bronchospasm, rhinitis, dyspnea, angioedema, nausea, and/or hypotension. Severe symptoms include pulmonary infiltrates, acute respiratory distress syndrome, myocardial infarction, ventricular fibrillation, and/or cardiogenic shock. Usually occur within 30 minutes to 2 hours after the start of the first infusion. Can be treated by slowing or interrupting the infusion and with supportive care.

TOXICITY 2

Myelosuppression with thrombocytopenia observed more frequently than neutropenia. The median duration of cytopenias ranges from 22 to 35 days, and the median time to nadir is 7–9 weeks. In <5% of patients, severe cytopenias remained beyond 12 weeks after therapy.

TOXICITY 3

Mild asthenia occurs in up to 40% of patients.

TOXICITY 4

Infections develop in nearly 30% of patients during the first 3 months after therapy.

TOXICITY 5

Mild nausea and vomiting.

TOXICITY 6

Cough, rhinitis, dyspnea, and sinusitis are observed in up to 35% of patients.

TOXICITY 7

Secondary malignancies occur in about 2% of patients. Acute myelogenous leukemia and myelodysplastic syndrome have been reported at a range of 8–34 months following therapy.

TOXICITY 8

Development of human anti-mouse (HAMA) and human anti-chimeric antibodies (HACA). Rare event in less than 1%–2% of patients.

Ibrutinib

TRADE NAME	Imbruvica	CLASSIFICATION	Signal transduction inhibitor, BTK inhibitor
CATEGORY	Targeted agent	DRUG MANUFACTURER	Pharmacyclics/Janssen Biotech

MECHANISM OF ACTION
- Irreversible small-molecule inhibitor of Bruton's tyrosine kinase (BTK).
- BTK is a key signaling molecule of the B-cell antigen receptor (BCR) and cytokine receptor pathways.

MECHANISM OF RESISTANCE
- Mutations in BTK that lead to reduced binding to ibrutinib.
- Mutations in the gene encoding phospholipase C-γ2 (PLCG2).
- Increased expression of kinases SYK and LYN, which are critical for activation of mutant PLCG2.

ABSORPTION
Absolute oral bioavailability has not been well characterized to date. Peak plasma drug levels are achieved in 1–2 hours after ingestion.

DISTRIBUTION
Extensive binding (97%) to plasma proteins. Steady-state drug levels are reached in approximately 8 days.

METABOLISM
Metabolism in the liver, primarily by CYP3A4 and to a minor extent by CYP2D6, with formation of several metabolites. PCI-45227 is a dihydrodiol metabolite with inhibitory activity against BTK, although significantly less than parent drug. Elimination is mainly hepatic (80%), with excretion in the feces. Renal elimination of parent drug and its metabolites accounts for only <10% of an administered dose. The terminal half-life of the parent drug is 7–8 hours.

INDICATIONS

1. FDA-approved for patients with mantle cell lymphoma (MCL) who have received at least one prior therapy.
2. FDA-approved for patients with CLL/small lymphocytic lymphoma who have received at least one prior therapy.
3. FDA-approved in combination with rituximab for the initial treatment of patients with CLL/small lymphocytic lymphoma.
4. FDA-approved for patients with CLL/small lymphocytic lymphoma and 17p deletion.
5. FDA-approved for patients with Waldenström's macroglobulinemia.
6. FDA-approved for patients with chronic graft-versus-host disease (cGVHD) after failure of one or more lines of systemic therapy.
7. FDA-approved for patients with marginal zone lymphoma (MZL) who require systemic therapy and who have received at least one prior anti-CD20-based therapy.

DOSAGE RANGE

1. MCL and MZL: recommended dose is 560 mg PO daily.
2. CLL, small lymphocytic lymphoma, Waldenström's macroglobulinemia, and cGVHD: recommended dose is 420 mg PO daily.

DRUG INTERACTION 1

Phenytoin and other drugs that stimulate the liver microsomal CYP3A4 enzymes, including carbamazepine, rifampin, phenobarbital, and St. John's Wort—These drugs may increase the metabolism of ibrutinib, resulting in its inactivation and lower effective drug levels.

DRUG INTERACTION 2

Drugs that inhibit the liver microsomal CYP3A4 enzymes, including ketoconazole, itraconazole, erythromycin, and clarithromycin—These drugs may decrease the metabolism of ibrutinib, resulting in increased drug levels and potentially increased toxicity.

DRUG INTERACTION 3

Warfarin—Patients receiving warfarin should be closely monitored for alterations in their clotting parameters (PT and INR) and/or bleeding, as ibrutinib may inhibit the metabolism of warfarin by the liver P450 system. Dose of warfarin may require careful adjustment in the presence of ibrutinib therapy.

SPECIAL CONSIDERATIONS

1. Ibrutinib capsules should be swallowed whole with water.
2. Monitor CBCs on a monthly basis.
3. Ibrutinib may increase the risk of bleeding in patients on antiplatelet or anticoagulant therapies.
4. Patients should be advised to maintain their hydration status.
5. Monitor renal function.
6. Monitor patients for fever and signs of infection.
7. Pregnancy category D. Breastfeeding should be avoided.

TOXICITY 1
Bleeding in the form of ecchymoses, GI bleeding, and hematuria.

TOXICITY 2
Infections.

TOXICITY 3
Myelosuppression with neutropenia, thrombocytopenia, and anemia.

TOXICITY 4
Renal toxicity with increases in serum creatinine. Serious and even fatal cases of renal failure have occurred.

TOXICITY 5
Second primary cancers with skin cancer and other solid tumors.

TOXICITY 6
Fatigue.

Idarubicin

TRADE NAME	Idamycin, 4-Demethoxydaunorubicin	**CLASSIFICATION**	Antitumor antibiotic, anthracycline
CATEGORY	Chemotherapy drug	**DRUG MANUFACTURER**	Pfizer

MECHANISM OF ACTION
- Semisynthetic anthracycline glycoside analog of daunorubicin.
- Inhibits topoisomerase II by forming a cleavable complex with topoisomerase II and DNA.
- In the presence of iron, drug forms oxygen free radicals, which cause single- and double-stranded DNA breaks.

- Intercalates into DNA, which results in inhibition of DNA synthesis and function.
- Specificity, in part, for the late S- and G2-phases of the cell cycle.

MECHANISM OF RESISTANCE
- Increased expression of the multidrug-resistant gene with enhanced drug efflux. This results in decreased intracellular drug accumulation.
- Decreased expression of topoisomerase II.
- Mutations in topoisomerase II, with decreased binding affinity to drug.
- Increased expression of sulfhydryl proteins, including glutathione and glutathione-associated enzymes.

ABSORPTION
Administered only via the IV route.

DISTRIBUTION
Rapid and extensive tissue distribution. Peak concentrations in nucleated blood and bone marrow cells are achieved within minutes of administration and are 100-fold greater than those in plasma. Parent drug and its major metabolite, idarubicinol, are extensively bound (>90%) to plasma proteins.

METABOLISM
Significant metabolism in liver and in extrahepatic tissues. Metabolism by the liver microsomal system yields the active metabolite idarubicinol, which may also be responsible for the cardiotoxic effects. Idarubicin is eliminated mainly by hepatobiliary excretion into feces, with renal clearance accounting for only about 15% of drug elimination. The half-life of the parent drug is on the order of 20 hours, while the half-life of drug metabolites may exceed 45 hours.

INDICATIONS
1. Acute myelogenous leukemia.
2. Acute lymphoblastic leukemia.
3. Chronic myelogenous leukemia in blast crisis.
4. Myelodysplastic syndromes.

DOSAGE RANGE
Acute myelogenous leukemia, induction therapy—12 mg/m^2 IV on days 1–3 in combination with cytarabine, 100 mg/m^2/day IV continuous infusion for 7 days.

DRUG INTERACTION 1
Probenecid and sulfinpyrazone—Avoid concomitant use of probenecid and sulfinpyrazone, as these are uricosuric agents and may lead to uric acid nephropathy.

DRUG INTERACTION 2
Heparin—Idarubicin is incompatible with heparin, as it forms a precipitate.

SPECIAL CONSIDERATIONS

1. Use with caution in patients with abnormal liver function. Dose modification should be considered in patients with liver dysfunction. Dose reduction by 50% is recommended for serum bilirubin in the range of 2.6–5.0 mg/dL. Absolutely contraindicated in patients with bilirubin >5.0 mg/dL.
2. Careful administration of drug, usually through a central venous catheter, is necessary, as it is a strong vesicant. If peripheral venous access is used, careful monitoring of drug administration is necessary to avoid extravasation. If extravasation is suspected, stop infusion immediately, withdraw fluid, elevate arm, and apply ice to site. In severe cases, consult a plastic surgeon.
3. Alkalinization of the urine, allopurinol, and vigorous IV hydration are recommended to prevent tumor lysis syndrome in patients with acute myelogenous leukemia.
4. Monitor cardiac function before (baseline) and periodically during therapy with either MUGA radionuclide scan or echocardiogram to assess LVEF. Risk of cardiac toxicity is higher in elderly patients >70 years of age, in patients with prior history of hypertension or pre-existing heart disease, in patients previously treated with anthracyclines, or in patients with prior radiation therapy to the chest. While maximum dose of idarubicin that may be administered safely is not known, cumulative doses of >150 mg/m^2 have been associated with decreased LVEF.
5. Caution patients against sun exposure and to wear sun protection when outside.
6. Caution patients about the potential for red discoloration of urine for 1–2 days after drug administration.
7. Pregnancy category D. Breastfeeding should be avoided.

TOXICITY 1
Myelosuppression is dose-limiting, with neutropenia and thrombocytopenia. Nadir typically occurs at 10–14 days after treatment, with recovery of counts by day 21. Risk of myelosuppression is greater in elderly patients and in those previously treated with chemotherapy and/or radiation therapy.

TOXICITY 2
Nausea and vomiting. Usually mild and occur in up to 80%–90% of patients.

TOXICITY 3
Cardiac toxicity. Cardiac effects are similar to but less severe than those of doxorubicin. Acute toxicity presents as atrial arrhythmias, chest pain, and myopericarditis syndrome that typically occur within the first 24–48 hours of drug administration. Dilated cardiomyopathy with congestive heart failure can occur, usually with higher cumulative doses above 150 mg/m^2.

TOXICITY 4
Alopecia is nearly universal but reversible.

TOXICITY 5

Generalized skin rash, increased sensitivity to sunlight, and hyperpigmentation of nails and at the injection site. Radiation-recall skin reactions can occur.

TOXICITY 6

Potent vesicant, and extravasation can lead to extensive tissue damage.

TOXICITY 7

Mucositis and diarrhea are common.

TOXICITY 8

Hepatotoxicity with alterations in SGOT and SGPT.

TOXICITY 9

Red discoloration of urine. Usually within the first 1–2 days after drug administration.

Idecabtagene vicleucel

TRADE NAME	Abecma, ide-cel, bb121	**CLASSIFICATION**	CAR T-cell therapy
CATEGORY	Cellular therapy, immunotherapy	**DRUG MANUFACTURER**	Bristol Myers Squibb

MECHANISM OF ACTION

- Idecabtagene vicleucel is a B-cell maturation antigen (BCMA)-directed, genetically modified, autologous T-cell immunotherapy that binds to BCMA-expressing target malignant plasma cells and normal B cells.
- Prepared from the patient's own peripheral blood mononuclear cells, which are enriched for T cells, and then genetically modified ex vivo by retroviral transduction to express a chimeric antigen receptor (CAR) made up of a murine anti-BCMA single-chain variable fragment-targeting domain for antigen specificity, a transmembrane domain, a CD3-zeta T-cell activation domain, and a 4-1BB co-stimulatory domain. The anti-BCMA CAR T cells are expanded ex vivo and infused back to the patient, where they target BCMA-expressing cells.
- Lymphocyte depletion conditioning regimen with cyclophosphamide and fludarabine leads to increased systemic levels of IL-15 and other pro-inflammatory cytokines and chemokines that enhance CAR T-cell activity.
- The conditioning regimen may also decrease immunosuppressive regulatory T cells, activate antigen-presenting cells, and induce pro-inflammatory tumor cell damage.

MECHANISM OF RESISTANCE
- Antigen loss or modulation.
- Insufficient reactivity against tumor cells with low antigen density.
- Emergence of an antigen-negative clone.

ABSORPTION
Administered only via the IV route.

DISTRIBUTION
Median time of maximum expansion of anti-BCMA CAR T cells are observed within 11 days after infusion.

METABOLISM
Metabolism of idecabtagene vicleucel has not been well characterized.

INDICATIONS
FDA-approved for the treatment of relapsed or refractory multiple myeloma after 4 or more lines of systemic therapy, including an immunomodulatory agent, a proteasome inhibitor, and an anti-CD38 monoclonal antibody.

DOSAGE RANGE
- A lymphodepleting chemotherapy regimen of cyclophosphamide 300 mg/m^2 IV and fludarabine 30 mg/m^2 IV should be administered for 3 days starting 5 days before infusion of idecabtagene vicleucel.
- Patients should be pre-medicated with acetaminophen 650 mg PO and diphenhydramine 12.5 mg IV 30–60 minutes before infusion of idecabtagene vicleucel.
- Dosing of idecabtagene vicleucel is based on a target dose of 300 to 460 × 10^6 CAR-positive T cells.

DRUG INTERACTIONS
None well characterized to date.

SPECIAL CONSIDERATIONS
1. Idecabtagene vicleucel is available only through a restricted program under a Risk Evaluation and Mitigation Strategy (REMS).
2. Monitor for hypersensitivity infusion reactions. Patients should be pre-medicated with acetaminophen 650 mg PO and diphenhydramine 12.5 mg IV at 30–60 minutes prior to CAR T-cell infusion. Prophylactic use of systemic corticosteroids should be avoided as they may interfere with the clinical activity of idecabtagene vicleucel.
3. Monitor patients at least daily for 7 days following infusion for signs and symptoms of cytokine release syndrome (CRS), which may be fatal or life-threatening in some cases. Patients need to be monitored for up to 4 weeks after infusion. Please see package insert for complete guidelines

regarding the appropriate management for CRS. This is a black-box warning.

4. Patients should be advised not to drive and not to engage in operating heavy or potentially dangerous machinery for at least 8 weeks following infusion.
5. Monitor for signs and symptoms of neurologic toxicities, which may be fatal or life-threatening in some cases. This is a black-box warning.
6. Monitor for evidence of hemaphagocytic lymphohistiocytosis (HLH)/macrophage activation syndrome (MAS), which manifests as hypotension, hypoxia, multiple organ function, renal dysfunction, and cytopenias. This is a black-box warning.
7. Monitor for signs and symptoms of infection.
8. Monitor CBCs periodically after infusion as prolonged cytopenias may result from treatment. This is a black-box warning.
9. Immunoglobulin levels should be monitored after treatment with idecabtagene vicleucel. Infection precautions, antibiotic prophylaxis, and immunoglobulin replacement may need to be instituted.
10. Patients will require lifelong monitoring for secondary malignancies.
11. The risk in pregnant women is currently unknown. Breastfeeding should be avoided.

TOXICITY 1
Hypersensitivity infusion reactions.

TOXICITY 2
CRS with fever, hypotension, tachycardia, chills, and hypoxia. More serious events include cardiac arrhythmias (both atrial and ventricular), decreased cardiac ejection fraction, cardiac arrest, capillary leak syndrome, hepatotoxicity, renal failure, and prolongation of coagulation parameters PT and partial thromboplastin time (PTT).

TOXICITY 3
Neurologic toxicity with headache, delirium, encephalopathy, tremors, dizziness, aphasia, imbalance and gait instability, and seizures.

TOXICITY 4
Myelosuppression with thrombocytopenia and neutropenia, which, in some cases, can be prolonged for several weeks after infusion.

TOXICITY 5
Infections, with non-specific pathogens, bacterial, and viral infections most common.

TOXICITY 6
Fatigue and anorexia.

TOXICITY 7
Hypogammaglobulinemia.

TOXICITY 8
Hepatitis B reactivation.

TOXICITY 9
Secondary malignancies.

Idelalisib

TRADE NAME	Zydelig	CLASSIFICATION	Signal transduction inhibitor, PI3K inhibitor
CATEGORY	Targeted agent	DRUG MANUFACTURER	Gilead

MECHANISM OF ACTION
- Small-molecule inhibitor of PI3Kδ kinase, which is expressed in normal and malignant B cells.
- Inhibits several key cell signaling pathways, including B-cell receptor signaling and CXCR4 and CXCR5 signaling.

MECHANISM OF RESISTANCE
- Mutations in PI3Kδ kinase.
- Mutations in other PI3Ks, including PIK3CA or PIK3CB.
- Mutations in MAPK/ERK pathway.
- Activation/upregulation of IGF2R pathway.
- Increased expression of survivin and MCL-1.

ABSORPTION

Absolute oral bioavailability has not been well characterized. Peak plasma drug levels are achieved in about 1.5 hours after ingestion. Ingestion of a high-fat meal may slightly increase idelalisib AUC.

DISTRIBUTION

Significant binding (>84%) to plasma proteins. Steady-state drug levels are reached in approximately 8 days.

METABOLISM

Metabolism in the liver primarily by CYP3A4 and to a minor extent by UGT1A4. GS-563117 is the major metabolite, and it is inactive against the phosphoinositide 3-kinase (PI3K) target. Elimination is mainly hepatic (approximately 80%), with excretion in feces. Renal elimination of parent drug and its metabolites accounts for only about 14% of an administered dose. The terminal half-life of the parent drug is approximately 8 hours.

INDICATIONS

1. FDA-approved for relapsed CLL in combination with rituximab, and in patients for whom rituximab alone would be considered appropriate therapy due to other comorbidities.
2. FDA-approved for relapsed follicular non-Hodgkin's lymphoma after at least 2 prior systemic therapies.
3. FDA-approved for relapsed small lymphocytic lymphoma (SLL) after at least 2 prior systemic therapies.

DOSAGE RANGE

Recommended dose is 150 mg PO bid.

DRUG INTERACTION 1

Phenytoin and other drugs that stimulate the liver microsomal CYP3A4 enzymes, including carbamazepine, rifampin, phenobarbital, and St. John's Wort—These drugs may increase the metabolism of idelalisib, resulting in its inactivation and lower effective drug levels.

DRUG INTERACTION 2

Drugs that inhibit the liver microsomal CYP3A4 enzymes, including ketoconazole, itraconazole, erythromycin, and clarithromycin—These drugs may decrease the metabolism of idelalisib, resulting in increased drug levels and potentially increased toxicity.

DRUG INTERACTION 3

Warfarin—Patients receiving warfarin should be closely monitored for alterations in their clotting parameters (PT and INR) and/or bleeding, as idelalisib may inhibit the metabolism of warfarin by the liver P450 system. Dose of warfarin may require careful adjustment in the presence of idelalisib therapy.

SPECIAL CONSIDERATIONS

1. Idelalisib tablets should be swallowed whole and can be taken with or without food.
2. Monitor liver function tests during treatment. Fatal and/or serious hepatoxicity occurs in 14% of patients, and this represents a black-box warning.
3. Monitor patients for severe diarrhea and/or colitis. Severe diarrhea and/or colitis occurs in 14% of patients, and this represents a black-box warning.
4. Monitor patients for pulmonary symptoms and bilateral interstitial infiltrates. Fatal and/or serious pneumonitis represents a black-box warning.
5. Idelalisib treatment can result in the development of intestinal perforations, which in some cases has resulted in death. These GI perforations represent a black-box warning.
6. Monitor CBCs every 2 weeks for the first 3 months of therapy.
7. Monitor patients for serious allergic reactions, as anaphylaxis has been reported. Idelalisib therapy should be discontinued permanently, and appropriate supportive measures need to be instituted.
8. Pregnancy category D. Breastfeeding should be avoided.

TOXICITY 1
Hepatotoxicity with elevations in LFTs and serum bilirubin.

TOXICITY 2
Diarrhea and/or colitis.

TOXICITY 3
Myelosuppression with neutropenia.

TOXICITY 4
GI perforations, which present as abdominal pain, diarrhea, fever, chills, and nausea/vomiting.

TOXICITY 5
Allergic reactions, including anaphylaxis.

TOXICITY 6
Skin toxicity, including erythema, pruritus, maculopapular rash, generalized skin rash.

Ifosfamide

TRADE NAME	Ifex, Isophosphamide	**CLASSIFICATION**	Alkylating agent
CATEGORY	Chemotherapy drug	**DRUG MANUFACTURER**	Teva

MECHANISM OF ACTION

- Inactive in its parent form.
- Activated by the liver cytochrome P450 microsomal system to various cytotoxic metabolites, including ifosfamide mustard and acrolein.
- Cytotoxic metabolites form cross-links with DNA, resulting in inhibition of DNA synthesis and function.
- Cell cycle–nonspecific agent, active in all phases of the cell cycle.

MECHANISM OF RESISTANCE

- Decreased cellular uptake of drug.
- Decreased expression of liver P450 activating enzymes.
- Increased expression of sulfhydryl proteins, including glutathione and glutathione-associated enzymes.
- Increased expression of aldehyde dehydrogenase, resulting in enhanced drug inactivation.
- Enhanced activity of DNA repair enzymes.

ABSORPTION

Administered only via the IV route.

DISTRIBUTION

Widely distributed into body tissues. About 20% of drug is bound to plasma proteins.

METABOLISM

Extensively metabolized in the liver by the cytochrome P450 system. Activated at a 4-fold slower rate than cyclophosphamide because of lower affinity to the liver P450 system. For this reason, about 4-fold more drug is required to produce equitoxic antitumor effects with cyclophosphamide. The half-life of the drug is 3–10 hours for standard therapy and up to 14 hours for high-dose therapy. Approximately 50%–70% of the drug and its metabolites is excreted in urine.

INDICATIONS
1. Recurrent germ cell tumors.
2. Soft tissue sarcoma, osteogenic sarcoma.
3. Non-Hodgkin's lymphoma.
4. Hodgkin's lymphoma.
5. SCLC and NSCLC.
6. Bladder cancer.
7. Head and neck cancer.
8. Cervical cancer.
9. Ewing's sarcoma.

DOSAGE RANGE
1. Testicular cancer: 1,200 mg/m^2 IV on days 1–5 every 21 days, as part of the VeIP salvage regimen.
2. Soft tissue sarcoma: 2,000 mg/m^2 IV continuous infusion on days 1–3 every 21 days, as part of the MAID regimen.
3. Non-Hodgkin's lymphoma: 1,000 mg/m^2 on days 1 and 2 every 28 days, as part of the ICE regimen.
4. Head and neck cancer: 1,000 mg/m^2 on days 1–3 every 21–28 days, as part of the TIC regimen.

DRUG INTERACTION 1
Phenobarbital, phenytoin, and other drugs that stimulate the liver P450 system—Increase the metabolic activation of ifosfamide to its toxic metabolites, resulting in enhanced toxicity.

DRUG INTERACTION 2
Cimetidine and allopurinol—Increase the formation of ifosfamide metabolites, resulting in increased toxicity.

DRUG INTERACTION 3
Cisplatin—Increases ifosfamide-associated renal toxicity.

DRUG INTERACTION 4
Warfarin—Ifosfamide may enhance the anticoagulant effects of warfarin. Need to monitor coagulation parameters, PT and INR.

SPECIAL CONSIDERATIONS
1. Administer prophylactic antiemetics to avoid nausea and vomiting.
2. Use with caution in patients with abnormal renal function. Dose reduction is recommended in this setting. Baseline CrCl must be obtained, and renal function should be monitored during therapy.
3. Uroprotection with mesna and hydration must be used to prevent bladder toxicity. Pre- and post-hydration (1,500–2,000 mL/day) or continuous

bladder irrigations are recommended to prevent hemorrhagic cystitis. Important to monitor urine for presence of gross and/or microscopic hematuria before each cycle of therapy.

4. Monitor coagulation parameters, including PT and INR, when ifosfamide is used concurrently with warfarin, as ifosfamide may enhance its anticoagulant effects.

5. Contraindicated in patients with peptic ulcer disease, severe liver disease, and/or cardiac disease.

6. Pregnancy category D. Breastfeeding should be avoided.

TOXICITY 1

Myelosuppression is dose-limiting. Mainly leukopenia and to a lesser extent thrombocytopenia. Nadir occurs at 10–14 days, with recovery in 21 days.

TOXICITY 2

Bladder toxicity can be dose-limiting and presents with hemorrhagic cystitis, dysuria, and increased urinary frequency. Chronic fibrosis of bladder leads to an increased risk of secondary bladder cancer. Uroprotection with mesna and hydration must be used to prevent bladder toxicity.

TOXICITY 3

Nausea and vomiting. Usually occurs within 3–6 hours of therapy and may last up to 3 days. Anorexia is fairly common.

TOXICITY 4

Neurotoxicity in the form of lethargy, confusion, seizure, cerebellar ataxia, weakness, hallucinations, cranial nerve dysfunction, and rarely stupor and coma. Incidence may be higher in patients receiving high-dose therapy and in those with impaired renal function.

TOXICITY 5

Skin toxicity with skin rash, hyperpigmentation, and nail changes are occasionally seen. Alopecia is common (>80%).

TOXICITY 6

Syndrome of inappropriate antidiuretic hormone secretion (SIADH).

TOXICITY 7

Amenorrhea, oligospermia, and infertility.

TOXICITY 8

Mutagenic, teratogenic, and carcinogenic.

Imatinib

TRADE NAME	STI571, Gleevec	CLASSIFICATION	Signal transduction inhibitor, Bcr-Abl inhibitor
CATEGORY	Targeted agent	DRUG MANUFACTURER	Novartis

MECHANISM OF ACTION

- Phenylaminopyrimidine methanesulfonate compound that occupies the ATP-binding site of the Bcr-Abl protein and only a very limited number of other tyrosine kinases. Binding in this ATP pocket results in subsequent inhibition of substrate phosphorylation.
- Potent and selective inhibitor of the P210 Bcr-Abl tyrosine kinase, resulting in inhibition of clonogenicity and tumorigenicity of Bcr-Abl and Ph+ cells.
- Induces apoptosis in Bcr-Abl–positive cells without causing cell differentiation.
- Inhibits other activated Abl tyrosine kinases, including P185 Bcr-Abl, and inhibits other receptor tyrosine kinases for platelet-derived growth factor receptor (PDGFR) and c-Kit.

MECHANISM OF RESISTANCE

- Increased expression of Bcr-Abl tyrosine kinase, through amplification of the Bcr-Abl gene.
- Mutations in the Bcr-Abl tyrosine kinase, resulting in altered binding affinity to the drug.
- Increased expression of P170 glycoprotein, resulting in enhanced drug efflux and decreased intracellular drug accumulation.
- Increased degradation and/or metabolism of the drug through as-yet-undefined mechanisms.
- Increased expression of c-Kit through amplification of the c-Kit gene.
- Mutations in the c-Kit tyrosine kinase, resulting in altered binding affinity to the drug.

ABSORPTION

Oral bioavailability is nearly 100%.

DISTRIBUTION

Extensive binding (95%) to plasma proteins, including albumin and α1-acid glycoprotein. Steady-state drug concentrations are reached in 2–3 days.

METABOLISM

Metabolism in the liver, primarily by CYP3A4 microsomal enzymes. Other cytochrome P450 enzymes play a minor role in its metabolism. The main metabolite is the N-demethylated piperazine derivative, and this metabolite shows in vitro potency similar to that of the parent drug. Elimination is mainly in the feces, predominantly as metabolites. The terminal half-life of the parent drug is 18 hours, while that of its main metabolite, the N-desmethyl derivative, is on the order of 40 hours.

INDICATIONS

1. Chronic phase of CML—FDA-approved first-line therapy in adult patients.
2. Chronic phase of CML after failure on interferon-α therapy—FDA-approved.
3. CML in accelerated phase and/or in blast crisis—FDA-approved.
4. Newly diagnosed pediatric patients with Ph+ acute lymphocytic leukemia (Ph+ ALL)—FDA-approved.
5. Chronic phase Ph+ CML in pediatric patients whose disease has recurred after stem cell transplant or is resistant to interferon-α.
6. Myelodysplastic/myeloproliferative diseases (MDS/MPD) associated with PDGFR gene rearrangements.
7. Hypereosinophilic syndrome/chronic eosinophilic leukemia (HES/CEL).
8. Relapsed/refractory adult Ph+ ALL.
9. Gastrointestinal stromal tumors (GIST) expressing c-Kit (CD117)—Unresectable and/or metastatic disease.
10. GIST expressing c-Kit (CD117)—Adjuvant therapy following resection of localized disease.

DOSAGE RANGE

1. Recommended starting dose is 400 mg/day for patients in chronic phase CML and 600 mg/day for patients in accelerated phase or blast crisis. Dose increases from 400 mg to 600 mg or 800 mg in patients with chronic phase disease, or from 600 mg to a maximum of 800 mg (given as 400 mg twice daily) in patients with accelerated phase or blast crisis, may be considered in the absence of severe adverse drug reaction and severe non–leukemia-related neutropenia or thrombocytopenia in the following circumstances: disease progression (at any time), failure to achieve a satisfactory hematologic response after at least 3 months of treatment, failure to achieve a cytogenetic response after 12 months of treatment, or loss of a previously achieved hematologic and/or cytogenetic response. Patients should be monitored closely following dose escalation given the potential for an increased incidence of adverse reactions at higher dosages.

2. Recommended starting dose is 400 mg/day for patients with unresectable and/or metastatic GIST. Limited data exist on the effect of dose increases from 400 mg to 600 mg or 800 mg in patients progressing at the lower dose.
3. Recommended dose is 400 mg/day for 3 years of adjuvant therapy of patients with early-stage GIST.
4. Recommended starting dose is 400 mg/day for patients with MDS/MPD.
5. Recommended starting dose is 400 mg/day for patients with HES/CEL.
6. Recommended starting dose is 600 mg/day for patients with Ph+ ALL.

DRUG INTERACTION 1
Phenytoin and other drugs that stimulate the liver microsomal CYP3A4 enzymes, including carbamazepine, rifampin, phenobarbital, and St. John's Wort—These drugs increase the metabolism of imatinib, resulting in its inactivation and lower effective drug levels.

DRUG INTERACTION 2
Drugs that inhibit the liver microsomal CYP3A4 enzymes, including ketoconazole, itraconazole, erythromycin, and clarithromycin—These drugs decrease the metabolism of imatinib, resulting in increased drug levels and potentially increased toxicity.

DRUG INTERACTION 3
Warfarin—Patients on warfarin should be closely monitored for alterations in their clotting parameters (PT and INR) and/or bleeding, as imatinib inhibits the metabolism of warfarin by the liver P450 system. Dose of warfarin may require careful adjustment in the presence of imatinib therapy.

SPECIAL CONSIDERATIONS
1. Patients should be weighed and monitored regularly for signs and symptoms of fluid retention. The risk of fluid retention and edema is increased with higher drug doses and in patients of age >65 years.
2. Use with caution in patients with underlying hepatic impairment. Dose adjustment is not required in patients with mild or moderate hepatic impairment. Patients with severe hepatic impairment should have a 25% reduction in the recommended starting dose.
3. Use with caution in patients with underlying renal impairment. For patients with moderate renal impairment (CrCL 20–39 mL/min), doses greater than 400 mg are not recommended, and patients should have a 50% reduction in the recommended starting dose. For patients with mild renal impairment (CrCL 40–59 mL/min), doses greater than 600 mg are not recommended.
4. Monitor CBC on a weekly basis for the first month, biweekly for the second month, and periodically thereafter.
5. Imatinib should be taken with food and a large glass of water to decrease the risk of GI irritation. Imatinib tablets can be dissolved in water or apple juice for patients who have difficulty swallowing.

6. Hematologic responses typically occur within 2 weeks after initiation of therapy, while complete hematologic responses are observed within 4 weeks after starting therapy.
7. Cytogenetic responses are observed as early as 2 months and up to 10 months after starting therapy. The median time to best cytogenetic response is about 5 months.
8. Monitor dose of drug when used in patients with seizure disorders on phenytoin. Dose of drug may need to be increased, as the metabolism of imatinib by the CYP3A4 enzyme is enhanced in the presence of phenytoin.
9. Patients who require anticoagulation should receive low-molecular-weight or standard heparin, as imatinib inhibits the metabolism of warfarin.
10. Monitor cardiac function before (baseline) and periodically during therapy with either MUGA radionuclide scan or echocardiogram to assess LVEF. The diagnosis of CHF should be considered in patients who experience edema while on imatinib.
11. Avoid Seville oranges, starfruit, pomelos, grapefruit juice, and grapefruit products while on imatinib therapy.
12. Patients should be closely monitored for depressive symptoms and suicidal ideation while on therapy.
13. Musculoskeletal pain may be a sign of potential withdrawal syndrome in patients who had stopped imatinib therapy after having been on treatment for more than 3 years. Pain sites include shoulder and hip regions, extremities, and hands and feet, along with muscle tenderness.
14. Screen all patients for hepatitis B (HBV) infection before initiation of imatinib therapy. Monitor HBV carriers for signs of active HBV infection during imatinib therapy. Imatinib therapy can increase the risk of HBV reactivation, and imatinib therapy should be permanently discontinued in the event of HBV reactivation.
15. Pregnancy category D. Breastfeeding should be avoided.

TOXICITY 1

Nausea and vomiting occur in 40%–50% of patients. Usually related to the swallowing of capsules and relieved when the drug is taken with food.

TOXICITY 2

Transient ankle and periorbital edema. Usually mild to moderate in nature.

TOXICITY 3

Occasional myalgias.

TOXICITY 4

Fluid retention with pleural effusion, ascites, pulmonary edema, and weight gain. Usually dose-related and more common in elderly patients and in those in blast crisis and the accelerated phase of CML. CHF is a rare but serious adverse event.

TOXICITY 5
Diarrhea is observed in 25%–30% of patients.

TOXICITY 6
Myelosuppression with neutropenia and thrombocytopenia.

TOXICITY 7
Mild, transient elevation in serum transaminases. Clinically asymptomatic in most cases.

TOXICITY 8
Skin toxicity in the form of bullous reactions, including erythema multiforme and Stevens-Johnson syndrome.

TOXICITY 9
Insomnia, depression, and suicidal ideation.

Infigratinib

TRADE NAME	Truseltiq, BGJ398	**CLASSIFICATION**	Signal transduction inhibitor, FGFR inhibitor
CATEGORY	Targeted agent	**DRUG MANUFACTURER**	Incyte

MECHANISM OF ACTION
- Orally bioavailable, selective, ATP-competitive pan-fibroblast growth factor receptor (FGFR) small molecule inhibitor.
- Leads to inhibition of FGFR-mediated signaling in tumors with activating FGFR amplification, mutations, fusions, and other rearrangements.
- FGFR signaling plays a critical role in tumor cell growth, proliferation, migration, angiogenesis, and survival.
- FGFR signaling pathway activated in 15%–20% of intrahepatic cholangiocarcinoma and in other tumor types, including bladder cancer, breast cancer, NSCLC, endometrial cancer, and head and neck cancer.

MECHANISM OF RESISTANCE
- Activation of receptor tyrosine kinase pathways, including EGFR, ErbB2, ErbB3, and MET.
- Activation of intracellular downstream cellular signaling pathways, for example, PI3K, AKT, mTOR, MAPK, and STAT3.
- Mutations in FGFR2 and FGFR3.
- Gatekeeper mutations in FGFR2, including V564F, that modify binding pocket with reduced binding to drug.

ABSORPTION
Median time to peak drug levels is 6 hours after oral ingestion. Food with high-fat/high-calorie content increases oral absorption.

DISTRIBUTION
Extensive binding (97%) of drug mainly to lipoproteins. Steady-state drug levels are reached in 15 days.

METABOLISM
Metabolized in the liver primarily by CYP3A4 (about 94%) and to a lesser extent by flavin-containing monooxygenase 3 (FMO3; 6%). BHS697 and CQM157 are the 2 main active metabolites. Approximately 77% of an administered dose is eliminated in feces (3.5% in parent form) and 7.2% is eliminated in urine, (2% in parent form). The mean terminal half-life of infigratinib is approximately 33.5 hours.

INDICATIONS
FDA-approved for previously treated, unresectable locally advanced or metastatic cholangiocarcinoma with an FGFR2 fusion or other rearrangement as detected by an FDA-approved test. Accelerated approval based on overall response rate and duration of response.

DOSAGE RANGE
Recommended dose is 125 mg PO once daily for 21 days followed by 7 days off in 28-day cycles.

DRUG INTERACTION 1
Drugs such as ketoconazole, itraconazole, erythromycin, clarithromycin, atazanavir, indinavir, nefazodone, nelfinavir, ritonavir, saquinavir, telithromycin, and voriconazole may decrease the metabolism of infigratinib, resulting in increased drug levels and potentially increased toxicity.

DRUG INTERACTION 2
Phenytoin and other drugs that stimulate the liver microsomal CYP3A4 enzymes, including carbamazepine, rifampin, phenobarbital, and St. John's Wort—These drugs may increase the metabolism of infigratinib, resulting in lower effective drug levels.

DRUG INTERACTION 3

Avoid concomitant use of agents that alter serum phosphate levels as infigratinib increases serum phosphate levels. Such drugs include potassium phosphate supplements, vitamin D supplements, antacids, phosphate-containing enemas or laxatives, and drugs known to have phosphate as an excipient.

DRUG INTERACTION 4

Avoid concomitant use of gastric acid-reducing agents, such as proton pump inhibitors, H2 blockers, and antacids as they may reduce oral bioavailability of infigratinib.

SPECIAL CONSIDERATIONS

1. Patients should be seen by a dietician and placed on a restricted phosphate diet to 600–800 mg daily.
2. Closely monitor serum phosphate levels while on therapy. The median time to onset of hyperphosphatemia is 8 days. Serum phosphate levels should be monitored on a monthly basis. If the serum phosphate level is >5.5 mg/dL, ensure that a restricted phosphate diet is being correctly followed. For serum phosphate levels >7.5 mg/dL, phosphate-lowering therapy, such as an oral phosphate binder, should be used, and the dose of drug should be held, reduced, or permanently discontinued based on duration and severity of the hyperphosphatemia.
3. Comprehensive eye exam, including optical coherence tomography (OCT), should be performed at baseline, at 1 month, at 3 months, and then every 3 months thereafter while on treatment. With the onset of new visual symptoms, patients should have an immediate evaluation with OCT, with follow-up every 3 weeks until resolution of symptoms or discontinuation of treatment.
4. For patients with mild hepatic impairment, the dose should be reduced to 100 mg PO daily for 21 days with 1-week off in a 28-day cycle. For patients with moderate hepatic impairment, the dose should be reduced to 75 mg PO daily for 21 days with 1 week off in a 28-day cycle. Has not been studied in the setting of severe hepatic impairment.
5. In the setting of mild and moderate renal impairment (CrCl, 30–89 mL/min), the dose should be reduced to 100 mg PO daily for 21 days with 1 week off in a 28-day cycle. Has not been studied in the setting of severe renal impairment or end-stage renal disease.
6. Concomitant use of a moderate or strong CYP3A inducer should be avoided.
7. Concomitant use of a gastric acid-reducing agent should be avoided. In the event that a co-administration cannot be avoided, the administration of infigratinib should be staggered with the proton pump inhibitor, H2 blocker, and/or antacid.
8. Embryo-fetal toxicity. Can cause fetal harm when administered to a pregnant woman. Females of reproductive potential should use effective contraception during drug therapy and for 1 month after the final dose. Breastfeeding should be avoided.

TOXICITY 1
Hyperphosphatemia.

TOXICITY 2
Ocular disorders with retinal pigment epithelial detachment (RPED) leading to blurred vision, visual floaters, or photopsia. Dry eye symptoms are common.

TOXICITY 3
Dysgeusia, diarrhea, mucositis, dry mouth, and nausea/vomiting.

TOXICITY 4
Fatigue and anorexia.

TOXICITY 5
Dry skin, palmar-plantar erythrodysesthesia, paronychia, and nail discoloration.

TOXICITY 6
Arthralgias.

Inotuzumab ozogamicin

TRADE NAME	Besponsa, CMC-544	**CLASSIFICATION**	Antibody-drug conjugate, anti-CD22 antibody
CATEGORY	Biologic response modifier agent, chemotherapy drug	**DRUG MANUFACTURER**	Pfizer

MECHANISM OF ACTION
- CD22-directed antibody-drug conjugate that is made up of inotuzumab, a humanized IgG4 κ antibody specific for the cell surface glycoprotein CD22, and N-acetyl-gamma-calicheamicin, a cytotoxic enediyne antibiotic derived from the soil microorganism *Micromonospora echinospora*.
- Upon binding to CD22, inotuzumab ozogamicin is rapidly internalized into lysosomes, and calicheamicin is then released inside the cell to interact with the minor groove of DNA, leading to site-specific double-strand DNA breaks. Calicheamicin causes cell cycle arrest in the G2-M phase, which is then followed by apoptosis.
- CD22 is expressed in >90% of patients with B-cell ALL and in most B-cell cancers but not expressed on other normal tissues, including hematopoietic stem cells.

MECHANISM OF RESISTANCE
None well characterized to date.

ABSORPTION
Administered only via the IV route.

DISTRIBUTION
Extensive binding (97%) of inotuzumab ozogamicin to plasma proteins. Steady-state drug concentrations are achieved by the fourth cycle of therapy.

METABOLISM
Inotuzumab ozogamicin is primarily metabolized by non-enzymatic reduction. The median terminal half-life is on the order of 12.3 days.

INDICATIONS
FDA-approved for adults with relapsed or refractory B-cell precursor ALL.

DOSAGE RANGE
1. Cycle 1 and subsequent cycles: 0.8 mg/m^2 IV on days 1, 8, and 15. Each cycle is given every 21 days.
2. For patients who achieved a complete response (CR) or CR with incomplete hematologic recovery (CRi): 0.5 mg/m^2 IV on days 1, 8, and 15. Each cycle is given every 28 days.
3. For patients who have not achieved a CR or CRi: 0.8 mg/m^2 IV on day 1 and 0.5 mg/m^2 IV on days 8 and 15. Each cycle is given every 28 days.

DRUG INTERACTIONS
None well characterized to date.

SPECIAL CONSIDERATIONS
1. Monitor for infusion-related reactions. Patients should be premedicated with a corticosteroid, antihistamine, and acetaminophen prior to all infusions. Patients should be monitored during and for at least 1 hour after the completion of the infusion.
2. Cytoreduction with a combination of hydroxyurea, steroids, and/or vincristine to a peripheral blast count of <10,000 is recommended prior to the first dose of therapy.
3. Monitor CBC prior to each treatment cycle. Please see package insert for details regarding dose modifications for hematologic toxicities.
4. Monitor LFTs and serum bilirubin levels closely, as hepatotoxicity, including hepatic veno-occlusive disease (VOD), has been observed. This is a black-box warning. The risk of VOD is greater in patients who undergo hematopoietic stem cell transplantation (HSCT) after inotuzumab ozogamicin treatment.
5. The use of HSCT conditioning regimens with two alkylating agents and total bilirubin > ULN before HSCT are associated with an increased risk of VOD. There are other risk factors for VOD, which include

ongoing or prior liver disease, prior HSCT, increased age, later salvage lines, and a higher number of inotuzumab ozogamicin treatment cycles.

6. There is an increased risk of post-HSCT non-disease relapse mortality rate in patients receiving inotuzumab ozogamicin.

7. ECGs should be obtained at baseline and periodically on treatment to assess QT interval. Monitoring should be more frequent when medications known to prolong the QT interval are used concomitantly with inotuzumab ozogamicin.

8. Dose reduction is not required for patients with mild, moderate, or severe renal dysfunction. Has not been studied in end-stage renal disease, and the effect of hemodialysis is not known.

9. Dose reduction is not required for patients with mild hepatic dysfunction. There is limited safety information for patients with moderate or severe hepatic dysfunction, and caution should be used in these patients.

10. Can cause fetal harm when given to a pregnant woman. Females of reproductive potential should use effective contraception during treatment and for at least 8 months after the last dose. Males with female partners of reproductive potential should use effective contraception while on treatment and for at least 5 months after the last dose. Breastfeeding should be avoided.

TOXICITY 1
Myelosuppression with thrombocytopenia and neutropenia.

TOXICITY 2
Infusion-related reactions.

TOXICITY 3
Hepatotoxicity with elevation in LFTs. Severe and sometimes fatal hepatic VOD observed in patients during or following treatment or following HSCT after completion of treatment.

TOXICITY 4
QT interval prolongation.

TOXICITY 5
Asthenia, fatigue, and pyrexia.

Interferon-α

TRADE NAME	α-interferon, IFN-α, Interferon-α2a, Roferon Interferon-α2b, Intron A, Sylatron (Peginterferon-α2b)	**CLASSIFICATION**	Cytokine
CATEGORY	Biologic response modifier agent, immunotherapy	**DRUG MANUFACTURER**	Roche (Roferon), Merck (Intron A), Merck (Sylatron)

MECHANISM OF ACTION
- Precise mechanism of antitumor action remains unknown.
- Direct antiproliferative effects on tumor cell mediated by induction of 2′, 5′-oligoadenylate synthetase and protein kinase, leading to decreased translation and inhibition of tumor cell protein synthesis; induction of differentiation; prolongation of the cell cycle; and modulation of oncogene expression.
- Indirect induction of antitumor mechanisms mediated by induced activity of at least four immune effector cells, including cytotoxic T cells, helper T cells, NK cells, and macrophages; enhancement of tumor surface expression of critical antigens that are recognized by the immune system; and inhibition of angiogenesis through decreased expression of various angiogenic factors.

MECHANISM OF RESISTANCE
- Development of neutralizing antibodies to interferon-α.
- Decreased expression of cell surface receptors to interferon-α.

ABSORPTION
Administered only via the parenteral route. Approximately 80%–90% of interferon-α is absorbed into the systemic circulation after IM or SC injection. Peak plasma levels are achieved in 4 hours after intramuscular injection and 7 hours after subcutaneous administration.

DISTRIBUTION
Does not cross the blood-brain barrier. Binding to plasma proteins has not been well characterized.

METABOLISM
Interferon-α is catabolized by renal tubule cells to various breakdown products. The major route of elimination is through the kidneys by both glomerular filtration and tubular secretion. Hepatic metabolism and biliary excretion play only a minor role in drug clearance. The elimination half-life is approximately 2–7 hours and depends on the specific route of drug administration.

INDICATIONS
1. Malignant melanoma—Adjuvant therapy.
2. Chronic myelogenous leukemia—Chronic phase.
3. Hairy cell leukemia.
4. AIDS-related Kaposi's sarcoma.
5. Cutaneous T-cell lymphoma.
6. Multiple myeloma.
7. Low-grade, non-Hodgkin's lymphoma.
8. Renal cell cancer.
9. Hemangioma.

DOSAGE RANGE
1. Chronic myelogenous leukemia: 9 million IU SC or IM daily.
2. Hairy cell leukemia: 3 million IU SC or IM daily for 16–24 weeks.
3. Malignant melanoma: 20 million IU/m^2 IV, 5 times weekly for 4 weeks, then 10 million IU/m^2 SC, 3 times weekly for 48 weeks.
4. Malignant melanoma (Peginterferon-α2b): 6 mg/kg/week SC for 8 doses followed by 3 mg/kg/week SC for up to 5 years.
5. Kaposi's sarcoma: 36 million IU SC or IM daily for 12 weeks.

DRUG INTERACTION 1
Phenytoin, phenobarbital—Effects of phenytoin and phenobarbital may be increased, as interferon-α inhibits the liver P450 system. Drug levels should be monitored closely, and dose adjustments made accordingly.

DRUG INTERACTION 2
Live vaccines—Vaccination with live vaccines is contraindicated during and for at least 3 months after completion of interferon-α therapy.

SPECIAL CONSIDERATIONS
1. Use with caution in patients with pre-existing cardiac, pulmonary, CNS, hepatic, and/or renal impairment, as they are at increased risk for developing serious and sometimes fatal reactions.
2. Contraindicated in patients with history of autoimmune disease, autoimmune hepatitis, or in those who have received immunosuppressive therapy for organ transplants.
3. Contraindicated in patients with a known allergy to benzyl alcohol, as the injectable solution form contains benzyl alcohol.
4. Use with caution in patients with myelosuppression or those who are receiving concurrent agents known to cause myelosuppression.
5. Use with caution in patients with a history of depression and/or other neuropsychiatric disorders. Routine neuropsychiatric monitoring of all patients on interferon-α is recommended. Therapy should be permanently discontinued in patients with persistently severe or worsening signs or symptoms of depression, psychosis, or encephalopathy.

6. Use with caution in older patients (>65 years of age), as they are at increased risk for developing fatigue and neurologic toxicities secondary to interferon-α.
7. Premedicate patient with acetaminophen to reduce the risk and/or severity of flu-like symptoms, including fever and chills. If acetaminophen is unsuccessful in controlling these symptoms, indomethacin can be used.
8. Pregnancy category C. Breastfeeding should be avoided.

TOXICITY 1
Flu-like symptoms with fever, chills, headache, myalgias, and arthralgias. Occur in 80%–90% of patients, usually beginning a few hours after the first injection and lasting for up to 8–9 hours. Incidence decreases with subsequent injections. Can be controlled with acetaminophen and/or indomethacin.

TOXICITY 2
Fatigue and anorexia are dose-limiting with chronic administration.

TOXICITY 3
Somnolence, confusion, or depression. Patients >65 years of age are more susceptible to the neurologic sequelae of interferon-α.

TOXICITY 4
Myelosuppression with mild leukopenia and thrombocytopenia. Reversible upon discontinuation of therapy.

TOXICITY 5
Mild, transient elevations in serum transaminases. Dose-dependent toxicity observed more frequently in the presence of pre-existing liver abnormalities.

TOXICITY 6
Renal toxicity is uncommon and usually manifested by mild proteinuria and hypocalcemia. Acute renal failure and nephrotic syndrome have been reported in rare instances.

TOXICITY 7
Alopecia, skin rash, pruritus with dry skin, and irritation at the injection site.

TOXICITY 8
Cardiac toxicity in the form of chest pain, arrhythmias, and congestive heart failure. Uncommon and almost always reversible.

TOXICITY 9
Impotence, decreased libido, menstrual irregularities, and an increased incidence of spontaneous abortions.

TOXICITY 10

Rare cases of autoimmune disorders, including thrombocytopenia, vasculitis, Raynaud's disease, lupus, rheumatoid arthritis, and rhabdomyolysis.

TOXICITY 11

Retinopathy with macular edema, retinal artery or vein thrombosis, optic neuritis, retinal detachment, cotton-wool spots, and small hemorrhages.

Ipilimumab

TRADE NAME	Yervoy	**CLASSIFICATION**	Anti-CTLA4 monoclonal antibody
CATEGORY	Immunotherapy, immune checkpoint inhibitor	**DRUG MANUFACTURER**	Bristol-Myers Squibb

MECHANISM OF ACTION

- Human IgGI kappa antibody that binds to cytotoxic T-lymphocyte-associated antigen 4 (CTLA-4), which is expressed on the surface of activated CD4 and CD8 T lymphocytes, resulting in inhibition of the interaction between CTLA-4 and its target ligands CD80/CD86.
- Blockade of CTLA-4 enhances T-cell immune responses, including T-cell activation and proliferation.

MECHANISM OF RESISTANCE

- Increased expression and/or activity of other immune checkpoint pathways (e.g., TIGIT, TIM3, and LAG3).
- Increased expression of other immune escape mechanisms.
- Increased infiltration of immune suppressive populations within the tumor microenvironment, which include Tregs, myeloid-derived suppressor cells (MDSCs), and M2 macrophages.
- Release of various cytokines, chemokines, and metabolites within the tumor microenvironment, including CSF-1, tryptophan metabolites, TGF-β, and adenosine.

ABSORPTION

Administered only via the IV route.

DISTRIBUTION

Distribution is not well characterized. Steady-state concentrations are generally reached by the third dose.

METABOLISM

Metabolism of ipilimumab has not been extensively characterized. The terminal half-life is on the order of 16–17 days.

INDICATIONS

1. FDA-approved for the treatment of adult and pediatric patients with unresectable or metastatic malignant melanoma as a single agent or in combination with nivolumab.
2. FDA-approved for the adjuvant treatment of adult patients with cutaneous melanoma with pathologic involvement of regional lymph nodes of more than 1 mm who have undergone complete resection, including total lymphadenectomy.
3. FDA-approved in combination with nivolumab for intermediate- or poor-risk previously untreated advanced renal cell cancer.
4. FDA-approved in combination with nivolumab for adult and pediatric patients 12 years of age or older with microsatellite instability-high (MSI-H) or mismatch repair deficient (dMMR) metastatic colorectal cancer that has progressed following treatment with a fluoropyrimidine, oxaliplatin, and irinotecan.
5. FDA-approved in combination with nivolumab for hepatocellular cancer (HCC) that has been previously treated with sorafenib. Approved under accelerated approval based on overall response rate and duration of response.
6. FDA-approved in combination with nivolumab as first-line treatment of adult patients with metastatic NSCLC expressing PD-L1 (>1%) with no EGFR or ALK mutations.
7. FDA-approved in combination with nivolumab and 2 cycles of platinum-doublet chemotherapy as first-line treatment of adult patients with metastatic or recurrent NSCLC with no EGFR or ALK mutations.
8. FDA-approved in combination with nivolumab as first-line treatment of adult patients with unresectable malignant pleural mesothelioma.
9. FDA-approved in combination with nivolumab as first-line treatment of adult patients with unresectable advanced or metastatic esophageal squamous cell cancer.

DOSAGE RANGE

1. Metastatic melanoma: Recommended dose is 3 mg/kg IV every 3 weeks for a total of 4 doses.
2. Adjuvant melanoma: Recommended dose is 10 mg/kg IV every 3 weeks for 4 doses, followed by 10 mg/kg IV every 12 weeks for up to 3 years.
3. Advanced renal cell cancer: Recommended dose is 1 mg/kg IV every 3 weeks for 4 doses in combination with nivolumab 3 mg/kg IV every 3 weeks, followed by single-agent nivolumab 240 mg IV every 2 weeks or 480 mg IV every 4 weeks.

4. MSI-H or dMMR metastatic colorectal cancer: Recommended dose is 1 mg/kg IV with nivolumab 3 mg/kg IV on the same day every 3 weeks for 4 doses, followed by single-agent nivolumab 240 mg IV every 2 weeks or 480 mg IV every 4 weeks.
5. HCC: Recommended dose is 3 mg/kg IV with nivolumab 1 mg/kg IV on the same day every 3 weeks for 4 doses, followed by single-agent nivolumab 240 mg IV every 2 weeks or 480 mg IV every 4 weeks.
6. NSCLC: Recommended dose is 1 mg/kg IV every 6 weeks with nivolumab 3 mg/kg IV every 2 weeks.
7. NSCLC: Recommended dose is 1 mg/kg IV every 6 weeks with nivolumab 360 mg IV every 3 weeks and 2 cycles of platinum-doublet chemotherapy.
8. Pleural mesothelioma: Recommended dose is 1 mg/kg IV every 6 weeks with nivolumab 360 mg IV every 3 weeks.
9. Esophageal squamous cell cancer: Recommended dose is 1 mg/kg IV every 6 weeks with nivolumab 360 mg IV every 3 weeks or 360 mg IV every 3 weeks.

DRUG INTERACTIONS
None well characterized to date.

SPECIAL CONSIDERATIONS
1. Ipilimumab can result in severe and fatal immune-mediated adverse reactions due to T-cell activation and proliferation. These immune-mediated reactions may involve any organ system, with the most common reactions being enterocolitis, hepatitis, dermatitis, neuropathy, and endocrinopathy. They typically occur during treatment, although some of these reactions may occur weeks to months after completion of therapy. These reactions represent a black-box warning.
2. Ipilimumab should be permanently discontinued for any of the following:
   - Persistent moderate adverse reactions or inability to reduce daily steroid dose to 7.5 mg prednisone
   - Failure to complete the full treatment course within 16 weeks from administration of first dose
   - Grade ¾ colitis
   - Grade ¾ pneumonitis
   - SGOT/SGPT $>5 \times$ ULN or total bilirubin $>3 \times$ ULN
   - Grade 4 nephritis with renal dysfunction
   - Grades 2, 3, or 4 myocarditis
   - Stevens-Johnson syndrome, toxic epidermal necrolysis, or rash complicated by full-thickness dermal ulceration or necrotic, bullous, or hemorrhagic manifestations
   - Severe motor or sensory neuropathy, Guillain-Barré syndrome, or myasthenia gravis
   - Severe immune-mediated reactions involving any organ system
   - Immune-mediated ocular disease that is unresponsive to topical immunosuppressive therapy
3. Ipilimumab should be withheld for any moderate immune-mediated adverse reaction or for symptomatic endocrinopathy. For patients with partial or complete resolution of symptoms (grades 0–1) and who are

receiving less than 7.5 mg prednisone, ipilimumab may be resumed at a dose of 3 mg/kg every 3 weeks until administration of all 4 planned doses or 16 weeks from first dose, whichever occurs earlier.

4. Closely monitor for signs and symptoms of enterocolitis, such as diarrhea and abdominal pain. Patients with inflammatory bowel disease may not be appropriate candidates for ipilimumab.

5. In patients with moderate enterocolitis, withhold ipilimumab therapy and administer antidiarrheal treatment. If symptoms persist for more than 1 week, administer prednisone at 0.5 mg/kg. In patients with severe enterocolitis, permanently discontinue ipilimumab and administer prednisone at 1–2 mg/kg/day.

6. Administer steroid eye drops to patients who develop uveitis, iritis, or episcleritis. Permanently discontinue ipilimumab for immune-mediated ocular disease that is unresponsive to local immunosuppressive therapy. In this setting, administer prednisone at 1–2 mg/kg/day.

7. FDA-approved Risk Evaluation and Mitigation Strategy (REMS) program has been developed to inform healthcare providers about the risk of serious immune-mediated adverse reactions caused by ipilimumab.

8. Monitor thyroid function tests at the start of treatment and before each dose.

9. Pregnancy category C. Breastfeeding should be avoided.

TOXICITY 1
Infusion-related reactions.

TOXICITY 2
Immune-mediated enterocolitis presenting as diarrhea, abdominal pain, fever, and ileus.

TOXICITY 3
Immune-mediated hepatotoxicity that can range from moderate to severe life-threatening hepatotoxicity.

TOXICITY 4
Immune-mediated dermatitis with rash and pruritis. Severe, life-threatening dermatitis in the form of Stevens-Johnson syndrome; toxic epidermal necrolysis; full-thickness dermal ulceration; or necrotic, bullous, or hemorrhagic skin lesions occurs rarely.

TOXICITY 5
Endocrinopathies with hypophysitis, adrenal insufficiency, hypopituitarism, hypogonadism, hyperthyroidism or hypothyroidism, and diabetes.

TOXICITY 6
Neurotoxicity with motor weakness, sensory alterations, myositis, myasthenia gravis, and Guillain-Barré–like syndromes.

TOXICITY 7
Ocular toxicities in the form of uveitis, iritis, conjunctivitis, blepharitis, or episcleritis.

TOXICITY 8
Cardiac toxicity with myocarditis, pericarditis, and vasculitis.

TOXICITY 9
Renal toxicity with nephritis.

Irinotecan

TRADE NAME	Camptosar, CPT-11	CLASSIFICATION	Topoisomerase I inhibitor
CATEGORY	Chemotherapy drug	DRUG MANUFACTURER	Pfizer

MECHANISM OF ACTION

- Semisynthetic derivative of camptothecin, an alkaloid extract from the *Camptotheca acuminata* tree.
- Inactive in its parent form. Converted by a carboxylesterase enzyme in the liver to the active SN-38 metabolite.
- SN-38 binds to and stabilizes the topoisomerase I-DNA complex and prevents the religation of DNA after it has been cleaved by topoisomerase I. The collision between this stable, cleavable complex and the advancing replication fork results in double-strand DNA breaks and cellular death.
- Antitumor activity of drug requires the presence of ongoing DNA synthesis.
- Cell cycle–nonspecific agent with activity in all phases of the cell cycle.
- Colorectal tumors express higher levels of topoisomerase I than normal colonic mucosa, making this an attractive target for chemotherapy.

MECHANISM OF RESISTANCE

- Decreased expression of topoisomerase I.
- Mutations in topoisomerase I enzyme, with decreased affinity for the drug.
- Increased expression of the multidrug-resistant phenotype, with over-expression of P170 glycoprotein. Results in enhanced efflux of drug and decreased intracellular accumulation of drug.
- Decreased formation of the cytotoxic metabolite SN-38 through decreased activity and/or expression of the carboxylesterase enzyme.
- Decreased accumulation of drug into cells by mechanisms not well identified.

ABSORPTION

Administered only via the IV route.

DISTRIBUTION

Widely distributed in body tissues. Irinotecan exhibits moderate binding to plasma proteins (30%–60%). In contrast, SN-38 shows extensive plasma protein binding (95%). Peak levels of SN-38 are achieved within 1 hour after drug administration.

METABOLISM

Conversion of irinotecan to the active metabolite SN-38 occurs primarily in the liver. This conversion can also take place in plasma and in intestinal mucosa. SN-38 subsequently undergoes conjugation in the liver to the glucuronide metabolite, which is essentially inactive. In aqueous solution, the lactone ring undergoes rapid hydrolysis to the carboxylate form. Only about 34%–44% of CPT-11 and 45%–64% of the active metabolite SN-38 are present in the active lactone form at 1 hour after drug administration. The major route of elimination of both irinotecan and SN-38 is via the hepatobiliary route with elimination in bile and feces, accounting for 50%–70% of drug clearance. Only 10%–14% of CPT-11 and <1% of SN-38 is cleared in urine. The half-lives of irinotecan and SN-38 are 6–12 and 10–20 hours, respectively.

INDICATIONS

1. Colorectal cancer—FDA-approved in combination with 5-FU and leucovorin (5-FU/LV) as first-line treatment of patients with metastatic colorectal cancer.
2. Colorectal cancer—FDA-approved as a single agent for second-line treatment of patients with metastatic colorectal cancer after failure of 5-FU–based chemotherapy.
3. NSCLC.
4. SCLC.

DOSAGE RANGE

1. Irinotecan can be administered at 180 mg/m^2 IV as monotherapy or in combination with infusional 5-FU/LV on an every-2-week schedule.
2. An alternative regimen is 300–350 mg/m^2 IV on an every-3-week schedule.

DRUG INTERACTION 1

Phenytoin and other drugs that stimulate the liver microsomal CYP3A4 enzyme, including carbamazepine, rifampin, phenobarbital, and St. John's Wort— These drugs increase the metabolism of irinotecan and SN-38, resulting in its inactivation and lower effective drug levels.

DRUG INTERACTION 2

Drugs that inhibit the liver microsomal CYP3A4 enzymes, including ketoconazole, itraconazole, erythromycin, and clarithromycin—These drugs decrease the metabolism of irinotecan and SN-38, resulting in increased drug levels and potentially increased toxicity.

SPECIAL CONSIDERATIONS

1. Irinotecan is a moderate emetogenic drug. Patients should routinely receive antiemetic prophylaxis with a 5-HT3 antagonist, such as ondansetron or granisetron, in combination with dexamethasone.
2. Treatment with irinotecan is complicated by a syndrome of "early diarrhea," which is a cholinergic response and consists of diarrhea, diaphoresis, and abdominal cramping during the infusion or within 24 hours of drug administration. The recommended treatment is atropine (0.25–1.0 mg) administered IV unless clinically contraindicated. The routine use of atropine for prophylaxis is not recommended. However, atropine prophylaxis should be administered if a cholinergic event has been experienced.
3. Instruct patients about the possibility of late diarrhea (starting after 24 hours of drug administration), which can lead to serious dehydration and/or electrolyte imbalances if not managed promptly. This side effect is thought to be due to a direct irritation of the gastrointestinal mucosa by SN-38, although other as-yet-unidentified mechanisms may be involved. Loperamide should be taken immediately after the first loose bowel movement. The recommended dose is 4 mg PO as a loading dose, followed by 2 mg every 2 hours around the clock (4 mg every

4 hours during the night). Loperamide can be discontinued once the patient is diarrhea-free for 12 hours. If diarrhea should continue without improvement in the first 24 hours, an oral fluoroquinolone should be added. Hospitalization with IV antibiotics and IV hydration should be considered with continued diarrhea.

4. Irinotecan should be held for grade 3 (7–9 stools/day, incontinence, or severe cramping) and/or grade 4 (<10 stools/day, grossly bloody stool, or need for parenteral support) diarrhea. Dose of drug must be reduced upon recovery by the patient.

5. Patients should be warned against taking laxatives while on therapy.

6. Carefully monitor administration of drug, as it is a moderate vesicant. The site of infusion should be carefully inspected for extravasation, in which case flushing with sterile water, elevation of the extremity, and local application of ice are recommended.

7. Use with caution in patients >65 years of age, in patients with poor performance status, and in those previously treated with pelvic and/or abdominal irradiation, as they are at increased risk for myelosuppression and diarrhea.

8. Careful monitoring of patients on a weekly basis, especially during the first treatment cycle. Monitor complete blood cell count and platelet count on a weekly basis.

9. Patients with the UGT1A1 7/7 (UGT1A1*28) genotype are at increased risk for developing GI toxicity and myelosuppression. Approximately 10% of the North American population is homozygous for this genotype. Dose reduction should be considered in this setting.

10. Patients should be warned to be off of St. John's Wort for at least 2 weeks before starting irinotecan therapy and should remain off until after the completion of irinotecan therapy. St. John's Wort has been shown to reduce the efficacy of irinotecan chemotherapy by inhibiting conversion of irinotecan to the active SN-38 metabolite.

11. Pregnancy category D. Breastfeeding should be avoided.

TOXICITY 1

Myelosuppression with neutropenia. Patients with prior history of abdominal/pelvic irradiation are particularly prone to developing myelosuppression after treatment with irinotecan. Typical nadir occurs at days 7–10, with full recovery by days 21–28.

TOXICITY 2

Diarrhea can be dose-limiting with two different forms: early and late. Early form occurs within 24 hours of drug treatment and is characterized by flushing, diaphoresis, abdominal pain, and diarrhea. Late-form diarrhea occurs after 24 hours, typically at 3–10 days after treatment; can be severe and prolonged; and can lead to dehydration and electrolyte imbalance. Up to 80%–90% of patients may experience some aspect of late diarrhea, although only 10%–20% of patients will experience grades 3 or 4 diarrhea. Anorexia, nausea, and vomiting are usually mild and dose-related.

TOXICITY 3
Mild alopecia.

TOXICITY 4
Transient elevation in serum transaminases, alkaline phosphatase, and bilirubin.

TOXICITY 5
Asthenia and anorexia.

Irinotecan liposome

TRADE NAME	Onivyde	CLASSIFICATION	Topoisomerase I inhibitor
CATEGORY	Chemotherapy drug	DRUG MANUFACTURER	Merrimack

MECHANISM OF ACTION
- Semisynthetic derivative of camptothecin, an alkaloid extract from the *Camptotheca acuminata* tree that is encapsulated in a liposome.
- Inactive in its parent form. Converted by a carboxylesterase enzyme in the liver to the active SN-38 metabolite.
- SN-38 binds to and stabilizes the topoisomerase I-DNA complex and prevents the religation of DNA after it has been cleaved by topoisomerase I. The collision between this stable, cleavable complex and the advancing replication fork results in double-strand DNA breaks and cellular death.
- Antitumor activity of drug requires the presence of ongoing DNA synthesis.
- Cell cycle–nonspecific agent with activity in all phases of the cell cycle.

MECHANISM OF RESISTANCE
- Decreased expression of topoisomerase I.
- Mutations in topoisomerase I enzyme with decreased affinity for the drug.

- Increased expression of the multidrug-resistant phenotype with over-expression of P170 glycoprotein. Results in enhanced efflux of drug and decreased intracellular accumulation of drug.
- Decreased formation of the cytotoxic metabolite SN-38 through decreased activity and/or expression of the carboxylesterase enzyme.

ABSORPTION
Administered only via the IV route.

DISTRIBUTION
Approximately 95% of irinotecan remains liposome-encapsulated. Plasma protein binding is <0.44% of the total irinotecan in the liposome preparation.

METABOLISM
Metabolism of irinotecan liposome has not been well characterized. Conversion of irinotecan to the active metabolite SN-38 occurs primarily in the liver. However, this conversion can also take place in plasma and in intestinal mucosa. SN-38 subsequently undergoes conjugation in the liver to form the inactive glucuronide metabolite. The metabolic clearance of irinotecan liposome has not been well characterized. The major route of elimination of both irinotecan and SN-38 is in bile and feces, accounting for 50%–70% of drug clearance. Only 11%–20% of CPT-11 and <1% of SN-38 is cleared in urine. The half-lives of irinotecan and SN-38 are about 26 and 68 hours, respectively.

INDICATIONS
FDA-approved in combination with 5-FU and leucovorin (5-FU/LV) for patients with metastatic pancreatic cancer after disease progression following gemcitabine-based therapy.

DOSAGE RANGE
1. Recommended dose is 70 mg/m^2 IV in combination with 5-FU/LV every 2 weeks.
2. A lower dose of 50 mg/m^2 IV is recommended every 2 weeks for patients found to be homozygous for UGT1A1*28.

DRUG INTERACTION 1
Phenytoin and other drugs that stimulate the liver microsomal CYP3A4 enzyme, including carbamazepine, rifampin, phenobarbital, and St. John's Wort—These drugs increase the metabolism of irinotecan and SN-38, resulting in its inactivation and lower effective drug levels.

DRUG INTERACTION 2
Drugs that inhibit the liver microsomal CYP3A4 enzymes, including ketoconazole, itraconazole, erythromycin, and clarithromycin—These drugs decrease the metabolism of irinotecan and SN-38, resulting in increased drug levels and potentially increased toxicity.

DRUG INTERACTION 3

Drugs that inhibit UGT1A1, including atazanavir, gemfibrozil, and indinavir—These drugs may increase the systemic exposure to irinotecan and SN-38, resulting in increased drug levels and potentially increased toxicity.

SPECIAL CONSIDERATIONS

1. Irinotecan is a moderate emetogenic drug. Patients should routinely receive antiemetic prophylaxis with a 5-HT3 antagonist, such as ondansetron or granisetron, in combination with dexamethasone.
2. Treatment with irinotecan can be complicated by an acute cholinergic effect, which consists of diarrhea, diaphoresis, and abdominal cramping during the infusion or within 24 hours of drug administration. The recommended treatment is atropine (0.25–1.0 mg) administered IV unless clinically contraindicated. The routine use of atropine for prophylaxis is not recommended. However, atropine prophylaxis should be administered if a cholinergic event has been experienced.
3. Instruct patients about the possibility of late diarrhea (starting after 24 hours of drug administration), which can lead to serious dehydration and/or electrolyte imbalances if not managed promptly. This represents a black-box warning. This side effect is thought to be due to a direct irritation of the gastrointestinal mucosa by SN-38, although other as-yet-unidentified mechanisms may be involved. Loperamide should be taken immediately after the first loose bowel movement. The recommended dose is 4 mg PO as a loading dose, followed by 2 mg every 2 hours around the clock (4 mg every 4 hours during the night). Loperamide can be discontinued once the patient is diarrhea-free for 12 hours. If diarrhea should continue without improvement in the first 24 hours, an oral fluoroquinolone should be added. Hospitalization with IV antibiotics and IV hydration should be considered with continued diarrhea.
4. Irinotecan liposome should **NOT** be given to patients with bowel obstruction.
5. Patients should be warned against taking laxatives while on therapy.
6. Monitor CBCs on days 1 and 8 of every cycle, as irinotecan liposome can cause severe, life-threatening neutropenia and neutropenic sepsis. This represents a black-box warning.
7. Irinotecan liposome should be withheld for ANC $<1,500/mm^3$ or neutropenic fever.
8. Patients with the UGT1A1 7/7 (UGT1A1*28) genotype are at increased risk for developing GI toxicity and myelosuppression. Approximately 10% of the North American population is homozygous for this genotype. Dose reduction to 50 mg/m^2 is recommended in this setting.
9. Patients should be warned to be off St. John's Wort for at least 2 weeks before starting irinotecan therapy and should remain off until after the completion of irinotecan therapy. St. John's Wort has been shown to reduce the efficacy of irinotecan chemotherapy by inhibiting metabolism of irinotecan to the active SN-38 metabolite.
10. Pregnancy category D. Breastfeeding should be avoided.

TOXICITY 1

Myelosuppression with neutropenia. Severe neutropenia occurs in 20% of patients, and neutropenic fever or sepsis occurs in 3% of patients.

TOXICITY 2

Diarrhea with two different forms: early and late. Early form occurs within 24 hours of drug treatment and is characterized by flushing, diaphoresis, abdominal pain, and diarrhea. Late-form diarrhea occurs after 24 hours, typically at 3–10 days after treatment, can be severe and prolonged, and can lead to dehydration and electrolyte imbalance. Severe late diarrhea occurs in 13% of patients.

TOXICITY 3

Interstitial lung disease with dyspnea, cough, and fever.

TOXICITY 4

Hypersensitivity reactions.

TOXICITY 5

Fatigue and anorexia.

Isatuximab

TRADE NAME	Sarclisa	CLASSIFICATION	Anti-CD38-directed monoclonal antibody
CATEGORY	Biologic response modifier agent, targeted agent	DRUG MANUFACTURER	Sanofi and Immunogen

MECHANISM OF ACTION

- IgG1 monoclonal antibody directed against CD38, which is a cell surface glycoprotein that is highly expressed on hematopoietic and tumor cells, including multiple myeloma cells. CD38 is expressed at low levels on normal lymphoid and myeloid cells.
- Inhibits the growth of CD38-expressing tumor cells by inducing apoptosis directly through Fc-mediated cross-linking as well as by immune-mediated tumor cell lysis through complement-dependent cytotoxicity (CDC), antibody-dependent cell-mediated cytotoxicity (ADCC), and antibody-dependent cellular phagocytosis.
- Targets a completely different epitope on human CD38 than daratumumab.

MECHANISM OF RESISTANCE
- Reduced expression of the CD38 target on myeloma cells.
- Increased expression of membrane-associated complement-inhibitory proteins, such as CD46, CD55, and CD59, in myeloma cells localized in the bone marrow and in peripheral blood.
- Increased expression of the anti-apoptotic proteins survivin and MCL-1 in bone marrow stromal cells.
- Activation of various immune checkpoint signaling pathways, including PD-1, LAG3, and TIGIT.

ABSORPTION
Administered only via the IV route.

DISTRIBUTION
Steady-state drug levels are achieved in 8 weeks.

METABOLISM
Metabolism has not been well-characterized, although the drug is expected to be broken down into small peptides by various catabolic pathways. Mean elimination of drug from plasma after the last dose is approximately 2 months.

INDICATIONS
1. FDA-approved in combination with pomalidomide and dexamethasone for patients with multiple myeloma who have received at least 2 prior lines of therapy, including lenalidomide and a proteasome inhibitor.
2. FDA-approved in combination with carfilzomib and dexamethasone for patients with relapsed or refractory multiple myeloma who have received 1–3 prior lines of therapy.

DOSAGE RANGE
Recommended dose is 10 mg/kg IV on a weekly basis for 4 weeks followed by every 2 weeks in combination with pomalidomide and dexamethasone or in combination with carfilzomib and dexamethasone.

DRUG INTERACTION
None well characterized to date.

SPECIAL CONSIDERATIONS
1. Isatuximab should be administered by IV infusion at the appropriate infusion rate. Consider increasing infusion rate only in the absence of infusion reactions. Please see package insert for specific details on the appropriate infusion rate.
2. The large majority of infusion reactions occur with the first infusion, and nearly all reactions occur during the infusion or within 4 hours of completing the infusion.
3. Premedication with antihistamines (diphenhydramine 25–50 mg PO or IV), antipyretics (acetaminophen 650–1,000 mg), H2 antagonists, and corticosteroids (dexamethasone 40 mg PO or IV) is required to reduce

the risk of infusion reactions. Interrupt the infusion for any reaction and manage as appropriate. Administer isatuximab in a clinical facility with immediate access to resuscitative measures (e.g., glucocorticoids, epinephrine, bronchodilators, and/or oxygen).

4. Administer oral corticosteroids (20 mg methylprednisolone) on the first and second days after all infusions to reduce the risk of delayed infusion reactions. For patients with chronic obstructive pulmonary disease, consider short- and long-acting bronchodilators and inhaled corticosteroids.

5. Blood transfusion centers should be informed that a patient has received isatuximab, as this drug can bind to CD38 on red blood cells. This binding may result in a false positive indirect antiglobulin test (Coombs test).

6. Patients should be typed and screened for red blood cell transfusions prior to starting isatuximab therapy.

7. Isatuximab may interfere with an accurate assessment of the myeloma response, as the drug may be detected on serum protein electrophoresis and immunofixation assays that are used to monitor for endogenous M-protein levels.

8. No dose adjustments are recommended for patients with renal dysfunction.

9. No dose adjustments are recommended for patients with mild hepatic dysfunction. Has not been studied in the setting of moderate or severe hepatic dysfunction.

10. Closely monitor CBCs on a periodic basis.

11. Prophylaxis for herpes zoster virus reactivation is recommended.

12. Can cause fetal harm when administered to a pregnant woman. Females of reproductive potential should use effective contraception during drug therapy and for at least 5 months after the final dose. Breastfeeding should be avoided.

TOXICITY 1
Myelosuppression with neutropenia, thrombocytopenia, and anemia.

TOXICITY 2
Infusion reactions presenting with bronchospasm, cough, wheezing, dyspnea, laryngeal edema, and hypertension.

TOXICITY 3
Infections with URIs and pneumonia.

TOXICITY 4
Fatigue, anorexia, and asthenia

TOXICITY 5
GI side effects with mild nausea/vomiting, diarrhea, and constipation.

TOXICITY 6
Secondary malignancies with squamous cell skin cancer, MDS, and breast angiosarcoma.

Ivosidenib

TRADE NAME	Tibsovo	CLASSIFICATION	Signal transduction inhibitor, IDH1 inhibitor
CATEGORY	Targeted agent	DRUG MANUFACTURER	Agios and Celgene

MECHANISM OF ACTION
- Inhibits the mutant isocitrate dehydrogenase 1 (IDH1) enzyme.
- Inhibition of mutant IDH1 leads to decreased 2-hydroxyglutarate (2-HG) levels, which then results in induced myeloid differentiation with an increase in mature myeloid cells.

MECHANISM OF RESISTANCE
None well characterized to date.

ABSORPTION
Oral bioavailability is 77%. Median time to peak drug levels is 1.3–1.8 hours after ingestion. Food with high-fat content reduces AUC and C_{max} by 16% and 31%, respectively.

DISTRIBUTION
Extensive binding (91%) of drug to plasma proteins. Steady-state drug levels are achieved in approximately 8 days.

METABOLISM
Metabolized in the liver primarily by CYP3A4 microsomal enzymes with minor contributions by CYP2C8 and UGT1A9. Following an administered dose, 49% of the dose is eliminated in urine and 42% is eliminated in feces. The terminal half-life is approximately 17.4 hours.

INDICATIONS
1. FDA-approved for newly diagnosed AML with an IDH1 mutation in patients who are >75 years of age or who have comorbidities that preclude the use of intensive induction chemotherapy.

2. FDA-approved for relapsed or refractory AML with an IDH1 mutation.
3. FDA-approved for previously treated, locally advanced or metastatic cholangiocarcinoma with an IDH1 mutation.

DOSAGE RANGE
Recommended dose is 500 mg PO once daily.

DRUG INTERACTION 1
Drugs such as ketoconazole, itraconazole, erythromycin, clarithromycin, atazanavir, indinavir, nefazodone, nelfinavir, ritonavir, saquinavir, telithromycin, and voriconazole may decrease the metabolism of ivosidenib, resulting in increased drug levels and potentially increased toxicity.

DRUG INTERACTION 2
Drugs such as rifampin, phenytoin, phenobarbital, carbamazepine, and St. John's Wort may increase the metabolism of ivosidenib, resulting in lower effective drug levels.

SPECIAL CONSIDERATIONS
1. Dose adjustment is not required for patients with mild or moderate hepatic impairment. Has not been studied in patients with severe hepatic impairment, and there are no formal recommendations for dosing in this setting.
2. Dose adjustment is not required for patients with mild or moderate renal impairment (CrCl >30 mL/min). Has not been studied in patients with severe renal impairment or in those on hemodialysis, and there are no formal recommendations for dosing in these settings.
3. Monitor CBCs and blood chemistries at baseline, and at least once weekly for the first month, once every other week for the second month, and once monthly for the duration of therapy.
4. Monitor serum CPK levels weekly for the first month of therapy.
5. Monitor ECGs at baseline, at least once per week for the first 3 weeks of therapy, and then at least once monthly for the duration of therapy, as ivosidenib therapy can result in QTc interval prolongation.
6. Avoid concomitant use of other drugs that can prolong the QTc interval.
7. Reduce the dose of ivosidenib if a strong CYP3A4 inhibitor must be co-administered.
8. Differentiation syndrome is a complication of ivosidenib therapy and may be life-threatening or fatal if not treated appropriately. Can present as early as 10 days and up to 5 months after start of therapy. Dexamethasone 10 mg IV every 12 hours should be initiated, and patients must undergo hemodynamic monitoring until improvement. In the presence of non-infectious leukocytosis, treatment with hydroxyurea or leukapheresis should be instituted. This is a black-box warning.
9. Monitor patients for signs or symptoms of motor and/or sensory neuropathy as ivosidenib therapy is associated with Guillain-Barre syndrome.
10. Patients should be selected based on the presence of IDH1 mutations in the blood or bone marrow.

11. Patients should be told to avoid a high-fat meal as this can increase drug levels.
12. Can cause fetal harm when administered to a pregnant woman. Females of reproductive potential should use effective contraception during drug therapy and for at least 30 days after the final dose. Breastfeeding should be avoided.

TOXICITY 1
Myelosuppression with anemia, thrombocytopenia, and neutropenia.

TOXICITY 2
Diarrhea, nausea/vomiting, abdominal pain.

TOXICITY 3
IDH differentiation syndrome with dyspnea, hypoxia, pulmonary infiltrates, pleural effusion, fever, bone pain, peripheral edema, and pericardial effusion. Hepatic, renal, and multi-organ dysfunction have also been observed.

TOXICITY 4
Fatigue and anorexia.

TOXICITY 5
QTc prolongation.

TOXICITY 6
Guillain-Barré syndrome.

Ixabepilone

TRADE NAME	Ixempra, BMS-247550	CLASSIFICATION	Epothilone, antimicrotubule agent
CATEGORY	Chemotherapy drug	DRUG MANUFACTURER	Bristol-Myers Squibb

MECHANISM OF ACTION
- Semisynthetic analog of epothilone B.
- Cell cycle–specific, active in the mitosis (M) phase of the cell cycle.

- Binds directly to β-tubulin subunits on microtubules, leading to inhibition of normal microtubule dynamics.
- Exhibits activity in drug-resistant tumors that overexpress P-glycoprotein, MRP-1, βIII tubulin isoforms, and tubulin mutations.

MECHANISM OF RESISTANCE
- Mutations in β-tubulin.
- Increased expression of galectin-1, a β-galactose–binding lectin that mediates tumor invasion and metastasis.

ABSORPTION
Administered only via the IV route.

DISTRIBUTION
Distributes widely to all body tissues. Moderate binding (60%–70%) to plasma proteins.

METABOLISM
Metabolized extensively by the hepatic P450 microsomal system via oxidation by CYP3A4. About 85% of drug is excreted in stool via hepatobiliary elimination. Less than 10% is eliminated as the parent form, with the majority being eliminated as metabolites. Renal clearance is relatively minor, with less than 10% of drug cleared via the kidneys. The terminal elimination half-life is on the order of 52 hours. Gender, race, and age do not impact drug pharmacokinetics.

INDICATIONS
1. FDA-approved in combination with capecitabine for metastatic or locally advanced breast cancer resistant to treatment with an anthracycline and a taxane, or in patients whose cancer is taxane-resistant and for whom further anthracycline therapy is contraindicated.
2. FDA-approved as monotherapy for metastatic or locally advanced breast cancer in patients whose tumors are resistant or refractory to anthracyclines, taxanes, and capecitabine.

DOSAGE RANGE
Recommended dose is 40 mg/m^2 IV every 3 weeks.

DRUG INTERACTION 1
Drugs such as ketoconazole, fluconazole, itraconazole, erythromycin, clarithromycin, and verapamil may decrease the metabolism of ixabepilone, resulting in increased drug levels and potentially increased toxicity.

DRUG INTERACTION 2
Drugs such as rifampin, phenytoin, phenobarbital, and carbamazepine may increase the metabolism of ixabepilone, resulting in its inactivation and lower effective drug levels.

DRUG INTERACTION 3

St. John's Wort may alter the metabolism of ixabepilone and should be avoided while on therapy.

DRUG INTERACTION 4

Ixabepilone does not appear to affect the metabolism of drugs that are substrates of liver microsomal enzymes.

SPECIAL CONSIDERATIONS

1. Contraindicated in patients with history of severe hypersensitivity reaction to paclitaxel or to other drugs formulated in Cremophor EL.
2. Use with caution in patients with abnormal liver function. When used as monotherapy, dose reduction is required in the setting of mild-to-moderate hepatic impairment. Contraindicated when used in combination with capecitabine in patients with SGOT or SGPT $>2.5 \times$ ULN or bilirubin $>1 \times$ ULN.
3. Contraindicated in patients with a neutrophil count $<1,500$ cells/mm^3 or a platelet count $<100,000$ cells/mm^3.
4. Use with caution in patients with prior history of diabetes mellitus and chronic alcoholism or prior therapy with known neurotoxic agents such as cisplatin.
5. Patients should receive premedication prior to treatment to prevent the incidence of hypersensitivity reactions. Give an H1-antagonist (diphenhydramine 50 mg PO) and an H2-antagonist (cimetidine 300 mg) 1 hour prior to drug administration. Patients experiencing a hypersensitivity reaction require premedication with dexamethasone 20 mg IV 30 minutes before drug treatment, along with diphenhydramine 50 mg IV and cimetidine 300 mg IV.
6. Medical personnel should be available at the time of drug administration. Emergency equipment, including Ambu bag, ECG machine, IV fluids, pressors, and other drugs for resuscitation, must be at bedside before initiation of treatment.
7. Pregnancy category D. Breastfeeding should be avoided.

TOXICITY 1

Myelosuppression with neutropenia and thrombocytopenia. Neutropenia typically occurs on days 10–14, with recovery by day 21.

TOXICITY 2

Hypersensitivity reaction characterized by generalized skin rash, flushing, erythema, hypotension, dyspnea, and/or bronchospasm. Premedication regimen, as outlined in Special Considerations, has significantly decreased incidence.

TOXICITY 3

Neurotoxicity, mainly in the form of peripheral sensory neuropathy with numbness and paresthesias. Occurs in up to 20% of patients.

TOXICITY 4
Fatigue and asthenia.

TOXICITY 5
GI toxicity in the form of nausea/vomiting, mucositis, and/or diarrhea.

TOXICITY 6
Myalgias, arthralgias, and musculoskeletal pain.

Ixazomib

TRADE NAME	Ninlaro	CLASSIFICATION	Proteasome inhibitor
CATEGORY	Targeted agent	DRUG MANUFACTURER	Millennium and Takeda Oncology

MECHANISM OF ACTION
- Reversible proteasome inhibitor that preferentially binds and inhibits the chymotrypsin-like activity of the β5 subunit of the 20S proteasome, which then results in activation of signaling cascades, cell-cycle arrest, and apoptosis.
- In vitro cytotoxicity against myeloma-derived cell lines from patients who had progressed on previous therapies, including bortezomib, lenalidomide, and dexamethasone.
- Combination of ixazomib and lenalidomide has synergistic cytotoxicity in multiple myeloma cell lines and in vitro and in vivo antitumor activity in myeloma tumor xenograft models.

MECHANISM OF RESISTANCE
None well characterized to date.

ABSORPTION
Absolute oral bioavailability is 58%, and the median T_{max} is 1 hour. Food with a high fat content reduces AUC by 28% and C_{max} by 69%, respectively.

DISTRIBUTION
Highly bound to plasma proteins (99%).

METABOLISM
Metabolized primarily in the liver by multiple liver microsomal CYP enzymes, with CYP3A4 being the major metabolizing enzyme. Non-CYP proteins are also involved in ixazomib metabolism. After drug administration, approximately 60% is excreted in urine, with <3.5% as unchanged drug, and 22% is excreted in feces. The terminal half-life is 9.5 days.

INDICATIONS
FDA-approved in combination with lenalidomide and dexamethasone for the treatment of patients with multiple myeloma who have received at least one prior therapy.

DOSAGE RANGE
Recommended dose is 4 mg PO on days 1, 8, and 15 of a 28-day cycle. Used in combination with lenalidomide 25 mg/day PO on days 1 through 21 and dexamethasone 40 mg PO on days 1, 8, 15, and 22.

DRUG INTERACTION
Phenytoin and other drugs that stimulate the liver microsomal CYP3A4 enzymes, including carbamazepine, rifampin, phenobarbital, and St. John's Wort—These drugs may increase the metabolism of ixazomib, resulting in reduced effective drug levels in the blood.

SPECIAL CONSIDERATIONS
1. Monitor CBCs on a periodic basis, with more frequent monitoring during the first three cycles.
2. Need to monitor for thrombocytopenia, with platelet nadirs usually occurring between days 14 and 21 of each 28-day cycle, with recovery to baseline by the start of the next cycle. Thrombocytopenia should be managed with dose modification as per the package insert as well as with platelet transfusion.
3. No dose adjustment is needed for mild hepatic dysfunction. Dose of ixazomib should be reduced to 3 mg in patients with moderate (total bilirubin >1.5–3 × ULN) or severe (total bilirubin >3 × ULN) hepatic dysfunction.
4. No dose reduction is needed for mild or moderate renal dysfunction. Dose of ixazomib should be reduced to 3 mg in patients with severe renal dysfunction (CrCl <30 mL/min) or in those with end-stage renal disease. In contrast to bortezomib and carfilzomib, ixazomib is not dialyzable, and as such, it may be administered without regard to the timing of dialysis.
5. LFTs should be monitored periodically, with dose adjustments for grades 3 and 4 liver toxicity.

6. Patients should avoid taking green tea products and supplements, as they may inhibit the clinical efficacy of ixazomib, similar to what is observed with bortezomib.
7. Patients should be followed for the development of skin rash and other cutaneous reactions, with dose adjustments as needed.

TOXICITY 1

Myelosuppression with thrombocytopenia and neutropenia.

TOXICITY 2

Neurologic toxicity with peripheral neuropathy most common and rare cases of peripheral motor neuropathy.

TOXICITY 3

GI toxicity with diarrhea, constipation, and nausea/vomiting.

TOXICITY 4

Dermatologic toxicity with maculopapular and macular skin rash.

TOXICITY 5

Hepatotoxicity with drug-induced liver injury, hepatic steatosis, and cholestatic hepatitis.

TOXICITY 6

Fatigue.

TOXICITY 7

Peripheral edema.

Lapatinib

TRADE NAME	Tykerb, GW572016	**CLASSIFICATION**		Signal transduction inhibitor, ErbB inhibitor
CATEGORY	Targeted agent	**DRUG MANUFACTURER**		GlaxoSmithKline

MECHANISM OF ACTION

- Potent small-molecule inhibitor of the tyrosine kinases associated with epidermal growth factor receptor (ErbB1; EGFR) and HER2 (ErbB2), resulting in inhibition of ErbB phosphorylation and downstream ErbB signaling.
- Inhibition of the EGFR and HER2 tyrosine kinases results in inhibition of critical mitogenic and antiapoptotic signals involved in proliferation, growth, invasion/metastasis, angiogenesis, and response to chemotherapy and/or radiation therapy.

MECHANISM OF RESISTANCE

- Mutations in the EGFR and HER2/neu growth factor receptors, leading to reduced binding affinity to lapatinib.
- Increased expression and/or activation of HER3.
- Activation of a heregulin (HRG)-driven HER3-EGFR-PI3K signaling axis.
- Increased ERα transcription and ER signaling.
- Increased expression/activation of c-Met.
- Increased expression of RON.
- Increased expression and activation of AXL.
- Activation/induction of alternative cellular signaling pathways, such as PI3K, resulting from activating PIK3CA mutations or loss of PTEN.

ABSORPTION

Oral absorption is incomplete and variable and is increased when administered with food. Peak plasma levels are achieved 4 hours after ingestion.

DISTRIBUTION

Extensive binding (99%) to plasma proteins, including albumin and α1-acid glycoprotein, and extensive tissue distribution. Steady-state drug concentrations are reached in 6–7 days.

METABOLISM

Metabolism in the liver primarily by the CYP3A4 and CYP3A5 microsomal enzymes and by CYP2C19 and CYP2C8 to a lesser extent. Elimination is mainly hepatic, with excretion in feces. Renal elimination of parent drug and its metabolites accounts for less than 2% of an administered dose. The terminal half-life of the parent drug is 14 hours, and with repeat dosing, the effective half-life is 24 hours.

INDICATIONS

FDA-approved in combination with capecitabine for patients with advanced or metastatic breast cancer whose tumors overexpress HER2 and who have received prior therapy, including an anthracycline, a taxane, and trastuzumab.

DOSAGE RANGE

Recommended dose is 1,250 mg PO daily on days 1–21 continuously in combination with capecitabine 1,000 mg/m^2 PO bid on days 1–14, with each cycle repeated every 21 days.

DRUG INTERACTION 1

Phenytoin and other drugs that stimulate the liver microsomal CYP3A4 enzymes, including carbamazepine, rifampin, phenobarbital, and St. John's Wort. These drugs may increase the metabolism of lapatinib, resulting in its inactivation and lower effective drug levels.

DRUG INTERACTION 2

Drugs that inhibit the liver microsomal CYP3A4 enzymes, including ketoconazole, itraconazole, erythromycin, and clarithromycin. These drugs may decrease the metabolism of lapatinib, resulting in increased drug levels and potentially increased toxicity.

DRUG INTERACTION 3

Warfarin—Patients receiving warfarin should be closely monitored for alterations in their clotting parameters (PT and INR) and/or bleeding, as lapatinib may inhibit the metabolism of warfarin by the liver P450 system. The dose of warfarin may require careful adjustment in the presence of lapatinib therapy.

SPECIAL CONSIDERATIONS

1. Use with caution in patients with hepatic impairment, and dose reduction and/or interruption should be considered.
2. Monitor cardiac function at baseline and periodically during therapy with either MUGA or echocardiogram to assess LVEF. The reduction in LVEF usually occurs within the first 9 weeks of therapy. Use with caution in patients with pre-existing conditions that could impair LVEF.

3. Monitor ECG with QT measurement at baseline and periodically during therapy, as QT prolongation has been observed. Use with caution in patients at risk of developing QT prolongation, including hypokalemia, hypomagnesemia, congenital long QT syndrome, patients taking antiarrhythmic medications or any other products that may cause QT prolongation, and cumulative high-dose anthracycline therapy.
4. Lapatinib should be taken 1 hour before or after a meal, and the daily dose should not be divided. When capecitabine is co-administered, capecitabine should be taken with a glass of water within 30 minutes after a meal.
5. Avoid Seville oranges, starfruit, pomelos, and grapefruit products while on therapy.
6. Monitor patients for diarrhea, as severe diarrhea may develop while on therapy. Aggressive management with antidiarrheal agents as well as replacement of fluids. Electrolyte status should be closely followed.
7. Pregnancy category D. Breastfeeding should be avoided.

TOXICITY 1
Diarrhea is the most common dose-limiting toxicity and occurs in 65% of patients. Mild nausea/vomiting may also occur.

TOXICITY 2
Cardiac toxicity with reduction in LVEF. QT prolongation occurs rarely.

TOXICITY 3
Myelosuppression with anemia more common than thrombocytopenia or neutropenia.

TOXICITY 4
Fatigue and anorexia.

TOXICITY 5
Hepatotoxicity with mild-to-moderate elevation of serum transaminases and serum bilirubin.

TOXICITY 6
Hand-foot syndrome (palmar-plantar erythrodysesthesia) and skin rash.

Larotrectinib

TRADE NAME	Vitrakvi	CLASSIFICATION	Signal transduction inhibitor, TRK inhibitor
CATEGORY	Targeted agent	DRUG MANUFACTURER	Loxo Oncology

MECHANISM OF ACTION
- Inhibits tropomyosin receptor kinases (TRK), TRKA, TRKB, and TRKC, which are encoded by NTRK1, NTRK2, and NTRK3, respectively.
- NTRK gene fusions involve chromosomal rearrangements between an expressed 5' partner and a 3' partner encoding a tyrosine kinase. These oncogenic fusions represent a novel oncogenic driver and have been identified in up to 1% of all solid cancers.

MECHANISM OF RESISTANCE
- Mutations in the TRK kinase domain, including TRKA-G595R, TRKA-G667C, and TRKC-G623R.
- Mutations in IGF1R, which leads to activation of the IGF1R signaling pathway.

ABSORPTION
Oral bioavailability is modest at 34%. The median time to C_{max} is 1 hour after ingestion.

DISTRIBUTION
Approximately 70% of drug is bound to plasma proteins. Steady-state drug levels are achieved in approximately 3 days.

METABOLISM
Metabolized in the liver primarily by CYP3A4 microsomal enzymes. Elimination is nearly equal with excretion in feces (41%) and urine (48%), with only <10% eliminated as unchanged parent drug. The terminal half-life of larotrectinib is approximately 2.9 hours.

INDICATIONS
FDA-approved for the treatment of adult and pediatric patients with metastatic solid tumors that have an NTRK gene fusion without a known acquired

resistance mutation and who have no satisfactory alternative treatments or that have progressed following treatment.

DOSAGE RANGE
1. Recommended dose for patients with a BSA of at least 1.0 m^2 is 100 mg PO bid.
2. Recommended dose for pediatric patients with a BSA of < 1.0 m^2 is 100 mg/m^2 PO bid.

DRUG INTERACTION 1
Drugs such as ketoconazole, itraconazole, erythromycin, clarithromycin, atazanavir, indinavir, nefazodone, nelfinavir, ritonavir, saquinavir, telithromycin, and voriconazole may decrease the metabolism of larotrectinib, resulting in increased drug levels and potentially increased toxicity.

DRUG INTERACTION 2
Drugs such as rifampin, phenytoin, phenobarbital, carbamazepine, and St. John's Wort may increase the metabolism of larotrectinib, resulting in its inactivation and lower effective drug levels.

SPECIAL CONSIDERATIONS
1. No dose adjustment is needed for patients with mild hepatic dysfunction. The dose of drug should be reduced by 50% in patients with moderate or severe hepatic dysfunction.
2. No dose adjustment is needed for patients with mild, moderate, or severe renal dysfunction.
3. Larotrectinib should be avoided in patients taking strong CYP3A4 inducers. If strong CYP3A4 inducers are required, the dose of larotrectinib should be doubled.
4. Larotrectinib should be avoided in patients taking strong CYP3A4 inhibitors. If strong CYP3A4 inhibitors are required, the dose of larotrectinib should be reduced by 50%.
5. Patients should be warned not to drive or operate hazardous machinery if experiencing neurotoxicity.
6. Monitor LFTs every 2 weeks during the first month of therapy, then monthly thereafter as clinically indicated.
7. NTRK testing using an FDA-approved test is required to confirm the presence of NTRK gene fusions.
8. Can cause fetal harm when administered to a pregnant woman. Females of reproductive potential should use effective contraception during drug therapy and for at least 1 week after the final dose. Breastfeeding should be avoided.

TOXICITY 1
Neurotoxicity with dizziness, delirium, dysarthria, gait abnormalities, and memory impairment.

TOXICITY 2

Hepatotoxicity with elevations in SGOT and SGPT.

TOXICITY 3

GI toxicity with nausea/vomiting, constipation, diarrhea, and abdominal pain.

TOXICITY 4

Fatigue and anorexia.

TOXICITY 5

Arthralgias, myalgias, and back pain.

Lenalidomide

TRADE NAME	Revlimid, CC-5013	**CLASSIFICATION**	Immunomodulatory thalidomide analog, anti-angiogenic agent
CATEGORY	Unclassified therapeutic agent, immunomodulatory agent	**DRUG MANUFACTURER**	Celgene

MECHANISM OF ACTION
- Mechanism of action is not fully characterized.
- Immunomodulatory drug that stimulates T-cell proliferation as well as IL-2 and IFN-γ production.
- Inhibition of TNF-α and IL-6 synthesis and down-modulation of cell surface adhesion molecules similar to thalidomide.
- May exert anti-angiogenic effect by inhibition of basic fibroblast growth factor (bFGF) and vascular endothelial growth factor (VEGF) through as yet undefined mechanisms.
- Overcomes cellular drug resistance to thalidomide.

MECHANISM OF RESISTANCE
- Increased activation of the Wnt/β-catenin signaling pathway.
- Increased expression of CD44, a hyaluronan (HA)-binding protein involved in cell adhesion.

ABSORPTION
Rapidly absorbed following oral administration, with peak plasma concentrations at 60–90 minutes post-ingestion. Co-administration with food does not alter the extent of absorption (AUC) but does reduce maximal plasma concentration (C_{max}) by 36%.

DISTRIBUTION
None well characterized.

METABOLISM
Does not appear to be metabolized or induced by the cytochrome P450 pathway. Approximately 66% of an administered dose is excreted unchanged in the urine. The elimination half-life of the drug is approximately 3 hours.

INDICATIONS
1. FDA-approved for low- or intermediate-1-risk myelodysplastic syndromes (MDS) associated with the deletion 5q (del 5q) cytogenetic abnormality with or without additional cytogenetic abnormalities.
2. FDA-approved for multiple myeloma in combination with dexamethasone for patients who have received at least one prior therapy.
3. FDA-approved for patients with mantle cell lymphoma whose disease has relapsed or progressed after two prior therapies, one of which included bortezomib.
4. FDA-approved as maintenance therapy for patients with multiple myeloma following autologous stem cell transplantation.
5. FDA-approved for patients with previously treated follicular lymphoma in combination with rituximab.
6. FDA-approved for patients with previously treated marginal zone lymphoma in combination with rituximab.

DOSAGE RANGE
1. Myelodysplastic syndrome: 10 mg PO daily.
2. Multiple myeloma: 25 mg PO daily on days 1–21 and 40 mg dexamethasone PO on days 1–4, 9–12, and 17–20 of a 28-day cycle. An alternative regimen is to use 40 mg dexamethasone PO on days 1, 8, 15, and 22 of a 28-day cycle.
3. Multiple myeloma maintenance therapy: 10 mg PO daily on days 1–28 of a 28-day cycle.
4. Mantle cell lymphoma: 25 mg PO daily on days 1–21 of a 28-day cycle.
5. Follicular lymphoma or marginal zone lymphoma: 25 mg PO daily on days 1–21 of a 28-day cycle for up to 12 cycles.

DRUG INTERACTIONS
None well characterized to date.

SPECIAL CONSIDERATIONS
1. Pregnancy category X. Lenalidomide is a thalidomide analog, a known human teratogen that causes severe or life-threatening birth defects. As such, women who are pregnant or who wish to become pregnant should not take lenalidomide. Severe fetal malformations can occur if even one capsule is taken by a pregnant woman. All women should have a baseline β-human chorionic gonadotropin (β-HCG) before starting lenalidomide therapy. Women of reproductive age must have two negative pregnancy tests before starting therapy: one should be 10–14 days before therapy is begun, and the second should be 24 hours before therapy.
2. All women of childbearing potential should practice two forms of birth control throughout therapy with lenalidomide: one highly effective form (intrauterine device, hormonal contraception [patch, implant, pill, injection], partner's vasectomy, or tubal ligation) and one additional barrier method (latex condom, diaphragm, or cervical cap). It is strongly recommended that these precautionary measures be taken 1 month before initiation of therapy, continued while on therapy, and continued at least 1 month after therapy is discontinued.
3. Lenalidomide is only available under a special restricted distribution program called "RevAssist®." Only prescribers and pharmacists registered with the RevAssist® program are able to prescribe and dispense the drug. Lenalidomide should only be dispensed to those patients who are registered and meet all the conditions of the RevAssist® program.
4. Breastfeeding while on therapy should be avoided, as it remains unknown if lenalidomide is excreted in breast milk.
5. Men taking lenalidomide must use latex condoms for every sexual encounter with a woman of childbearing potential, as the drug may be present in semen.
6. Patients taking lenalidomide should not donate blood or semen while receiving treatment and for at least 1 month after stopping this drug.
7. Monitor CBCs while on therapy, as lenalidomide has hematologic toxicity, especially in patients with del 5q MDS.
8. Use with caution in patients with impaired renal function, as the risk of toxicity may be increased. Starting dose should be adjusted based on the creatinine clearance.
9. There is a significantly increased risk of thromboembolic complications, including deep venous thrombosis (DVT) and pulmonary embolism (PE), especially in patients treated with lenalidomide and dexamethasone. Prophylaxis with low-molecular-weight heparin or aspirin (325 mg PO qd) can help prevent and/or reduce this risk.

TOXICITY 1
Potentially severe or fatal teratogenic effects.

TOXICITY 2
Myelosuppression with neutropenia and thrombocytopenia that is usually reversible.

TOXICITY 3
Increased risk of thromboembolic complications, such as DVT and PE.

TOXICITY 4
Nausea/vomiting, diarrhea, and constipation are most common GI side effects.

TOXICITY 5
Neurotoxic side effects are rare, with almost no sedation.

TOXICITY 6
Increased risk for second primary tumors, including AML, myelodysplastic syndrome, and solid tumors.

Lenvatinib

TRADE NAME	Lenvima, E7080	**CLASSIFICATION**	Signal transduction inhibitor, anti-angiogenic agent
CATEGORY	Targeted agent	**DRUG MANUFACTURER**	Eisai

MECHANISM OF ACTION
- Small-molecule, multitargeted receptor tyrosine kinase inhibitor (TKI) that inhibits the kinase activities of vascular endothelial growth factor receptor 1 (VEGFR-1), VEGFR-2, and VEGFR-3.
- Inhibits other tyrosine kinase inhibitors, including fibroblast growth factor receptor 1 (FGFR-1), FGFR-2, FGFR-3, FGFR-4, platelet-derived growth

factor receptor-α (PDGFR-α), Kit, and RET, which are involved in tumor angiogenesis, tumor growth, and cancer progression.

MECHANISM OF RESISTANCE
- Increased expression of the target receptor tyrosine kinases (RTKs), such as VEGFR.
- Alterations in binding affinity of the drug to the RTKs resulting from mutations in the tyrosine kinase domain.
- Activation of the hepatocyte growth factor pathway through its cognate receptor c-Met.
- Activation/induction of alternative cellular signaling pathways, such as IGF-1R.

ABSORPTION
Oral absorption is relatively fast, with peak plasma concentrations achieved within 1–4 hours after ingestion. Food does not affect the extent of absorption but decreases the rate of absorption and delays the median T_{max} from 2–4 hours.

DISTRIBUTION
Extensive binding of lenvatinib to human plasma proteins (98% to 99%).

METABOLISM
Metabolized to a large extent by the liver CYP3A enzymes and aldehyde oxidase as well as by non-enzymatic processes. Approximately 64% and 25% of drug is eliminated in feces and urine, respectively. The terminal elimination half-life of lenvatinib is approximately 28 hours.

INDICATIONS
1. FDA-approved for patients with locally recurrent or metastatic, progressive, radioactive iodine-refractory differentiated thyroid cancer.
2. FDA-approved in combination with everolimus for patients with advanced renal cell cancer following one prior anti-angiogenic therapy.
3. FDA-approved for first-line treatment of patients with unresectable hepatocellular cancer (HCC).
4. FDA-approved in combination with pembrolizumab for treatment of patients with advanced endometrial cancer that is not MSI-H or dMMR and who have disease progression following prior systemic therapy in any setting and not candidates for curative surgery or radiation.

DOSAGE RANGE
1. Thyroid cancer: 24 mg PO once daily with or without food.
2. Renal cell cancer: 18 mg PO once daily in combination with everolimus 5 mg PO once daily.
3. HCC: 12 mg PO once daily for patients >60 kg and 8 mg PO once daily for patients <60 kg.
4. Endometrial cancer: 20 mg PO once daily in combination with pembrolizumab 200 mg IV every 3 weeks.

DRUG INTERACTION 1

Drugs that stimulate liver microsomal CYP3A4 enzymes, including phenytoin, carbamazepine, rifampin, phenobarbital, and St. John's Wort—These drugs may increase the metabolism of lenvatinib, resulting in lower drug levels and potentially reduced clinical activity.

DRUG INTERACTION 2

Drugs that inhibit liver microsomal CYP3A4 enzymes, including ketoconazole, itraconazole, erythromycin, and clarithromycin—These drugs may reduce the metabolism of lenvatinib, resulting in increased drug levels and potentially increased toxicity.

SPECIAL CONSIDERATIONS

1. Dose modification is not required in patients with mild or moderate hepatic impairment. Dose reduction is recommended in the setting of severe hepatic impairment (Child-Pugh Class C), and the recommended dose is 14 mg PO daily for thyroid cancer and 10 mg PO daily for renal cell cancer.
2. Dose modification is not required in patients with mild or moderate renal impairment. Dose reduction is recommended in the setting of severe renal impairment (CrCl <30 mL/min), and the recommended dose is 14 mg PO daily for thyroid cancer and 10 mg PO daily for renal cancer.
3. Monitor blood pressure while on therapy and treat as needed with standard oral antihypertensive medication. Should be discontinued in patients who develop hypertensive crisis.
4. Baseline and periodic evaluation of LVEF should be performed while on lenvatinib therapy. Dose should be held if grade 3 cardiac dysfunction occurs, until improved to grades 0 or 1 or baseline. Either resume at a reduced dose or discontinue depending on the severity and persistence of cardiac dysfunction. Should be discontinued for grade 4 cardiac dysfunction.
5. Patients should be warned of the risk of arterial thromboembolic events. The drug should be discontinued following an arterial thrombotic event.
6. Monitor liver function tests prior to initiation of therapy and every 2 weeks thereafter for the first 2 months, and then at least monthly during treatment. Should be held for the development of grade 3 or greater liver impairment until resolved to grades 0 to 1 or baseline. Should be discontinued in the setting of liver failure.
7. Monitor renal function while on therapy, as renal impairment has been observed in up to 14% of patients treated with lenvatinib therapy.
8. Monitor urine for protein at baseline and periodically throughout treatment. If urine dipstick proteinuria is greater than or equal to 2+, a 24-hour urine collection for protein needs to be obtained. Should be withheld for ≥2 g of proteinuria/24 hours and resumed at a reduced dose when proteinuria is <2 g/24 hours. Should be terminated in patients who develop the nephrotic syndrome.

9. Monitor ECG with QTc measurement at baseline and periodically during therapy, as QTc prolongation has been observed in nearly 10% of patients. Use with caution in patients at increased risk of developing QT prolongation, including hypokalemia, hypomagnesemia, congenital QT syndrome, and in patients on antiarrhythmic medications or any other products that may cause QT prolongation.

10. Monitor patients for neurologic symptoms as lenvatinib treatment can result in RPLS, as manifested by headache, seizure, lethargy, confusion, blindness and other visual side effects, as well as other neurologic disturbances. Brain MRI is helpful in confirming the diagnosis. Once confirmed by MRI, the drug should be withheld until RPLS is fully resolved. Upon resolution, resume at a reduced dose or discontinue depending on the severity and persistence of neurologic symptoms.

11. Monitor electrolyte status and especially serum calcium levels on at least a monthly basis.

12. Monitor TSH levels on a monthly basis, and adjust thyroid replacement medication as needed.

13. Pregnancy category D.

TOXICITY 1
Hypertension.

TOXICITY 2
GI toxicity with nausea/vomiting, anorexia, diarrhea, and mucositis.

TOXICITY 3
Mild to moderate bleeding complications, with epistaxis being most commonly observed.

TOXICITY 4
Increased risk of arterial thromboembolic events, including MI, angina, stroke, and transient ischemic attack (TIA).

TOXICITY 5
Hepatotoxicity.

TOXICITY 6
Renal toxicity with impairment of renal function and proteinuria.

TOXICITY 7
Cardiac toxicity in the form of cardiac dysfunction and/or cardiac failure. QTc prolongation may also occur.

TOXICITY 8
Hypocalcemia.

TOXICITY 9

GI perforation, fistula formation, and wound-healing complications.

TOXICITY 10

Impairment of thyroid-stimulating hormone suppression.

TOXICITY 11

RPLS with seizures, headache, visual disturbances, confusion, or altered mental function.

Letrozole

TRADE NAME	Femara	CLASSIFICATION	Aromatase inhibitor
CATEGORY	Hormonal agent	DRUG MANUFACTURER	Novartis

MECHANISM OF ACTION

- Nonsteroidal, competitive inhibitor of aromatase. Nearly 200-fold more potent than aminoglutethimide.
- Inhibits synthesis of estrogens by inhibiting the conversion of adrenal androgens (androstenedione and testosterone) to estrogens (estrone, estrone sulfate, and estradiol). Serum estradiol levels are suppressed by 90% within 14 days and nearly completely suppressed after 6 weeks of therapy.
- No inhibitory effect on adrenal corticosteroid biosynthesis.

MECHANISM OF RESISTANCE

- Decreased expression of ER.
- Mutations in the ER leading to decreased binding affinity to letrozole.
- Overexpression of growth factor receptors, such as EGFR, HER2/neu, IGF-1R, or TGF-β, that counteract the inhibitory effects of letrozole.
- Presence of ESR1 mutations.

ABSORPTION
Rapidly and completely absorbed after oral administration. Food does not interfere with oral absorption.

DISTRIBUTION
Significant uptake in peripheral tissues and in breast cancer cells.

METABOLISM
Metabolism occurs in the liver by the cytochrome P450 system. Process of glucuronidation leads to inactive metabolites. Parent drug and metabolites are excreted via the kidneys, with over 75%–90% cleared in urine.

INDICATIONS
1. First-line treatment of postmenopausal women with hormone-receptor-positive or hormone-receptor-unknown locally advanced or metastatic breast cancer.
2. Second-line treatment of postmenopausal women with advanced breast cancer after progression on antiestrogen therapy.
3. Adjuvant treatment of postmenopausal women with hormone-receptor-positive early-stage breast cancer.
4. Extended adjuvant treatment of early-stage breast cancer in postmenopausal women who have received 5 years of adjuvant tamoxifen therapy.

DOSAGE RANGE
1. Metastatic disease: 2.5 mg PO qd until disease progression.
2. Adjuvant setting: 2.5 mg PO qd until disease relapse.

DRUG INTERACTION 1
Phenytoin and other drugs that stimulate the liver microsomal CYP3A4 enzymes, including carbamazepine, rifampin, phenobarbital, and St. John's Wort. These drugs may increase the metabolism of letrozole, resulting in its inactivation and lower effective drug levels.

DRUG INTERACTION 2
Drugs that inhibit the liver microsomal CYP3A4 enzymes, including ketoconazole, itraconazole, erythromycin, and clarithromycin. These drugs may decrease the metabolism of letrozole, resulting in increased drug levels and potentially increased toxicity.

DRUG INTERACTION 3
Warfarin—Patients receiving coumarin-derived anticoagulants should be closely monitored for alterations in their clotting parameters (PT and INR) and/or bleeding, as letrozole may inhibit the metabolism of warfarin by the liver P450 system. The dose of warfarin may require careful adjustment in the presence of letrozole therapy.

DRUG INTERACTION 4

Clopidogrel (Plavix)—Letrozole therapy may reduce the clinical efficacy of clopidogrel, as it is an inhibitor of CYP2C19, which is required for activation of clopidogrel.

SPECIAL CONSIDERATIONS

1. Letrozole is indicated only for postmenopausal women. Efficacy in premenopausal women has not been established. There may be an increased risk of benign ovarian tumors and cystic ovarian disease in this population.
2. Use with caution in patients with abnormal liver function. Monitor liver function at baseline and periodically during therapy. The dose should be reduced by 50% in patients with cirrhosis and severe hepatic dysfunction. In this setting, the recommended dose is 2.5 mg PO every other day.
3. No need for glucocorticoid and/or mineralocorticoid replacement.
4. Monitor women with osteoporosis or at risk of osteoporosis by performing bone densitometry at the start of therapy and at regular intervals. Treatment or prophylaxis for osteoporosis should be initiated when appropriate.
5. Letrozole can be taken with or without food.
6. Pregnancy category D. Breastfeeding should be avoided.

TOXICITY 1

Mild musculoskeletal pains and arthralgias are the most common adverse events.

TOXICITY 2

Headache and fatigue.

TOXICITY 3

Mild nausea with less frequent vomiting and anorexia.

TOXICITY 4

Hot flashes occur in less than 10% of patients.

TOXICITY 5

Hepatotoxicity with mild elevation in serum transaminases and serum bilirubin.

TOXICITY 6

Thromboembolic events are rarely observed.

Leuprolide

TRADE NAME	Lupron	CLASSIFICATION	LHRH agonist
CATEGORY	Hormonal agent	DRUG MANUFACTURER	TAP Pharmaceuticals

MECHANISM OF ACTION
Administration of this LHRH agonist leads to initial release of FSH and LH followed by suppression of gonadotropin secretion as a result of desensitization of the pituitary to gonadotropin-releasing hormone. This eventually leads to decreased secretion of LH and FSH from the pituitary, resulting in castration levels of testosterone. Plasma levels of testosterone fall to castrate levels after 2–4 weeks of therapy.

ABSORPTION
Leuprolide is not orally absorbed. After SC injection, approximately 90% of a dose is absorbed into the systemic circulation.

DISTRIBUTION
Distribution is not well characterized. Leuprolide is slowly released over a 28-day period. Peak serum concentrations are achieved 10–15 days after drug administration. About 45%–50% of drug is bound to plasma proteins.

METABOLISM
Metabolism of leuprolide occurs mainly via hydrolysis of the C-terminal amino acids. Leuprolide is nearly completely eliminated in its parent form in urine (>90%), with an elimination half-life of 3–4 hours. Half-life is prolonged in patients with impaired renal function.

INDICATIONS
1. Advanced prostate cancer.
2. Neoadjuvant therapy of early-stage prostate cancer.

DOSAGE RANGE

Administer 22.5 mg SC every 3 months. Can also be given at a dose of 30 mg SC every 4 months.

DRUG INTERACTIONS

None well characterized to date.

SPECIAL CONSIDERATIONS

1. Initiation of treatment with leuprolide may induce a transient tumor flare due to the initial release of LH and FSH. Patients with impending ureteral obstruction and/or spinal cord compression or those with painful bone metastases are at especially high risk. To prevent tumor flare, patients should be started on antiandrogen therapy at least 2 weeks before starting leuprolide.
2. Serum testosterone levels decrease to castrate levels within 2–4 weeks after initiation of therapy.
3. Use with caution in patients with abnormal renal function.
4. Caution patients about the possibility of hot flashes. Consider the use of clonidine 0.1–0.2 mg PO daily, megestrol acetate 20 mg PO bid, or soy tablets 1 tablet PO tid for prevention and/or treatment.

TOXICITY 1

Hot flashes, impotence, and gynecomastia. Decreased libido occurs less commonly.

TOXICITY 2

Tumor flare may occur in up to 20% of patients, usually within the first 2 weeks of starting therapy. In this setting, may observe increased bone pain, urinary retention, or back pain with spinal cord compression. May be prevented by pretreating with an antiandrogen agent such as flutamide, bicalutamide, or nilutamide.

TOXICITY 3

Local discomfort at the site of injection.

TOXICITY 4

Elevated serum cholesterol levels.

TOXICITY 5

Nausea and vomiting.

TOXICITY 6

Hypersensitivity reaction.

TOXICITY 7

Peripheral edema. Results from sodium retention.

TOXICITY 8

Asthenia.

Lisocabtagene maraleucel

TRADE NAME	Breyanzi, liso-cel	**CLASSIFICATION**	CAR T-cell therapy
CATEGORY	Cellular therapy, immunotherapy	**DRUG MANUFACTURER**	Juno

MECHANISM OF ACTION
- Lisocabtagene maraleucel is a CD19-directed genetically modified autologous T-cell immunotherapy that binds to CD19-expressing target cells and normal B cells.
- Prepared from the patient's own peripheral blood mononuclear cells, which are enriched for T cells, and then genetically modified ex vivo by retroviral transduction to express a chimeric antigen receptor (CAR) made up of an FMC63 monoclonal antibody-derived single-chain variable fragment (scFv), IgG4 hinge region, CD28 transmembrane domain, 4-1BB (CD1370 co-stimulatory domain, and CD3-zeta activation domain. Also includes a non-functional epidermal growth factor receptor that is co-expressed on the cell surface with the CD19-specific CAR. The anti-CD19 CAR T cells are expanded ex vivo and infused back to the patient, where they target CD19-expressing cells.
- Lymphocyte depletion conditioning regimen with cyclophosphamide and fludarabine leads to increased systemic levels of IL-15 and other pro-inflammatory cytokines and chemokines that enhance CAR T-cell activity.
- The conditioning regimen may also decrease immunosuppressive regulatory T cells, activate antigen-presenting cells, and induce pro-inflammatory tumor cell damage.
- Clinical studies have shown an association between higher CAR T-cell levels in peripheral blood and clinical response.

MECHANISM OF RESISTANCE
- Selection of alternatively spliced CD19 isoforms that lack the CD19 epitope recognized by the CAR T cells.
- Antigen loss or modulation.
- Insufficient reactivity against tumors cells with low antigen density.
- Emergence of an antigen-negative clone.
- Lineage switching from lymphoid to myeloid leukemia phenotype.

ABSORPTION
Administered only via the IV route.

DISTRIBUTION
Peak levels of anti-CD19 CAR T cells are observed within 12 days after infusion. Present in peripheral blood for up to 2 years.

METABOLISM
Metabolism of lisocabtagene maraleucel has not been well characterized.

INDICATIONS
FDA-approved for the treatment of relapsed or refractory large B-cell lymphoma after 2 or more lines of systemic therapy, including diffuse large B-cell lymphoma (DLBCL) not otherwise specified (including DLBCL arising from follicular lymphoma), primary mediastinal large B-cell lymphoma, high-grade B-cell lymphoma, and follicular lymphoma grade 3B.

DOSAGE RANGE
- A lymphodepleting chemotherapy regimen of cyclophosphamide 300 mg/m^2 IV and fludarabine 30 mg/m^2 IV for 3 days should be administered 2–7 days before infusion of lisocabtagene maraleucel.
- Patients should be pre-medicated with acetaminophen 650 mg PO and diphenhydramine 12.5 mg IV 30–60 minutes before infusion of lisocabtagene maraleucel.
- Dosing of lisocabtagene maraleucel is based on a target dose of 50–110 × 10^6 CAR-positive viable T cells.

DRUG INTERACTIONS
None well characterized to date.

SPECIAL CONSIDERATIONS
1. Lisocabtagene maraleucel is available only through a restricted program under a Risk Evaluation and Mitigation Strategy (REMS).
2. Monitor for hypersensitivity infusion reactions. Patients should be pre-medicated with acetaminophen 650 mg PO and diphenhydramine 12.5 mg IV at 1 hour prior to CAR T-cell infusion. Prophylactic use of systemic corticosteroids should be avoided as they may interfere with the clinical activity of lisocabtagene maraleucel.
3. Monitor patients at least daily for 7 days following infusion for signs and symptoms of cytokine release syndrome (CRS), which may be fatal or life-threatening in some cases. Patients should be monitored for up to 4 weeks after infusion. Please see package insert for complete guidelines regarding the appropriate management for CRS. This is a black-box warning.
4. Monitor for signs and symptoms of neurologic toxicities, which may be fatal or life-threatening in some cases. This is a black-box warning.
5. Monitor for signs and symptoms of infection.
6. Monitor CBCs periodically after infusion as patients may experience prolonged and significant myelosuppression.

7. Immunoglobulin levels should be monitored after treatment with lisocabtagene maraleucel. Infection precautions, antibiotic prophylaxis, and immunoglobulin replacement may need to be instituted.
8. Patients should be advised not to drive and not to engage in operating heavy or potentially dangerous machinery for at least 8 weeks after receiving lisocabtagene maraleucel.
9. Patients will require lifelong monitoring for secondary malignancies.
10. The risk in pregnant women is currently unknown. Breastfeeding should be avoided.

TOXICITY 1
Hypersensitivity infusion reactions.

TOXICITY 2
CRS with fever, hypotension, tachycardia, chills, and hypoxia. More serious events include cardiac arrhythmias (both atrial and ventricular), decreased cardiac ejection fraction, cardiac arrest, capillary leak syndrome, hepatotoxicity, renal failure, and prolongation of coagulation parameters PT and partial thromboplastin time (PTT).

TOXICITY 3
Neurologic toxicity with headache, delirium, encephalopathy, tremors, dizziness, aphasia, imbalance and gait instability, and seizures.

TOXICITY 4
Myelosuppression with thrombocytopenia and neutropenia, which, in some cases, can be prolonged for several weeks after infusion.

TOXICITY 5
Infections with non-specific pathogen, bacterial, and viral infections most common.

TOXICITY 6
Hypogammaglobulinemia.

TOXICITY 7
Hepatitis B reactivation.

TOXICITY 8
Secondary malignancies.

TOXICITY 9
Fatigue and anorexia.

L

Lomustine

$$Cl-CH_2-CH_2-N-\overset{\overset{\displaystyle O}{\parallel}}{C}-NH-\bigcirc$$
$$\underset{NO}{|}$$

TRADE NAME	CCNU	**CLASSIFICATION**	Alkylating agent, nitrosourea analog
CATEGORY	Chemotherapy drug	**DRUG MANUFACTURER**	Bristol-Myers Squibb

MECHANISM OF ACTION
- Cell cycle–nonspecific nitrosourea analog.
- Alkylation and carbamoylation by lomustine metabolites interfere with the synthesis and function of DNA, RNA, and proteins.
- Antitumor activity appears to correlate best with formation of intrastrand cross-linking of DNA.

MECHANISM OF RESISTANCE
- Decreased cellular uptake of drug.
- Increased intracellular thiol content due to glutathione and/or glutathione-related enzymes.
- Enhanced activity of DNA repair enzymes.

ABSORPTION
Readily and completely absorbed orally. Peak plasma concentrations are observed within 3 hours after oral administration.

DISTRIBUTION
Lipid-soluble drug with broad tissue distribution. Well-absorbed after oral administration and crosses the blood-brain barrier. CNS levels approach 15%–30% of plasma levels.

METABOLISM
Metabolized by the liver microsomal P450 system to active metabolites. The elimination half-life of the drug is about 72 hours, and excretion mainly occurs via the kidneys. Approximately 50% of a dose is excreted in urine within the first 12–24 hours, while 60% of a dose is excreted after 48 hours.

INDICATIONS
1. Brain tumors—Early stage or metastatic.
2. Hodgkin's lymphoma.
3. Non-Hodgkin's lymphoma.

DOSAGE RANGE

Recommended dose as a single agent in previously untreated patients is 130 mg/m^2 PO every 6 weeks. In patients with compromised bone marrow function, the dose should be reduced to 100 mg/m^2 PO every 6 weeks.

DRUG INTERACTION 1

Cimetidine—Cimetidine enhances the toxicity of lomustine.

DRUG INTERACTION 2

Alcohol—Ingestion of alcohol should be avoided for at least 1 hour before and after administration of lomustine.

SPECIAL CONSIDERATIONS

1. Monitor CBC while on therapy. Subsequent cycles should not be given before 6 weeks, given the delayed and potentially cumulative effects of the drug. Platelet and neutrophil counts must return to normal before starting the next course of therapy.
2. PFTs should be obtained at baseline and monitored periodically during therapy. There is an increased risk of pulmonary toxicity in patients with a prior history of lung disease and a baseline FVC or DLCO below 70% of predicted.
3. Administer lomustine on an empty stomach, as food may inhibit absorption.
4. Pregnancy category D. Breastfeeding should be avoided.

TOXICITY 1

Myelosuppression is dose-limiting. Nadirs are delayed and typically occur 4–6 weeks after therapy and may persist for 1–3 weeks.

TOXICITY 2

Nausea and vomiting may occur within 2–6 hours after a dose of drug and can last for up to 24 hours. Mucositis is unusual.

TOXICITY 3

Anorexia.

TOXICITY 4

Impotence, male sterility, amenorrhea, ovarian suppression, menopause, and infertility. Gynecomastia is occasionally observed.

TOXICITY 5

Pulmonary toxicity is uncommon at doses lower than 1,100 mg/m^2.

TOXICITY 6

ILD and pulmonary fibrosis in the form of an insidious cough, dyspnea, pulmonary infiltrates, and/or respiratory failure may be observed.

TOXICITY 7
Renal toxicity is uncommon at total cumulative doses of lower than 1,000 mg/m^2. Usually manifested by progressive azotemia and decrease in kidney size, which can progress to renal failure.

TOXICITY 8
Neurotoxicity in the form of confusion, lethargy, dysarthria, and ataxia.

TOXICITY 9
Increased risk of secondary malignancies with long-term use, especially AML and MDS.

TOXICITY 10
Alopecia is rarely seen.

Loncastuximab tesirine-lpyl

TRADE NAME	Zynlonta, ADCT-402	CLASSIFICATION	Antibody drug conjugate, anti-CD19 monoclonal antibody
CATEGORY	Targeted agent	DRUG MANUFACTURER	ADC Therapeutics

MECHANISM OF ACTION
- Antibody-drug conjugate that is composed of a humanized anti-CD-19 monoclonal antibody conjugated to SG3199, a novel pyrrolobenzodiazepine (PBD) dimer toxin that is made up of PBD monomers (antitumor antibiotics).
- Upon binding to CD19, the molecule is internalized, followed by release of SG3199 via proteolytic cleavage. Once inside the cell, SG3199 then binds to the DNA minor groove, forming DNA interstrand crosslinks, leading to cell death.
- CD19 is expressed in B-cell malignancies but not on normal hematopoietic cells and inhibits B-cell receptor signaling and tumor cell proliferation.

MECHANISM OF RESISTANCE
None well characterized to date.

ABSORPTION
Administered only via the IV route.

DISTRIBUTION

Mean volume of distribution is 7.11 L.

METABOLISM

The loncastuximab antibody is expected to be metabolized via catabolism to small peptides and amino acids. The small molecule SG3199 is metabolized by liver microsomal CYP3A4 and CYP3A5 enzymes. Although the main elimination pathways have not been well characterized, it is presumably eliminated in stool via the hepatobiliary route. SG3199 is not expected to be eliminated by the kidneys.

INDICATIONS

FDA-approved for treatment of relapsed or refractory large B-cell lymphoma, including DLBCL not otherwise specified, DLBCL arising from low-grade lymphoma, and high-grade B-cell lymphoma, after 2 or more lines of systemic therapy.

DOSAGE RANGE

Recommended dose is 0.15 mg/kg IV every 3 weeks for 2 cycles and then 0.075 mg/kg IV every 3 weeks for all subsequent cycles.

DRUG INTERACTIONS

None well characterized to date.

SPECIAL CONSIDERATIONS

1. Monitor for infusion-related reactions, which is most frequently seen during cycle 1 or 2. Premedication with antihistamines (diphenhydramine), antipyretics (acetaminophen), and glucocorticoids (dexamethasone or methylprednisolone) administered 30 minutes to 2 hours before drug infusion can prevent and/or reduce the severity of the infusion reaction.
2. Monitor for signs and symptoms of infection.
3. Monitor CBC prior to each cycle and periodically while on therapy. Patients may need G-CSF for support.
4. Embryo-fetal toxicity. Females of reproductive potential should use effective contraception during drug therapy and for 3 months after the final dose. Breastfeeding should be avoided.

TOXICITY 1

Myelosuppression with neutropenia, thrombocytopenia, and anemia.

TOXICITY 2

Fatigue and anorexia.

TOXICITY 3

Nausea and vomiting.

TOXICITY 4
Peripheral edema, pleural effusion, pericardial effusion, ascites, and generalized edema.

TOXICITY 5
Hepatotoxicity with elevation in LFTs

TOXICITY 6
Skin toxicities with rash, erythema, maculopapular rash, pruritis, including photosensitivity reactions.

TOXICITY 7
Infections with URI and pneumonia.

Lorlatinib

TRADE NAME	Lorbrena	CLASSIFICATION	Signal transduction inhibitor, ALK and ROS1 inhibitor
CATEGORY	Targeted agent	DRUG MANUFACTURER	Pfizer

MECHANISM OF ACTION
- Inhibits multiple receptor tyrosine kinases (RTKs), including anaplastic lymphoma kinase (ALK) and ROS1.
- Retains activity in NSCLC tumors resistant to crizotinib, including ALK mutations at L1196M, G1202R, C1156Y, F1174L, and R1275Q.
- Specifically designed to cross the blood-brain barrier.

MECHANISM OF RESISTANCE
- L1198F mutation in ALK kinase domain.
- Increased expression of miR-100-5p.
- Epithelial-to-mesenchymal transition (EMT) with decreased expression of miR-200c and increased expression of ZEB1.

ABSORPTION

Oral bioavailability is relatively high at 81%. The median time to C_{max} is 1.2–2 hours, and there is no food effect on oral absorption.

DISTRIBUTION

Approximately 66% of drug is bound to plasma proteins. Steady-state drug levels are achieved in approximately 15 days.

METABOLISM

Metabolized in liver primarily by CYP3A4 and UGT1A4 microsomal enzymes, with relatively minor contribution from CYP3A5, CYP2C8, CYP2C9, and UGT1A3. Elimination is nearly equal, with excretion in feces (41%) and urine (48%), and only <10% eliminated as unchanged parent drug. The terminal half-life of lorlatinib is approximately 24 hours.

INDICATIONS

FDA-approved for treatment of patients with ALK-positive metastatic NSCLC.

DOSAGE RANGE

Recommended dose is 100 mg PO once daily.

DRUG INTERACTION 1

Drugs such as ketoconazole, itraconazole, erythromycin, clarithromycin, atazanavir, indinavir, nefazodone, nelfinavir, ritonavir, saquinavir, telithromycin, and voriconazole may decrease the metabolism of lorlatinib, resulting in increased drug levels and potentially increased toxicity.

DRUG INTERACTION 2

Drugs such as rifampin, phenytoin, phenobarbital, carbamazepine, and St. John's Wort may increase the metabolism of lorlatinib, resulting in its inactivation and lower effective drug levels.

SPECIAL CONSIDERATIONS

1. No dose adjustment is needed for patients with mild hepatic dysfunction. Has not been evaluated in patients with moderate or severe hepatic dysfunction.
2. No dose adjustment is needed for patients with mild or moderate renal dysfunction. The dose should be reduced to 75 mg PO daily for patients with severe renal dysfunction. Has not been evaluated in patients on hemodialysis.
3. Contraindicated in patients taking strong CYP3A4 inducers. If strong CYP3A4 inducers are required, discontinue for at least 3 plasma half-lives prior to starting drug therapy.
4. Monitor patients for new or progressive pulmonary symptoms, including cough, dyspnea, and fever.
5. Baseline and periodic evaluations of ECG should be performed while on therapy as the drug can cause PR interval prolongation and atrioventricular (AV) block.

6. ALK testing using an FDA-approved test is required to confirm the presence of ALK-positive NSCLC.
7. Monitor serum cholesterol and triglyceride levels during treatment. Lipid-lowering agents may be required to treat hyperlipidemia.
8. Can cause fetal harm when administered to a pregnant woman. Females of reproductive potential should use an effective non-hormonal method of contraception during drug therapy and for at least 6 months after the final dose. Breastfeeding should be avoided.

TOXICITY 1
Hyperlipidemia with increased serum cholesterol and triglycerides.

TOXICITY 2
CNS effects with changes in cognitive function, mental status, mood, speech, and sleep. Seizures and hallucinations have also been observed.

TOXICITY 3
Peripheral edema and weight gain.

TOXICITY 4
ECG abnormalities with PR interval prolongation and AV block

TOXICITY 5
Hepatotoxicity with elevations in serum transaminases (SGOT, SGPT).

TOXICITY 6
Diarrhea and nausea/vomiting are the most common GI side effects.

TOXICITY 7
Fatigue.

TOXICITY 8
Interstitial lung disease and pneumonitis.

TOXICITY 9
Elevations in serum lipase.

TOXICITY 10
Peripheral edema.

TOXICITY 11
Arthralgias, myalgias, and back pain.

Lurbinectedin

TRADE NAME	Zepzelca, PM01183	CLASSIFICATION	Alkylating agent
CATEGORY	Chemotherapy drug	DRUG MANUFACTURER	Pharma Mar and Jazz

MECHANISM OF ACTION
- Synthetic tetrahydroisoquinoline alkylating agent that binds to guanine residues in the minor groove of DNA, leading to formation of DNA adducts.
- DNA adduct formation results in single- and double-strand breaks and inhibition of DNA synthesis and function.
- Binding to CG rich sequences on DNA results in irreversible stalling of elongating RNA polymerase II, leading to inhibition of transcription.
- Antitumor activity may also relate to inhibitory effects on the tumor microenvironment.
- Inhibits tumor-associated macrophages and inhibits production of inflammatory cytokines in the tumor microenvironment.
- Cell cycle nonspecific. Active in all phases of the cell cycle.

MECHANISM OF RESISTANCE
- None well characterized to date.

ABSORPTION
Administered only via the IV route.

DISTRIBUTION
Extensive binding (99%) of drug is bound to plasma proteins, to both albumin and α-1-acid glycoprotein.

METABOLISM

Rapidly and extensively metabolized by CYP3A liver microsomal enzymes. There is negligible unchanged drug in feces and urine following drug administration. Elimination is mainly hepatic with excretion in feces (89%), with renal elimination accounting for only 6% of an administered dose. The terminal elimination half-life is approximately 51 hours.

INDICATIONS

FDA-approved for the treatment of metastatic SCLC following disease progression on or after platinum-based chemotherapy.

DOSAGE RANGE

Recommended dose is 3.25 mg/m^2 IV every 3 weeks.

DRUG INTERACTION 1

Drugs such as ketoconazole, itraconazole, erythromycin, clarithromycin, atazanavir, indinavir, nefazodone, nelfinavir, ritonavir, saquinavir, telithromycin, and voriconazole may decrease the metabolism of lurbinectedin, resulting in increased drug levels and potentially increased toxicity.

DRUG INTERACTION 2

Drugs such as rifampin, phenytoin, phenobarbital, carbamazepine, and St. John's Wort may increase the metabolism of lurbinectedin, resulting in its inactivation and lower effective drug levels.

SPECIAL CONSIDERATIONS

1. Dose reduction is not recommended in patients with mild hepatic dysfunction. Has not been studied in the setting of moderate or severe hepatic dysfunction.
2. Dose reduction is not required in patients with mild or moderate renal dysfunction. Has not been studied in patients with severe renal dysfunction and end-stage renal disease.
3. Monitor CBCs on a periodic basis with a particular focus on WBC and ANC.
4. Monitor LFTs periodically during treatment. The median time to onset of altered LFTs is 8 days, and the median duration is 7 days.
5. Monitor patients for signs and symptoms of extravasation reaction during infusion. Central venous catheter should be used for drug administration.
6. Monitor CPK levels at baseline and periodically during treatment.
7. Can cause fetal harm when administered to a pregnant woman. Females of reproductive potential should use effective contraception during drug therapy and for at least 6 months after the final dose. Breastfeeding should be avoided.

TOXICITY 1

Myelosuppression with neutropenia, thrombocytopenia, and anemia. Severe and fatal neutropenic sepsis may occur.

TOXICITY 2
Hepatotoxicity with elevations in SGOT, SGPT, and serum bilirubin.

TOXICITY 3
Potent vesicant and extravasation can lead to skin and soft tissue injury.

TOXICITY 4
Fatigue and anorexia.

TOXICITY 5
GI toxicity with nausea/vomiting, constipation, and diarrhea.

TOXICITY 6
Rhabdomyolysis.

Lutetium Lu 177 dotatate

TRADE NAME	Lutathera	CLASSIFICATION	Somatostatin analog
CATEGORY	Radionuclide agent, targeted agent	DRUG MANUFACTURER	Advanced Accelerator Applications

MECHANISM OF ACTION
- First-in-class peptide receptor radionuclide therapy.
- Radiolabeled somatostatin analog that binds to somatostatin receptors, with highest affinity for subtype 2 receptors.
- The somatostatin analog is then internalized, and the beta-emission from Lu 177 induces damage by formation of free radicals in the somatostatin receptor–positive cells and in neighboring cells.
- Ionizing radiation from the Lu 177 radioisotope results in cell death.

ABSORPTION
Administered only via the IV route.

DISTRIBUTION
Distributes to tumor lesions, kidneys, liver, spleen, and in some patients, thyroid and pituitary gland within 4 hours after administration. The non-radioactive form of lutetium dotatate is 43% bound to plasma proteins.

METABOLISM
Does not undergo liver metabolism. Mainly eliminated via renal excretion, and >99% eliminated in urine within 14 days after drug administration. The mean terminal half-life is prolonged at 71 hours.

INDICATIONS

FDA-approved for adult patients with somatostatin receptor–positive gastroenteropancreatic neuroendocrine tumors, including foregut, midgut, and hindgut neuroendocrine tumors.

DOSAGE RANGE

- Administer 200 mCi of lutetium Lu 177 dotatate every 8 weeks for a total of 4 doses.
- Administer long-acting octreotide 30 mg IM at 4–24 hours after each dose of lutetium Lu 177 dotatate.
- Long-acting octreotide 30 mg IM should be continued every 4 weeks after completion of lutetium Lu 177 dotatate until disease progression or for up to 18 months following initiation of treatment.
- An IV amino acid solution of L-lysine and L-arginine is administered 30 minutes before administration of lutetium Lu 177 dotatate. The amino acid infusion should be continued during and for at least 3 hours after completion of the lutetium Lu 177 dotatate infusion. The dose of the amino acid infusion should not be reduced if the dose of lutetium Lu 177 dotatate is reduced for toxicity.

DRUG INTERACTIONS

Somatostatin analogs—Somatostatin and its analogs can bind competitively to somatostatin receptors and may interfere with the clinical activity of lutetium Lu 177 dotatate.

SPECIAL CONSIDERATIONS

1. No dose adjustment is recommended for patients with mild or moderate hepatic dysfunction. Has not been studied in patients with severe hepatic dysfunction (total bilirubin >3 × ULN, any AST), and caution should be used in this setting.
2. No dose adjustment is recommended for patients with mild or moderate renal dysfunction. Has not been studied in patients with severe renal dysfunction or end-stage renal disease, and caution should be used in these settings.
3. Monitor CBCs closely, and treatment should be withheld, reduced, or permanently discontinued depending on the severity of the myelosuppression. Please see package insert for details on dose modifications based on blood cell counts.
4. Monitor LFTs and serum bilirubin at baseline and periodically while on therapy. Patients with metastatic liver disease may be at increased risk of hepatotoxicity as a result of radiation exposure.
5. Monitor patients for evidence of neuroendocrine hormonal crisis, which usually occurs during or within 24 hours after the initial dose of therapy.
6. Patients should be advised to urinate frequently during and after administration of lutetium Lu 177 dotatate.
7. Monitor renal function at baseline and on a periodic basis while on therapy. Patients with mild or moderate renal dysfunction at baseline may be at increased risk of toxicity.

8. Lutetium Lu 177 dotatate increases the patient's overall long-term radiation exposure, which is associated with an increased risk of secondary cancers.

9. Radiation exposure to patients, medical personnel, and household contacts should be minimized during and after treatment with lutetium Lu 177 dotatate, as radiation can be detected in patient's urine for up to 30 days after drug administration.

10. Long-acting somatostatin analogs should be stopped for at least 4 weeks prior to each dose of lutetium Lu 177 dotatate, and short-acting octreotide should be stopped for at least 24 hours before each treatment dose.

11. May cause fetal harm in women who are pregnant. Females of reproductive potential should use effective contraception during treatment and for 7 months after the final dose. Males with female partners of reproductive potential should use effective contraception during treatment and for 4 months after the final dose.

TOXICITY 1
Infusion-related symptoms, including fever, chills, urticaria, flushing, fatigue, headache, bronchospasm, rhinitis, dyspnea, angioedema, nausea, and/or hypotension. Usually resolve upon slowing and/or interrupting the infusion and with supportive care.

TOXICITY 2
Myelosuppression is most common side effect, with anemia, thrombocytopenia, and neutropenia. Time to platelet nadir is at about 5 weeks, and the duration of thrombocytopenia is 2 months.

TOXICITY 3
Mild fatigue and asthenia.

TOXICITY 4
Nausea and vomiting.

TOXICITY 5
Hepatotoxicity with elevations in LFTs and serum bilirubin.

TOXICITY 6
Infertility.

TOXICITY 7
Neuroendocrine hormonal crisis with flushing, diarrhea, bronchospasm, and hypotension.

TOXICITY 8
Secondary malignancies with MDS and AML.

Margetuximab-cmkb

TRADE NAME	Margenza, Anti-HER2-antibody	**CLASSIFICATION**	Signal transduction inhibitor, anti-HER2 monoclonal antibody
CATEGORY	Biologic response modifier agent, targeted agent	**DRUG MANUFACTURER**	MacroGenics

MECHANISM OF ACTION

- Recombinant chimeric Fc-engineered IgG1-κ monoclonal antibody directed against the extracellular domain (IV) of the HER2 growth factor receptor. This receptor is overexpressed in several human cancers, including 25%–30% of breast cancers and up to 20% of gastric cancers.
- Modified Fc region engineered to increase affinity for the activating Fcγreceptor CD16A (FCγRIIIa) and to reduce affinity for the inhibitory FCγR receptor CD32B (FCγRIIIb). These effects on Fc receptors are expected to increase activation of innate and adaptive immune-mediated responses, including antibody-dependent cellular cytotoxicity (ADCC) and/or complement-mediated cell lysis.
- Inhibits HER2 intracellular signaling pathways.

MECHANISM OF RESISTANCE

- Mutations in the HER2 growth factor receptor, leading to reduced binding affinity to the antibody.
- Reactivation of HER signaling through acquisition of the HER2 L755S mutation.
- Decreased expression of HER2.
- Expression of P95HER2, a constitutively active, truncated form of the HER2 receptor.
- Increased expression of HER3.
- Activation/induction of alternative cellular signaling pathways, such as the PI3K/AKT, IGF-1 receptor, and/or the c-MET receptor.

DISTRIBUTION

Distribution in the body has not been well characterized. Time to steady-state levels is on the order of 2 months.

METABOLISM

Margetuximab is expected to be metabolized via catabolic pathways to small peptides and amino acids. The mean terminal half-life is on the order of 19 days.

INDICATIONS

Treatment of adult patients with metastatic HER2-positive breast cancer who have received 2 or more prior anti-HER2 regimens, at least one of which was for metastatic disease.

DOSAGE RANGE

Recommended initial dose of 15 mg/kg IV administered over 120 minutes, followed by 15 mg/kg IV administered over at least 30 minutes every 3 weeks for all subsequent doses.

DRUG INTERACTIONS

None well characterized to date.

SPECIAL CONSIDERATIONS

1. Caution should be used in treating patients with pre-existing cardiac dysfunction. Careful baseline assessment of cardiac function (LVEF) before treatment and frequent monitoring (every 3 months) of cardiac function while on therapy. Margituximab should be held for >16% absolute decrease in LVEF from a normal baseline value and should be stopped immediately in patients who develop clinically significant congestive heart failure. This is a black-box warning.
2. Carefully monitor for infusion reactions, which typically occur during or within 24 hours of drug administration. May need to pre-medicate with diphenhydramine and acetaminophen. The rate of infusion needs to be reduced for mild or moderate infusion reactions. In severe cases, may need to treat with IV fluids and/or pressors. Drug therapy should be stopped in patients with severe or life-threatening reactions.
3. Although no formal drug-drug interaction studies have been conducted to date, as with other HER2-directed antibody therapies, should avoid anthracycline-based regimens for up to 4 months after stopping margituximab therapy.
4. Embryo-fetal toxicity (black-box warning). May cause fetal harm when administered to a pregnant woman. Females of reproductive potential should use effective contraception during drug therapy and for at least 4 months after the final dose. Breastfeeding should be avoided.

TOXICITY 1

Infusion-related symptoms occur in 40%–50% of patients with fever, chills, urticaria, flushing, fatigue, headache, bronchospasm, dyspnea, angioedema, and hypotension. Usually mild to moderate in severity.

TOXICITY 2

Mild GI toxicity in the form of nausea/vomiting, diarrhea, and constipation.

TOXICITY 3

Cardiac toxicity in the form of dyspnea, peripheral edema, and reduced left ventricular function (black-box warning). Significantly increased risk when used in combination with an anthracycline-based regimen. In most instances, cardiac dysfunction is readily reversible.

TOXICITY 4
Fatigue, asthenia, and anorexia.

TOXICITY 5
Myelosuppression with neutropenia and anemia.

TOXICITY 6
Pulmonary toxicity with increased cough, dyspnea, and fever.

Mechlorethamine

$$CH_3$$
$$ClCH_2CH_2{-}\overset{\oplus}{\underset{H}{N}}{-}CH_2CH_2Cl$$

TRADE NAME	Mustargen, Nitrogen mustard	CLASSIFICATION	Alkylating agent
CATEGORY	Chemotherapy drug	DRUG MANUFACTURER	Merck

MECHANISM OF ACTION
- Analog of mustard gas.
- Classic alkylating agent that forms interstrand and intrastrand cross-links with DNA, resulting in inhibition of DNA synthesis and function.
- Cell cycle–nonspecific, with activity in all phases of the cell cycle.

MECHANISM OF RESISTANCE
- Decreased cellular uptake of drug.
- Increased inactivation of cytotoxic species through increased expression of sulfhydryl proteins, including glutathione and glutathione-associated enzymes.
- Enhanced activity of DNA repair enzymes.

ABSORPTION
Administered only via the IV route.

DISTRIBUTION
Distribution is not well characterized.

METABOLISM
Undergoes rapid hydrolysis in plasma to reactive metabolites. Extremely short plasma half-life on the order of 15–20 minutes. No significant organ metabolism. Greater than 50% of inactive drug metabolites are excreted in urine within 24 hours.

INDICATIONS
1. Hodgkin's lymphoma.
2. Non-Hodgkin's lymphoma.
3. Cutaneous T-cell lymphoma (topical use).
4. Intrapleural, intrapericardial, and intraperitoneal treatment of metastatic disease resulting in pleural effusion.

DOSAGE RANGE
1. Hodgkin's lymphoma: 6 mg/m^2 IV on days 1 and 8 every 28 days, as part of the MOPP regimen.
2. Cutaneous T-cell lymphoma: Dilute 10 mg in 60 mL of sterile water and apply topically to skin lesions.
3. Intracavitary use: 0.2–0.4 mg/kg into the pleural and/or peritoneal cavity.

DRUG INTERACTIONS
Sodium thiosulfate—Sodium thiosulfate inactivates mechlorethamine.

SPECIAL CONSIDERATIONS
1. Mechlorethamine is a potent vesicant, and caution should be exercised in administering the drug.
2. Administer drug into either a new IV site or one that is less than 24 hours old to reduce the risk of extravasation.
3. Pregnancy category D. Breastfeeding should be avoided.

TOXICITY 1
Myelosuppression is dose-limiting, with leukopenia and thrombocytopenia. Nadirs occur at days 7–10 and recover by day 21.

TOXICITY 2
Nausea and vomiting usually occur within the first 3 hours after drug administration, lasting for 4–8 hours and up to 24 hours, and often severe. Can be dose-limiting in some patients.

TOXICITY 3
Potent vesicant. Pain, inflammation, erythema, induration, and necrosis can be observed at the injection site.

TOXICITY 4
Alopecia.

TOXICITY 5
Amenorrhea and azoospermia.

TOXICITY 6
Hyperuricemia.

TOXICITY 7
CNS toxicities, including weakness, sleepiness, and headache, are rare.

TOXICITY 8
Hypersensitivity reactions. Rarely observed.

TOXICITY 9
Increased risk of secondary malignancies, including AML with IV administration. Basal cell and squamous cell cancers of the skin with topical application.

Megestrol acetate

TRADE NAME	Megace	CLASSIFICATION	Progestational agent
CATEGORY	Hormonal agent	DRUG MANUFACTURER	Bristol-Myers Squibb

MECHANISM OF ACTION
- Synthetic derivative of the naturally occurring steroid hormone progesterone.
- Possesses antiestrogenic effects. Induces the activity of 17-hydroxysteroid dehydrogenase, which then oxidizes estradiol to the less active metabolite estrone. Also activates estrogen sulfotransferase, which metabolizes estrogen to less potent metabolites.
- Inhibits release of luteinizing hormone receptors, resulting in a decrease in estrogen levels.
- Inhibits stability, availability, and turnover of estrogen receptors.

MECHANISM OF RESISTANCE
None well characterized.

ABSORPTION
Rapidly and completely absorbed after an oral dose. Peak plasma concentration is reached within 1–3 hours after oral administration.

DISTRIBUTION
Large fraction of megestrol is distributed into body fat.

METABOLISM
About 70% of drug is metabolized in the liver to inactive steroid metabolites. Primarily eliminated in urine in the form of parent drug and metabolites, and 60%–80% of the drug is renally excreted within 10 days after administration. Elimination half-life is quite variable and ranges from 15 to 105 hours, with a mean of 34 hours.

INDICATIONS
1. Breast cancer.
2. Endometrial cancer.
3. Renal cell cancer.
4. Appetite stimulant in cancer and HIV patients.

DOSAGE RANGE
1. Breast cancer: 40 mg PO qid.
2. Endometrial cancer: 40 mg PO qid.
3. Appetite stimulant: 80–200 mg PO qid.

DRUG INTERACTIONS
Aminoglutethimide—Aminoglutethimide enhances the hepatic metabolism of megestrol, resulting in decreased serum levels.

SPECIAL CONSIDERATIONS
1. Use with caution in patients with a history of either thromboembolic or hypercoagulable disorders, as megestrol acetate has been associated with an increased incidence of thromboembolic events.
2. Use with caution in patients with diabetes mellitus, as megestrol may exacerbate this condition.
3. Use with caution in patients with abnormal liver function. Dose reduction is recommended in this setting.
4. Caution patients on the risk of weight gain and fluid retention. Patients should be advised to go on a low-salt diet.
5. Pregnancy category D. Breastfeeding should be avoided.

TOXICITY 1
Weight gain results from a combination of fluid retention and increased appetite.

TOXICITY 2
Thromboembolic events are rarely observed.

TOXICITY 3
Nausea and vomiting.

TOXICITY 4
Breakthrough menstrual bleeding.

TOXICITY 5
Tumor flare.

TOXICITY 6
Hyperglycemia.

TOXICITY 7
Hot flashes, sweating, and mood changes.

Melphalan

$$\text{Cl} \diagdown \text{N} \diagup \text{Cl} - \text{C}_6\text{H}_4 - \text{CH}_2\text{CHCO}_2\text{H} \text{ (NH}_2\text{)}$$

TRADE NAME	Alkeran, Phenylalanine mustard, L-PAM	CLASSIFICATION	Alkylating agent
CATEGORY	Chemotherapy drug	DRUG MANUFACTURER	GlaxoSmithKline

MECHANISM OF ACTION
- Analog of nitrogen mustard.
- Classic bifunctional alkylating agent that forms interstrand and intrastrand cross-links with DNA, resulting in inhibition of DNA synthesis and function.
- Cell cycle–nonspecific, as it acts at all stages of the cell cycle.

MECHANISM OF RESISTANCE

- Decreased cellular uptake of drug.
- Increased inactivation of cytotoxic species through increased expression of sulfhydryl proteins, including glutathione and glutathione-associated enzymes.
- Enhanced activity of DNA repair enzymes.

ABSORPTION

Oral absorption is poor and incomplete. Oral bioavailability ranges between 25% and 90%, with a mean of 60%, and oral absorption is decreased when taken with food.

DISTRIBUTION

Widely distributed in all tissues. Approximately 80%–90% of drug is bound to plasma proteins.

METABOLISM

Undergoes rapid hydrolysis in plasma to reactive metabolites. Short plasma half-life on the order of 60–90 minutes. No significant organ metabolism. About 25%–30% of drug is excreted in urine within 24 hours after administration, with the majority of the drug being excreted in feces (up to 50%) over 6 days.

INDICATIONS

1. Multiple myeloma.
2. Breast cancer.
3. Ovarian cancer.
4. High-dose chemotherapy and transplant setting.
5. Polycythemia vera.

DOSAGE RANGE

1. Multiple myeloma: 9 mg/m^2 IV on days 1–4 every 4 weeks as part of the melphalan-prednisone regimen.
2. Transplant setting: 140 mg/m^2 as a single agent in bone marrow/stem cell transplant setting.

DRUG INTERACTION 1

Cimetidine—Cimetidine decreases the oral bioavailability of melphalan by up to 30%.

DRUG INTERACTION 2

Steroids—Steroids enhance the antitumor effects of melphalan.

DRUG INTERACTION 3

Cyclosporine—Cyclosporine enhances the risk of renal toxicity secondary to melphalan.

SPECIAL CONSIDERATIONS

1. Use with caution in patients with abnormal renal function. Although the drug has been used in high doses in the transplant setting in the face of renal dysfunction without increased toxicity, dose reduction should be considered in the setting of renal dysfunction.
2. When administered orally, drug should be taken on an empty stomach to maximize absorption.
3. IV administration may cause hypersensitivity reaction.
4. Monitor CBC, as melphalan therapy is associated with delayed and prolonged nadir.
5. Monitor injection site for erythema, pain, and/or burning.
6. Pregnancy category D. Breastfeeding should be avoided.

TOXICITY 1

Myelosuppression is dose-limiting, with leukopenia and thrombocytopenia equally affected. Effect may be prolonged and cumulative, with a delayed nadir at 4–6 weeks after therapy.

TOXICITY 2

Nausea and vomiting, mucositis, and diarrhea. Generally mild with conventional doses but can be severe with high-dose therapy.

TOXICITY 3

Hypersensitivity reactions are rare with oral form. Observed in about 10% of patients treated with IV form of drug and manifested as diaphoresis, urticaria, skin rashes, bronchospasm, dyspnea, tachycardia, and hypotension.

TOXICITY 4

Alopecia is uncommon.

TOXICITY 5

Skin ulcerations and other skin reactions at the injection site are uncommon.

TOXICITY 6

Increased risk of secondary malignancies including AML and MDS with prolonged use.

Melphalan flufenamide

TRADE NAME	Melflufen, Pepaxto	CLASSIFICATION	Peptide-conjugated alkylating agent
CATEGORY	Chemotherapy drug	DRUG MANUFACTURER	Ocopeptides AB

MECHANISM OF ACTION
- Peptide conjugated alkylating agent.
- Highly lipophilic drug that passively enters cells and then enzymatically hydrolyzed to melphalan.
- Classic bifunctional alkylating agent that forms interstrand and intrastrand cross-links with DNA, resulting in inhibition of DNA synthesis and function.
- Synergistic activity in combination with dexamethasone in both melphalan-sensitive and melphalan-resistant cell lines.
- Cell cycle–nonspecific, as it acts at all stages of the cell cycle.

MECHANISM OF RESISTANCE
- Increased inactivation of cytotoxic species through increased expression of sulfhydryl proteins, including glutathione and glutathione-associated enzymes.
- Enhanced activity of DNA repair enzymes.

ABSORPTION
Administered only via the IV route.

DISTRIBUTION
Rapidly distributed to peripheral tissues. Peak drug levels reached during the 30-minute infusion.

METABOLISM
Metabolized in tissues to desethyl-melphalan flufenamide and melphalan. Melphalan is then metabolized by hydrolysis to the monohydroxy, dihydroxy, and parafluoro-phenylalanine metabolites. The mean half-life of the parent drug is 2.1 minutes and that of melphalan is 70 minutes.

INDICATIONS
Treatment of adult patients with relapsed or refractory multiple myeloma who have received at least 4 prior lines of therapy and whose disease is refractory to at least one proteasome inhibitor, one immunomodulatory agent, and one CD38-directed monoclonal antibody.

DOSAGE RANGE
Recommended dose is 40 mg IV on day 1 of a 28-day cycle.

DRUG INTERACTIONS
Have not been well characterized to date.

SPECIAL CONSIDERATIONS
1. Should not be used in patients with a history of serious hypersensitivity reactions to melphalan or melphalan flufenamide.
2. Monitor CBC, as therapy is associated with myelosuppression.
3. Recommended dose of drug should not be exceeded as higher doses may be associated with an increased risk of death.
4. Monitor patients long term for the risk of secondary malignancies.
5. Embryo-fetal toxicity. Females of reproductive potential need to use effective contraception while on treatment and for 6 months after the last dose. Breastfeeding should be avoided.

TOXICITY 1
Myelosuppression with neutropenia, thrombocytopenia, and anemia.

TOXICITY 2
Nausea and vomiting, diarrhea, and constipation.

TOXICITY 3
Fatigue, asthenia, and anorexia.

TOXICITY 4
Infections, with URIs and pneumonia.

TOXICITY 5
Increased risk of secondary malignancies including AML and MDS with prolonged use.

Mercaptopurine

TRADE NAME	6-MP, Purinethol, Purixan	**CLASSIFICATION**	Antimetabolite, purine analog
CATEGORY	Chemotherapy drug	**DRUG MANUFACTURER**	GlaxoSmithKline, Rare Disease Therapeutics

MECHANISM OF ACTION
- Cell cycle–specific purine analog with activity in the S-phase.
- Parent drug is inactive. Requires intracellular phosphorylation by the enzyme hypoxanthine-guanine phosphoribosyltransferase (HGPRT) to the cytotoxic monophosphate form, which is then eventually metabolized to the triphosphate metabolite.
- Inhibits de novo purine synthesis by inhibiting 5-phosphoribosyl-1 pyrophosphate (PRPP) amidotransferase.
- Incorporation of thiopurine triphosphate nucleotides into DNA, resulting in inhibition of DNA synthesis and function.
- Incorporation of thiopurine triphosphate nucleotides into RNA, resulting in alterations in RNA processing and/or mRNA translation.

MECHANISM OF RESISTANCE
- Decreased expression of the activating enzyme HGPRT.
- Increased expression of the catabolic enzyme alkaline phosphatase or the conjugating enzyme thiopurine methyltransferase (TPMT).
- Decreased expression of mismatch repair enzymes (e.g., hMLH1, hMSH2).
- Decreased transmembrane transport of drug.
- Cross-resistance observed between mercaptopurine and thioguanine.

ABSORPTION
Oral absorption of the tablet form is erratic and incomplete. Only 50% of an oral dose is absorbed. A new oral suspension is approved by the FDA with greater oral bioavailability than the tablet form.

DISTRIBUTION
Widely distributed in total body water. Does not cross the blood-brain barrier. About 20%–30% of drug is bound to plasma proteins.

METABOLISM

Metabolized in the liver by methylation to inactive metabolites and via oxidation by xanthine oxidase to inactive metabolites. About 50% of parent drug and metabolites is eliminated in urine within the first 24 hours. Plasma half-life after oral administration is 1.5 hours, in contrast to the plasma half-life after IV administration, which ranges between 20 and 50 minutes.

INDICATIONS

Acute lymphoblastic leukemia.

DOSAGE RANGE

1. Induction therapy: 2.5 mg/kg PO daily.
2. Maintenance therapy: 1.5–2.5 mg/kg PO daily.

DRUG INTERACTION 1

Warfarin—Anticoagulant effects of warfarin are inhibited by 6-MP through an unknown mechanism. Monitor coagulation parameters (PT/ INR), and adjust dose accordingly.

DRUG INTERACTION 2

Allopurinol—Allopurinol inhibits xanthine oxidase and the catabolic breakdown of 6-MP, resulting in enhanced toxicity. Dose of mercaptopurine must be reduced by 50%–75% when given concurrently with allopurinol.

DRUG INTERACTION 3

Trimethoprim/sulfamethoxazole (Bactrim DS) may enhance the myelosuppressive effects of 6-MP when given concurrently.

SPECIAL CONSIDERATIONS

1. Dose reduction of 50%–75% is required when 6-MP is given concurrently with allopurinol. This is because allopurinol inhibits the catabolic breakdown of 6-MP by xanthine oxidase.
2. Use with caution in patients with abnormal liver and/or renal function. Dose reduction should be considered in these settings.
3. Use with caution in the presence of other hepatotoxic drugs, as risk of 6-MP-associated hepatic toxicity is increased.
4. Patients with a deficiency in the metabolizing enzyme thiopurine methyltransferase (TPMT) are at increased risk for developing severe toxicities, with myelosuppression and GI toxicity. This enzyme deficiency is an autosomal recessive pharmacogenetic syndrome.
5. Administer on an empty stomach to facilitate oral absorption. Advise patient to take 6-MP at bedtime.
6. Pregnancy category D. Breastfeeding should be avoided.

TOXICITY 1

Myelosuppression. Mild to moderate, with neutropenia more common than thrombocytopenia. Leukopenia nadir at days 10–14, with recovery by day 21.

TOXICITY 2
Mucositis and/or diarrhea. Usually seen with higher doses.

TOXICITY 3
Hepatotoxicity with elevated serum bilirubin and transaminases. Usually occurs 2–3 months after initiation of therapy.

TOXICITY 4
Mild nausea and vomiting.

TOXICITY 5
Skin toxicity with dry skin, urticaria, and photosensitivity.

TOXICITY 6
Immunosuppression with increased risk of bacterial, fungal, and parasitic infections.

TOXICITY 7
Mutagenic, teratogenic, and carcinogenic.

Methotrexate

TRADE NAME	MTX, Amethopterin	CLASSIFICATION	Antimetabolite, antifolate analog
CATEGORY	Chemotherapy drug	DRUG MANUFACTURER	Lederle Laboratories and Immunex

MECHANISM OF ACTION
- Cell cycle–specific antifolate analog, active in S-phase of the cell cycle.
- Enters cells through specific transport systems mediated by the reduced folate carrier (RFC) and the folate receptor protein (FRP).
- Requires polyglutamation by the enzyme folylpolyglutamate synthase (FPGS) for its cytotoxic activity.
- Inhibition of dihydrofolate reductase (DHFR), resulting in depletion of critical reduced folates.
- Inhibition of de novo thymidylate synthesis.

- Inhibition of de novo purine synthesis.
- Incorporation of dUTP into DNA, resulting in inhibition of DNA synthesis and function.

MECHANISM OF RESISTANCE

- Decreased carrier-mediated transport of drug into cell through decreased expression and/or activity of reduced folate carrier (RFC) or folate-receptor protein (FRP).
- Decreased formation of cytotoxic methotrexate polyglutamates through either decreased expression of FPGS or increased expression of γ-glutamyl hydrolase (GGH).
- Increased expression of the target enzyme DHFR through either gene amplification or increased transcription, translation, and/or post-translational events.
- Reduced binding affinity of DHFR for methotrexate.

ABSORPTION

Oral bioavailability is saturable and erratic at doses greater than 25 mg/m^2. Peak serum levels are achieved within 1–2 hours of oral administration. Methotrexate is completely absorbed from parenteral routes of administration, and peak serum concentrations are reached in 30–60 minutes after IM injection.

DISTRIBUTION

Widely distributed throughout the body. At conventional doses, CSF levels are only about 5%–10% of those in plasma. High-dose methotrexate yields therapeutic concentrations in the CSF. Distributes into third-space fluid collections such as pleural effusion and ascites. Only about 50% of drug bound to plasma proteins, mainly to albumin.

METABOLISM

Extensive metabolism in liver and in cells by FPGS to higher polyglutamate forms. About 10%–20% of parent drug and the 7-hydroxymetabolite are eliminated in bile and then reabsorbed via enterohepatic circulation. Renal excretion is the main route of elimination and is mediated by glomerular filtration and tubular secretion. About 80%–90% of an administered dose is eliminated unchanged in urine within 24 hours. Terminal half-life of drug is on the order of 8–10 hours.

INDICATIONS

1. Breast cancer.
2. Head and neck cancer.
3. Osteogenic sarcoma.
4. Acute lymphoblastic leukemia.
5. Non-Hodgkin's lymphoma.
6. Primary CNS lymphoma.
7. Meningeal leukemia and carcinomatous meningitis.
8. Bladder cancer.
9. Gestational trophoblastic cancer.

DOSAGE RANGE

1. Low dose: 10–50 mg/m^2 IV every 3–4 weeks.
2. Low dose weekly: 25 mg/m^2 IV weekly.
3. Moderate dose: 100–500 mg/m^2 IV every 2–3 weeks.
4. High dose: 1–12 g/m^2 IV over a 3- to 24-hour period every 1–3 weeks.
5. Intrathecal: 10–15 mg IT two times weekly until CSF is clear, then weekly dose for 2–6 weeks, followed by monthly dose.
6. Intramuscular: 25 mg/m^2 IM every 3 weeks.

DRUG INTERACTION 1

Aspirin, penicillins, probenecid, NSAIDs, and cephalosporins—These drugs inhibit the renal excretion of methotrexate, leading to increased plasma drug levels and potentially increased toxicity.

DRUG INTERACTION 2

Warfarin—Methotrexate may enhance the anticoagulant effect of warfarin through competitive displacement from plasma proteins.

DRUG INTERACTION 3

5-FU—Methotrexate enhances the antitumor activity of 5-FU when given 24 hours before fluoropyrimidine treatment.

DRUG INTERACTION 4

Leucovorin—Leucovorin rescues the toxic effects of methotrexate but may also impair the antitumor activity. The active form of leucovorin is the L-isomer.

DRUG INTERACTION 5

Thymidine—Thymidine rescues the toxic effects of methotrexate and may also impair the antitumor activity.

DRUG INTERACTION 6

Folic acid supplements—These supplements may counteract the antitumor effects of methotrexate and should be discontinued while on therapy.

DRUG INTERACTION 7

Proton pump inhibitors—These agents may reduce the elimination of methotrexate, which can then result in increased serum methotrexate levels, leading to increased toxicity. This is an especially important issue for patients receiving high-dose methotrexate.

DRUG INTERACTION 8

L-Asparaginase—L-Asparaginase antagonizes the antitumor activity of methotrexate.

SPECIAL CONSIDERATIONS

1. Use with caution in patients with abnormal renal function. Dose should be reduced in proportion to the creatinine clearance. Important to obtain baseline creatinine clearance and to monitor renal status during therapy.

2. Instruct patients to stop folic acid supplements during therapy, as they may negate the antitumor effects of methotrexate.
3. Monitor CBCs on a weekly basis and more frequently with high-dose therapy.
4. Use with caution in patients with third-space fluid collections such as pleural effusion and ascites, as the half-life of methotrexate is prolonged, leading to enhanced clinical toxicity. Fluid collections should be drained before methotrexate therapy.
5. Use with caution in patients with bladder cancer status post-cystectomy and ileal conduit diversion, as they are at increased risk for delayed elimination of methotrexate and subsequent toxicity.
6. With high-dose therapy, methotrexate doses >1 g/m^2, important to vigorously hydrate the patient with 2.5–3.5 liters/m^2/day of IV 0.9% sodium chloride starting 12 hours before and for 24–48 hours after methotrexate infusion. Sodium bicarbonate (1–2 amps/L solution) should be included in the IV fluid to ensure that the urine pH is greater than 7.0 at the time of drug infusion and ideally for up to 48–72 hours after drug is given.
7. Methotrexate blood levels should be monitored in patients receiving high-dose therapy, patients with renal dysfunction (CrCl <60 mL/min) regardless of dose, and patients who have experienced increased toxicity with prior treatment with methotrexate.
8. With high-dose therapy, methotrexate blood levels should be monitored every 24 hours starting at 24 hours after methotrexate infusion. Rescue with leucovorin or L-leucovorin, the active isomer of leucovorin, should begin at 24 hours after drug infusion and should continue until the methotrexate drug level is <50 nM (5 × 10^{-8} M).
9. Glucarpidase is indicated for the treatment of significantly elevated plasma methotrexate concentrations (>1 mM) in patients with delayed drug clearance due to impaired renal function.
10. Patients should be instructed to lie on their side for at least 1 hour after intrathecal administration of methotrexate. This position will ensure adequate delivery of drug throughout the CSF.
11. Intrathecal administration of methotrexate may lead to myelosuppression and/or mucositis as therapeutic blood levels can be achieved.
12. Methotrexate overdose can be treated with leucovorin, L-leucovorin, and/or thymidine.
13. Instruct patients to avoid sun exposure for at least 1 month after therapy.
14. Caution patients about drinking carbonated beverages, as they can increase the acidity of urine, resulting in impaired drug elimination.
15. Pregnancy category D. Breastfeeding should be avoided.

TOXICITY 1

Myelosuppression is dose-limiting toxicity, with neutrophil nadir at days 4–7 and recovery usually by day 14.

TOXICITY 2
GI toxicity with mucositis can be dose-limiting. Typical onset is 3–7 days after methotrexate therapy and precedes the decrease in leukocyte and platelet count. Nausea and vomiting are dose-dependent.

TOXICITY 3
Acute renal failure, azotemia, urinary retention, and uric acid nephropathy. Renal toxicity results from the intratubular precipitation of methotrexate and its metabolites. Methotrexate, itself, may also exert a direct toxic effect on the renal tubules.

TOXICITY 4
Hepatotoxicity with transient elevation in serum transaminases and bilirubin may be observed with high-dose therapy. Usually occurs within the first 12–24 hours after start of infusion and returns to normal within 10 days.

TOXICITY 5
Pneumonitis characterized by fever, cough, and interstitial pulmonary infiltrates.

TOXICITY 6
Acute chemical arachnoiditis with headaches, nuchal rigidity, seizures, vomiting, fever, and an inflammatory cell infiltrate in the CSF observed immediately after intrathecal administration. Chronic, demyelinating encephalopathy observed in children months to years after intrathecal methotrexate and presents as dementia; limb spasticity; and, in advanced cases, coma.

TOXICITY 7
Acute cerebral dysfunction with paresis, aphasia, behavioral abnormalities, and seizures observed in 5%–15% of patients receiving high-dose methotrexate. Usually occurs within 6 days of treatment and resolves within 48–72 hours. A chronic form of neurotoxicity manifested as an encephalopathy with dementia and motor paresis can develop 2–4 months after treatment.

TOXICITY 8
Skin toxicity with erythematous skin rash, pruritus, urticaria, photosensitivity, and hyperpigmentation. Radiation-recall skin reaction is also observed.

TOXICITY 9
Menstrual irregularities, abortion, and fetal deaths in women. Reversible oligospermia with testicular failure reported in men with high-dose therapy.

Midostaurin

TRADE NAME	Rydapt	CLASSIFICATION	Signal transduction inhibitor, FLT3 inhibitor
CATEGORY	Targeted agent	DRUG MANUFACTURER	Novartis

MECHANISM OF ACTION

- Potent inhibitor of multiple receptor tyrosine kinases, including wild-type FLT3, FLT3 mutant kinases (ITD and TKD), KIT (wild-type and D816V mutant), PDGFR α/β, VEGFR-R2, and members of the serine/threonine protein kinase C (PKC) family.
- Inhibits FLT3 signaling and cell proliferation.
- Induces apoptosis in leukemic cells expressing ITD and TKD mutant FLT3 receptors or overexpressing FLT3 and PDGF receptors.
- Inhibits KIT signaling, cell proliferation, and histamine release and induces apoptosis in mast cells.

MECHANISM OF RESISTANCE

- Increased levels of FLT3 ligand (FL).
- Mutations in the FLT3 gene, leading to reduced binding affinity to drug.
- Increased expression of FLT3 receptor.
- Activation of signaling pathways downstream of FLT3 receptor, including STAT5 and MAPK pathways.
- Up-regulation of anti-apoptotic signals and down-regulation of pro-apoptotic pathways.
- Mutations in the c-Kit tyrosine kinase, resulting in altered binding affinity to the drug.

ABSORPTION

Rapidly absorbed with peak plasma drug levels reached in 1–3 hours in a fasting state.

DISTRIBUTION
Extensive binding (99.8%) of midostaurin and metabolites to plasma proteins, including albumin and α1-acid glycoprotein. Steady-state drug concentrations are reached in approximately 28 days.

METABOLISM
Metabolism in the liver primarily by CYP3A4 microsomal enzymes with formation of active metabolites CGP62221 and CGP52421. Elimination is mainly in feces (95%), predominantly as metabolites (91%) and only 4% of unchanged midostaurin. Approximately 5% of drug is eliminated in urine. The terminal half-life of the parent drug is 21 hours, while that of the CGP62221 metabolite is 32 hours and that of the CGP52421 metabolite is prolonged at 482 hours.

INDICATIONS
1. FDA-approved for AML that is FLT3 mutation-positive, as detected by an FDA-approved test, in combination with standard cytarabine and daunorubicin induction and cytarabine consolidation.
2. FDA-approved for aggressive systemic mastocytosis (ASM), systemic mastocytosis with associated hematologic neoplasm (SM-AHN), or mast cell leukemia (MCL).

DOSAGE RANGE
1. AML: 50 mg/day PO bid on days 8–21 of each cycle of cytarabine and daunorubicin induction therapy and on days 8–21 of each cycle of high-dose cytarabine consolidation therapy.
2. ASM, SM-AHN, MCL: 100 mg PO bid

DRUG INTERACTION 1
Phenytoin and other drugs that stimulate the liver microsomal CYP3A4 enzymes, including carbamazepine, rifampin, phenobarbital, and St. John's Wort—These drugs may increase the metabolism of midostaurin, resulting in its inactivation and lower effective drug levels.

DRUG INTERACTION 2
Drugs that inhibit the liver microsomal CYP3A4 enzymes, including ketoconazole, itraconazole, erythromycin, and clarithromycin—These drugs may decrease the metabolism of midostaurin, resulting in increased drug levels and potentially increased toxicity.

DRUG INTERACTION 3
Drugs that prolong the QT interval—Anti-arrhythmic drugs, including amiodarone, disopyramide, procainamide, quinidine and sotalol, and other drugs known to prolong the QT interval including, but not limited to, chloroquine, halofantrine, clarithromycin, haloperidol, methadone, moxifloxacin, bepridil, pimozide, and ondansetron.

SPECIAL CONSIDERATIONS

1. Patients should take midostaurin with food, twice daily at approximately 12-hour intervals. The drug capsules should not be opened or crushed.
2. Dose adjustment is not required in patients with mild or moderate hepatic impairment. Use with caution in patients with severe hepatic impairment, as the effect on midostaurin metabolism and elimination is not known.
3. Dose adjustment is not required in patients with mild or moderate renal impairment. Use with caution in patients with severe renal impairment, as the drug has not been studied in this setting.
4. Closely monitor for new signs or symptoms of pulmonary toxicity, and treatment should be stopped in this setting.
5. Monitor ECG with QT measurement at baseline and periodically during therapy, as QTc prolongation has been observed. Use with caution in patients at risk of developing QT prolongation, including hypokalemia, hypomagnesemia, congenital QT syndrome, and patients on anti-arrhythmic medications or any other agents that may prolong QT interval.
6. May cause fetal harm when given to a pregnant woman. Breastfeeding should be avoided and for at least 4 months after the completion of therapy.

TOXICITY 1
Myelosuppression with anemia, thrombocytopenia, and neutropenia.

TOXICITY 2
GI side effects with nausea, vomiting, abdominal pain, diarrhea, and constipation.

TOXICITY 3
Fatigue.

TOXICITY 4
Dyspnea, cough, interstitial lung disease, and pneumonitis.

TOXICITY 5
Hyperglycemia.

TOXICITY 6
Hepatotoxicity with elevation in serum transaminases, alkaline phosphatase, and serum bilirubin.

TOXICITY 7
Myalgias and arthralgias.

TOXICITY 8
Infections, with URI and UTI most common.

TOXICITY 9
QT prolongation.

Mirvetuximab soravtansine-gynx

TRADE NAME	Elahere	CLASSIFICATION	Antibody-drug conjugate, anti-FRα antibody
CATEGORY	Biologic response modifier agent, chemotherapy drug	DRUG MANUFACTURER	ImmunoGen

MECHANISM OF ACTION
- Antibody-drug conjugate made up of the chimeric IgG1 antibody directed against folate receptor alpha (FRα), conjugated to the maytansinoid microtubule inhibitor DM4.
- Upon binding to FRα, mirvetuximab soravtansine is rapidly internalized, and DM4 is then released inside the cell via proteolytic cleavage.
- FRα is a transmembrane glycoprotein that facilitates the unidirectional transport of folates into cells. It is expressed in about 80% of ovarian cancer and absent from normal ovarian epithelium.
- DM4 is a microtubule-disrupting agent that disrupts the microtubule network of actively dividing cells leading to cell cycle arrest and apoptosis.
- May also mediate antibody-dependent cellular phagocytosis and antibody-dependent cellular cytotoxicity.

MECHANISM OF RESISTANCE
None well characterized to date.

ABSORPTION
Administered only via the IV route.

DISTRIBUTION
Extensive binding (99%) of drug to plasma proteins. Steady-state drug levels are achieved within 24 days.

METABOLISM
The anti-FRα antibody is expected to undergo catabolism to small peptides and amino acids. DM4 undergoes metabolism by liver CYP3A4 enzymes. The elimination of mirvetuximab soravtansine has not been well characterized. The median terminal half-life is 5 days.

INDICATIONS
FDA-approved for patients with FRα, platinum-resistant epithelial ovarian, fallopian tube, or primary peritoneal cancer who have received 1-3 prior systemic therapies. Approved under accelerated approval based on tumor response rate and duration of response.

DOSAGE RANGE
Recommended dose is 6 mg/kg IV on day 1 of a 21-day schedule.

DRUG INTERACTION
None well characterized to date.

SPECIAL CONSIDERATIONS
1. Patients should undergo an eye exam that includes visual acuity and slit lamp exam at baseline, every other cycle for the first eight cycles, and as clinically indicated.
2. Topical corticosteroid eye drops should be administered in each eye six times daily starting the day prior to each infusion until day 4. Eye drops need to be continued in each eye four times daily for days 5–8 of each cycle.
3. Topical lubricating eye drops should be administered at least four times daily in each eye. Patients should be instructed to use lubricating eye drops and to wait until at least 10 min after ophthalmic topical steroid administration before instilling lubricating eye drops.
4. Patients should avoid wearing contact lenses for the entire duration of therapy.
5. Monitor patients for signs and symptoms of neurologic changes.
6. Monitor patients for new pulmonary symptoms, such as cough and dyspnea.
7. No dose adjustment for mild hepatic dysfunction. Should not be used in setting of moderate of severe hepatic dysfunction.
8. No dose adjustment for mild or moderate renal dysfunction. Has not been studied in setting of severe renal dysfunction or end-stage renal disease.
9. Can cause fetal harm when given to a pregnant woman. Females of reproductive potential should use effective contraception during treatment and for at least 7 months after the last dose. Breastfeeding should be avoided while on therapy and for 1 month after the last dose.

TOXICITY 1
Ocular toxicity with visual impairment, corneal disorders, keratopathy, dry eye, photophobia, eye pain, and uveitis. This is a black-box warning.

TOXICITY 2
Neurologic toxicity with peripheral neuropathy, paresthesia, motor neuropathy, neuralgia, and muscular weakness.

TOXICITY 3
Pneumonitis with cough, dyspnea, hypoxia, and interstitial infiltrates on imaging. Fatal interstitial lung disease (ILD) can occur rarely.

TOXICITY 5
Fatigue and anorexia.

TOXICITY 6
Mild nausea and vomiting

Mitomycin-C

$$H_2N-\overset{8}{\underset{6}{\overset{7}{\bigcirc}}}\quad CH_3\quad \overset{9}{\underset{5}{\bigcirc}}\quad \overset{10}{CH_2O-\overset{O}{\overset{\|}{C}}-NH_2}\quad OCH_3\quad \underset{3}{\overset{N}{\bigvee}}\underset{2}{\overset{1}{\bigtriangleup}}N-H$$

TRADE NAME	Mutamycin, Mitomycin	CLASSIFICATION	Antitumor antibiotic, alkylating agent
CATEGORY	Chemotherapy drug	DRUG MANUFACTURER	Bristol-Myers Squibb

MECHANISM OF ACTION
- Isolated from the broth of *Streptomyces caespitosus* species.
- Acts as an alkylating agent to cross-link DNA, resulting in inhibition of DNA synthesis and function.
- Inhibits transcription by targeting DNA-dependent RNA polymerase.
- Bioreductive activation by NADPH cytochrome P450 reductase, NADH cytochrome B450 reductase, and DT-diaphorase to oxygen free radical forms, semiquinone or hydroquinone species, which target DNA and inhibit DNA synthesis and function.
- Preferential activation of mitomycin-C in hypoxic tumor cells.

MECHANISM OF RESISTANCE

- Increased expression of the multidrug-resistant gene with elevated P170 protein levels. This leads to increased drug efflux and decreased intracellular drug accumulation. Cross-resistance to anthracyclines, vinca alkaloids, and other natural products.
- Decreased bioactivation through decreased expression of DT-diaphorase.
- Increased activity of DNA excision repair enzymes.
- Increased expression of glutathione and glutathione-dependent detoxifying enzymes.

ABSORPTION

Administered only via the IV route. There is a formulation for pylocalyceal use only where the drug is administered via ureteral catheter or nephrostomy tube.

DISTRIBUTION

Rapidly cleared from plasma after IV administration and widely distributed to tissues. Does not cross the blood-brain barrier.

METABOLISM

Metabolism in the liver with formation of both active and inactive metabolites. Mediated by the liver cytochrome P450 system and DT-diaphorase. Bioactivation can also occur in the spleen, kidney, and heart. Parent compound and its metabolites are excreted mainly through the hepatobiliary system into feces. Renal clearance accounts for only 8%–10% of drug elimination. Elimination half-life of about 50 minutes.

INDICATIONS

1. Gastric cancer.
2. Pancreatic cancer.
3. Breast cancer.
4. NSCLC.
5. Cervical cancer.
6. Head and neck cancer (in combination with radiation therapy).
7. Superficial bladder cancer.
8. Anal cancer.
9. FDA-approved for treatment of low-grade upper tract urothelial cancer (LG-UTUC).

DOSAGE RANGE

1. Gastric cancer: 10 mg/m^2 IV every 8 weeks, as part of the FAM regimen.
2. Breast cancer: Usual dose in various combination regimens is 10 mg/m^2 IV every 8 weeks.
3. Intravesicular therapy: Usual dose for intravesicular instillation is 40 mg administered in 20 mL of water.
4. Pyelocalyceal therapy: Usual dose is 4 mg/mL not to exceed 15 mL (60 mg of mitomycin) and instilled once weekly for 6 weeks. For patients with a complete response 3 months after initiation of therapy, instillations may be given once a month for a maximum of 11 additional months.

DRUG INTERACTIONS
None well characterized.

SPECIAL CONSIDERATIONS
1. Use with caution in patients with abnormal liver function. Dose reduction is recommended in the setting of liver dysfunction.
2. Because mitomycin-C is a potent vesicant, administer slowly over 30–60 minutes with a rapidly flowing IV. Administer drug carefully, usually through a central venous catheter. Careful monitoring is necessary to avoid extravasation. If extravasation is suspected, immediately stop infusion, withdraw fluid, elevate extremity, and apply ice to involved site. May administer topical DMSO. In severe cases, consult a plastic surgeon.
3. Monitor CBCs on a weekly basis. Mitomycin-C therapy results in delayed and cumulative myelosuppression. Risk of myelosuppression is increased when used in combination with other myelosuppressive agents.
4. Monitor patients for acute dyspnea and severe bronchospasm following drug administration. Bronchodilators, steroids, and/or oxygen may help to relieve symptoms. Risk of pulmonary toxicity increased with cumulative doses of mitomycin-C >50 mg/m^2.
5. FIO$_2$ concentrations in the perioperative period should be maintained below 50%, as patients receiving mitomycin-C concurrently with other anticancer agents are at increased risk for developing ARDS. Careful attention to fluid status is important.
6. Monitor for signs of hemolytic-uremic syndrome (anemia with fragmented cells on peripheral blood smear, thrombocytopenia, and renal dysfunction), especially when total cumulative doses of mitomycin-C are >50 mg/m^2.
7. Pregnancy category D. Breastfeeding should be avoided.

TOXICITY 1
Myelosuppression is dose-limiting, and cumulative toxicity with leukopenia is more common than thrombocytopenia. Nadir counts are delayed at about 4–6 weeks.

TOXICITY 2
Nausea and vomiting. Usually mild and occur within 1–2 hours of treatment, lasting for up to 3 days.

TOXICITY 3
GI toxicity with mucositis is common but not dose-limiting. Observed within the first week of treatment.

TOXICITY 4
Potent vesicant. Extravasation can lead to tissue necrosis and chemical thrombophlebitis at the site of injection.

TOXICITY 5
Anorexia and fatigue are common.

TOXICITY 6
Hemolytic-uremic syndrome. Consists of microangiopathic hemolytic anemia (hematocrit <25%), thrombocytopenia (<100,000/mm^3), and renal failure (serum creatinine >1.6 mg/dL). Other complications include pulmonary edema, neurologic abnormalities, and hypertension. Rare event seen in <2% of patients treated. May occur at any time during treatment but usually when cumulative doses >50 mg/m^2. In rare cases, syndrome can be fatal.

TOXICITY 7
Interstitial pneumonitis. Presents with dyspnea, non-productive cough, and interstitial infiltrates on chest X-ray. Occurs more frequently with total cumulative doses >50 mg/m^2.

TOXICITY 8
Hepatic veno-occlusive disease. Presents with abdominal pain, hepatomegaly, and liver failure. Occurs only with high-dose therapy in transplant setting.

TOXICITY 9
Chemical cystitis and bladder contraction. Observed only in the setting of pyelocalyceal therapy.

TOXICITY 10
Ureteric obstruction is observed only in the setting of pyelocalyceal instillation.

Mitotane

TRADE NAME	Lysodren	CLASSIFICATION	Adrenolytic agent
CATEGORY	Chemotherapy drug	DRUG MANUFACTURER	Bristol-Myers Squibb

MECHANISM OF ACTION
- Dichloro derivative of the insecticide DDD.
- Direct toxic effect on mitochondria of adrenal cortical cells, resulting in inhibition of adrenal steroid production.
- Alters the peripheral metabolism of steroids, resulting in decreased levels of 17-OH corticosteroid.

ABSORPTION
About 35%–45% of an oral dose is absorbed. Peak plasma levels are achieved in 3–5 hours.

DISTRIBUTION
Widely distributed to tissues. Highly fat-soluble, with large amounts of drug distributed in adipose tissues. Mitotane is slowly released, with drug levels being detectable for up to 10 weeks. Does not cross the blood-brain barrier.

METABOLISM
Metabolism in the liver with formation of both active and inactive metabolites. Parent compound and its metabolites are excreted mainly through the hepatobiliary system into feces (60%). Renal clearance accounts for only 10%–25% of drug elimination. Variable elimination half-life of up to 160 hours due to storage of drug in adipose tissue.

INDICATIONS
Adrenocortical cancer.

DOSAGE RANGE
Usual dose is 2–10 g/day PO in three or four divided doses.

DRUG INTERACTION 1
Warfarin—Mitotane alters the metabolism of warfarin, leading to an increased requirement for warfarin. Coagulation parameters, including PT and INR, should be monitored closely, and dose adjustments made accordingly.

DRUG INTERACTION 2
Barbiturates, phenytoin, cyclophosphamide—Mitotane alters the metabolism of various drugs that are metabolized by the liver microsomal P450 system, including barbiturates, phenytoin, and cyclophosphamide.

DRUG INTERACTION 3
Steroids—Mitotane interferes with steroid metabolism. If steroid replacement is required, doses higher than those for physiologic replacement may be needed.

SPECIAL CONSIDERATIONS
1. Use with caution in patients with abnormal liver function. Dose reduction is required in the setting of liver dysfunction.
2. Adrenal insufficiency may develop, and adrenal steroid replacement with glucocorticoid and/or mineralocorticoid therapy is indicated.
3. Stress-dose IV steroids are required in the event of infection, stress, trauma, and/or shock.
4. Patients should be cautioned about driving, operating complicated machinery, and/or other activities that require increased mental alertness, as mitotane causes lethargy and somnolence.

5. Concurrent use of mitotane and warfarin requires careful monitoring of coagulation parameters, including PT and INR, as mitotane can alter warfarin metabolism.
6. Pregnancy category C. Breastfeeding should be avoided.

TOXICITY 1
Mild nausea and vomiting occur in 80% of patients and is dose-limiting.

TOXICITY 2
Lethargy, somnolence, vertigo, and dizziness. CNS side effects observed in 40% of patients.

TOXICITY 3
Mucositis is common but not dose-limiting. Observed within the first week of treatment.

TOXICITY 4
Transient skin rash and hyperpigmentation.

TOXICITY 5
Adrenal insufficiency. Rarely occurs with steroid replacement therapy.

Mitoxantrone

TRADE NAME	Novantrone	CLASSIFICATION	Anthracycline
CATEGORY	Chemotherapy drug	DRUG MANUFACTURER	OSI

MECHANISM OF ACTION
- Synthetic planar anthracenedione analog.
- Inhibits topoisomerase II by forming a cleavable complex with topoisomerase II and DNA.
- Intercalates into DNA, resulting in inhibition of DNA synthesis and function.

MECHANISM OF RESISTANCE

- Increased expression of the multidrug-resistant gene with enhanced drug efflux, resulting in decreased intracellular drug accumulation.
- Decreased expression of topoisomerase II.
- Mutations in topoisomerase II with decreased binding affinity to drug.
- Increased expression of sulfhydryl proteins, including glutathione and glutathione-associated enzymes.

ABSORPTION

Administered only via the IV route.

DISTRIBUTION

Rapid and extensive distribution to formed blood elements and to body tissues. Distributes in high concentrations in liver, bone marrow, heart, lung, and kidney. Does not cross the blood-brain barrier. Extensively bound (about 80%) to plasma proteins. Peak plasma levels are achieved immediately after IV injection.

METABOLISM

Metabolism by the liver microsomal P450 system. Elimination is mainly through the hepatobiliary route, with 25% of the drug excreted in feces. Renal clearance accounts for only 6%–10% of drug elimination, mainly as unchanged drug. The elimination half-life ranges from 23 to 215 hours, with a median of 75 hours.

INDICATIONS

1. Advanced, hormone-refractory prostate cancer—Used in combination with prednisone as initial chemotherapy.
2. Acute myelogenous leukemia.
3. Breast cancer.
4. Non-Hodgkin's lymphoma.

DOSAGE RANGE

1. Acute myelogenous leukemia, induction therapy: 12 mg/m^2 IV on days 1–3, given in combination with ara-C, 100 mg/m^2/day IV continuous infusion for 5–7 days.
2. Prostate cancer: 12 mg/m^2 IV on day 1 every 21 days, given in combination with prednisone 5 mg PO bid.
3. Non-Hodgkin's lymphoma: 10 mg/m^2 IV on day 1 every 21 days, given as part of the CNOP or FND regimens.

DRUG INTERACTIONS

Heparin—Mitoxantrone is incompatible with heparin, as a precipitate will form.

SPECIAL CONSIDERATIONS

1. Use with caution in patients with abnormal liver function. Dose modification should be considered in patients with liver dysfunction.
2. Carefully monitor the IV injection site, as mitoxantrone is a potent vesicant. Skin may turn blue at site of injection. Avoid extravasation, but ulceration and tissue injury are rare when drug is properly diluted.

3. Alkalinization of the urine, allopurinol, and vigorous IV hydration are recommended to prevent tumor lysis syndrome in patients with acute myelogenous leukemia.

4. Monitor cardiac function prior to (baseline) and periodically during therapy with either MUGA radionuclide scan or echocardiogram to assess LVEF. Risk of cardiac toxicity is higher in elderly patients >70 years of age, in patients with prior history of hypertension or pre-existing heart disease, in patients previously treated with anthracyclines, or in patients with prior radiation therapy to the chest. Cumulative doses of 140 mg/m^2 in patients with no prior history of anthracycline therapy and 120 mg/m^2 in patients with prior anthracycline therapy are associated with increased risk for cardiac toxicity. A decrease in LVEF by 15%–20% is an indication to discontinue treatment.

5. Monitor CBCs while on therapy.

6. Patients may experience blue-green urine for up to 24 hours after drug administration.

7. Pregnancy category D. Breastfeeding should be avoided.

TOXICITY 1

Myelosuppression is dose-limiting, with neutropenia more common than thrombocytopenia. Nadir typically occurs at 10–14 days after treatment but may occur earlier in acute leukemia, with recovery of counts by day 21. Risk of myelosuppression is greater in elderly patients and in those previously treated with chemotherapy and/or radiation therapy.

TOXICITY 2

Nausea and vomiting are observed in 70% of patients. Usually mild, and occurs less frequently than with doxorubicin.

TOXICITY 3

GI toxicity with mucositis and diarrhea.

TOXICITY 4

Cardiac toxicity. Cardiac effects are similar to but less severe than those of doxorubicin. Acute toxicity presents as atrial arrhythmias, chest pain, and myopericarditis syndrome that typically occurs within the first 24–48 hours of drug administration. Transient and mostly asymptomatic.

Chronic toxicity is manifested in the form of a dilated cardiomyopathy with congestive heart failure. Cumulative doses of 140 mg/m^2 in patients with no prior history of anthracycline therapy and 120 mg/m^2 in patients with prior anthracycline therapy are associated with increased risk for developing congestive cardiomyopathy.

TOXICITY 5

Alopecia observed in 40% of patients but less severe than with doxorubicin.

TOXICITY 6
Hepatotoxicity with transient and reversible effects on liver enzymes, including SGOT and SGPT.

TOXICITY 7
Blue discoloration of fingernails, sclera, and urine for 1–2 days after treatment.

TOXICITY 8
Secondary AML.

Mobocertinib

TRADE NAME	Exkivity	CLASSIFICATION	Signal transduction inhibitor, EGFR-TKI
CATEGORY	Targeted agent	DRUG MANUFACTURER	Takeda

MECHANISM OF ACTION
- First-in-class oral irreversible inhibitor of EGFR exon 20 insertion mutation.
- Inhibition of the EGFR signaling pathway results in inhibition of critical mitogenic and anti-apoptotic signals involved in proliferation, growth, invasion/metastasis, and angiogenesis.

MECHANISM OF RESISTANCE
None well characterized to date.

ABSORPTION
Peak drug levels are achieved in 4 hours. Oral bioavailability is on the order of 37%. Food does not appear to alter oral absorption. Can be taken with or without food.

DISTRIBUTION
Extensive binding to plasma proteins.

METABOLISM

Metabolism in the liver mainly by CYP3A4 enzymes with formation of two active metabolites AP32960 and AP32914. The two active metabolites are equipotent to the parent compound and account for 36% and 4%, respectively, of the combined molar AUC. Half-life is on the order of 18 hours.

INDICATIONS

FDA-approved for the treatment of locally advanced or metastatic NSCLC with EGFR exon 20 insertion mutations whose disease has progressed on or after platinum-based chemotherapy This indication is approved under accelerated approval based on overall response rate and duration of response.

DOSAGE RANGE

Recommended dose is 160 mg PO once daily.

DRUG INTERACTION 1

Phenytoin and other drugs that stimulate the liver microsomal CYP3A4 enzymes, including carbamazepine, rifampin, phenobarbital, and St. John's Wort—These drugs may increase the metabolism of mobocertinib, resulting in its inactivation and potentially reduced clinical activity.

DRUG INTERACTION 2

Drugs that inhibit the liver microsomal CYP3A4 enzymes, including ketoconazole, itraconazole, erythromycin, and clarithromycin—These drugs may decrease the metabolism of mobocertinib, resulting in increased drug levels and potentially increased toxicity.

DRUG INTERACTION 3

Avoid the use of drugs known to prolong the QTc interval as co-administration with mobocertinib may increase the risk of QTc prolongation.

SPECIAL CONSIDERATIONS

1. Dose reduction is not recommended in patients with mild or moderate hepatic dysfunction. Has not been studied in patients with severe hepatic dysfunction, and caution should be used in this setting.
2. Dose reduction is not recommended in patients with mild or moderate renal dysfunction. Has not been studied in patients with severe renal dysfunction, and caution should be used in this setting.
3. Monitor patients for new or progressive pulmonary symptoms, including cough, dyspnea, and fever. Drug therapy should be interrupted pending further diagnostic evaluation.
4. Baseline and periodic evaluations of ECG and electrolyte status should be performed while on therapy. If the QTc >500 msec, therapy should be interrupted. Use with caution in patients at risk of developing QT prolongation, including hypokalemia, hypomagnesemia, congenital long QT syndrome, and in patients taking antiarrhythmic medications or any other drugs that may cause QT prolongation.

5. Baseline and periodic evaluations of LVEF should be performed while on therapy. If grade 2 decreased LVEF, the drug should be withheld until <grade 1 or baseline. If recovered to baseline within 2 weeks, can resume drug therapy at the same dose. If not recovered to baseline within 2 weeks, the drug should be permanently discontinued. If >grade 2 CHF or grade ¾ decreased LVEF, the drug should be permanently discontinued.
6. Monitor for diarrhea. Patients should be advised to start an anti-diarrheal agent at the first sign of diarrhea or increased stool frequency and to also increase fluid and electrolyte oral intake.
7. Avoid Seville oranges, starfruit, pomelos, grapefruit, and grapefruit juice while on mobocertinib therapy.
8. Advise females of potential of increased risk to a fetus and to use effective contraception during treatment and for one month after the last dose of drug.

TOXICITY 1
Diarrhea is most common GI toxicity. Mild nausea/vomiting, mucositis, and constipation are also observed.

TOXICITY 2
Pulmonary toxicity in the form of ILD manifested by increased cough, dyspnea, fever, and pulmonary infiltrates.

TOXICITY 3
QTc prolongation.

TOXICITY 4
Fatigue, anorexia, and reduced appetite.

TOXICITY 5
Cardiomyopathy and CHF. Atrial fibrillation, atrial dysrhythmias, and ventricular arrhythmias have been observed.

TOXICITY 6
Skin toxicity in the form of rash, dry skin, pruritus, and nail bed changes.

Mogamulizumab-kpkc

TRADE NAME	Poteligeo	**CLASSIFICATION**	Chemokine receptor antibody
CATEGORY	Biologic response modifier agent, immunotherapy	**DRUG MANUFACTURER**	Kyowa Kirin

MECHANISM OF ACTION

- Mogamulizumab-kcpc is a defucosylated, humanized IgG1 κ monoclonal antibody that binds to CCR4, which is a G protein-coupled receptor for CC chemokines involved in the trafficking of lymphocytes to various organs.
- CCR4 is expressed on the surface of T-cell malignancies, such as cutaneous T-cell lymphoma (CTCL), and is also expressed on regulatory T cells (Tregs) and a subset of Th2 T cells.

MECHANISM OF RESISTANCE

None well characterized to date.

ABSORPTION

Administered only via the IV route.

DISTRIBUTION

Steady-state drug levels are achieved after 12 weeks of therapy.

METABOLISM

Metabolism of this drug is not well characterized. Most likely undergoes proteolytic degradation, as with other antibodies, into small peptides and amino acids via catalytic pathways. The median terminal half-life is on the order of 17 days.

INDICATIONS

FDA-approved for adults with relapsed or refractory mycosis fungoides (CTCL) or Sezary syndrome after at least one prior systemic therapy.

DOSAGE RANGE

Recommended dose is 1 mg/kg IV on days 1, 8, 15, and 22 of the first 28-day cycle and on days 1 and 15 of each subsequent cycle.

DRUG INTERACTIONS

None well characterized to date.

SPECIAL CONSIDERATIONS

1. Monitor for infusion-related reactions, and interrupt the infusion for any grade reaction and treat accordingly. If an infusion reaction occurs, acetaminophen and an antihistamine should be administered for all subsequent infusions.
2. Monitor for skin rash throughout the entire treatment. May need to perform skin biopsy to differentiate between drug eruption and disease progression.
3. Patients should be warned of the increased risk for infections.
4. Patients who receive allogeneic HSCT after mogamulizumab treatment have an increased risk of transplant complications, including acute GVHD, steroid-refractory GVHD, and transplant-related death.

5. Can cause fetal harm when given to a pregnant woman. Females of reproductive potential should use effective contraception during treatment and for at least 30 days after the last dose. Breastfeeding should be avoided.

TOXICITY 1
Skin toxicity with maculopapular rash, lichenoid dermatitis, scaly plaques, pustular eruption, folliculitis, non-specific dermatitis, and psoriasiform dermatitis.

TOXICITY 2
Infusion-related reactions.

TOXICITY 3
Infections with URIs and skin infections.

TOXICITY 4
Musculoskeletal pain.

TOXICITY 5
Autoimmune complications with myositis, myocarditis, hepatitis, pneumonitis, Guillain-Barré syndrome, and hypothyroidism.

TOXICITY 6
Transplant complications with acute GVHD, steroid-refractory GVHD, and even transplant-related death.

Mosunetuzumab

TRADE NAME	Lunsumio, JNJ-64007957	CLASSIFICATION	BiTE antibody, anti-CD20 monoclonal antibody
CATEGORY	Biologic response modifier agent, immunotherapy	DRUG MANUFACTURER	Genentech

MECHANISM OF ACTION
- Bispecific T-cell engaging (BiTE) humanized IgG1 antibody that binds to CD20 antigen expressed on malignant B cells and CD3 expressed on surface of T cells.
- This bispecific binding causes cytotoxic T cells to be physically linked to malignant CD20-positive lymphoma cells and triggers the signaling

cascade, leading to upregulation of cell adhesion molecules, production of cytolytic proteins, release of inflammatory cytokines, and proliferation of T cells, ultimately resulting in lysis of CD20-positive malignant B cells.

- CD20 is expressed on more than 90% of all B-cell non-Hodgkin's lymphomas and leukemias.
- CD20 is not expressed on early pre–B cells, plasma cells, normal bone marrow stem cells, antigen-presenting dendritic reticulum cells, or other normal tissues.
- Mechanism of action differs from classic anti-CD20 monoclonal antibodies that induce direct cell death by inhibition of CD20 intracellular signaling and by antibody-dependent cellular cytotoxicity and complement-mediated cellular cytotoxicity.

ABSORPTION
Administered via the IV and SC routes. Mean bioavailability is approximately 70% when administered SC. Time to reach maximal concentrations occurs at days 3–8 after SC injection. Peak drug levels are achieved at the end of the IV infusion in cycle 2.

DISTRIBUTION
Following SC administration, steady-state levels are reached after 12 weekly treatments.

METABOLISM
Metabolism has not been well characterized. As with other antibodies, it is assumed that mosunetuzumab is degraded to small peptides and amino acids via catabolic pathways. The terminal half-life is approximately 16 days.

INDICATIONS
FDA-approved for the treatment of adult patients with relapsed or refractory follicular lymphoma after 2 or more lines of therapy. Approved under accelerated approval based on response rate.

DOSAGE RANGE
1. Administered only as IV infusion
2. Cycle 1, Day 1 – 2 mg; Cycle 1, Day 8 – 2 mg; Cycle 1, Day 15 – 60 mg. For cycle 1, drug should be infused over a minimum of 4 hours.
3. Cycle 2, Day 1 – 60 mg. For cycle 2 and beyond, drug should be infused over 2 hours if infusion from Cycle 1 were well tolerated.
4. Cycle 3 and thereafter – 30 mg.

DRUG INTERACTION
Mosunetuzumab treatment results in release of cytokines that may suppress the activity of CYP3A4 enzymes. This may then lead to increased exposure of drugs that are CYP3A4 substrates.

SPECIAL CONSIDERATIONS

1. Patients should be premedicated one to three hours prior to each step-up dose and first treatment dose to reduce the risk of CRS with 16 mg dexamethasone (oral or IV), H1 receptor antagonist (oral or IV diphenhydramine), and an antipyretic (oral or IV acetaminophen).
2. Monitor for infusion-related events. These events may be clinically indistinguishable from the signs and symptoms of cytokine release syndrome (CRS), with life-threatening or fatal consequences.
3. Monitor for CRS, which occurs most frequently with the first two cycles of therapy. This is a black-box warning.
4. Monitor for neurologic toxicity, presenting as encephalopathy, convulsions, speech disorders, disturbances in consciousness, confusion and disorientation, and coordination and balance disorders.
5. Monitor for signs and symptoms of infection.
6. Monitor CBCs while on therapy.
7. Monitor LFTs and serum bilirubin while on therapy.
8. Dose reduction is not required in patients with mild hepatic dysfunction. Has not been studied in setting of moderate or severe hepatic dysfunction.
9. Dose reduction is not required in patients with mild or moderate renal dysfunction. Has not been studied in setting of severe renal dysfunction or end-stage renal disease.
10. Monitor for signs and symptoms of tumor flare, especially in patents with bulky tumors or in those whose disease is located close to airways or other vital organs.
11. May cause fetal harm. Women should be advised to use effective contraception during treatment and for 3 months after the last dose of treatment. Breastfeeding should be avoided while on therapy and for 3 months after the last dose.

TOXICITY 1
Infusion-related symptoms.

TOXICITY 2
Cytokine release syndrome (CRS) with fever, chills, hypotension, tachycardia, hypoxia, and headache.

TOXICITY 3
Myelosuppression with neutropenia, anemia, and thrombocytopenia.

TOXICITY 4
Neurological toxicities with headache, motor dysfunction, sensory neuropathy, and encephalopathy. ICANS can present with confusional state and dysgraphia.

TOXICITY 5
Hepatotoxicity.

TOXICITY 6
Increased risk of viral, bacterial, fungal, and opportunistic infections. Can cause severe or fatal infections.

TOXICITY 7
Hypophosphatemia.

TOXICITY 8
Tumor flare.

TOXICITY 9
Tumor lysis syndrome.

Moxetumomab pasudotox

TRADE NAME	Lumoxiti	**CLASSIFICATION**	Anti-CD22 immunotoxin
CATEGORY	Biologic response modifier agent	**DRUG MANUFACTURER**	AstraZeneca

MECHANISM OF ACTION
- CD22-directed immunotoxin that is made up of the Fv fragment of a recombinant murine anti-CD22 monoclonal antibody fused to a 38 kDa fragment of Pseudomonas exotoxin A (PE38).
- The Fv portion of moxetumomab pasudotox binds to CD22 on the cell surface of B cells, and the PE38 Pseudomonas exotoxin is then internalized. The process of internalization leads to PE38 catalyzing the ADP-ribosylation of the dipthamide residue in elongation factor 2, which then leads to inhibition of protein synthesis of the anti-apoptotic protein myeloid cell leukemia (Mcl-1) and eventual apoptotic cell death.
- CD22 is expressed in >90% of patients with B-cell ALL and in most B-cell cancers but not expressed on other normal tissues, including hematopoietic stem cells.

MECHANISM OF RESISTANCE
None well characterized to date.

ABSORPTION
Administered only via the IV route.

DISTRIBUTION

Mean volume of distribution is estimated to be 6.5 L. High exposure to moxetumomab pasudotox is significantly associated with low baseline CD19+ B-cell levels.

METABOLISM

Metabolism is not well characterized. It is presumed that moxetumomab pasudotox undergoes proteolytic degradation into small peptides and amino acids via catalytic pathways. The median terminal half-life is on the order of 1.4 days.

INDICATIONS

FDA-approved for adults with relapsed or refractory hairy cell leukemia who received at least 2 prior systemic therapies, including a purine nucleoside analog.

DOSAGE RANGE

Recommended dose is 0.04 mg/kg IV on days 1, 3, and 5 of a 28-day cycle.

DRUG INTERACTIONS

None well characterized to date.

SPECIAL CONSIDERATIONS

1. Monitor for infusion-related reactions. Patients should be premedicated with acetaminophen, antihistamine, and H2-receptor antagonist prior to all infusions. Patients should be monitored during and for at least 1 hour after the completion of the infusion. Patients may need to take oral antihistamines and acetaminophen and even oral steroids for up to 24 hours after drug infusion.
2. Monitor for evidence of capillary leak syndrome (CLS). This is a black-box warning.
3. Monitor for evidence of hemolytic-uremic syndrome (HUS). This is a black-box warning.
4. Patients should be advised to have adequate oral hydration with up to 3 liters of oral fluid per 24 hours on days 1–8 of each 28-day cycle.
5. Consider low-dose aspirin on days 1–8 of each 28-day cycle as thromboprophylaxis to reduce the risk of thrombosis.
6. Dose reduction is not required for patients with mild, moderate, or severe hepatic dysfunction.
7. Dose reduction is not required for patients with mild or moderate renal dysfunction. Has not been studied in patients with severe renal dysfunction, end-stage renal disease, and in setting of hemodialysis, and caution should be used in these patients.

8. Approximately 75% of patient will have detectable neutralizing antibodies at the end of treatment, regardless of response status. Patients who achieve complete or partial response usually have anti-drug antibody titers <10,000.
9. Can cause fetal harm when given to a pregnant woman. Females of reproductive potential should use effective contraception during treatment and for at least 30 days after the last dose. Breastfeeding should be avoided.

TOXICITY 1
Peripheral edema.

TOXICITY 2
Infusion-related reactions.

TOXICITY 3
Fatigue, headache, and pyrexia.

TOXICITY 4
Nausea/vomiting.

TOXICITY 5
Capillary leak syndrome.

TOXICITY 6
Hemolytic-uremic syndrome.

TOXICITY 7
Renal toxicity with elevated serum creatinine.

TOXICITY 8
Hypocalcemia.

Nadofaragene firadenovec-vcng

TRADE NAME	Adstiladrin	**CLASSIFICATION**	Gene therapy
CATEGORY	Biologic response modifier agent, immunotherapy	**DRUG MANUFACTURER**	Ferring

MECHANISM OF ACTION
- Non-replicating adenoviral vector-based gene therapy designed to deliver a copy of a gene encoding human interferon-α2b (IFNα2b) to the bladder urothelium.
- Intravesical instillation results in cell transduction and transient local expression of IFNα2b in the bladder urothelium.

MECHANISM OF RESISTANCE
None well characterized to date.

ABSORPTION
Administered only via the intravesical route.

DISTRIBUTION
Confined to the bladder urothelium. Detectable levels of vector DNA at day 12 after intravesical administration. Measurable levels of IFNα2b in urine at day 12 post-dose.

METABOLISM
Expected to be metabolized by nucleases throughout the body.

INDICATIONS
FDA-approved for treatment of adult patients with high-risk BCG-unresponsive non-muscle invasive bladder cancer with carcinoma in situ with or without papillary tumors.

DOSAGE RANGE
Recommended dose is 75 mL at a concentration of 3×10^{11} viral particles (vp)/mL once every 3 months.

DRUG INTERACTION
None well characterized.

SPECIAL CONSIDERATIONS
1. Contraindicated in patient with prior hypersensitivity to interferon-α or to any component of the product.
2. Patient's bladder must be completely emptied prior to instillation.

3. After intravesical instillation, nadofaragene firadenovec should be retained in the bladder for 1 hour.
4. Voided urine should be disinfected for 30 min with a virucidal agent before flushing of the toilet.
5. Immunocompromised patients may be at increased risk for disseminated adenovirus infection.
6. Individuals who are immunosuppressed should not come into contact with nadofaragene firadenovec.
7. Females of reproductive potential should use effective contraception during treatment with nadofaragene firadenovec and for 6 months following the last dose. Male patients with female partners of reproductive potential should use effective contraception during treatment with nadofaragene firadenovec and for 3 months following the last dose.

TOXICITY 1
Instillation site discharge.

TOXICITY 2
Bladder spasm, micturition urgency, hematuria, and dysuria.

TOXICITY 3
Fever and chills.

TOXICITY 4
Fatigue.

Necitumumab

TRADE NAME	Portrazza, IMC-11F8	CLASSIFICATION	Anti-EGFR monoclonal antibody
CATEGORY	Targeted agent	DRUG MANUFACTURER	Eli Lilly

MECHANISM OF ACTION
- Recombinant fully human IgG1 monoclonal antibody directed against the epidermal growth factor receptor (EGFR). EGFR is overexpressed in a broad range of human solid tumors, including colorectal cancer, head and neck cancer, NSCLC, pancreatic cancer, and breast cancer.

- Binds with higher affinity to EGFR than normal ligands EGF and TGF-α, which then results in inhibition of EGFR. Prevents both homodimerization and heterodimerization of the EGFR, leading to inhibition of autophosphorylation and inhibition of EGFR signaling.
- Inhibition of the EGFR signaling pathway results in inhibition of critical mitogenic and antiapoptotic signals involved in proliferation, growth, invasion/metastasis, and angiogenesis.
- Inhibition of the EGFR pathway enhances the response to chemotherapy and/or radiation therapy.
- Immunologic mechanisms may also be involved in antitumor activity, and they include recruitment of ADCC and/or complement-mediated cell lysis.

MECHANISM OF RESISTANCE

- Mutations in EGFR, leading to decreased binding affinity to necitumumab.
- Decreased expression of EGFR.
- Increased expression of TGF-α ligand.
- Presence of KRAS mutations.
- Presence of BRAF mutations.
- Presence of NRAS mutations.
- Increased expression of HER2 through gene amplification.
- Increased HER3 expression.
- Activation/induction of alternative cellular signaling pathways, such as PI3K/Akt and IGF-1R.

ABSORPTION

Administered only via the IV route.

DISTRIBUTION

Distribution in the body is not well characterized. Time to reach steady state is 100 days.

METABOLISM

Metabolism of necitumumab has not been extensively characterized. Half-life is on the order of 14 days.

INDICATIONS

FDA-approved in combination with gemcitabine and cisplatin for first-line treatment of metastatic squamous NSCLC. Necitumumab is **NOT** recommended for the treatment of non-squamous NSCLC.

DOSAGE RANGE

Recommended dose is 800 mg IV on days 1 and 8 on an every-21-day cycle.

DRUG INTERACTIONS

None well characterized to date.

SPECIAL CONSIDERATIONS

1. Level of EGFR expression does not accurately predict for necitumumab clinical activity. As such, EGFR testing should not be required for the clinical use of necitumumab.

2. Electrolyte status should be closely monitored prior to each infusion, especially serum magnesium, as hypomagnesemia has been observed with necitumumab treatment. This represents a black-box warning. Electrolyte status should continue to be monitored for at least 8 weeks following completion of therapy.

3. Increased risk of cardiopulmonary arrest or sudden death in patients treated with necitumumab plus gemcitabine and cisplatin. This represents a black-box warning. Caution should be used in patients with significant coronary artery disease, MI within the previous 6 months, history of CHF, and/or arrhythmias.

4. In patients who develop a skin rash, topical antibiotics such as clindamycin gel or erythromycin cream or either oral clindamycin, oral doxycycline, or oral minocycline may help. Patients should be warned to avoid sunlight exposure.

5. Most infusion reactions occur with the first or second infusion. For patients who have experienced a prior grades 1 or 2 infusion reaction, patients should be premedicated with diphenhydramine prior to all subsequent infusions. For patients who have experienced a second-grade 1 or 2 infusion reaction, a more aggressive premedication regimen is required with diphenhydramine, acetaminophen, and dexamethasone prior to each infusion.

6. Necitumumab should **NOT** be used in the setting of non-squamous NSCLC, as it is associated with increased toxicity and increased mortality.

7. Can cause fetal harm. Advise females of reproductive potential to use effective contraception during treatment and for 3 months after the last dose. Breastfeeding should be avoided while on therapy and for 3 months after the last dose.

TOXICITY 1

Infusion-related symptoms with fever, chills, urticaria, flushing, fatigue, headache, bronchospasm, dyspnea, angioedema, and hypotension. Usually mild to moderate in severity and observed most commonly after the first or second infusion.

TOXICITY 2

Skin toxicity with pruritus, dry skin, and a pustular, acneiform skin rash. Presents mainly on the face, neck region, and upper trunk. Improves with continued treatment and resolves upon cessation of therapy. Nailbed changes may also be observed with prolonged use.

TOXICITY 3

Cardiopulmonary arrest and/or sudden death. Occurs in about 3% of patients.

TOXICITY 4
Hypomagnesemia occurs in approximately 80% of patients, with severe cases observed in 20% of patients.

TOXICITY 5
Increased risk of venous and arterial thromboembolic events.

Nelarabine

TRADE NAME	Arranon, 2-amino-9-β-D-arabinofuranosyl-6-methoxy-9H-purine	CLASSIFICATION	Antimetabolite, Deoxyguanosine analog
CATEGORY	Chemotherapy drug	DRUG MANUFACTURER	GlaxoSmithKline

MECHANISM OF ACTION
- Prodrug of the deoxyguanosine analog 9-β-D-arabinofuranosylguanosine (ara-G).
- Ara-G is transported into the cell via a nucleoside transport protein.
- Cell cycle–specific with activity in the S-phase.
- Requires intracellular activation to the triphosphate nucleotide metabolite ara-GTP.
- Incorporation of ara-GTP into DNA, resulting in chain termination and inhibition of DNA synthesis and function.

MECHANISM OF RESISTANCE
- Decreased activation of drug through decreased expression and/or activity of the anabolic enzyme deoxycytidine kinase.
- Decreased nucleoside transport of drug into cells.

ABSORPTION
Administered only via the IV route, as the drug has poor oral bioavailability.

DISTRIBUTION

Extensively distributed in the body. Binding to plasma proteins has not been well characterized.

METABOLISM

Undergoes metabolism by adenosine deaminase to form ara-G, which is subsequently phosphorylated to the active ara-GTP form. A minor route of nelarabine metabolism is via hydrolysis to form methylguanine, which is then demethylated to form guanine. Nelarabine and ara-G are rapidly eliminated from plasma, with a half-life in adults of approximately 30 minutes and 3 hours, respectively. Nelarabine (5%–10%) and ara-G (20%–30%) are eliminated, to a minor extent, by the kidneys. The mean clearance of nelarabine is approximately 30% higher in pediatric patients than adult patients, while the clearance of ara-G is similar in the two patient populations. Age and gender have no effects on nelarabine or ara-G pharmacokinetics.

INDICATIONS

1. FDA-approved for T-cell acute lymphoblastic leukemia (T-ALL) that has not responded to or has relapsed following treatment with at least two chemotherapy regimens.
2. FDA-approved for T-cell lymphoblastic lymphoma (T-LBL) that has not responded to or has relapsed following treatment with at least two chemotherapy regimens.

DOSAGE RANGE

1. Pediatric patients: 650 mg/m^2/day IV over 1 hour on days 1–5 every 21 days.
2. Adult patients: 1,500 mg/m^2/day IV over 2 hours on days 1, 3, and 5 every 28 days.

DRUG INTERACTIONS

None well characterized to date.

SPECIAL CONSIDERATIONS

1. Monitor CBCs on a regular basis during therapy.
2. Monitor for neurologic events, as this represents a black-box warning.
3. Patients treated previously or concurrently with intrathecal chemotherapy and/or previously with craniospinal radiation therapy may be at increased risk for developing neurotoxicity.
4. Patients should be advised against performing activities that require mental alertness, including operating hazardous machinery and driving.
5. Alkalinization of the urine (pH >7.0), allopurinol, and vigorous IV hydration are recommended to prevent tumor lysis syndrome.
6. Pregnancy category D. Breastfeeding should be avoided.

TOXICITY 1

Myelosuppression is the most common toxicity, with neutropenia, thrombocytopenia, and anemia.

TOXICITY 2
Nausea and vomiting. Mild to moderate emetogenic agent.

TOXICITY 3
Neurotoxicity is dose-limiting, with headache, altered mental status, seizures, and peripheral neuropathy with numbness, paresthesias, motor weakness, and paralysis. Rare events of demyelination and ascending peripheral neuropathies similar to Guillain-Barré syndrome have been reported.

TOXICITY 4
Mild hepatotoxicity, with elevation of serum transaminases and bilirubin.

TOXICITY 5
Fatigue and asthenia.

Neratinib

TRADE NAME	Nerlynx, HKI-272	CLASSIFICATION	Signal transduction inhibitor, Pan-ErB inhibitor
CATEGORY	Targeted agent	DRUG MANUFACTURER	Puma/Pfizer

MECHANISM OF ACTION
- Potent irreversible small-molecule inhibitor of the tyrosine kinases associated with epidermal growth factor receptor (ErbB1; EGFR), HER2 (ErbB2), and HER4 (ErbB4), resulting in inhibition of ErbB tyrosine kinase phosphorylation and downstream signaling.
- Inhibition of the ErbB tyrosine kinases results in inhibition of critical mitogenic and anti-apoptotic signals involved in proliferation, growth, invasion/metastasis, angiogenesis, and response to chemotherapy and/or radiation therapy.

MECHANISM OF RESISTANCE

- Gatekeeper mutation in HER2/neu growth factor receptor, T798I, leading to reduced binding affinity to neratinib.
- Increased activity of CYP3A4 liver microsomal enzymes.

ABSORPTION

Oral absorption is relatively slow, with peak plasma levels achieved in 3–6.5 hours after ingestion, and is increased with food.

DISTRIBUTION

Extensive binding (99%) to plasma proteins, including albumin and α1-acid glycoprotein, along with extensive tissue distribution.

METABOLISM

Metabolism in the liver primarily by CYP3A4 microsomal enzymes, with formation of 4 main metabolites, M3, M6, M7, and M11, and by flavin-containing mono-oxygenase (FMO) to a lesser extent. Elimination is mainly hepatic, with excretion in feces. Renal elimination of parent drug and its metabolites accounts for only about 1% of an administered dose. The terminal half-life of the parent drug is 14 hours, while the half-lives of the M3, M6, and M7 metabolites are 21.6, 13.8, and 10.4 hours, respectively.

INDICATIONS

1. FDA-approved as monotherapy for the extended adjuvant treatment of adult patients with early-stage HER2-overexpressed/amplified breast cancer to follow adjuvant trastuzumab-based therapy.
2. FDA-approved in combination with capecitabine for advanced or metastatic HER2-positive breast cancer following 2 or more prior anti-HER2-based regimens in the metastatic setting.

DOSAGE RANGE

1. Breast cancer adjuvant therapy: recommended dose is 240 mg PO daily for 1 year.
2. Metastatic breast cancer: recommended dose is 240 mg PO on days 1–21 in combination with capecitabine (750 mg/m^2 PO bid on days 1–14) of a 21-day cycle.

DRUG INTERACTION 1

Phenytoin and other drugs that stimulate the liver microsomal CYP3A4 enzymes, including carbamazepine, rifampin, phenobarbital, and St. John's Wort—These drugs may increase the metabolism of neratinib, resulting in its inactivation and lower effective drug levels.

DRUG INTERACTION 2

Drugs that inhibit the liver microsomal CYP3A4 enzymes, including ketoconazole, itraconazole, erythromycin, and clarithromycin—These drugs may decrease the metabolism of neratinib, resulting in increased drug levels and potentially increased toxicity.

DRUG INTERACTION 3

Warfarin—Patients receiving warfarin should be closely monitored for alterations in their clotting parameters (PT and INR) and/or bleeding, as neratinib may inhibit the metabolism of warfarin by the liver P450 system. The dose of warfarin may require careful adjustment in the presence of neratinib therapy.

DRUG INTERACTION 4

Gastric acid reducing agents—Gastric acid reducing agents, including proton pump inhibitors and H2-receptor blockers, should be avoided, as their concomitant use may reduce the effective concentrations of neratinib, leading to reduced activity. Antacids may be used if clinically indicated, but it is important to space out dosing of neratinib by 3 hours after ingestion of antacids.

SPECIAL CONSIDERATIONS

1. No dose modification is required in patients with mild or moderate hepatic impairment (Child-Pugh Class A or B). Dose reduction to 80 mg is recommended in patients with severe hepatic impairment (Child-Pugh Class C).
2. Dose reduction is not required in patients with renal impairment.
3. Monitor patients for diarrhea, as severe diarrhea may develop while on therapy. Anti-diarrheal prophylaxis with loperamide is recommended during the first 2 cycles of therapy and should be initiated with the first dose.
4. Important to aggressively manage diarrhea with additional anti-diarrheals, fluids, and close monitoring of electrolyte status. Therapy should be held in patients experiencing severe and/or persistent diarrhea.
5. Specific dose modifications are recommended in the setting of diarrhea. Please see package insert for specific details.
6. Specific dose modifications are in place for drug-induced hepatotoxicity.
7. Neratinib should be taken with food at the same time each day. The drug tablets should be swallowed whole and not crushed or chewed.
8. Avoid Seville oranges, starfruit, pomelos, and grapefruit products while on therapy.
9. Monitor liver function tests for the first 3 months of therapy, then 3 months thereafter while on therapy, and as clinically indicated.
10. Pregnancy category D. Breastfeeding should be avoided.

TOXICITY 1

Diarrhea is the most common dose-limiting toxicity, and all-grade diarrhea occurs in 95% of patients. Grade 3 diarrhea occurs in 40% of patients. Mild nausea/vomiting, abdominal pain, and mucositis may also occur.

TOXICITY 2

Fatigue and anorexia.

TOXICITY 3

Hepatotoxicity with elevations in serum transaminases (SGOT, SGPT) and serum bilirubin.

TOXICITY 4
Muscle spasms.

TOXICITY 5
Skin rash, dry skin, and nail disorders.

Nilotinib

TRADE NAME	Tasigna, AMN107	**CLASSIFICATION**	Signal transduction inhibitor, Brc-Abl inhibitor, c-Kit inhibitor
CATEGORY	Targeted agent	**DRUG MANUFACTURER**	Novartis

MECHANISM OF ACTION
- Second-generation phenylaminopyrimidine inhibitor of the Bcr-Abl, c-Kit, and PDGFR-β tyrosine kinases.
- Higher binding affinity (up to 20- to 50-fold) and selectivity for Abl kinase domain when compared to imatinib and overcomes imatinib resistance resulting from Bcr-Abl mutations.

MECHANISM OF RESISTANCE
1. Gatekeeper mutation within the ATP-binding pocket of the Abl tyrosine kinase (T3151).
2. Increased expression of P170 glycoprotein, resulting in enhanced drug efflux and reduced intracellular drug accumulation.
3. Increased expression of the ATP Binding Cassette family efflux protein ABCG2.
4. Increased expression of ATP Binding Cassette family efflux protein ABBC6.

ABSORPTION
Rapidly absorbed following oral administration with good oral bioavailability. Peak plasma concentrations are observed within 3 hours of oral ingestion.

DISTRIBUTION
Extensive binding of parent drug to plasma proteins in the range of 95%–98%.

METABOLISM
Metabolized in the liver primarily by CYP3A4 microsomal enzymes. Other liver P450 enzymes, such as UGT, play a relatively minor role in metabolism. None of the metabolites is biologically active. Approximately 90% of an administered dose is eliminated in feces within 7 days. The terminal half-life of the parent drug is on the order of 15–17 hours.

INDICATIONS
1. FDA-approved for adults with chronic phase (CP) and accelerated phase (AP) Ph+ CML with resistance or intolerance to prior therapy that included imatinib.
2. FDA-approved for the front-line treatment of adult and pediatric patients with newly diagnosed CP Ph+ CML.
3. FDA-approved for pediatric patients older than or equal to 1 year of age with CP Ph+ CML resistant or intolerant to prior TKI therapy.

DOSAGE RANGE
1. Resistant or intolerant adult Ph+ CML-CP and CML-AP: 400 mg PO bid.
2. Newly diagnosed adult Ph+ CML-CP: 300 mg PO bid.
3. Pediatric dosing: 230 mg/m^2 PO bid, rounded to the nearest 50-mg dose (maximum single dose of 400 mg).

DRUG INTERACTION 1
Nilotinib is an inhibitor of CYP3A4 and may decrease the metabolic clearance of drugs that are metabolized by CYP3A4.

DRUG INTERACTION 2
Drugs such as ketoconazole, itraconazole, erythromycin, and clarithromycin may decrease the metabolism of nilotinib, resulting in increased drug levels and potentially increased toxicity.

DRUG INTERACTION 3
Drugs such as rifampin, phenytoin, phenobarbital, carbamazepine, and St. John's Wort may increase the metabolism of nilotinib, resulting in its inactivation and lower effective drug levels.

DRUG INTERACTION 4
Nilotinib is a substrate of the P-glycoprotein transporter. Caution should be used in patients on medications that inhibit P-glycoprotein (e.g., verapamil), as this may lead to increased concentrations of nilotinib.

SPECIAL CONSIDERATIONS

1. Nilotinib tablets should not be taken with food for at least 2 hours before a dose and for at least 1 hour after a dose.
2. Important to review patient's list of medications, as nilotinib has several potential drug–drug interactions.
3. Monitor CBC every 2 weeks for the first 2 months and monthly thereafter.
4. Use with caution in patients with a prior history of pancreatitis. Serum lipase levels should be checked periodically.
5. Nilotinib should not be used in patients with hypokalemia, hypomagnesemia, or long QT syndrome. Electrolyte abnormalities must be corrected prior to initiation of therapy, and electrolyte status should be monitored periodically during therapy.
6. ECGs should be performed at baseline, 7 days after initiation of therapy, and periodically thereafter.
7. Patients should be warned about not taking St. John's Wort while on nilotinib therapy.
8. Avoid Seville oranges, starfruit, pomelos, grapefruit juice, and grapefruit products while on therapy.
9. Pregnancy category D. Breastfeeding should be avoided.

TOXICITY 1
Myelosuppression with thrombocytopenia, neutropenia, and anemia.

TOXICITY 2
Prolongation of QT interval, which, on rare occasions, may lead to sudden death.

TOXICITY 3
Elevations in serum lipase.

TOXICITY 4
Electrolyte abnormalities with hypophosphatemia, hypokalemia, hypocalcemia, and hyponatremia.

TOXICITY 5
Fatigue, asthenia, and anorexia.

TOXICITY 6
Hepatotoxicity with elevations in serum transaminases and/or bilirubin (usually indirect bilirubin).

Nilutamide

TRADE NAME	Nilandron	CLASSIFICATION	Antiandrogen
CATEGORY	Hormonal agent	DRUG MANUFACTURER	Sanofi-Aventis

MECHANISM OF ACTION
Nonsteroidal, antiandrogen agent that binds to androgen receptor and inhibits androgen uptake. Also inhibits androgen binding in the nucleus of androgen-sensitive prostate cancer cells.

MECHANISM OF RESISTANCE
- Decreased expression of androgen receptor.
- Mutation in androgen receptor, leading to decreased binding affinity to nilutamide.

ABSORPTION
Rapidly and completely absorbed by the GI tract. Absorption is not affected by food.

DISTRIBUTION
Distribution is not well characterized. Moderate binding of nilutamide to plasma proteins.

METABOLISM
Extensive metabolism occurs in the liver to both active and inactive metabolites. About 60% of drug is excreted in urine, mainly in metabolite form, and only minimal clearance in feces. The elimination half-life is approximately 41–49 hours.

INDICATIONS
Stage D2 metastatic prostate cancer in combination with surgical castration.

DOSAGE RANGE
Recommended dose is 300 mg PO daily for 30 days, then 150 mg PO daily.

DRUG INTERACTION 1
Warfarin—Nilutamide can inhibit metabolism of warfarin by the liver P450 system, leading to increased anticoagulant effect. Coagulation parameters, PT and INR, must be followed routinely, and dose adjustments may be needed.

DRUG INTERACTION 2
Drugs metabolized by the liver P450 system—Nilutamide inhibits the activity of liver cytochrome P450 enzymes and may therefore reduce the metabolism of various compounds, including phenytoin and theophylline. Increased drug levels resulting in enhanced toxicity of these agents may be observed, and dose adjustment may be required.

DRUG INTERACTION 3
Alcohol—Increased risk of alcohol intolerance following treatment with nilutamide.

SPECIAL CONSIDERATIONS
1. Should be given on the same day as or on the day after surgical castration to achieve maximal benefit.
2. Nilutamide can be taken with or without food.
3. Should be used with caution in patients with abnormal liver function and is contraindicated in patients with severe liver impairment. Monitor LFTs at baseline and during therapy.
4. Contraindicated in patients with severe respiratory insufficiency. Baseline PFTs and chest X-ray should be obtained in all patients and periodically during therapy. If findings of interstitial pneumonitis appear on chest X-ray or there is a significant decrease by 20%–25% in DLCO and FVC on PFTs, treatment with nilutamide should be terminated.
5. Caution patients about the potential for hot flashes. Consider the use of clonidine 0.1–0.2 mg PO daily, megestrol acetate 20 mg PO bid, or soy tablets 1 tablet PO tid for prevention and/or treatment.
6. Instruct patients on the potential risk of altered sexual function and impotence.
7. Patients should be advised to abstain from alcohol while on nilutamide, as there is an increased risk of intolerance (facial flushes, malaise, hypotension) to alcohol.
8. Pregnancy category C. Breastfeeding should be avoided.

TOXICITY 1
Hot flashes, decreased libido, impotence, gynecomastia, nipple pain, and galactorrhea.

TOXICITY 2
Visual disturbances in the form of impaired adaptation to dark, abnormal vision, and alterations in color vision. Occurs in up to 60% of patients and results in treatment discontinuation in 1%–2% of patients.

TOXICITY 3
Anorexia, nausea, and constipation. Transient elevations in serum transaminases are uncommon.

TOXICITY 4
Cough, dyspnea, and interstitial pneumonitis occur rarely in about 2% of patients. Usually observed within the first 3 months of treatment. Incidence may be higher in patients of Asian descent.

Niraparib

TRADE NAME	Zejula	**CLASSIFICATION**	Signal transduction inhibitor, PARP inhibitor
CATEGORY	Targeted agent	**DRUG MANUFACTURER**	Tesaro

MECHANISM OF ACTION
- Small-molecule inhibitor of poly (ADP-ribose) polymerase (PARP) enzymes, including PARP1 and PARP2.
- Inhibition of PARP enzymatic activity, with increased formation of PARP-DNA complexes, results in cell death.
- Enhanced antitumor activity in tumors that are BRCA-deficient.
- Potentiates the effects of radiation therapy in a p53-independent manner.

MECHANISM OF RESISTANCE
- Increased expression of the P-glycoprotein drug efflux transporter protein.
- Reduced expression of p53-binding protein 1 (53BP1), which is a critical component of DNA double-strand break (DSB) signaling and repair in mammalian cells.
- Reversion mutations in BRCA1 or BRCA2 that result in restoration of BRCA function.

- Loss of REV7 expression and function leads to restoration of homologous recombination, resulting in PARP resistance.
- Reduced expression of PARP enzymes.
- Increased stabilization of replication forks.

ABSORPTION
Oral bioavailability is approximately 73%. Oral absorption is rapid, with peak plasma concentrations achieved within 3 hours after administration. Food with high fat content can slow the rate of absorption but does not alter systemic drug exposure.

DISTRIBUTION
Fairly extensive binding of niraparib to plasma proteins (83%). With daily dosing, steady-state blood levels are achieved in about 3–4 days.

METABOLISM
Metabolized in the liver primarily by CYP3A4 microsomal enzymes. A large fraction of an administered dose of drug is metabolized by carboxylesterases to form a major inactive metabolite (M1), which undergoes subsequent glucuronidation. With respect to drug elimination, approximately 39% of drug is recovered in feces and nearly 48% in urine, with the majority of drug being in metabolite form. The terminal half-life is on the order of 36 hours.

INDICATIONS
1. FDA-approved for the maintenance treatment of advanced epithelial ovarian, fallopian tube, or primary peritoneal cancer in complete or partial response to platinum-based chemotherapy.
2. FDA-approved for the maintenance treatment of deleterious or suspected deleterious germline BRCA-mutated recurrent epithelial ovarian, fallopian tube, or primary peritoneal cancer in complete or partial response to platinum-based chemotherapy.

DOSAGE RANGE
1. First-line maintenance treatment of advanced ovarian, fallopian tube, or primary peritoneal cancer: For patients weighing >77 kg (>170 lbs) and a platelet count of >150,000, recommended dose is 300 mg PO daily. For patients weighing <77 kg (<170 lbs) and a platelet count of <150,000, the recommended dose is 200 mg PO daily.

DRUG INTERACTIONS
No formal drug interaction studies have been performed to date with niraparib.

SPECIAL CONSIDERATIONS
1. Patients should start treatment no later than 8 weeks after their most recent platinum-containing chemotherapy regimen.

2. No dose modification is needed in patients with mild hepatic impairment. Has not been studied in patients with moderate or severe hepatic impairment, and caution should be used in these settings.
3. No dose modification is needed in patients with mild or moderate renal impairment (CrCl 30–89 mL/min). Has not been studied in patients with severe renal impairment, end-stage renal disease, or those on hemodialysis, and there are no formal recommendations for dosing in these settings.
4. Niraparib capsules should be swallowed whole and should not be chewed, dissolved, or crushed.
5. Closely monitor blood pressure and heart rate monthly for the first year and periodically thereafter while on therapy. Patients with underlying cardiovascular disorders, including hypertension and cardiac arrhythmias, are at increased risk for developing the cardiac toxicities associated with niraparib.
6. Closely monitor blood counts weekly for the first month, monthly for the next 11 months of therapy, and periodically thereafter. For prolonged hematologic toxicities, interrupt therapy, and monitor CBCs on a weekly basis until recovery. If blood counts have not recovered within 4 weeks, bone marrow analysis and peripheral blood for cytogenetics should be performed to rule out the possibility of MDS/AML.
7. Pregnancy category D. Females of reproductive potential should be advised to use effective contraception during treatment and for 6 months after the last dose of niraparib.

TOXICITY 1
Myelosuppression with anemia, thrombocytopenia, and neutropenia.

TOXICITY 2
Fatigue, anorexia, and asthenia.

TOXICITY 3
GI side effects in the form of nausea/vomiting, abdominal pain, diarrhea, constipation, and mucositis.

TOXICITY 4
Arthralgias, myalgias, and back pain.

TOXICITY 5
Increased risk of infections, with UTI most common.

TOXICITY 6
MDS and AML.

Niraparib and Abiraterone

TRADE NAME	Akeega	**CLASSIFICATION**	Signal transduction inhibitor, PARP inhibitor
CATEGORY	Targeted agent	**DRUG MANUFACTURER**	Janssen

MECHANISM OF ACTION

- Small-molecule inhibitor of poly (ADP-ribose) polymerase (PARP) enzymes, including PARP1 and PARP2.
- Inhibition of PARP enzymatic activity, with increased formation of PARP-DNA complexes, results in cell death.
- Enhanced antitumor activity in tumors that are BRCA-deficient.
- Potentiates the effects of radiation therapy in a p53-independent manner.
- Selective inhibition of 17α-hydroxylase/C17, 20-lyase (CYP17). This enzyme is expressed in testicular, adrenal, and prostatic tumor tissues and is required for androgen biosynthesis.
- Inhibition of CYP17 leads to inhibition of the conversion of pregnenolone and progesterone to their 17α-hydroxy derivatives.
- Inhibition of CYP17 leads to inhibition of subsequent formation of dehydroepiandrosterone (DHEA) and androstenedione.

MECHANISM OF RESISTANCE

- Increased expression of the P-glycoprotein drug efflux transporter protein.
- Reduced expression of p53-binding protein 1 (53BP1), which is a critical component of DNA double-strand break (DSB) signaling and repair in mammalian cells.
- Reversion mutations in BRCA1 or BRCA2 that result in restoration of BRCA function.
- Loss of REV7 expression and function leads to restoration of homologous recombination, resulting in PARP resistance.
- Reduced expression of PARP enzymes.
- Increased stabilization of replication forks.
- Upregulation of CYP17.

- Induction of androgen receptor (AR) and AR splice variants that result in ligand-independent AR transactivation.
- Expression of truncated androgen receptors.

ABSORPTION

Oral absorption of niraparib is rapid, with peak plasma concentrations achieved within 3 hours after administration. Oral bioavailability is approximately 73%. Food with high fat content can slow the rate of absorption but does not alter systemic drug exposure.

Following oral administration, of abiraterone maximum drug levels are reached within 1.5 hours. Oral absorption is increased with food and, in particular, food with high fat content.

DISTRIBUTION

Fairly extensive binding of niraparib to plasma proteins (83%). With daily dosing, steady-state blood levels are achieved in about 3–4 days. Abiraterone is highly protein bound (>99%) to albumin and α1-acid glycoprotein.

METABOLISM

Metabolized in the liver primarily by CYP3A4 microsomal enzymes. A large fraction of an administered dose of drug is metabolized by carboxylesterases to form a major inactive metabolite (M1), which undergoes subsequent glucuronidation. With respect to drug elimination, approximately 39% of drug is recovered in feces and nearly 48% in urine, with the majority of drug being in metabolite form. The terminal half-life of niraparib when given in combination with abiraterone is on the order of 62 hours.

Following oral administration, abiraterone acetate is rapidly hydrolyzed to abiraterone, the active metabolite. The two main circulating metabolites of abiraterone are abiraterone sulphate and N-oxide abiraterone sulphate, both of which are inactive. Nearly 90% of an administered dose is recovered in feces, while only 5% is eliminated in urine. The terminal half-life of abiraterone when given in combination with niraparib is 20 hours.

INDICATIONS

FDA-approved in combination with abiraterone for treatment of deleterious or suspected deleterious BRCA-mutated metastatic castration-resistant prostate cancer.

DOSAGE RANGE

BRCA-mutated prostate cancer: 200 mg niraparib/1,000 mg abiraterone PO once daily in combination with 10 mg prednisone PO daily.

DRUG INTERACTIONS

- Use with caution in the presence of CYP2D6 substrates as abiraterone is a CYP2D6 moderate inhibitor.
- Use with caution in the presence of CYP2C8 substrates as abiraterone is a CYP2C8 inhibitor.

- Use with caution in the presence of CYP3A4 inhibitors and inducers as abiraterone is a CYP3A4 substrate.
- No formal drug interaction studies have been performed to date with niraparib.

SPECIAL CONSIDERATIONS

1. Monitor CBC weekly for the first month, every 2 weeks for the next 2 months, monthly for the remainder of the first year, then every other month, and as clinically indicated.
2. Monitor for hypertension, hypokalemia, and fluid retention at least weekly for the first 2 months, then once a month, and as clinically indicated.
3. Monitor liver function tests periodically while on therapy.
4. Monitor for signs and symptoms of adrenal insufficiency.
5. Monitor blood glucose levels especially in patients with underlying diabetes.
6. No dose modification is needed in patients with mild hepatic impairment. Use with caution in patients with moderate or severe hepatic impairment.
7. No dose modification is needed in patients with mild or moderate renal impairment (CrCl 30–90 mL/min). Has not been studied in patients with severe renal impairment, end-stage renal disease, or those on hemodialysis.
8. May cause fetal harm. Males with female partners of reproductive potential should be advised to use effective contraception during treatment and for 4 months after the last dose of niraparib/abiraterone.

TOXICITY 1
Myelosuppression with anemia, thrombocytopenia, and neutropenia.

TOXICITY 2
Hepatotoxicity with elevations in LFTs and serum bilirubin.

TOXICITY 3
Hypertension, fluid retention, and hypokalemia.

TOXICITY 4
Adrenocortical insufficiency.

TOXICITY 5
Hypoglycemia.

TOXICITY 6
MDS and AML.

TOXICITY 7
Posterior reversible encephalopathy syndrome (PRES).

Nivolumab

TRADE NAME	Opdivo, MDX-1106, BMS-936558	CLASSIFICATION	Anti-PD1 monoclonal antibody
CATEGORY	Immunotherapy, immune checkpoint inhibitor	DRUG MANUFACTURER	Bristol-Myers Squibb

MECHANISM OF ACTION
- Fully human IgG4 monoclonal antibody that binds to the programmed death (PD)-1 receptor, which is expressed on T cells, and inhibits the interaction between the PD-L1 and PD-L2 ligands and the PD-1 receptor.
- Blockade of the PD-1 pathway-mediated immune checkpoint enhances T-cell immune response, leading to T-cell activation and proliferation.

MECHANISM OF RESISTANCE
- Increased expression and/or activity of other immune checkpoint pathways (e.g., TIGIT, TIM3, and LAG3).
- Increased expression of other immune escape mechanisms.
- Increased infiltration of immune suppressive populations within the tumor microenvironment, which include Tregs, myeloid-derived suppressor cells (MDSCs), and M2 macrophages.
- Release of various cytokines, chemokines, and metabolites within the tumor microenvironment, including CSF-1, tryptophan metabolites, TGF-β, and adenosine.

DISTRIBUTION
Steady-state concentrations are achieved by 12 weeks.

METABOLISM
Metabolism of nivolumab has not been extensively characterized. The mean elimination half-life is on the order of 26.7 days.

INDICATIONS
1. FDA-approved as a single agent or in combination with ipilimumab for unresectable or metastatic melanoma.
2. FDA-approved for the adjuvant treatment of melanoma with lymph node involvement or following complete surgical resection of metastatic disease.
3. FDA-approved for the first-line treatment of metastatic NSCLC expressing PD-L1 (>1%) with no EGFR or ALK mutations in combination with ipilimumab.

4. FDA-approved for the first-line treatment of metastatic or recurrent NSCLC with no EGFR or ALK mutations in combination with ipilimumab and 2 cycles of platinum-doublet chemotherapy.
5. FDA-approved for metastatic NSCLC with progression on or after platinum-based chemotherapy. Patients with EGFR or ALK mutations should have disease progression on FDA-approved targeted therapy prior to receiving nivolumab.
6. FDA-approved in combination with platinum-doublet chemotherapy in neoadjuvant treatment of resectable (tumors>4 cm or node positive) NSCLC.
7. Activity in metastatic small cell lung cancer (SCLC) following progression after platinum-based chemotherapy and at least one other line of therapy.
8. FDA-approved in combination with ipilimumab for first-line treatment of unresectable malignant pleural mesothelioma.
9. FDA-approved for advanced renal cell cancer following prior anti-angiogenic therapy.
10. FDA-approved in combination with ipilimumab for first-line treatment of intermediate- or poor-risk, advanced renal cell cancer.
11. FDA-approved in combination with cabozantinib for first-line treatment of advanced renal cell cancer.
12. FDA-approved for Hodgkin's lymphoma that has relapsed or progressed after autologous stem cell transplantation and post-transplantation brentuximab therapy or after 3 or more lines of systemic therapy that include autologous stem cell transplantation.
13. FDA-approved for recurrent or metastatic squamous cell cancer of the head and neck with disease progression on or after platinum-based chemotherapy.
14. FDA-approved for locally advanced or metastatic urothelial cancer with disease progression during or following platinum-based chemotherapy or with disease progression within 12 months of neoadjuvant or adjuvant treatment with platinum-based chemotherapy.
15. FDA-approved for adjuvant treatment of urothelial cancer at high risk of recurrence after undergoing radical surgical resection.
16. FDA-approved as a single agent or in combination with ipilimumab for adult and pediatric patients 12 years of age and older with microsatellite instability-high (MSI-H) or mismatch repair deficient (dMMR) mCRC that has progressed on treatment with a fluoropyrimidine, oxaliplatin, and irinotecan.
17. FDA-approved in combination with ipilimumab for hepatocellular cancer that has been previously treated with sorafenib.
18. FDA-approved as a single agent for unresectable advanced, recurrent, or metastatic esophageal squamous cell cancer after prior fluoropyrimidine- and platinum-based chemotherapy.
19. FDA-approved as a single agent for completely resected esophageal or gastroesophageal junction (GEJ) cancer with residual pathologic disease who have received neoadjuvant chemoradiotherapy.
20. FDA-approved in combination with fluoropyrimidine- and platinum-containing chemotherapy as first-line treatment for unresectable advanced or metastatic esophageal squamous cell cancer.

21. FDA-approved in combination with ipilimumab as first-line treatment for unresectable advanced or metastatic esophageal squamous cell cancer.
22. FDA-approved as a single agent in patients with completely resected esophageal or gastroesophageal junction (GEJ) cancer with residual pathologic disease and who have received neoadjuvant chemoradiotherapy.
23. FDA-approved in combination with fluoropyrimidine- and platinum-containing chemotherapy in advanced or metastatic gastric cancer, GEJ, and esophageal adenocarcinoma.

DOSAGE RANGE

1. Unresectable or metastatic melanoma: 240 mg IV every 2 weeks or 480 mg IV every 4 weeks.
2. Unresectable or metastatic melanoma: Recommended dose in combination with ipilimumab is nivolumab at 1 mg/kg IV followed by ipilimumab 3 mg/kg IV every 3 weeks for 4 doses, then nivolumab at 240 mg IV every 2 weeks or 480 mg IV every 4 weeks as a single agent.
3. Adjuvant therapy of melanoma: 240 mg IV every 2 weeks or 480 mg IV every 4 weeks.
4. Metastatic NSCLC: 240 mg IV every 2 weeks or 480 mg IV every 4 weeks.
5. Metastatic NSCLC: 3 mg/kg IV every 2 weeks with ipilimumab 1 mg/kg every 6 weeks.
6. Metastatic NSCLC: 360 mg IV every 3 weeks with ipilimumab 1 mg/kg every 6 weeks and 2 cycles of platinum-doublet chemotherapy.
7. Neoadjuvant therapy of NSCLC: 360 mg IV every 3 weeks with platinum-doublet chemotherapy for 3 cycles.
8. SCLC: 240 mg IV every 2 weeks or 480 mg IV every 4 weeks.
9. Malignant pleural mesothelioma: 360 mg IV every 3 weeks with ipilimumab 1 mg/kg every 6 weeks.
10. Advanced renal cell cancer: 240 mg IV every 2 weeks or 480 mg IV every 4 weeks.
11. Advanced renal cell cancer: 3 mg/kg IV followed by ipilimumab 1 mg/kg every 3 weeks for 4 doses. Nivolumab is then administered as a single agent at 240 mg IV every 2 weeks or 480 mg IV every 4 weeks.
12. Advanced renal cell cancer: 240 mg IV every 2 weeks or 480 mg IV every 4 weeks in combination with cabozantinib 40 mg PO daily.
13. Hodgkin's lymphoma: 240 mg IV every 2 weeks or 480 mg IV every 4 weeks.
14. Recurrent or metastatic squamous cell cancer of the head and neck: 240 mg IV every 2 weeks or 480 mg IV every 4 weeks.
15. Locally advanced or metastatic urothelial cancer: 240 mg IV every 2 weeks or 480 mg IV every 4 weeks.
16. Adjuvant treatment of urothelial cancer: 240 mg IV every 2 weeks or 480 mg IV every 4 weeks.
17. Metastatic colorectal cancer: 240 mg IV every 2 weeks or 480 mg IV every 4 weeks.
18. Metastatic colorectal cancer: 3 mg/kg IV in combination with ipilimumab 1 mg/kg IV on same day every 3 weeks for 4 doses, and then 240 mg IV every 2 weeks or 480 mg IV every 4 weeks.

19. Hepatocellular cancer: 1 mg/kg IV in combination with ipilimumab 3 mg/kg IV on same day every 3 weeks for 4 doses, and then 240 mg IV every 2 weeks or 480 mg IV every 4 weeks.
20. Metastatic esophageal squamous cell cancer: 240 mg IV every 2 weeks or 480 mg IV every 4 weeks.
21. Locally advanced or metastatic esophageal squamous cell cancer: 240 mg IV every 2 weeks or 480 mg IV every 4 weeks in combination with chemotherapy.
22. Locally advanced or metastatic esophageal squamous cell cancer: 360 mg IV every 3 weeks with ipilimumab 1 mg/kg every 6 weeks.
23. Gastric cancer, GEJ, and esophageal adenocarcinoma: 360 mg IV every 3 weeks with fluoropyrimidine- and platinum-containing chemotherapy every 3 weeks or 240 mg IV every 2 weeks with fluoropyrimidine- and platinum-containing chemotherapy every 2 weeks.

DRUG INTERACTIONS
None well characterized to date.

SPECIAL CONSIDERATIONS
1. Nivolumab can result in significant immune-mediated adverse reactions due to T-cell activation and proliferation. These immune-mediated reactions may involve any organ system, with the most common reactions being pneumonitis, enterocolitis, hepatitis, dermatitis, hypophysitis, nephritis, and thyroid dysfunction.
2. Nivolumab should be withheld for any of the following:
   - Grade 2 pneumonitis
   - Grades 2 or 3 colitis
   - SGOT/SGPT >3 × ULN and up to 5 × ULN or total bilirubin >1.5 × ULN and up to 3 × ULN
   - Serum creatinine >1.5 × ULN and up to 6 × ULN or >1.5 × baseline
   - Any other severe or grade 3 treatment-related toxicity
3. Nivolumab should be permanently discontinued for any of the following:
   - Any life-threatening or grade 4 toxicity
   - Grades 3 or 4 pneumonitis
   - Grade 4 colitis
   - SGOT/SGPT >5 × ULN or total bilirubin >3 × ULN
   - Serum creatinine >6 × ULN
   - Any severe or grade 3 toxicity that recurs
   - Inability to reduce steroid dose to 10 mg or less of prednisone or equivalent per day within 12 weeks
   - Persistent grades 2 or 3 toxicity that does not recover to grade 1 or resolve within 12 weeks after the last dose of drug
4. Monitor thyroid function prior to and during therapy.
5. Immune-mediated reactions may occur even after discontinuation of therapy.
6. Pregnancy category D.

TOXICITY 1
GI toxicity with colitis, diarrhea, and abdominal pain.

TOXICITY 2
Pneumonitis with dyspnea and cough.

TOXICITY 3
Hepatotoxicity with elevations in SGOT/SGPT, alkaline phosphatase, and serum bilirubin.

TOXICITY 4
GI side effects with nausea/vomiting and dry mouth. Pancreatitis is also observed.

TOXICITY 5
Fatigue, anorexia, and asthenia.

TOXICITY 6
Endocrinopathies, including hypophysitis, thyroid disorders, adrenal insufficiency, and diabetes.

TOXICITY 7
Neurologic toxicity with neuropathy, myositis, and myasthenia gravis.

TOXICITY 8
Renal toxicity with nephritis.

TOXICITY 9
Musculoskeletal symptoms with arthralgias, oligoarthritis, polyarthritis, tenosynovitis, polymyalgia rheumatica, and myalgias.

TOXICITY 10
Maculopapular skin rash, erythema, dermatitis, and pruritus.

O

Obinutuzumab

TRADE NAME	Gazyva	CLASSIFICATION	Anti-CD20 monoclonal antibody
CATEGORY	Biologic response modifier agent, targeted agent	DRUG MANUFACTURER	Genentech/Roche

MECHANISM OF ACTION
- Glycoengineered type II anti-CD20 monoclonal antibody with a higher affinity for the CD20 epitope than rituximab. Type II antibody that binds to CD20 in a different orientation without forming cross-links to CD tetramers and remains dispersed throughout the entire surface of the B cell when compared type I anti-CD20 antibodies.
- More potent anti-CD20 antibody when compared to rituximab.
- CD20 is expressed on more than 90% of all B-cell, non-Hodgkin's lymphomas and leukemias.
- CD20 is not expressed on early pre–B cells, plasma cells, normal bone marrow stem cells, antigen-presenting dendritic reticulum cells, or other normal tissues.
- Enhanced binding affinity to natural killer cells, macrophages/dendritic cells, and neutrophils.
- More effectively mediates antibody-dependent cellular cytotoxicity (ADCC) and direct cell death when compared to rituximab.

ABSORPTION
Administered only via the IV route.

DISTRIBUTION
Volume of distribution at steady state is approximately 3.8 L.

METABOLISM
Eliminated through both a linear clearance mechanism and a time-dependent, non-linear clearance mechanism. The mean terminal half-life of obinutuzumab is approximately 28.4 days.

INDICATIONS
1. FDA-approved in combination with chlorambucil for previously untreated CLL.
2. FDA-approved in combination with bendamustine followed by obinutuzumab monotherapy for patients with follicular lymphoma (NHL) who relapsed after or are refractory to a rituximab-containing regimen.

3. FDA-approved in combination with chemotherapy followed by obinutuzumab monotherapy for patients with previously untreated stage II bulky, stage III, or stage IV follicular lymphoma (NHL).

DOSAGE RANGE

Recommended dose for 6 cycles (28-day cycles) is as follows:

CLL:
- 100 mg on cycle 1, day 1
- 900 mg on cycle 1, day 2
- 1,000 mg on cycle 1, days 8 and 15
- 1,000 mg on cycles 2–6, day 1

NHL:
- 1,000 mg on cycle 1, days 1, 8, and 15
- 1,000 mg on cycles 2–6, day 1
- and then 1,000 mg on day 1 every 2 months for 2 years

DRUG INTERACTIONS

None well characterized to date.

SPECIAL CONSIDERATIONS

1. Closely monitor patients for infusion reactions, which usually occur during the infusion, but infusion reactions have been observed within 24 hours of receiving obinutuzumab. Patients should be premedicated 30 min to 2 hours with oral acetaminophen (1,000 mg), oral or IV diphenhydramine, and IV corticosteroid (prednisolone 100 mg) to prevent the development of infusion-related reactions.

2. Monitor for infusion-related events, especially during the first two infusions. Infusions should be immediately stopped if signs or symptoms of an allergic reaction are observed. Immediate institution of diphenhydramine, corticosteroids, albuterol, IV fluids, and/or vasopressors may be necessary. For grade 1/2 reactions, the infusion rate can be reduced or the infusion interrupted and the symptoms treated; if the patient's symptoms have resolved, the infusion rate escalation may resume at the increments and intervals as appropriate for the treatment cycle dose. For grade 3 reactions, the infusion should be interrupted, and if the reaction symptoms resolve, the infusion can be resumed at a rate no more than half the previous rate; if no further infusion reactions are experienced, the infusion rate escalation may resume at the increments and intervals as appropriate for the treatment cycle dose. For grade 4 reactions, the infusion should be stopped immediately and permanently discontinued.

3. Consider holding off on antihypertensive treatments for 12 hours prior to and throughout each obinutuzumab infusion given the potential risk of hypotension.

4. Monitor for tumor lysis syndrome, especially in patients with high numbers of peripheral circulating cells ($>25,000/mm^3$). In this setting,

patients should be premedicated with allopurinol starting 12–24 hours prior to the start of therapy as well as be adequately hydrated.

5. Monitor CBCs at regular intervals during therapy.
6. Consider the diagnosis of progressive multifocal leukoencephalopathy (PML) in patients who present with new onset of or changes in pre-existing neurological signs or symptoms. This is a black-box warning.
7. Obinutuzumab should not be given to patients with active infection, as serious bacterial, fungal, and new or reactivated viral infections can occur during and following treatment.
8. Screen all patients for hepatitis B (HBV) infection before initiation of obinutuzumab therapy. Closely monitor hepatitis B carriers for signs of active HBV infection during treatment with obinutuzumab and for 6–12 months following the last infusion. Obinutuzumab therapy should be permanently discontinued in the event of HBV reactivation. This is a black-box warning.
9. Pregnancy category C. Breastfeeding should be avoided.

TOXICITY 1
Infusion-related symptoms occur, usually during the first cycle of therapy, and present as nausea/vomiting, flushing, headache, fever, and chills. More serious symptoms include bronchospasm, dyspnea, laryngeal edema, and pulmonary edema.

TOXICITY 2
Myelosuppression with neutropenia and thrombocytopenia.

TOXICITY 3
Progressive multifocal leukoencephalopathy (PML).

TOXICITY 4
Hepatitis B reactivation.

TOXICITY 5
Increased risk of bacterial, viral, and fungal infections.

TOXICITY 6
Mild nausea.

TOXICITY 7
Headache.

TOXICITY 8
Musculoskeletal disorders, including pain.

Ofatumumab

TRADE NAME	Arzerra, HuMax-CD20	**CLASSIFICATION**	Monoclonal antibody, anti-CD20 antibody
CATEGORY	Biologic response modifier agent, targeted agent	**DRUG MANUFACTURER**	GlaxoSmithKline and Genman A/S

MECHANISM OF ACTION

- Fully human IgG1-κ immunoglobulin monoclonal antibody that binds specifically to both the small and large extracellular loops of the CD20 antigen on B cells.
- Targets a different CD20 epitope and binds CD20 with a reduced off-rate when compared to rituximab, resulting in prolonged antitumor activity.
- Maintains activity in rituximab-resistant tumors, which express low levels of CD20 and/or high levels of complement-regulatory proteins.
- CD20 is expressed on more than 90% of all B-cell, non-Hodgkin's lymphomas and leukemias.
- CD20 is not expressed on early pre–B cells, plasma cells, normal bone marrow stem cells, antigen-presenting dendritic reticulum cells, or other normal tissues.
- Mediates antibody-dependent cellular cytotoxicity (ADCC) and stronger complement-dependent cellular cytotoxicity (CDCC) when compared to rituximab.

ABSORPTION

Administered only via the IV route.

DISTRIBUTION

Mean volume of distribution at steady-state ranges from 1.7 to 5.1 L. The volume of distribution increases with body weight and male gender, but dose adjustment is not required based on body weight or gender.

METABOLISM

Eliminated through both a B-cell-mediated and a target-independent route. Due to the depletion of B cells, the clearance of ofatumumab is reduced significantly after subsequent infusions compared to the first infusion. The mean half-life of ofatumumab between the 4th and 12th infusions is approximately 14 days.

INDICATIONS

1. Refractory CLL—FDA-approved for CLL that is refractory to fludarabine and alemtuzumab.
2. FDA-approved for previously untreated CLL where fludarabine-based therapy is considered not appropriate.

3. FDA-approved for extended treatment of patients who are in complete or partial response after at least two lines of therapy for recurrent or progressive CLL.
4. FDA-approved in combination with fludarabine and cyclophosphamide for relapsed CLL.
5. Relapsed and/or refractory follicular, CD20+, B-cell non-Hodgkin's lymphoma.
6. Intermediate- and/or high-grade, CD20+, B-cell non-Hodgkin's lymphoma.

DOSAGE RANGE
Previously untreated CLL:
- 300 mg on day 1 followed by 1,000 mg on day 8 (cycle 1)
- 1,000 mg on day 1 of subsequent 28-day cycles for a minimum of 3 cycles until best response or a maximum of 12 cycles

Extended treatment of CLL:
- 300 mg on day 1, followed by
- 1,000 mg 1 week later on day 8, followed by
- 1,000 mg 7 weeks later and every 8 weeks thereafter for up to a maximum of 2 years

Refractory CLL:
- 300 mg initial dose on day 1, followed 1 week later by
- 2,000 mg weekly for 7 doses, followed 4 weeks later by
- 2,000 mg every 4 weeks for 4 doses

DRUG INTERACTIONS
None well characterized to date.

SPECIAL CONSIDERATIONS
1. Patients should be premedicated 30 minutes to 2 hours with oral acetaminophen (1,000 mg), oral or IV diphenhydramine, and IV corticosteroid (prednisolone 100 mg) to prevent the incidence of infusion-related reactions. The steroid dose for doses 1, 2, and 9 should not be reduced. If grade 3 or greater infusion reaction did not occur with the preceding dose, the steroid dose may be gradually reduced for doses 3 through 8.
2. Infusion should be started at an initial rate of 3.6 mg/hr (12 mL/hr). If no toxicity observed, rate may be escalated in 2-fold increments at 30-minute intervals to a maximum of 200 mL/hr. Second dose infusion should be started at an initial rate of 24 mg/hr (12 mL/hr). If no toxicity is observed, rate may be escalated in 2-fold increments at 30-minute intervals to a maximum of 200 mL/hr. For doses 3 through 12, infusion should be started at an initial rate of 50 mg/hr (25 mL/hr). If infusion is well tolerated, rate may be escalated in 2-fold increments at 30-minute intervals to a maximum of 400 mL/hr. Ofatumumab should **NOT** be given by IV push.
3. Monitor for infusion-related events, especially during the first two infusions. Infusions should be immediately stopped if signs or symptoms of an allergic reaction are observed. Immediate institution

of diphenhydramine, corticosteroids, albuterol, IV fluids, and/or vasopressors may be necessary. For grade 1/2 reactions, the infusion can be restarted at a reduced rate (50%) once symptoms have completely resolved. For grade 3 reactions, interrupt infusion, and if reaction resolves or remains less than or equal to grade 2, resume infusion at a rate of 12 mL/hr; resume infusion at normal escalation as tolerated. For grade 4 reactions, the infusion should be discontinued.

4. Use with caution in patients with moderate-to-severe chronic obstructive pulmonary disease.
5. Do not administer live viral vaccines to patients who have recently received ofatumumab. The ability to generate an immune response to any vaccine following administration of ofatumumab has not been studied.
6. Monitor CBCs at regular intervals during therapy.
7. Consider the diagnosis of progressive multifocal leukoencephalopathy (PML) in patients who present with new onset of or changes in pre-existing neurological signs or symptoms.
8. Use with caution in patients with renal or hepatic impairment, as no formal studies of ofatumumab have been conducted in these patient populations.
9. Screen patients at high risk of hepatitis B infection before initiation of ofatumumab therapy. Closely monitor hepatitis B carriers for signs of active HBV infection during treatment with ofatumumab and for 6–12 months following the last infusion.
10. Pregnancy category C. Breastfeeding should be avoided.

TOXICITY 1
Infusion-related symptoms occur, especially during the first two infusions, and present as bronchospasm, dyspnea, laryngeal edema, pulmonary edema, angioedema, syncope, back pain, abdominal pain, rash, and cardiac ischemia/infarction.

TOXICITY 2
Myelosuppression with neutropenia and thrombocytopenia.

TOXICITY 3
Progressive multifocal leukoencephalopathy (PML), with rare cases resulting in death.

TOXICITY 4
Hepatitis B reactivation.

TOXICITY 5
Increased risk of bacterial, viral, and fungal infections. Nasopharyngitis and upper respiratory infections are most commonly observed.

TOXICITY 6
Skin reactions, including macular and vesicular rash with or without urticaria.

TOXICITY 7
Mild nausea and diarrhea.

TOXICITY 8
Cough and dyspnea.

TOXICITY 9
Fatigue.

Olaparib

TRADE NAME	Lynparza	**CLASSIFICATION**	Signal transduction inhibitor, PARP inhibitor
CATEGORY	Targeted agent	**DRUG MANUFACTURER**	AstraZeneca

MECHANISM OF ACTION
- Small-molecule inhibitor of poly (ADP-ribose) polymerase (PARP) enzymes, including PARP1, PARP2, and PARP3.
- Inhibition of PARP enzymatic activity, with increased formation of PARP-DNA complexes, results in cell death.
- Enhanced antitumor activity in tumors that are BRCA-deficient.

MECHANISM OF RESISTANCE
- Increased expression of the P-glycoprotein drug efflux transporter protein.
- Reduced expression of p53-binding protein 1 (53BP1), which is a critical component of DNA double-strand break (DSB) signaling and repair in mammalian cells.
- Reversion mutations in BRCA1 or BRCA2 that result in restoration of BRCA function.

- Loss of REV7 expression and function leads to restoration of homologous recombination, resulting in PARP resistance.
- Reduced expression of PARP enzymes.
- Increased stabilization of replication forks.

ABSORPTION

Oral absorption is rapid, with peak plasma concentrations achieved between 1 and 3 hours after administration. Food with high-fat content can slow the rate of absorption but does not alter systemic drug exposure.

DISTRIBUTION

Fairly extensive binding of olaparib to plasma proteins (82%). With daily dosing, steady-state blood levels are achieved in about 3–4 days.

METABOLISM

Metabolized in the liver primarily by CYP3A4 microsomal enzymes. A large fraction of an administered dose of drug is metabolized by oxidation reactions, with several of the metabolites undergoing subsequent glucuronide or sulfate conjugation. Nearly 90% of drug is recovered, with 42% in feces and 44% in urine, with the majority of drug being in metabolite form. The terminal half-life is on the order of 12 hours.

INDICATIONS

1. FDA-approved for the maintenance treatment of recurrent epithelial ovarian, fallopian tube, or primary peritoneal cancer in complete or partial response to platinum-based chemotherapy.
2. FDA-approved for the maintenance treatment of deleterious or suspected deleterious germline or somatic BRCA-mutated advanced epithelial ovarian, fallopian tube, or primary peritoneal cancer in complete or partial response to first-line platinum-based chemotherapy.
3. FDA-approved in combination with bevacizumab for the maintenance treatment of advanced epithelial ovarian, fallopian tube, or primary peritoneal cancer in complete or partial response to first-line platinum-based chemotherapy.
4. FDA-approved for the treatment of deleterious or suspected deleterious germline BRCA-mutated, HER2-negative metastatic breast cancer that has been treated with chemotherapy in the neoadjuvant, adjuvant, or metastatic setting. Patients with hormone receptor–positive breast cancer should have been treated with prior endocrine therapy or be considered inappropriate for endocrine therapy.
5. FDA-approved for the adjuvant treatment of deleterious or suspected deleterious germline BRCA-mutated, HER2-negative high-risk early-stage breast cancer that has been treated with neoadjuvant or adjuvant chemotherapy.
6. FDA-approved for the maintenance treatment of deleterious or suspected deleterious germline or somatic BRCA-mutated metastatic pancreatic cancer whose disease has not progressed on at least 16 weeks of a first-line platinum-based chemotherapy regimen.

7. FDA-approved for the maintenance treatment of deleterious or suspected deleterious germline or somatic homologous recombination repair (HRR) gene-mutated metastatic castration-resistant prostate cancer following progression on prior treatment with enzalutamide or abiraterone.

DOSAGE RANGE

1. Advanced ovarian cancer: 300 mg PO bid. The previous recommended capsule dose was 400 mg PO bid.
2. Ovarian cancer maintenance therapy: 300 mg PO bid.
3. Metastatic breast cancer, pancreatic cancer, and prostate cancer maintenance therapy: 300 mg PO bid.
4. Early-stage breast cancer: 300 mg PO bid.

DRUG INTERACTION 1

Drugs that stimulate liver microsomal CYP3A4 enzymes, including phenytoin, carbamazepine, rifampin, phenobarbital, and St. John's Wort—These drugs may increase the metabolism of olaparib, resulting in lower drug levels and potentially reduced clinical activity.

DRUG INTERACTION 2

Drugs that inhibit liver microsomal CYP3A4 enzymes, including ketoconazole, itraconazole, erythromycin, and clarithromycin—These drugs may reduce the metabolism of olaparib, resulting in increased drug levels and potentially increased toxicity.

SPECIAL CONSIDERATIONS

1. Olaparib has not been studied in patients with liver impairment, and there are no formal recommendations for dosing in this setting.
2. No dose modification is needed in patients with mild renal impairment (CrCl 50–80 mL/min). Olaparib has not been studied in patients with moderate or severe renal impairment. There are no formal recommendations for dosing in this setting.
3. Olaparib capsules should be swallowed whole and should not be chewed, dissolved, or crushed.
4. Olaparib capsules are in the process of being phased out, and only olaparib tablets will be available. Patients need to be educated that olaparib tablets and capsules are **NOT** interchangeable.
5. Closely monitor for new onset of pulmonary symptoms, and if pneumonitis is confirmed, olaparib therapy should be stopped.
6. Closely monitor blood counts at monthly intervals. For prolonged hematologic toxicities, interrupt therapy and monitor CBCs on a weekly basis until recovery. If blood counts have not recovered within 4 weeks, bone marrow analysis and peripheral blood for cytogenetics should be performed to rule out the possibility of MDS/AML.
7. Pregnancy category D.

TOXICITY 1
Fatigue, anorexia, and asthenia.

TOXICITY 2
Increased risk of infections, with nasopharyngitis, pharyngitis, and URI.

TOXICITY 3
Pneumonitis with dyspnea, fever, cough, and wheezing.

TOXICITY 4
GI side effects in the form of nausea/vomiting, abdominal pain, diarrhea, and constipation.

TOXICITY 5
Arthralgias and myalgias.

TOXICITY 6
Myelosuppression with anemia, thrombocytopenia, and neutropenia.

TOXICITY 7
MDS and AML.

Olutasidenib

TRADE NAME	Rezlidhia	CLASSIFICATION	Signal transduction inhibitor, IDH inhibitor
CATEGORY	Targeted agent	DRUG MANUFACTURER	Rigel Pharmaceuticals and Forma Therapeutics

MECHANISM OF ACTION
- Highly potent, orally bioavailable small-molecule inhibitor of isocitrate dehydrogenase 1 (IDH1). Specifically targets the mutant IDH2 variants R140Q, R172S, and R172K at significantly lower concentrations than the wild-type IDH enzyme.
- IDH1 mutations occur in about 10% of AML patients. These mutations are associated with an increased level of an oncometabolite

2-hydroxyglutarate (2-HG), which induces a block in cell differentiation, epigenetic dysregulation with aberrant histone and DNA methylation, and inhibition of apoptosis through BCL-2.
- Treatment leads to reduced 2-HG levels, induces myeloid differentiation, and reduces abnormal histone hypermethylation.

MECHANISM OF RESISTANCE
- Second-site IDH1 mutations.
- IDH2 mutations through trans or cis dimer-interface mutations.
- Mutations in NRAS and MAPK genes leading to activation of NRAS and MAPK signaling.
- Mutations in other receptor tyrosine kinase (RTK) pathway genes, such as KRAS, PTPN11, KIT, and FLT3.

ABSORPTION
Oral bioavailability is approximately 57%. Peak plasma drug levels are achieved in 4 hours after ingestion. Food with high fat content significantly increases AUC and C_{max}.

DISTRIBUTION
Extensive binding (93%) to plasma proteins. Steady-state drug levels are reached in approximately 14 days.

METABOLISM
Metabolism in the liver primarily by CYP3A4 and minor contribution by CYP2C8, CYP2C9, CYP1A2, and CYP2C19. Following drug administration, 75% of an administered dose is eliminated in feces and 17% is eliminated in urine. The terminal half-life is approximately 67 hours.

INDICATIONS
FDA-approved for relapsed or refractory AML with an IDH1 mutation as detected by an FDA-approved diagnostic test.

DOSAGE RANGE
Recommended dose is 100 mg PO daily.

DRUG INTERACTION 1
Drugs such as ketoconazole, itraconazole, erythromycin, clarithromycin, atazanavir, indinavir, nefazodone, nelfinavir, ritonavir, saquinavir, telithromycin, and voriconazole may decrease the metabolism of olutasidenib, resulting in increased drug levels and potentially increased toxicity.

DRUG INTERACTION 2
Drugs such as rifampin, phenytoin, phenobarbital, carbamazepine, and St. John's Wort may increase the metabolism of olutasidenib, resulting in lower effective drug levels.

SPECIAL CONSIDERATIONS

1. Dose reduction is not required in the setting of mild or moderate hepatic impairment (Child-Pugh Class A and B). Has not been studied in the setting of severe hepatic impairment.
2. Dose reduction is not required in patients with mild or moderate renal impairment (CrCl >30 mL/min). Has not been studied in the setting of severe renal impairment or in patients with end-stage renal disease or on dialysis.
3. Monitor for the development of the differentiation syndrome, which may be fatal if not appropriately treated. Can present as early as 10 days and up to 5 months after start of therapy. Steroids (dexamethasone 10 mg IV every 12 hours) should be initiated if differentiation syndrome is suspected with hemodynamic monitoring. This is a black-box warning.
4. Monitor CBCs and blood chemistries at baseline and at least once weekly for the first 2 months, once every other week for the third month, once in the fourth month, and once every other month thereafter for the duration of therapy.
5. Patients should be selected based on the presence of IDH1 mutations in the blood or bone marrow.
6. May cause fetal harm when administered to a pregnant woman. Breastfeeding should be avoided.

TOXICITY 1
Hepatotoxicity with elevations in LFTs and serum bilirubin.

TOXICITY 2
Differentiation syndrome with dyspnea, hypoxia, pulmonary infiltrates, pleural effusion, fever, pericardial effusion, and peripheral edema. Hepatic, renal, and multi-organ dysfunction have also been observed.

TOXICITY 3
Myelosuppression with neutropenia, anemia, and thrombocytopenia.

TOXICITY 4
Nausea/vomiting and diarrhea.

TOXICITY 5
Fatigue and anorexia.

TOXICITY 6
Non-infectious leukocytosis.

TOXICITY 7
QT prolongation is a rare event.

Omacetaxine mepesuccinate

TRADE NAME	Synribo	CLASSIFICATION	Protein synthesis inhibitor, Bcr-Abl inhibitor
CATEGORY	Targeted agent	DRUG MANUFACTURER	Cephalon/Teva

MECHANISM OF ACTION
- Precise mechanism of action not fully characterized but is independent of direct binding to Bcr-Abl.
- Inhibits protein translation by preventing the initial elongation step. It does so by interacting with the ribosomal A-site and preventing the correct positioning of amino acid side chains of incoming aminoacyl-tRNAs.
- Reduces protein expression of Bcr-Abl and Mcl-1 independent of direct Bcr-Abl binding.
- Induces apoptosis through mitochondrial disruption and cytochrome c release, leading to caspase-9 and caspase-3 activation.
- Has preclinical in vivo activity against wild-type and T315I-mutated Bcr-Abl CML.

MECHANISM OF RESISTANCE
None well characterized to date.

ABSORPTION
Following SC administration, maximum drug concentrations are achieved within 30 minutes. The absolute SC bioavailability has not yet been determined.

DISTRIBUTION
Binding to plasma proteins is <50%.

METABOLISM
Omacetaxine mepesuccinate is primarily hydrolyzed to 4'-DMHHT by plasma esterases, with minimal hepatic microsomal oxidative and/or esterase-mediated metabolism. The major route of drug elimination is unknown at this time. Less than 15% of an administered dose of drug is excreted unchanged in the urine. The mean half-life is approximately 6 hours.

INDICATIONS

FDA-approved for adult patients with chronic or accelerated phase chronic myeloid leukemia (CML) with resistance and/or intolerance to two or more tyrosine kinase inhibitors.

DOSAGE RANGE

1. Recommended induction dose is 1.25 mg/m^2 SC bid for 14 consecutive days every 28 days until patients achieve a hematologic response.
2. Maintenance schedule is 1.25 mg/m^2 SC bid for 7 consecutive days every 28 days.

DRUG INTERACTIONS

None well characterized to date.

SPECIAL CONSIDERATIONS

1. Patients should be weighed and monitored regularly for symptoms and signs of fluid retention, especially when using higher drug doses and in patients age >65 years.
2. Monitor CBC on a weekly basis during induction and early maintenance cycles and every 2 weeks during later maintenance cycles.
3. Patients should be warned of the risk of increased bleeding.
4. Patients should avoid anticoagulants, aspirin, and NSAIDs while on therapy.
5. Monitor blood glucose levels frequently in patients with diabetes or in patients with risk factors for diabetes. Omacetaxine should be avoided in patients with poorly controlled diabetes until good glycemic control has been established.
6. Pregnancy category D. Breastfeeding should be avoided.

TOXICITY 1

Myelosuppression with thrombocytopenia, neutropenia, and anemia. Febrile neutropenia observed in 20% of patients.

TOXICITY 2

Impaired glucose tolerance with severe hyperglycemia in up to 10% of patients.

TOXICITY 3

Increased risk of bleeding complications in the setting of thrombocytopenia. Severe, nonfatal GI bleeding occurs rarely (2%), as well as cerebral bleeding leading to death (2%).

TOXICITY 4

Gastrointestinal toxicity with diarrhea, nausea/vomiting, abdominal pain, and anorexia.

TOXICITY 5

Mild to moderate headaches occur in nearly 20%.

TOXICITY 6
Fatigue and asthenia.

TOXICITY 7
Injection site reactions.

Osimertinib

TRADE NAME	Tagrisso	**CLASSIFICATION**	Signal transduction inhibitor, EGFR TKI
CATEGORY	Targeted agent	**DRUG MANUFACTURER**	AstraZeneca

MECHANISM OF ACTION
- Potent and selective small-molecule inhibitor of the EGFR, which binds irreversibly to specific mutant forms of EGFR, including T790M, L858R, and exon 19 deletion.
- Inhibition of these EGFR mutants results in inhibition of critical mitogenic and antiapoptotic signals involved in proliferation, growth, invasion/metastasis, angiogenesis, and response to chemotherapy and/or radiation therapy.

MECHANISM OF RESISTANCE
- Loss of T790M mutation.
- EGFR C797S mutation.
- KRAS mutations.
- Amplification of the c-Met gene, with increased gene copy number.
- BRAF mutations.
- Activation/induction of alternative cellular signaling pathways such as PI3K/Akt.
- Small cell transformation.

ABSORPTION

Oral bioavailability is on the order of 92%. Peak plasma drug levels are achieved in 2–5 hours after ingestion. Can be taken with or without food.

DISTRIBUTION

Extensive binding to plasma proteins. Steady-state drug levels are reached in approximately 15 days.

METABOLISM

Metabolism in the liver primarily by CYP3A4 microsomal enzymes, with formation of two active metabolites, AZ7550 and AZ5104. Elimination is mainly hepatic (approximately 70%), with excretion in the feces. The mean exposure of each of these metabolites was approximately 10% of the exposure of parent drug at steady state. Renal elimination of parent drug and its metabolites account for only about 14% of an administered dose. The terminal half-life of the parent drug is 48 hours.

INDICATIONS

1. FDA-approved for metastatic NSCLC with EGFR T790M mutation as detected by an FDA-approved test following progression on or after EGFR TKI therapy.
2. FDA-approved for first-line treatment of metastatic NSCLC with EGFR exon 19 deletions or exon 21 L858R mutations as detected by an FDA-approved test.
3. FDA-approved for adjuvant therapy of early-stage NSCLC with EGFR exon 19 deletions or exon 21 L858R mutation.

DOSAGE RANGE

1. Adjuvant therapy: recommended dose is 80 mg/day PO for up to 3 years.
2. Metastatic NSCLC: recommended dose is 80 mg/day PO

DRUG INTERACTION 1

Phenytoin and other drugs that stimulate the liver microsomal CYP3A4 enzymes, including carbamazepine, rifampin, phenobarbital, and St. John's Wort—These drugs may increase the metabolism of osimertinib, resulting in its inactivation and potentially reduced clinical activity.

DRUG INTERACTION 2

Drugs that inhibit the liver microsomal CYP3A4 enzymes, including ketoconazole, itraconazole, erythromycin, and clarithromycin—These drugs may decrease the metabolism of osimertinib, resulting in increased drug levels and potentially increased toxicity.

DRUG INTERACTION 3

Warfarin—Patients receiving warfarin should be closely monitored for alterations in their clotting parameters (PT and INR) and/or bleeding, as osimertinib may inhibit the metabolism of warfarin by the liver P450 system. Dose of warfarin may require careful adjustment in the presence of osimertinib therapy.

SPECIAL CONSIDERATIONS

1. Dose reduction is not recommended in patients with mild hepatic dysfunction. Has not been studied in patients with moderate or severe hepatic dysfunction, and caution should be used in this setting.
2. Dose reduction is not recommended in patients with mild or moderate renal dysfunction. Has not been studied in patients with severe renal dysfunction, and caution should be used in this setting.
3. Closely monitor patients for new or progressive pulmonary symptoms, including cough, dyspnea, and fever. Osimertinib therapy should be interrupted pending further diagnostic evaluation.
4. Patients should be educated on the increased risk of cardiac toxicities when compared to other EGFR TKIs.
5. Baseline and periodic evaluations of ECG and electrolyte status should be performed while on therapy. If the QTc >500 msec, therapy should be interrupted. Use with caution in patients at risk of developing QT prolongation, including hypokalemia, hypomagnesemia, congenital long QT syndrome, and in patients taking antiarrhythmic medications or any other drugs that may cause QT prolongation.
6. Baseline and periodic evaluations of LVEF should be performed while on therapy. If there is an absolute decrease in LVEF of 10% from baseline and below 50%, therapy should be interrupted for up to 4 weeks. If the LVEF improves to baseline, therapy can resume. However, if the LVEF does not return to baseline, therapy should be terminated. In the setting of symptomatic CHF, therapy should be permanently discontinued.
7. Patients should be warned to avoid sunlight exposure.
8. Avoid Seville oranges, starfruit, pomelos, grapefruit, and grapefruit juice while on osimertinib therapy.
9. Pregnancy category D. Breastfeeding should be avoided.

TOXICITY 1
Skin toxicity in the form of rash, dry skin, pruritus, and nail bed changes.

TOXICITY 2
Diarrhea is most common GI toxicity. Mild nausea/vomiting, mucositis, and constipation are also observed.

TOXICITY 3
Pulmonary toxicity in the form of ILD manifested by increased cough, dyspnea, fever, and pulmonary infiltrates. Observed in approximately 3% of patients.

TOXICITY 4
QTc prolongation.

TOXICITY 5
Fatigue, anorexia, and reduced appetite.

TOXICITY 6
Cardiomyopathy and CHF. Atrial fibrillation has also been observed.

Oxaliplatin

TRADE NAME	Eloxatin, Diaminocyclohexane platinum	**CLASSIFICATION**	Platinum analog
CATEGORY	Chemotherapy drug	**DRUG MANUFACTURER**	Sanofi-Aventis

MECHANISM OF ACTION
- Third-generation platinum compound.
- Cell cycle–nonspecific, with activity in all phases of the cell cycle.
- Covalently binds to DNA, with preferential binding to the N-7 position of guanine and adenine.
- Reacts with two different sites on DNA to produce cross-links, either intrastrand (<90%) or interstrand (<5%). Formation of DNA adducts results in inhibition of DNA synthesis and function as well as inhibition of transcription.
- DNA mismatch repair enzymes are unable to recognize oxaliplatin-DNA adducts in contrast with other platinum-DNA adducts as a result of their bulkier size.
- Binding to nuclear and cytoplasmic proteins may result in additional cytotoxic effects.

MECHANISM OF RESISTANCE
- Decreased drug accumulation due to alterations in cellular transport.
- Increased inactivation by thiol-containing proteins such as glutathione and glutathione-related enzymes.
- Increased DNA repair enzyme activity (e.g., ERCC-1).
- Non–cross-resistant to cisplatin and carboplatin in tumor cells that are deficient in MMR enzymes (e.g., hMHL1, hMSH2).

ABSORPTION
Administered only via the IV route.

DISTRIBUTION
Widely distributed to all tissues, with a 50-fold higher volume of distribution than cisplatin. About 40% of drug is sequestered in red blood cells within 2–5 hours of infusion. Extensive binding to plasma proteins in time-dependent manner (up to 98%).

METABOLISM
Undergoes extensive non-enzymatic conversion to its active cytotoxic species. As observed with cisplatin, oxaliplatin undergoes aquation reaction in the presence of low concentrations of chloride. The major species are monochloro-DACH, dichloro-DACH, and mono-diaquo-DACH platinum. Renal excretion accounts for >50% of oxaliplatin clearance. More than 20 different metabolites have been identified in the urine. Only 2% of drug is excreted in feces. Prolonged terminal half-life of up to 240 hours.

INDICATIONS
1. Metastatic colorectal cancer—FDA-approved in combination with infusional 5-FU/LV in patients with advanced, metastatic disease.
2. Early-stage colon cancer—FDA-approved as adjuvant therapy in combination with infusional 5-FU/LV in patients with stage III colon cancer and also effective in patients with high-risk stage II disease.
3. Metastatic pancreatic cancer.
4. Metastatic gastric cancer and gastroesophageal cancer.

DOSAGE RANGE
Recommended dose is 85 mg/m^2 IV over 2 hours, on an every-2-week schedule. Can also be administered at 100–130 mg/m^2 IV on an every-3-week schedule.

DRUG INTERACTIONS
None well characterized.

SPECIAL CONSIDERATIONS
1. Use with caution in patients with abnormal renal function, especially when CrCl <20 mL/min. Baseline creatinine clearance should be obtained, and renal status should be closely monitored during treatment.
2. Oxaliplatin should not be administered with basic solutions (e.g., solutions containing 5-FU), as it may be partially degraded.
3. Careful neurologic evaluation should be performed before starting therapy and at the beginning of each cycle, as the dose-limiting toxicity of oxaliplatin is neurotoxicity.
4. Caution patients to avoid exposure to cold following drug administration, which can trigger and/or worsen acute neurotoxicity.
5. Calcium/magnesium infusions (1 g calcium gluconate/1 g magnesium sulfate) prior to and at the completion of the oxaliplatin infusion can be used to reduce the incidence of acute neurotoxicity. There is no evidence that these infusions impair the clinical activity of oxaliplatin.
6. May lengthen oxaliplatin infusion from 2 to up to 4 hours to reduce the development of acute neurotoxicity.
7. Anaphylactic reactions to oxaliplatin have been reported and may occur within minutes of drug administration. This hypersensitivity reaction represents a black-box warning.
8. Monitor EKGs at baseline and periodically during therapy to assess QT interval.
9. Pregnancy category D. Breastfeeding should be avoided.

TOXICITY 1

Neurotoxicity with acute and chronic forms. Acute toxicity seen in up to 80%–85% of patients and characterized by a peripheral sensory neuropathy with distal paresthesia and visual and voice changes, often triggered or exacerbated by cold. Dysesthesias in the upper extremities and laryngopharyngeal region with episodes of difficulty breathing or swallowing can be observed and usually within hours or 1–3 days after therapy. Risk increases upon exposure to cold and usually is spontaneously reversible. Chronic toxicity is dose-dependent, with a 15% and >50% risk of impairment in proprioception and neurosensory function at cumulative doses of 850 and 1,200 mg/m^2, respectively. Oxaliplatin-induced neuropathy appears to be reversible and returns to normal usually within 3–4 months of discontinuation of oxaliplatin. Gait abnormalities and cognitive dysfunction can also occur.

TOXICITY 2

Nausea/vomiting occurs in majority of patients treated with the combination of 5-FU/LV and oxaliplatin. Usually well controlled with antiemetic therapy.

TOXICITY 3

Diarrhea.

TOXICITY 4

Myelosuppression is relatively mild, with thrombocytopenia and anemia more common than neutropenia. Autoimmune thrombocytopenia, autoimmune hemolytic anemia, and TTP also observed, albeit rarely.

TOXICITY 5

Allergic reactions with facial flushing; rash; urticaria; and, less frequently, bronchospasm and hypotension. In rare cases, anaphylactic-like reactions can occur.

TOXICITY 6

Hepatotoxicity with sinusoidal injury resulting in portal hypertension, ascites, splenomegaly, thrombocytopenia, and varices.

TOXICITY 7

RPLS has been observed, with headache, lethargy, seizures, visual disturbances, and encephalopathy.

TOXICITY 8

Rare cases of bronchiolitis obliterans organizing pneumonia (BOOP), acute ILD, and pulmonary fibrosis.

TOXICITY 9

QT prolongation.

TOXICITY 10

Rhabdomyolysis is a rare occurrence.

Paclitaxel

TRADE NAME	Taxol	CLASSIFICATION	Taxane, antimicrotubule agent
CATEGORY	Chemotherapy drug	DRUG MANUFACTURER	Bristol-Myers Squibb

MECHANISM OF ACTION
- Isolated from the bark of the Pacific yew tree, *Taxus brevifolia*.
- Cell cycle–specific, active in the mitosis (M) phase of the cell cycle.
- High-affinity binding to microtubules enhances tubulin polymerization. Normal dynamic process of microtubule network is inhibited, leading to inhibition of mitosis and cell division.

MECHANISM OF RESISTANCE
- Alterations in tubulin with decreased binding affinity for drug.
- Multidrug-resistant phenotype, with increased expression of P170 glycoprotein. Results in enhanced drug efflux, with decreased intracellular accumulation of drug. Cross-resistant to other natural products, including vinca alkaloids, anthracyclines, taxanes, and etoposide.

ABSORPTION
Administered only via the IV route.

DISTRIBUTION
Widely distributed to all body tissues, including third-space fluid collections such as ascites. Negligible penetration into the CNS. Extensive binding (>90%) to plasma and cellular proteins.

METABOLISM

Metabolized extensively by the hepatic P450 microsomal system. About 70%–80% of drug is excreted via fecal elimination. Less than 10% is eliminated as the parent form, with the majority being eliminated as metabolites. Renal clearance is relatively minor, with less than 10% of drug cleared via the kidneys. Terminal elimination half-life ranges from 9 to 50 hours depending on the schedule of administration.

INDICATIONS

1. Ovarian cancer.
2. Breast cancer.
3. SCLC and NSCLC.
4. Head and neck cancer.
5. Esophageal cancer.
6. Prostate cancer.
7. Bladder cancer.
8. AIDS-related Kaposi's sarcoma.

DOSAGE RANGE

1. Ovarian cancer: 135–175 mg/m^2 IV as a 3-hour infusion every 3 weeks.
2. Breast cancer: 175 mg/m^2 IV as a 3-hour infusion every 3 weeks.
3. Bladder cancer, head and neck cancer: 250 mg/m^2 IV as a 24-hour infusion every 3 weeks.
4. Weekly schedule: 80–100 mg/m^2 IV each week for 3 weeks with 1 week of rest.
5. Infusional schedule: 140 mg/m^2 as a 96-hour infusion.

DRUG INTERACTION 1

Radiation therapy—Paclitaxel is a radiosensitizing agent.

DRUG INTERACTION 2

Concomitant use of inhibitors and/or activators of the liver P450 CYP3A4 enzyme system may affect paclitaxel metabolism and its subsequent antitumor and toxic effects.

DRUG INTERACTION 3

Phenytoin, phenobarbital—These drugs accelerate the metabolism of paclitaxel, resulting in lower plasma levels of drug and potentially reduced clinical activity.

DRUG INTERACTION 4

Cisplatin—Myelosuppression is greater when cisplatin is administered before paclitaxel as cisplatin inhibits plasma clearance of paclitaxel. When cisplatin is used in combination, paclitaxel must be given first. No such sequence interaction holds for carboplatin and paclitaxel.

DRUG INTERACTION 5
Cyclophosphamide—Myelosuppression is greater when cyclophosphamide is administered before paclitaxel.

DRUG INTERACTION 6
Doxorubicin—Paclitaxel reduces the plasma clearance of doxorubicin by about 30%, resulting in increased severity of myelosuppression.

SPECIAL CONSIDERATIONS
1. Contraindicated in patients with history of severe hypersensitivity reaction to paclitaxel or to other drugs formulated in Cremophor EL, including cyclosporine, etoposide, or teniposide.
2. Use with caution in patients with abnormal liver function. Dose reduction is recommended in this setting. Patients with abnormal liver function are at higher risk for toxicity. Contraindicated in patients with severe hepatic dysfunction.
3. Use with caution in patients with prior history of diabetes mellitus and chronic alcoholism or prior therapy with known neurotoxic agents such as cisplatin.
4. Use with caution in patients with previous history of ischemic heart disease, with MI within the preceding 6 months, conduction system abnormalities, or on medications known to alter cardiac conduction (beta blockers, calcium channel blockers, and digoxin).
5. Patients should receive premedication to prevent the incidence of hypersensitivity reactions (HSRs). Administer dexamethasone 20 mg PO at 12 and 6 hours before drug administration, diphenhydramine 50 mg IV, and cimetidine 300 mg IV at 30 minutes before drug administration. Patients experiencing major hypersensitivity reaction may be rechallenged after receiving multiple high doses of steroids, dexamethasone 20 mg IV every 6 hours for 4 doses. Patients should also be treated with diphenhydramine 50 mg IV and cimetidine 300 mg IV 30 minutes before the rechallenge. HSRs usually not observed with prolonged drug infusion.
6. Medical personnel should be readily available at the time of drug administration. Emergency equipment, including Ambu bag, ECG machine, IV fluids, pressors, and other drugs for resuscitation, must be at bedside before initiation of treatment.
7. Monitor patient's vital signs every 15 minutes during the first hour of drug administration. Hypersensitivity reaction usually occurs within 2–3 minutes of start of infusion and almost always within the first 10 minutes.
8. Patients who have received >6 courses of weekly paclitaxel should be advised to avoid sun exposure of their skin as well as their fingernails and toenails, as they are at increased risk for developing onycholysis. This side effect is not observed with the every-3-week schedule.
9. Pregnancy category D. Breastfeeding should be avoided.

TOXICITY 1

Myelosuppression with neutropenia is dose-limiting. Decreased incidence of neutropenia with 3-hour schedule when compared to 24-hour schedule.

TOXICITY 2

Infusion reactions occur in up to 20%–40% of patients. Characterized by generalized skin rash, flushing, erythema, hypotension, dyspnea, and/or bronchospasm. Usually occurs within the first 2–3 minutes of an infusion and almost always within the first 10 minutes. Incidence of infusion reaction is the same with 3- and 24-hour schedules.

TOXICITY 3

Neurotoxicity mainly in the form of sensory neuropathy with numbness and paresthesias. Dose-dependent effect. Other risk factors include prior exposure to known neurotoxic agents (e.g., cisplatin) and pre-existing medical disorders such as diabetes mellitus and chronic alcoholism. More frequent with longer infusions and at doses >175 mg/m^2. Motor and autonomic neuropathy observed at high doses. Optic nerve disturbances with scintillating scotomata observed rarely.

TOXICITY 4

Transient asymptomatic sinus bradycardia is most common cardiotoxicity. Occurs in 30% of patients. Other rhythm disturbances are seen, including Mobitz type I, Mobitz type II, and third-degree heart block, as well as ventricular arrhythmias.

TOXICITY 5

Alopecia occurs in nearly all patients with loss of total body hair.

TOXICITY 6

Mucositis and/or diarrhea seen in 30%–40% of patients. Mucositis is more common with the 24-hour schedule. Mild to moderate nausea and vomiting, usually of brief duration.

TOXICITY 7

Transient elevations in serum transaminases, bilirubin, and alkaline phosphatase.

TOXICITY 8

Onycholysis. Mainly observed in patients receiving >6 courses on the weekly schedule. Not usually seen with the every-3-week schedule.

Palbociclib

TRADE NAME	Ibrance, PD 0332991	CLASSIFICATION	Signal transduction inhibitor, CDK inhibitor
CATEGORY	Targeted agent	DRUG MANUFACTURER	Pfizer

MECHANISM OF ACTION
- Inhibitor of cyclin-dependent kinase (CDK) 4 and 6.
- Inhibition of CDK 4/6 leads to inhibition of cell proliferation and growth by blocking progression of cells from G1 to the S-phase of the cell cycle.
- Decreased retinoblastoma (Rb) protein phosphorylation, resulting in reduced E2F expression and signaling.
- Induces cell senescence.

MECHANISM OF RESISTANCE
- Acquired CDK6 amplification resulting in increased CDK6 expression.
- Increased expression of CDK2 and CDK4.
- Loss of pRb expression.
- Overexpression of cyclins A and E.
- FGFR1 gene amplification.
- Increased expression of 3-phosphoinositide-dependent protein kinase 1 (PDK1) with activation of AKT pathway and other AGC kinases.

ABSORPTION
Oral bioavailability is on the order of 46%. Food intake appears to reduce the interpatient variability of drug exposure.

DISTRIBUTION
Significant binding (85%) to plasma proteins and extensive tissue distribution. Steady-state drug levels are achieved within 8 days following repeat daily dosing.

METABOLISM
Extensively metabolized in the liver primarily by CYP3A4 microsomal enzymes, with oxidation and sulfonation reactions being most important. Acylation and glucuronidation play only minor roles in drug metabolism. Nearly 92% of drug is recovered, with 74% in feces and 17.5% in urine, with the majority of drug being in metabolite form. The elimination half-life of the drug is 26 hours.

INDICATIONS

1. FDA-approved in combination with an aromatase inhibitor as initial endocrine-based therapy in postmenopausal women with hormone receptor (HR)–positive, HER2-negative advanced or metastatic breast cancer.
2. FDA-approved in combination with fulvestrant for patients with HR-positive, HER2-negative advanced or metastatic breast cancer in women with disease progression following endocrine therapy.

DOSAGE RANGE

Recommended dose is 125 mg PO daily for 21 days followed by 7 days off.

DRUG INTERACTION 1

Drugs that stimulate liver microsomal CYP3A4 enzymes, including phenytoin, carbamazepine, rifampin, phenobarbital, and St. John's Wort—These drugs may increase the metabolism of palbociclib, resulting in lower drug levels and potentially reduced clinical activity.

DRUG INTERACTION 2

Drugs that inhibit liver microsomal CYP3A4 enzymes, including ketoconazole, itraconazole, erythromycin, and clarithromycin—These drugs may reduce the metabolism of palbociclib, resulting in increased drug levels and potentially increased toxicity.

SPECIAL CONSIDERATIONS

1. Dose reduction is not required in the setting of mild hepatic impairment. Use with caution in patients with moderate or severe hepatic impairment, although no specific dose recommendations have been provided.
2. Dose reduction is not required in the setting of mild and moderate renal impairment. Use with caution in patients with severe renal impairment, as palbociclib has not been studied in this setting.
3. Closely monitor CBC and platelet count every 2 weeks during the first 2 months of therapy and at monthly intervals thereafter.
4. Monitor for signs and symptoms of infection.
5. Monitor for signs and symptoms of pulmonary embolism.
6. Pregnancy category D.

TOXICITY 1

Myelosuppression with neutropenia, anemia, and thrombocytopenia.

TOXICITY 2

Fatigue and anorexia.

TOXICITY 3

Increased risk of infections, with URI being most common.

TOXICITY 4
Nausea/vomiting, abdominal pain, and diarrhea.

TOXICITY 5
Increased risk of pulmonary emboli.

TOXICITY 6
Alopecia.

Panitumumab

TRADE NAME	Vectibix	**CLASSIFICATION**	Monoclonal antibody, anti-EGFR antibody
CATEGORY	Targeted agent	**DRUG MANUFACTURER**	Amgen

MECHANISM OF ACTION
- Fully human IgG2 monoclonal antibody directed against the EGFR.
- Binds with nearly 40-fold higher affinity to EGFR than normal ligands EGF and TGF-α, which results in inhibition of EGFR. Prevents both homodimerization and heterodimerization of the EGFR, which leads to inhibition of autophosphorylation and inhibition of EGFR signaling.
- Inhibition of the EGFR pathway results in inhibition of critical mitogenic and anti-apoptotic signals involved in proliferation, growth, invasion/metastasis, and angiogenesis.
- Inhibition of the EGFR pathway enhances the response to chemotherapy and/or radiation therapy.
- In contrast to cetuximab, immunologic-mediated mechanisms are not involved in antitumor activity as the antibody is of the IgG2 isotype.

MECHANISM OF RESISTANCE
- Mutations in EGFR, leading to reduced binding affinity to panitumumab.
- Reduced expression of EGFR.
- KRAS mutations, which mainly occur in codons 12 and 13.
- BRAF mutations.
- NRAS mutations.
- Increased expression of HER2 through gene amplification.
- Increased expression of HER3.
- Activation/induction of alternative cellular signaling pathways, such as PI3K/Akt and IGF-1R.
- Increased expression of lncRNA MIR100HG and two embedded miRNAs, miR-100 and miR-125, that leads to activation of Wnt signaling.

DISTRIBUTION
Distribution in the body is not well characterized.

METABOLISM
Metabolism of panitumumab has not been extensively characterized. Pharmacokinetic studies showed clearance of antibody was saturated at a weekly dose of 2 mg/kg. Half-life is on the order of 6–7 days.

INDICATIONS
1. FDA-approved as monotherapy for the treatment of wild-type RAS metastatic colorectal cancer (mCRC) following prior therapy with fluoropyrimidine-, oxaliplatin-, and irinotecan-containing regimens.
2. FDA-approved for the first-line treatment of wild-type RAS mCRC in combination with FOLFOX chemotherapy.
3. Approved in Europe in first-line treatment of wild-type RAS mCRC in combination with FOLFOX or FOLFIRI; in second-line treatment in combination with FOLFIRI for mCRC patients who have progressed on first-line oxaliplatin-based chemotherapy; and as monotherapy after progression on fluoropyrimidine-, oxaliplatin-, and irinotecan-containing regimens.

DOSAGE RANGE
1. Recommended dose for mCRC is 6 mg/kg IV on an every-2-week schedule.
2. An alternative schedule is 2.5 mg/kg IV every week.

DRUG INTERACTIONS
No formal drug interactions have been characterized to date.

SPECIAL CONSIDERATIONS
1. The incidence of infusion reactions is lower when compared with cetuximab, as panitumumab is a fully human antibody. Reduce infusion rate by 50% in patients who experience grade 1/2 infusion reaction for the duration of that infusion. The infusion should be terminated in patients who experience a severe infusion reaction.
2. The level of EGFR expression does not correlate with clinical activity, and as such, EGFR testing is required for clinical use.
3. Extended RAS testing should be performed in all patients to determine KRAS and NRAS status. Only patients whose tumors express wild-type KRAS and NRAS should receive panitumumab, either as monotherapy or in combination with chemotherapy.
4. Development of skin toxicity appears to be a surrogate marker for panitumumab clinical activity. Refer to the prescribing information for dose modifications in the setting of skin toxicity.
5. Use with caution in patients with underlying ILD, as these patients are at increased risk for developing worsening of their ILD.

6. In patients who develop a skin rash, topical antibiotics such as clindamycin gel or erythromycin cream/gel or oral clindamycin, oral doxycycline, or oral minocycline may help. Patients should be warned to avoid sunlight exposure. This represents a black-box warning.
7. Electrolyte status (magnesium and calcium) should be closely monitored during therapy and for up to 8 weeks after completion of therapy.
8. May cause fetal harm. Females of reproductive potential should be advised of the potential risk to the fetus. Should also be advised to use effective contraception during treatment and for 2 months after the last dose. Breastfeeding should be avoided while on therapy and for 2 months after the last dose.

TOXICITY 1
Pruritus, dry skin with mainly a pustular, acneiform skin rash. Presents mainly on the face and upper trunk. Improves with continued treatment and resolves upon cessation of therapy. Skin toxicity occurs in up to 90% of patients, with grade 3/4 toxicity occurring in 15% of patients.

TOXICITY 2
Infusion-related symptoms with fever, chills, urticaria, flushing, and headache. Usually minor in severity and observed most commonly with administration of the first infusion.

TOXICITY 3
Pulmonary toxicity in the form of ILD manifested by increased cough, dyspnea, and pulmonary infiltrates. Observed rarely in less than 1% of patients and more frequent in patients with underlying pulmonary disease.

TOXICITY 4
Hypomagnesemia.

TOXICITY 5
Diarrhea.

TOXICITY 6
Asthenia and generalized malaise in up to 10%–15% of patients.

TOXICITY 7
Paronychial inflammation with swelling of the lateral nail folds of the toes and fingers. Usually occurs with prolonged use of panitumumab.

Panobinostat

TRADE NAME	Farydak, LBH 589	CLASSIFICATION	Histone deacetylase (HDAC) inhibitor
CATEGORY	Chemotherapy drug	DRUG MANUFACTURER	Novartis

MECHANISM OF ACTION
- Potent pan-inhibitor of histone deacetylase (HDAC) enzymes.
- Inhibition of HDAC activity leads to accumulation of acetyl groups on the histone lysine residues, resulting in open chromatin structure and transcriptional activation.
- HDAC inhibition activates differentiation, inhibits the cell cycle, and induces cell cycle arrest and apoptosis.
- Increased expression of HDAC in human tumors, including multiple myeloma.

MECHANISM OF RESISTANCE
- Increased expression and activity of the chemokine receptor CXCR4.
- Activation of mTOR signaling.

DISTRIBUTION
Approximately 90% of drug is bound to plasma proteins. Oral bioavailability is on the order of 21%, and peak plasma levels are achieved within 2 hours after ingestion.

METABOLISM
Extensively metabolized in the liver by microsomal enzymes, with CYP3A4 accounting for about 40% of drug metabolism. Only 2% of parent drug is recovered in urine. The drug is a P-glycoprotein substrate and a CYP2D6 inhibitor. Approximately equal amounts of an administered dose of drug are excreted in feces and in urine, and only less than 2% of parent drug is recovered in urine. The elimination half-life is on the order of 30 hours.

INDICATIONS

FDA-approved for patients with multiple myeloma who have received at least two prior regimens, including bortezomib and an immunomodulatory agent.

DOSAGE RANGE

Recommended dose is 20 mg PO on days 1, 3, 5, 8, 10, and 12 of weeks 1 and 2, with cycles repeated every 21 days for 8 cycles.

DRUG INTERACTION 1

Drugs that stimulate liver microsomal CYP3A4 enzymes, including phenytoin, carbamazepine, rifampin, phenobarbital, and St. John's Wort—These drugs may increase the metabolism of panobinostat, resulting in lower drug levels and potentially reduced clinical activity.

DRUG INTERACTION 2

Drugs that inhibit liver microsomal CYP3A4 enzymes, including ketoconazole, itraconazole, erythromycin, and clarithromycin—These drugs may reduce the metabolism of panobinostat, resulting in increased drug levels and potentially increased toxicity.

DRUG INTERACTION 3

Drugs that serve as substrates of CYP2D6, including perphenazine, atomoxetine, desipramine, dextromethorphan, metoprolol, nebivolol, tolterodine, and venlafaxine—Panobinostat is a CYP2D6 inhibitor, and co-administration with CYP2D6 substrates may result in higher drug levels and potentially increased toxicity.

SPECIAL CONSIDERATIONS

1. Dose modification is recommended in the setting of mild or moderate hepatic impairment. Should not be administered to patients with severe hepatic impairment, as the drug has not been studied in this setting.
2. Can be used safely in patients with mild, moderate, or severe renal dysfunction. It has not been studied in patients with end-stage renal disease or in those undergoing dialysis.
3. Closely monitor patients for diarrhea, which can occur at any time. Important to monitor the hydration status of the patient and closely follow serum electrolytes, including potassium, magnesium, and phosphate. Anti-diarrheal medication should be started at the onset of diarrhea, and panobinostat should be interrupted with the onset of moderate diarrhea. This represents a black-box warning.
4. Closely monitor for cardiac toxicities, which include ECG changes, arrhythmias, and cardiac ischemic events. Should not be given to patients with history of recent MI or unstable angina. This represents a black-box warning.

5. Monitor CBC and platelet count on a weekly basis during treatment.
6. Monitor liver function tests before treatment and before the start of each cycle. Interrupt and/or adjust dosage until recovery, or permanently discontinue based on the severity of the hepatic toxicity.
7. Monitor ECG with QTc measurement at baseline and periodically during therapy, as QTc prolongation has been observed.
8. Monitor patients for infections, as pneumonia, bacterial infections, fungal infections, and viral infections have been observed. Therapy should be interrupted and/or terminated with the development of active infections.
9. Pregnancy category D.

TOXICITY 1
Diarrhea and nausea/vomiting are the most common GI side effects.

TOXICITY 2
Myelosuppression with thrombocytopenia and neutropenia more common than anemia.

TOXICITY 3
Cardiac toxicity with ECG changes, arrhythmias, and cardiac ischemic events. QTc prolongation has been observed.

TOXICITY 4
Hepatotoxicity.

TOXICITY 5
Increased risk of infections with pneumonia, bacterial infections, fungal infections, and viral infections.

TOXICITY 6
Electrolyte abnormalities with hypokalemia, hypomagnesemia, and hypophosphatemia.

TOXICITY 7
Peripheral neuropathy.

Pazopanib

TRADE NAME	Votrient	**CLASSIFICATION**	Signal transduction inhibitor, TKI
CATEGORY	Targeted agent	**DRUG MANUFACTURER**	GlaxoSmithKline

MECHANISM OF ACTION
- Oral multikinase inhibitor of angiogenesis.
- Inhibits VEGFR-1, VEGFR-2, VEGFR-3, platelet-derived growth factor receptor (PDGFR)-α and PDGFR–β, fibroblast growth factor receptor (FGFR)-1 and FGFR-3, c-Kit, interleukin-2 receptor inducible T-cell kinase (Itk), leukocyte-specific protein tyrosine kinase (Lck), and transmembrane glycoprotein receptor tyrosine kinase (c-Fms).

MECHANISM OF RESISTANCE
- Increased expression of VEGFR-1, VEGFR-2, VEGFR-3, PDGFR, FGFR, and c-Kit.
- Mutations in target receptors, resulting in alterations in drug-binding affinity.
- Activation of angiogenic switch, with increased expression of alternative pro-angiogenic pathways.
- Increased pericyte coverage to tumor vessels, with increased expression of VEGF and other pro-angiogenic factors.
- Recruitment of pro-angiogenic inflammatory cells from bone marrow, such as tumor-associated macrophages, monocytes, and myeloid-derived suppressor cells (MDSCs).

ABSORPTION
Oral bioavailability ranges from 14% to 39% with median time to peak concentrations of 2–4 hours. Systemic exposure to pazopanib is increased when administered with food.

DISTRIBUTION
Extensive binding (>99%) of pazopanib to plasma proteins.

METABOLISM

Pazopanib undergoes oxidative metabolism primarily by CYP3A4 microsomal enzymes and to a lesser extent by CYP1A2 and CYP2C8 isoenzymes. Pazopanib is a weak inhibitor of CYP2C8 and CYP2D6, as well as UGT1A1 and OATP1B1, and it is a substrate for P-glycoprotein. Elimination is primarily via the hepatobiliary route with excretion in feces, with renal elimination accounting for less than 4% of the administered dose. In patients with moderate hepatic impairment, clearance is decreased by 50%. A plateau in steady-state drug exposure is observed at doses of ≥800 mg once daily, and the half-life is 31 hours.

INDICATIONS

1. FDA-approved for advanced renal cell carcinoma.
2. FDA-approved for advanced soft tissue sarcoma (STS) following treatment with prior chemotherapy. The efficacy of pazopanib has not been documented in adipocytic STS or GIST.

DOSAGE RANGE

Recommended dose is 800 mg PO once daily without food at least 1 hour before or 2 hours after a meal.

DRUG INTERACTION 1

Concomitant administration of CYP3A4 inhibitors such as ketoconazole, itraconazole, clarithromycin, atazanavir, indinavir, nefazodone, nelfinavir, ritonavir, saquinavir, telithromycin, and voriconazole decreases pazopanib metabolism, resulting in increased drug levels and potentially increased toxicity.

DRUG INTERACTION 2

Concomitant administration of CYP3A4 inducers such as phenytoin, carbamazepine, rifampin, phenobarbital, and St. John's Wort increases pazopanib metabolism, resulting in its inactivation and reduced effective drug levels.

SPECIAL CONSIDERATIONS

1. Baseline and periodic evaluation of liver function tests (at weeks 3, 5, 7, and 9 and at months 3 and 4) should be performed while on pazopanib therapy. Patients with isolated SGOT elevations between 3 × ULN and 8 × ULN may be continued on therapy with weekly monitoring of LFTs until they return to grade 1 or baseline. In this setting, the dose of pazopanib should be reduced to 200 mg PO once daily. Patients with isolated SGOT elevations of more than 8 × ULN should have pazopanib therapy interrupted.
2. Use with caution in patients with moderate hepatic impairment, as drug clearance is reduced by at least 50% in this setting. Should not be used in patients with severe hepatic impairment.
3. Closely monitor ECG with QT measurement at baseline and periodically during therapy, as QT prolongation has been observed. Use with caution in patients at risk of developing QT prolongation, including hypokalemia, hypomagnesemia, and congenital long QT syndrome; patients taking

antiarrhythmic medications or any other products that may cause QT prolongation; and in those with pre-existing cardiac disease.

4. Avoid use in patients with a prior history of hemoptysis and cerebral or clinically significant GI hemorrhage within 6 months of initiation of pazopanib.
5. Use with caution in patients with cardiovascular and cerebrovascular disease, especially those with prior MI, angina, stroke, and TIA.
6. Closely monitor blood pressure while on therapy.
7. Blood pressure should be well controlled prior to initiation of pazopanib.
8. Closely monitor thyroid function tests, as pazopanib therapy results in hypothyroidism.
9. Baseline and periodic urinalysis during treatment is recommended, and pazopanib should be discontinued in the setting of grade 4 proteinuria.
10. Avoid Seville oranges, starfruit, pomelos, grapefruit, and grapefruit products while on pazopanib therapy, as they can inhibit CYP3A4 activity, resulting in increased drug levels.
11. Pregnancy category D. Breastfeeding should be avoided.

TOXICITY 1
Hypertension occurs in nearly 50% of patients. Usually occurs within the first 18 weeks of therapy and usually well controlled with oral antihypertensive medications.

TOXICITY 2
Diarrhea, nausea/vomiting, and abdominal pain are the most common GI side effects. Elevations in serum lipase have been observed in up to 30% of patients. Increased risk of GI fistulas and/or perforations.

TOXICITY 3
Fatigue, asthenia, and anorexia.

TOXICITY 4
Hair color changes with depigmentation.

TOXICITY 5
Bleeding complications with hematuria, epistaxis, and hemoptysis.

TOXICITY 6
Increased risk of arterial thromboembolic events, including MI, angina, TIA, and stroke.

TOXICITY 7
Proteinuria develops in 8% of patients.

TOXICITY 8
Myelosuppression with neutropenia and thrombocytopenia. Usually mild to moderate in severity.

TOXICITY 9

Hypothyroidism.

TOXICITY 10

Elevations in serum transaminases usually observed within the first 18 weeks of therapy. Indirect hyperbilirubinemia may occur in patients with underlying Gilbert's syndrome.

TOXICITY 11

Cardiac toxicity with QT prolongation (≥500 msec) and Torsades de Pointes.

TOXICITY 12

Electrolyte abnormalities with hyperglycemia, hypophosphatemia, hyponatremia, hypomagnesemia, and hypoglycemia.

Pegaspargase

TRADE NAME	Oncaspar	CLASSIFICATION	Enzyme
CATEGORY	Chemotherapy drug	DRUG MANUFACTURER	Servier Pharmarceuticals

MECHANISM OF ACTION

- Pegylated form of native *E. coli*–derived L-asparaginase that is conjugated to polyethylene glycol.
- Pegaspargase has a prolonged circulation time when compared to *E. coli* L-asparaginase, which offers less frequent administration, and has potentially reduced immunogenicity.
- Tumor cells lack asparagine synthetase and thus require exogenous sources of L-asparagine.
- Asparaginase hydrolyzes circulating L-asparagine to aspartic acid and ammonia.
- Depletion of the essential amino acid L-asparagine results in rapid inhibition of protein synthesis as well as inhibition of DNA- and RNA-mediated synthesis. Cytotoxicity of drug correlates with inhibition of protein synthesis.

MECHANISM OF RESISTANCE

- Increased expression of the L-asparagine synthetase gene, which facilitates the cellular production of L-asparagine from endogenous sources.
- Formation of antibodies against L-asparaginase, resulting in inhibition of function.

ABSORPTION
Administered only via the intramuscular (IM) and IV routes. The mean relative bioavailability is 82% following the first IM dose and increases to 98% following repeat dosing.

DISTRIBUTION
After IM injection, peak plasma levels of asparaginase activity are reached on day 5.

METABOLISM
Metabolism is expected to be mediated via catabolic pathways into small peptides and amino acids. The mean elimination half-life is 5.8 days following IM injection and 5.3 days after IV infusion.

INDICATIONS
1. FDA-approved for first-line treatment of ALL
2. FDA-approved for ALL and hypersensitivity to asparaginase.

DOSAGE RANGE
1. Patients <21 years of age: 2,500 IU/m^2 IM or IV no more frequently than every 14 days
2. Patients >21 years of age: 2,000 IU/m^2 IM or IV no more frequently than every 14 days

DRUG INTERACTION 1
Methotrexate—Asparaginase can inhibit the cytotoxic effects of methotrexate and thus reduce methotrexate antitumor activity and toxicity. It is recommended that these drugs be administered 24 hours apart.

DRUG INTERACTION 2
Vincristine—Asparaginase inhibits the clearance of vincristine, resulting in increased toxicity, especially neurotoxicity. Vincristine should be administered 12–24 hours before asparaginase.

SPECIAL CONSIDERATIONS
1. Monitor patient for allergic reactions and/or anaphylaxis. Observe patients for 1 hour after drug administration. Should be administered in a setting with resuscitation equipment and medications to treat anaphylaxis, including oxygen, epinephrine, intravenous steroids, and antihistamines.
2. Induction treatment of acute lymphoblastic leukemia with asparaginase may induce rapid lysis of blast cells. Prophylaxis against tumor lysis syndrome with vigorous IV hydration, urinary alkalinization, and allopurinol is recommended for all patients.

3. Monitor for signs and symptoms of pancreatitis. Contraindicated in patients with either active pancreatitis or a history of pancreatitis. If pancreatitis develops while on therapy, asparaginase should be stopped immediately.
4. Monitor LFTs and serum bilirubin at baseline and every 2–3 weeks.
5. Monitor serum glucose levels as glucose intolerance can occur while on pegaspargase therapy. In some cases, glucose intolerance can be irreversible.
6. Monitor for evidence of bleeding complications, and monitor coagulation parameters (PT, PTT, INR) and fibrinogen levels.
7. Asparaginase can interfere with thyroid function tests. This effect is probably due to a marked reduction in serum concentration of thyroxine-binding globulin, which is observed within 2 days after the first dose. Levels of thyroxine-binding globulin return to normal within 4 weeks of the last dose.
8. The effect of hepatic and renal impairment on pegaspargase has not been studied.
9. Potential risk to a fetus. Women of reproductive potential should use effective non-hormonal contraception while on treatment with pegaspargase and for at least 3 months after the last dose. Breastfeeding should be avoided.

TOXICITY 1
Hypersensitivity reactions. Risk is higher in patients with known hypersensitivity to *E. coli* asparaginase. Mild form manifested by skin rash and urticaria. Anaphylactic reaction may be life-threatening and presents as bronchospasm, respiratory distress, and hypotension.

TOXICITY 2
Pancreatitis with increases in serum amylase and lipase levels.

TOXICITY 3
Glucose intolerance.

TOXICITY 4
Hepatotoxicity with mild elevation in SGOT/SGPT, serum bilirubin, and alkaline phosphatase.

TOXICITY 5
Increased risk of both bleeding and clotting. Alterations in clotting with decreased levels of clotting factors, including fibrinogen, factors IX and XI, antithrombin III, proteins C and S, plasminogen, and α-2-antiplasmin. Observed in over 50% of patients.

Pembrolizumab

TRADE NAME	Keytruda, MK-3475	**CLASSIFICATION**	Anti-PD-1 antibody
CATEGORY	Immunotherapy, immune checkpoint inhibitor	**DRUG MANUFACTURER**	Merck

MECHANISM OF ACTION
- Humanized IgG4 antibody that binds to the PD-1 receptor, which is expressed on T cells, and inhibits the interaction between the PD-L1 and PD-L2 ligands and the PD-1 receptor.
- Blockade of the PD-1 pathway-mediated immune checkpoint enhances T-cell immune response, leading to T-cell activation and proliferation.

MECHANISM OF RESISTANCE
- Increased expression and/or activity of other immune checkpoint pathways (e.g., TIGIT, TIM3, and LAG3).
- Increased expression of other immune escape mechanisms.
- Increased infiltration of immune suppressive populations within the tumor microenvironment, which include Tregs, myeloid-derived suppressor cells (MDSCs), and M2 macrophages.
- Release of various cytokines, chemokines, and metabolites within the tumor microenvironment, including CSF-1, tryptophan metabolites, TGF-β, and adenosine.

DISTRIBUTION
Distribution in body has not been well characterized. Steady-state levels are achieved by 18 weeks.

METABOLISM
Metabolism of pembrolizumab has not been extensively characterized. The terminal half-life is on the order of 26 days.

INDICATIONS
1. FDA-approved for unresectable or metastatic melanoma.
2. FDA-approved for adjuvant treatment of adult and pediatric patients with Stage IIb, IIC, or III melanoma following complete resection.
3. FDA-approved for patients with metastatic NSCLC whose tumors express PD-L1 as determined by an FDA-approved test and who have disease progression on or after platinum-based chemotherapy. Patients with EGFR or ALK genomic alterations should have disease progression on FDA-approved targeted therapy prior to receiving pembrolizumab.
4. FDA-approved in combination with pemetrexed and platinum chemotherapy as first-line treatment of patients with metastatic non-squamous NSCLC with no EGFR or ALK genomic alterations.

5. FDA-approved in combination with carboplatin and either paclitaxel or nab-paclitaxel as first-line treatment of patients with metastatic squamous NSCLC.
6. FDA-approved as a single agent for first-line treatment of patients with NSCLC expressing PD-L1 (Tumor Proportion Score (TPS) >1%), as determined by an FDA-approved test, with no EGFR or ALK genomic alterations and is either metastatic or stage III where patients are not candidates for surgical resection or definitive chemoradiation.
7. FDA-approved as a single agent for adjuvant treatment following resection and platinum-based chemotherapy for patients with Stage IB(T2a>4 cm), II, IIIA NSCLC.
8. FDA-approved as a single agent for recurrent or metastatic head and neck cancer with disease progression on or after platinum-based chemotherapy.
9. FDA-approved as a single agent for first-line treatment of patients with metastatic or unresectable, recurrent head and neck cancer whose tumors express PD-L1 (Combined Positive Score (CPS) >1) as determined by an FDA-approved test.
10. FDA-approved in combination with platinum and 5-FU for first-line treatment of patients with metastatic or unresectable, recurrent head and neck cancer.
11. Clinical activity for metastatic SCLC with disease progression on or after platinum-based chemotherapy and at least 1 other prior line of therapy.
12. FDA-approved for adult and pediatric patients with relapsed or refractory classical Hodgkin's lymphoma or who have relapsed after 2 or more prior lines of therapy.
13. FDA-approved for adult and pediatric patients with refractory primary mediastinal large B-cell lymphoma (PMBCL) or who have relapsed after 2 or more prior lines of therapy.
14. FDA-approved in combination with enfortumab vedotin for patients with locally advanced or metastatic urothelial cancer who are not eligible for cisplatin-containing chemotherapy.
15. FDA-approved for patients with locally advanced or metastatic urothelial cancer who are not eligible for platinum-containing chemotherapy .
16. FDA-approved as a single agent for locally advanced or metastatic urothelial cancer with disease progression during or following platinum-containing chemotherapy or within 12 months of neoadjuvant or adjuvant treatment with platinum-based chemotherapy.
17. FDA-approved for patients with BCG-unresponsive, high-risk, non-muscle invasive bladder cancer with carcinoma in situ with or without papillary tumors who are ineligible for or who have elected not to undergo cystectomy.
18. FDA-approved for adult and pediatric patients with unresectable or metastatic, microsatellite instability-high (MSI-H) or mismatch repair deficient (dMMR) solid tumors that have progressed following prior treatment and/or who have no satisfactory alternative treatment options.
19. FDA-approved for first-line treatment of unresectable or metastatic, MSI-H or dMMR CRC.

20. FDA-approved in combination with trastuzumab, fluoropyrimidine- and platinum-containing chemotherapy for first-line treatment of locally advanced unresectable or metastatic HER2-positive gastric or GEJ adenocarcinoma.
21. FDA-approved for patients with locally advanced or metastatic esophageal or GEJ carcinoma that is not amenable to surgical resection or definitive chemoradiation either in combination with fluoropyrimidine- and platinum-containing chemotherapy or as a single agent after one or more lines of systemic therapy for patients with squamous cell cancer.
22. FDA-approved as a single agent for patients with recurrent locally advanced or metastatic squamous cell cancer of the esophagus whose tumors express PD-L1 (CPS >10) as determined by an FDA-approved test, with disease progression after 1 or more prior lines of systemic therapy.
23. FDA-approved in combination with chemotherapy, with or without bevacizumab, for patients with persistent, recurrent or metastatic cervical cancer whose tumors express PD-L1 (CPS ≥ 1) as determined by an FDA-approved test.
24. FDA-approved as a single agent for patients with recurrent or metastatic cervical cancer with disease progression on or after chemotherapy whose tumors express PD-L1 (CPS ≥ 1) as determined by an FDA-approved test.
25. FDA-approved for patients with hepatocellular cancer (HCC) who have been previously treated with sorafenib.
26. FDA-approved for adult and pediatric patients with recurrent locally advanced or metastatic Merkel cell cancer (MCC).
27. FDA-approved in combination with axitinib for first-line treatment of patients with advanced renal cell cancer (RCC).
28. FDA-approved in combination with lenvatinib for first-line treatment of patients with advanced RCC.
29. FDA-approved for adjuvant therapy of patients with RCC at intermediate-high or high risk of recurrence following nephrectomy, or following nephrectomy and resection of metastatic lesions.
30. FDA-approved in combination with lenvatinib for patients with advanced endometrial cancer that is mismatch repair proficient (pMMR) or not MSI-H and who have disease progression following prior systemic therapy and are not candidates for curative surgery or radiation.
31. FDA-approved as a single agent for patients with advanced endometrial cancer that is MSI-H or dMMR and who have disease progression following prior systemic therapy and who are not candidates for curative surgery or radiation.
32. FDA-approved for adult and pediatric patients with unresectable or metastatic tumor mutational burden-high (TMB-H) (10 mutations/megabase) solid tumors, as determined by an FDA-approved test, that have progressed following prior therapy and who have no satisfactory alternative treatment options.
33. FDA-approved for patients with recurrent or metastatic cutaneous squamous cell cancer (cSCC) that is not curable by surgery or radiation.

34. FDA-approved for patients with high-risk early-stage triple-negative breast cancer (TNBC) in combination with chemotherapy as neoadjuvant treatment and then continued as single agent as adjuvant treatment after surgery.
35. FDA-approved in combination with chemotherapy for patients with locally recurrent unresectable TNBC whose tumors express PD-L1 (CPS >10) as determined by an FDA-approved test.

DOSAGE RANGE

1. Melanoma: 200 mg IV every 3 weeks or 400 mg IV every 6 weeks.
2. NSCLC: 200 mg IV every 3 weeks or 400 mg IV every 6 weeks. For adjuvant therapy, treatment up to 12 months or until disease recurrence or unacceptable toxicity.
3. SCLC: 200 mg IV every 3 weeks or 400 mg IV every 6 weeks.
4. Head and neck cancer: 200 mg IV every 3 weeks or 400 mg IV every 6 weeks.
5. Hodgkin's lymphoma and PMBCL: 200 mg IV every 3 weeks or 400 mg IV every 6 weeks for adults and 2 mg/kg (up to 200 mg) IV every 3 weeks for children.
6. Urothelial cancer: 200 mg IV every 3 weeks or 400 mg IV every 6 weeks.
7. MSI-H cancers: 200 mg IV every 3 weeks or 400 mg IV every 6 weeks for adults and 2 mg/kg (up to 200 mg) IV every 3 weeks for children.
8. MSI-H CRC: 200 mg IV every 3 weeks or 400 mg IV every 6 weeks.
9. Gastric cancer: 200 mg IV every 3 weeks or 400 mg IV every 6 weeks.
10. Esophageal cancer: 200 mg IV every 3 weeks or 400 mg IV every 6 weeks.
11. Cervical cancer: 200 mg IV every 3 weeks or 400 mg IV every 6 weeks.
12. HCC: 200 mg IV every 3 weeks or 400 mg IV every 6 weeks.
13. MCC: 200 mg IV every 3 weeks or 400 mg IV every 6 weeks.
14. RCC: 200 mg IV every 3 weeks or 400 mg IV every 6 weeks as a single agent in the adjuvant setting or in combination with axitinib 5 mg PO bid or lenvatinib 20 mg PO once daily in the advance setting.
15. Endometrial cancer: 200 mg IV every 3 weeks or 400 mg IV every 6 weeks with lenvatinib 20 mg PO once daily.
16. TMB-H: 200 mg IV every 3 weeks or 400 mg IV every 6 weeks.
17. cSCC: 200 mg IV every 3 weeks or 400 mg IV every 6 weeks.
18. TNBC: 200 mg IV every 3 weeks or 400 mg IV every 6 weeks.

DRUG INTERACTIONS
None well characterized to date.

SPECIAL CONSIDERATIONS

1. Can result in significant immune-mediated adverse reactions due to T-cell activation and proliferation. These immune-mediated reactions may involve any organ system, with the most common reactions being pneumonitis, colitis, hepatitis, hypophysitis, nephritis, and thyroid dysfunction.
2. Should be withheld for any of the following:
   - Grade 2 pneumonitis
   - Grade 2 or 3 colitis

- SGOT/SGPT >3 × ULN and up to 5 × ULN or total bilirubin >1.5 × ULN and up to 3 × ULN
- Grade 2 nephritis
- Symptomatic hypophysitis
- Grade 3 hyperthyroidism
- Any other severe or grade 3 treatment-related toxicity

3. Should be permanently discontinued for any of the following:
   - Any life-threatening toxicity
   - Grades 3 or 4 pneumonitis
   - SGOT/SGPT >5 × ULN or total bilirubin >3 × ULN
   - Grades 3 or 4 infusion-related reactions
   - Grades 3 or 4 nephritis
   - Any severe or grade 3 toxicity that recurs
   - Inability to reduce steroid dose to 10 mg or less of prednisone or equivalent per day within 12 weeks
4. Monitor thyroid function prior to and during therapy.
5. Dose modification is not needed for patients with renal dysfunction.
6. Dose modification is not needed for patients with mild hepatic dysfunction. Has not been studied in patients with moderate or severe hepatic dysfunction.
7. Pregnancy category D.

TOXICITY 1
Colitis with diarrhea and abdominal pain.

TOXICITY 2
Pneumonitis with dyspnea and cough.

TOXICITY 3
Hepatotoxicity with elevations in SGOT/SGPT, alkaline phosphatase, and serum bilirubin.

TOXICITY 4
GI side effects with nausea/vomiting and dry mouth. Pancreatitis can be observed.

TOXICITY 5
Fatigue, anorexia, and asthenia.

TOXICITY 6
Neurologic toxicity with neuropathy, myositis, and myasthenia gravis.

TOXICITY 7
Renal toxicity with nephritis.

TOXICITY 8
Musculoskeletal symptoms, which may present with arthralgias, oligoarthritis, polyarthritis, tenosynovitis, polymyalgia rheumatica, and myalgias.

TOXICITY 9
Endocrinopathies, including hypophysitis, thyroid disorders, adrenal insufficiency, and diabetes.

TOXICITY 10
Maculopapular skin rash, erythema, dermatitis, and pruritus.

Pemetrexed

TRADE NAME	Alimta, LY231514	**CLASSIFICATION**	Antimetabolite
CATEGORY	Chemotherapy drug	**DRUG MANUFACTURER**	Eli Lilly

MECHANISM OF ACTION
- Pyrrolopyrimidine antifolate analog with activity in the S-phase of the cell cycle.
- Transported into the cell primarily via the RFC and to a smaller extent by the folate receptor protein (FRP).
- Metabolized intracellularly to higher polyglutamate forms by the enzyme folylpolyglutamate synthase (FPGS). The pentaglutamate form is the predominant intracellular species. Pemetrexed polyglutamates are approximately 60-fold more potent than the parent monoglutamate compound, and they exhibit prolonged cellular retention.
- Inhibition of the folate-dependent enzyme thymidylate synthase (TS), resulting in inhibition of de novo thymidylate and DNA synthesis. This represents the main site of action of the drug.
- Inhibition of TS leads to accumulation of dUMP and subsequent incorporation of dUTP into DNA, resulting in inhibition of DNA synthesis and function.
- Inhibition of DHFR, resulting in depletion of reduced folates and of critical one-carbon carriers for cellular metabolism.
- Inhibition of de novo purine biosynthesis through inhibition of glycinamide ribonucleotide formyltransferase (GART) and aminoimidazole carboxamide ribonucleotide formyltransferase (AICART).

MECHANISM OF RESISTANCE
- Increased expression of the target enzyme TS.
- Alterations in the binding affinity of TS for pemetrexed.
- Decreased transport of drug into cells through decreased expression of the RFC and/or FRP.
- Decreased polyglutamation of drug, resulting in decreased formation of cytotoxic metabolites.

ABSORPTION
Administered only via the IV route.

DISTRIBUTION
Peak plasma levels are reached in less than 30 minutes. Widely distributed throughout the body. Tissue concentrations highest in liver, kidneys, small intestine, and colon.

METABOLISM
Significant intracellular metabolism to the polyglutamated species. Metabolism in the liver through as yet undefined mechanisms. Principally cleared by renal excretion, with as much as 90% of the drug in the urine unchanged during the first 24 hours after administration. Short distribution half-life in plasma, with a mean of 3 hours. Relatively prolonged terminal half-life of about 20 hours and a prolonged intracellular half-life as a result of pemetrexed polyglutamates.

INDICATIONS
1. Mesothelioma—FDA-approved in combination with cisplatin for treatment of locally advanced or metastatic non-squamous NSCLC.
2. NSCLC—FDA-approved in combination with cisplatin for the initial treatment of locally advanced or metastatic non-squamous NSCLC.
3. NSCLC—FDA-approved as second-line monotherapy for locally advanced or metastatic non-squamous NSCLC.
4. NSCLC—FDA-approved as maintenance treatment of locally advanced or metastatic non-squamous NSCLC whose disease has not progressed after four cycles of platinum-based first-line chemotherapy.
5. Should not be used in patients with squamous cell NSCLC.

DOSAGE RANGE
1. Recommended dose as a single agent is 500 mg/m^2 IV every 3 weeks.
2. When used in combination with cisplatin, recommended dose is 500 mg/m^2 IV every 3 weeks.

DRUG INTERACTION 1
Thymidine—Thymidine rescues against the host toxic effects of pemetrexed.

DRUG INTERACTION 2
5-FU—Pemetrexed may enhance the antitumor activity of 5-FU. Precise mechanism of interaction remains unknown.

DRUG INTERACTION 3
Leucovorin—Administration of leucovorin may decrease the antitumor activity of pemetrexed.

DRUG INTERACTION 4
NSAIDs and aspirin—Concomitant administration of NSAIDs and aspirin may inhibit the renal excretion of pemetrexed, resulting in enhanced drug toxicity.

SPECIAL CONSIDERATIONS
1. Use with caution in patients with abnormal renal function. Important to obtain baseline CrCl and to monitor renal function before each cycle of therapy. Should not be given if CrCl <45 mL/min.
2. Dose reduction is not necessary in patients with mild or moderate liver impairment.
3. Monitor CBCs on a periodic basis.
4. Use with caution in patients with third-space fluid collections such as pleural effusion and ascites, as the half-life of pemetrexed may be prolonged, leading to enhanced toxicity. Should consider draining of fluid collections prior to initiation of therapy.
5. Dietary folate status of patient is an important factor in determining risk for clinical toxicity. Patients with insufficient folate intake are at increased risk for toxicity. Evaluation of serum homocysteine and folate levels at baseline and during therapy may be helpful. A baseline serum homocysteine level >10 is a good predictor for the development of grade ¾ toxicities.
6. All patients should receive vitamin supplementation with 350 µg/day of folic acid PO and 1,000 µg of vitamin B12 IM every 3 cycles to reduce the risk and incidence of toxicity while on drug therapy. Folic acid supplementation should begin 7 days prior to initiation of pemetrexed treatment, and the first vitamin B12 injection should be administered at least 1 week prior to the start of pemetrexed. No evidence has been found to suggest that vitamin supplementation reduces clinical efficacy.
7. Prophylactic use of steroids may ameliorate and/or completely eliminate the development of skin rash. Dexamethasone can be given at a dose of 4 mg PO bid for 3 days beginning the day before therapy.
8. NSAIDs and aspirin should be discontinued for at least 2 days before therapy with pemetrexed and should not be restarted for at least 2 days after a drug dose. These agents may inhibit the renal clearance of pemetrexed, resulting in enhanced toxicity.
9. Pregnancy category D. Breastfeeding should be avoided.

TOXICITY 1
Myelosuppression is dose-limiting with neutropenia and thrombocytopenia most commonly observed.

TOXICITY 2
Skin rash, usually in the form of hand-foot syndrome.

TOXICITY 3
Mucositis, diarrhea, and nausea and vomiting.

TOXICITY 4
Hepatotoxicity with elevation in SGOT/SGPT and bilirubin. Occurs in 10%–15% of patients, and clinically asymptomatic in most cases.

TOXICITY 5
Fatigue.

Pemigatinib

TRADE NAME	Pemazyre	CLASSIFICATION	Signal transduction inhibitor, FGFR inhibitor
CATEGORY	Targeted agent	DRUG MANUFACTURER	Incyte

MECHANISM OF ACTION
- Small molecule inhibitor of FGFR1, FGFR2, and FGFR3. Weak inhibitor of FGFR4. Leads to inhibition of FGFR-mediated signaling, which involves tumor cell growth, proliferation, migration, angiogenesis, and survival.
- Broad spectrum activity against a wide range of solid tumors, including cholangiocarcinoma, hepatocellular cancer, NSCLC, prostate cancer, and esophageal cancer.

MECHANISM OF RESISTANCE
- Acquired FGFR2 mutations, including N549K/H, E565A, K659M, and L617V
- Activation of WNT3A-TCF7-SOX9 signaling axis.

ABSORPTION
Median time to peak drug levels is 1.1 hours after oral ingestion. Food does not affect oral absorption. Steady-state drug levels are achieved in 4 days.

DISTRIBUTION
Extensive binding (90%) of drug to plasma proteins, mainly α-1-acid glycoprotein.

METABOLISM
Metabolized in the liver primarily by CYP3A4 microsomal enzymes. Approximately 82% of an administered dose is eliminated in feces (1.4% in parent form), and 12.6% is eliminated in urine (1% in parent form). The terminal half-life of pemigatinib is approximately 15.4 hours.

INDICATIONS
1. FDA-approved for patients with previously treated, unresectable locally advanced or metastatic cholangiocarcinoma with a fibroblast growth factor receptor 2 (FGFR2) fusion or other rearrangement as detected by an FDA-approved test.
2. FDA-approved for patients with relapsed or refractory myeloid/lymphoid neoplasms (MLNs) with FGFR1 rearrangement.

DOSAGE RANGE
1. Cholangiocarcinoma: Recommended dose is 13.5 mg PO once daily for 14 days followed by 7 days off in 21-day cycles.
2. MLNs: Recommended dose is 13.5 mg PO once daily.

DRUG INTERACTION 1
Drugs such as ketoconazole, itraconazole, erythromycin, clarithromycin, atazanavir, indinavir, nefazodone, nelfinavir, ritonavir, saquinavir, telithromycin, and voriconazole may decrease the pemigatinib metabolism, resulting in increased drug levels and potentially increased toxicity.

DRUG INTERACTION 2
Phenytoin and other drugs that stimulate the liver microsomal CYP3A4 enzymes, including carbamazepine, rifampin, phenobarbital, and St. John's Wort—These drugs may increase pemigatinib metabolism, resulting in lower effective drug levels and potentially reduced clinical activity.

DRUG INTERACTION 3
Avoid concomitant use of agents that alter serum phosphate levels as pemigatinib increases serum phosphate levels. Such drugs include potassium phosphate supplements, vitamin D supplements, antacids, phosphate-containing enemas or laxatives, and drugs known to have phosphate as an excipient.

SPECIAL CONSIDERATIONS

1. Patients should be seen by a dietician and should be placed on a restricted phosphate diet to 600–800 mg daily.
2. Closely monitor serum phosphate levels while on therapy. The median time to onset of hyperphosphatemia is 8 days. Serum phosphate levels should be monitored on a monthly basis. If the serum phosphate level is >5.5 mg/dL, ensure that a restricted phosphate diet is being correctly followed. For serum phosphate levels >7.0 mg/dL, phosphate-lowering therapy, such as an oral phosphate binder, should be used, and the dose of drug should be held, reduced, or permanently discontinued based on duration and severity of the hyperphosphatemia.
3. Comprehensive eye exam, including optical coherence tomography (OCT), should be performed at baseline and every 2 months for the first 6 months of therapy and every 3 months thereafter. With the onset of new visual symptoms, patients should have an immediate evaluation with OCT, with follow-up every 3 weeks until resolution of symptoms or discontinuation of treatment.
4. If concomitant use of a moderate or strong CYP3A inhibitor can not be avoided, the dose of pemigatinib should be reduced from 13.5 mg to 9 mg.
5. Concomitant use of a moderate or strong CYP3A inducer should be avoided.
6. Can cause fetal harm when administered to a pregnant woman. Females of reproductive potential should use effective contraception during drug therapy and for 1 week after the final dose. Breastfeeding should be avoided.

TOXICITY 1
Hyperphosphatemia.

TOXICITY 2
Ocular disorders with retinal pigment epithelial detachment (RPED) leading to blurred vision, visual floaters, or photopsia. Dry eye symptoms occur in nearly 30% of patients.

TOXICITY 3
Dysgeusia, diarrhea, mucositis, dry mouth, and nausea/vomiting.

TOXICITY 4
Fatigue and anorexia.

TOXICITY 5
Dry skin, palmar-plantar erythrodysesthesia, paronychia, and nail discoloration.

TOXICITY 6
Arthralgias.

Pertuzumab

TRADE NAME	Perjeta	**CLASSIFICATION**	Monoclonal antibody, anti-HER2 antibody
CATEGORY	Biologic response modifier agent, targeted agent	**DRUG MANUFACTURER**	Genentech/Roche

MECHANISM OF ACTION

- Recombinant humanized IgG1 monoclonal antibody directed against the extracellular dimerization domain (subdomain II) of the HER2/neu growth factor receptor. Binds to a different HER2 epitope than trastuzumab (domain IV).
- Binding of pertuzumab to HER2 leads to inhibition of heterodimerization of HER2 with other HER family members, including EGFR, HER3, and HER4.
- Inhibition of these heterodimerization processes leads to the inhibition of downstream signaling pathways, which includes mitogen-activated protein (MAP) kinase, PI3K, and initiation of cell apoptosis.
- Immunologic mechanisms may also be involved in antitumor activity, including ADCC.

MECHANISM OF RESISTANCE

- Mutations in HER2/neu receptor, leading to reduced binding affinity to pertuzumab.
- Loss of expression of HER2.
- HER2 reactivation through acquisition of the HER2L755S mutation.
- Activation/induction of alternative cellular signaling pathways, such as IGF-1R, c-MET, PIK3CA/AKT, Ras/Raf MEK/ERK.
- Loss of PTEN.

ABSORPTION

Administered only via the IV route.

DISTRIBUTION

Steady-state drug levels are generally achieved after the first maintenance dose.

METABOLISM

Metabolism of pertuzumab has not been extensively evaluated. The terminal half-life is approximately 18 days using an every-3-week infusion schedule.

INDICATIONS

1. FDA-approved in combination with trastuzumab and docetaxel for patients with HER2-positive metastatic breast cancer who have not received prior anti-HER2 therapy or chemotherapy for metastatic disease.

2. FDA-approved in combination with trastuzumab and chemotherapy as neoadjuvant therapy for patients with HER2-positive, locally advanced, inflammatory, or early-stage breast cancer as part of a complete treatment regimen for early breast cancer.

3. FDA-approved in combination with trastuzumab and chemotherapy as adjuvant therapy for patients with HER2-positive early breast cancer at high risk of recurrence.

4. Patients must have tumors that express HER2/neu protein to be treated with this monoclonal antibody.

DOSAGE RANGE

1. Recommended initial dose is 840 mg IV administered over 60 minutes, followed by a maintenance dose of 420 mg over 30–60 minutes every 3 weeks.

2. Metastatic breast cancer: Administer pertuzumab, trastuzumab, and docetaxel by IV infusion every 3 weeks.

3. Neoadjuvant setting: Administer pertuzumab, trastuzumab, and chemotherapy by IV infusion every 3 weeks. Should administer 3–6 cycles before surgery and then give up to a total of 1 year (up to 18 cycles) of pertuzumab, trastuzumab, and chemotherapy following surgical resection.

4. Adjuvant setting: Administer pertuzumab, trastuzumab, and chemotherapy by IV infusion every 3 weeks for a total of 1 year (up to 18 cycles).

DRUG INTERACTIONS

No drug–drug interactions have been observed between pertuzumab and trastuzumab or between pertuzumab and docetaxel. No other drug interactions have been formally investigated to date.

SPECIAL CONSIDERATIONS

1. Pertuzumab is associated with reduced LVEF. Patients with prior exposure to anthracyclines or radiotherapy to the chest may be at increased risk of developing a decline in LVEF. Caution should be exercised in treating patients with pre-existing cardiac disease such as congestive heart failure, ischemic heart disease, myocardial infarction, valvular heart disease, or arrhythmias.

2. Careful baseline assessment of cardiac function (LVEF) before treatment and frequent monitoring (every 3 months) of cardiac function while on therapy. Pertuzumab should be held for at least 3 weeks if there is a drop in LVEF <45% or an LVEF of 45%–49% with a 10% or greater absolute decline from baseline. If cardiac function does not improve after 3 weeks of withholding therapy, consider permanently discontinuing therapy.

3. Carefully monitor for infusion-related and hypersensitivity reactions. Monitor patients 60 minutes after the first infusion and for 30 minutes after subsequent infusions for infusion reactions or cytokine release syndrome. If an infusion reaction occurs, slow and/or interrupt treatment. Immediate institution of diphenhydramine, acetaminophen, corticosteroids, IV fluids, and/or vasopressors may be necessary. Resuscitation equipment should be readily available at bedside.

4. The pregnancy status of a female patient must be verified prior to the start of pertuzumab therapy. Patients should be advised of the risks of embryo-fetal deaths and birth defects and the need for contraception during and after treatment.

5. May cause fetal harm. Women of reproductive potential should be advised to use effective contraception during treatment and for 7 months following the last dose. Breastfeeding should be avoided while on therapy and for 7 months after the last dose.

TOXICITY 1
Embryo-fetal deaths and/or severe birth defects.

TOXICITY 2
Cardiac toxicity with a reduced LVEF.

TOXICITY 3
Infusion-related symptoms with fever, chills, urticaria, flushing, fatigue, headache, hypersensitivity, and myalgia. Occurs in up to 13% of patients. Most commonly observed with administration of first infusion.

TOXICITY 4
Fatigue.

TOXICITY 5
Diarrhea and nausea/vomiting.

Pirtobrutinib

TRADE NAME	Jaypirca, LOXO-305	CLASSIFICATION	Signal transduction inhibitor, BTK inhibitor
CATEGORY	Targeted agent	DRUG MANUFACTURER	Eli Lilly

MECHANISM OF ACTION

- Highly selective, non-covalent small-molecule inhibitor of Bruton's tyrosine kinase (BTK). Greater than 300-fold selectivity for BTK versus 98% of other tyrosine kinases.
- Differs from covalent irreversible BTK inhibitors such as ibrutinib, acalabrutinib, and zanubrutinib.
- Binds to both wild-type BTK and BTK harboring C481 mutations.
- BTK is a key signaling protein of the B-cell antigen receptor (BCR) and cytokine receptor pathways.

MECHANISM OF RESISTANCE

- Non-Cys481 BTK mutations including V416L, A428D, M437R, T474I, T474L, and L528W leading to reduced binding affinity to drug.
- Non-Cys481 BTK mutations confer resistance to covalent BTK inhibitors.
- Mutations in the gene encoding phospholipase C-γ2 (PLCG2).
- Activation of B-cell receptor signaling.
- Activation of AKT signaling.

ABSORPTION

Oral bioavailability is approximately 85%. Peak plasma drug levels are achieved in 2 hours after ingestion, and food does not appear to alter bioavailability. Steady-state levels reached within 5 days of daily dosing.

DISTRIBUTION

Extensive binding (96%) to plasma proteins.

METABOLISM

Metabolism in the liver primarily by CYP3A4 and by UGT1A8 and UGT1A9 glucuronidation. Elimination of parent drug and metabolites in urine (57%) and in feces (37%). Terminal half-life is approximately 19 hours.

INDICATIONS

FDA-approved under accelerated approval based on overall response rate and duration of response for relapsed or refractory mantle cell lymphoma (MCL) after at least 2 prior lines of systemic therapy, including a covalent BTK inhibitor.

DOSAGE RANGE

Recommended dose is 200 mg PO daily with or without food.

DRUG INTERACTION 1

Phenytoin and other drugs that stimulate the liver microsomal CYP3A4 enzymes, including carbamazepine, rifampin, phenobarbital, and St. John's Wort—These drugs may increase the metabolism of pirtobrutinib, resulting in its inactivation and lower effective drug levels.

DRUG INTERACTION 2

Drugs that inhibit the liver microsomal CYP3A4 enzymes, including ketoconazole, itraconazole, erythromycin, and clarithromycin—These drugs may decrease the metabolism of pirtobrutinib, resulting in increased drug levels and potentially increased toxicity.

SPECIAL CONSIDERATIONS

1. Dose reduction is not required in the setting of mild to severe hepatic impairment.
2. Dose reduction is not required in the setting of mild or moderate renal impairment. Dose reduction is recommended in the setting of severe renal impairment, with dose reduced from 200 mg to 100 mg. The effects of end-stage renal disease and dialysis have not been studied.
3. Pirtobrutinib tablets should be swallowed whole with water.
4. Monitor CBCs on a monthly basis.
5. Monitor for bleeding, especially in patients on antiplatelet or anticoagulant therapies.
6. Monitor patients for fever and signs of infection.
7. Patients should be advised to avoid sun exposure.
8. May cause fetal harm when administered to a pregnant woman. Females should use effective contraception during treatment and for 1 week after the last dose. Breastfeeding should be avoided while on treatment and for 1 week after the last dose.

TOXICITY 1

Bleeding with bruising and petechiae. GI and CNS bleeding occur rarely.

TOXICITY 2

Infections with pneumonia are most common. Bacterial, viral, or fungal infections along with opportunistic infections, such as PJP.

TOXICITY 3

Myelosuppression with neutropenia, thrombocytopenia, and anemia.

TOXICITY 4

Abdominal pain, diarrhea, and nausea/vomiting are the most common GI side effects.

TOXICITY 5

Second primary cancers with non-melanoma skin cancer and other solid tumors, such as GU and breast cancers.

TOXICITY 6

Fatigue and anorexia.

TOXICITY 7

Cardiac toxicity with atrial fibrillation/atrial flutter.

Polatuzumab vedotin

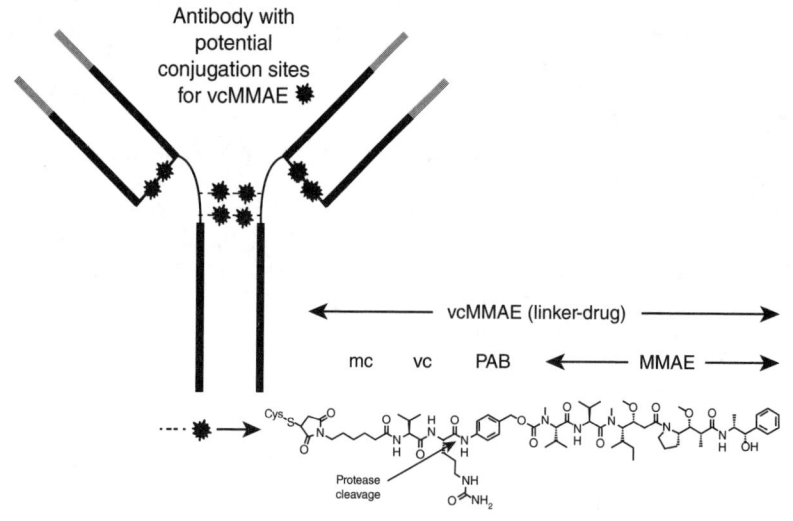

TRADE NAME	Polivy	**CLASSIFICATION**	Antibody-drug conjugate
CATEGORY	Biologic response modifier agent, chemotherapy drug	**DRUG MANUFACTURER**	Genentech

MECHANISM OF ACTION

- Antibody-drug conjugate made up of a monoclonal antibody directed against CD79b, a B-cell receptor component expressed in a majority of malignant lymphomas, covalently linked to the microtubule-disrupting anti-mitotic agent monomethyl auristatin E (MMAE).
- Upon binding to CD79b, polatuzumab vedotin is rapidly internalized into lysosomes, and MMAE is then released to bind to microtubules, which inhibits mitosis and cell division, resulting in cell death. The MMAE biological activity is similar to that of other anti-microtubule inhibitors and works in the M-phase of the cell cycle.
- CD79b is a component of the B-cell receptor and expressed on normal B cells and in most mature B-cell malignancies, including >95% of DLBCL NHL and CLL.

MECHANISM OF RESISTANCE

None well characterized to date.

ABSORPTION
Administered only via the IV route.

DISTRIBUTION
Moderate binding (77%) of drug to plasma proteins.

METABOLISM
Expected to undergo catabolism to small peptides, amino acids, unconjugated MMAE, and unconjugated MMAE-related catabolites. MMAE serves as a substrate for CYP3A4 liver microsomal enzymes. The median terminal half-life of the antibody-conjugated MMAE is about 12 days, while the unconjugated MMAE terminal half-life is about 4 days after the first dose of the antibody-drug conjugate.

INDICATIONS
1. FDA-approved in combination with bendamustine and rituximab for relapsed or refractory diffuse large B-cell lymphoma after at least 2 prior therapies.
2. FDA-approved in combination with a rituximab product, cyclophosphamide, doxorubicin, and prednisone (R-CHP) for previously untreated diffuse large B-cell lymphoma (DLBCL) or high-grade B-cell lymphoma with an International Prognostic Index (IPI) score of 2 or greater.

DOSAGE RANGE
Recommended dose is 1.8 mg/kg IV every 21 days for 6 cycles.

DRUG INTERACTIONS
None well characterized to date.

SPECIAL CONSIDERATIONS
1. Monitor for infusion-related reactions. Patients should be premedicated with an antihistamine and acetaminophen at least 30 min prior to all infusions. Patients should be monitored during and for at least 90 min after the completion of the infusion.
2. Monitor for tumor lysis syndrome, especially in patients with high tumor burden and/or rapidly growing disease.
3. Monitor CBC prior to each treatment cycle. See package insert for details regarding dose modifications for hematologic toxicities. Patients should receive prophylactic GSF.
4. Monitor LFTs and serum bilirubin levels closely, especially in patients with pre-existing liver disease and elevated baseline LFTs and on medications that may increase the risk of hepatotoxicity.
5. Dose reduction is not required for patients with mild or moderate renal dysfunction. Has not been studied in patients with severe renal impairment, end-stage renal disease, and/or on hemodialysis.

6. Dose reduction is not required for patients with mild hepatic dysfunction. Limited safety information for patients with moderate or severe hepatic dysfunction, and caution should be used in these patients.
7. Monitor for signs and symptoms of infection. Prophylaxis for PJP and HSV should be administered.
8. Monitor for new or worsening behavioral, cognitive, or neurological changes as PML has been reported in patients treated with polatuzumab vedotin.
9. May cause fetal harm when given to a pregnant woman. Females of reproductive potential should use effective contraception during treatment and for at least 3 months after the last dose. Males with female partners of reproductive potential should use effective contraception while on treatment and for at least 5 months after the last dose. Breastfeeding should be avoided.

TOXICITY 1
Myelosuppression with neutropenia, thrombocytopenia, and anemia.

TOXICITY 2
Infusion-related reactions.

TOXICITY 3
Peripheral neuropathy. Can occur with the first cycle of treatment and cumulative in nature.

TOXICITY 4
Hepatotoxicity with elevation in LFTs.

TOXICITY 5
Increased risk of serious and opportunistic infections, including PJP and other fungal pneumonias, HSV, and CMV.

TOXICITY 6
Tumor lysis syndrome in the setting of large tumor burden or rapidly growing tumors.

TOXICITY 7
Progressive multifocal leukoencephalopathy (PML).

Pomalidomide

TRADE NAME	Pomalyst	**CLASSIFICATION**	Immunomodulatory analog of thalidomide, anti-angiogenic agent
CATEGORY	Unclassified therapeutic agent, biologic response modifier agent	**DRUG MANUFACTURER**	Celgene

MECHANISM OF ACTION
- Mechanism of action is not fully characterized.
- More potent antiproliferative immunomodulating agent than thalidomide and lenalidomide.
- Immunomodulatory drug that stimulates T-cell proliferation as well as IL-2 and IFN-γ production.
- Inhibition of TNF-α and IL-6 synthesis and down-modulation of cell surface adhesion molecules similar to thalidomide.
- May exert anti-angiogenic effect by inhibition of basic fibroblast growth factor (bFGF) and vascular endothelial growth factor (VEGF) and through as-yet-undefined mechanisms.
- Overcomes cellular drug resistance to thalidomide and lenalidomide.

MECHANISM OF RESISTANCE
- Reduced expression of cereblon, a member of the cullin 4 ring ligase complex (CRL4).
- Increased genome-wide DNA methylation with increased expression of DNA methyltransferases and EZH2.
- Reduced chromatin accessibility.

ABSORPTION
Well absorbed following oral administration with 73% oral bioavailability. Peak plasma concentrations at 2–3 hours.

DISTRIBUTION
Binding to plasma proteins ranges from 12%–44%. Distributed in male semen at concentrations of approximately 67% of plasma levels after 4 days of treatment.

METABOLISM
Primarily metabolized in the liver by CYP1A2 and CYP3A4, with minor effects by CYP2C19 and CYP2D6. Approximately 75% of an administered dose is excreted in urine, primarily in the form of drug metabolites, while 15% of an administered dose is eliminated in feces. The elimination half-life of the drug is approximately 7.5 hours.

INDICATIONS
1. FDA-approved for patients with multiple myeloma who have received at least two prior therapies, including lenalidomide and bortezomib, and who have disease progression on or within 60 days of completion of the previous therapy.
2. FDA-approved for adult patients with AIDS-related Kaposi's sarcoma after failure of highly active antiretroviral therapy and Kaposi's sarcoma in adult patients who are HIV-negative.

DOSAGE RANGE
1. Multiple myeloma: Recommended dose is 4 mg PO daily on days 1–21 of a 28-day cycle.
2. Multiple myeloma: May be given in combination with dexamethasone 40 mg PO daily on days 1, 8, 15, and 22 of a 28-day cycle.
3. Kaposi's sarcoma: Recommended dose is 5 mg PO daily on days 1–21 of a 28-day cycle.

DRUG INTERACTIONS
None well characterized to date.

SPECIAL CONSIDERATIONS
1. Pregnancy category X. Pomalidomide is a thalidomide analog, a known human teratogen that causes severe or life-threatening birth defects. Women who are pregnant or who wish to become pregnant should not take pomalidomide. Severe fetal malformations can occur if even one capsule is taken by a pregnant woman. All women should have a baseline β-human chorionic gonadotropin (β-HCG) before starting pomalidomide therapy. Women of reproductive age must have two negative pregnancy tests before starting therapy: the first test should be performed 10–14 days before therapy is begun, and the second should be 24 hours before therapy. This is a black-box warning.
2. All women of childbearing potential should practice two forms of birth control throughout therapy with pomalidomide: one highly effective form (intrauterine device, hormonal contraception [patch, implant, pill, injection], partner's vasectomy, or tubal ligation) and one additional barrier method (latex condom, diaphragm, or cervical cap). It is strongly recommended that these precautionary measures be taken 1 month before initiation of therapy, continue while on therapy, and continue at least 1 month after therapy is discontinued.

3. Pomalidomide is only available under a special restricted distribution program called "POMALYST REMS." Only prescribers and pharmacists registered with this program are able to prescribe and dispense the drug. Pomalidomide should only be dispensed to those patients who are registered and meet all the conditions of this program.
4. Breastfeeding while on therapy should be avoided, as it remains unknown if pomalidomide is excreted in breast milk.
5. Men taking pomalidomide must use latex condoms for every sexual encounter with a woman of childbearing potential, as the drug may be present in semen.
6. Patients taking pomalidomide should not donate blood or semen while receiving treatment and for at least 1 month after stopping this drug.
7. Monitor CBCs while on therapy, as pomalidomide has hematologic toxicity.
8. Use with caution in patients with impaired renal function, as pomalidomide and its metabolites are mainly excreted by the kidneys. Although no formal renal dysfunction studies have been performed, pomalidomide should be avoided in patients with a serum creatinine >3 mg/dL.
9. Increased risk of thromboembolic complications, including DVT and PE. This represents a black-box warning. Prophylaxis with low-molecular-weight heparin or aspirin (325 mg PO qd) is recommended to prevent and/or reduce this risk.
10. Smoking should be avoided while on therapy, as cigarette smoking may reduce pomalidomide exposure secondary to CYP1A2 induction.

TOXICITY 1
Potentially severe or fatal teratogenic effects.

TOXICITY 2
Myelosuppression with neutropenia and thrombocytopenia that is usually reversible.

TOXICITY 3
Increased risk of thromboembolic complications, such as DVT and PE.

TOXICITY 4
Hepatotoxicity.

TOXICITY 5
Skin toxicity with skin rash, Steven-Johnson syndrome (SJS), exfoliative dermatitis, and toxic epidermal necrolysis (TEN).

TOXICITY 6
Dizziness and confusion are the two most common neurologic side effects.

TOXICITY 7
Hypersensitivity reactions. More likely to occur in patients with a prior history of hypersensitivity reactions to thalidomide or lenalidomide.

TOXICITY 8
Neuropathy observed in nearly 20% of patients, with approximately 10% in the form of peripheral neuropathy. Usually mild, with no grade 3 or higher neuropathy reported.

Ponatinib

TRADE NAME	Iclusig, AP24534	CLASSIFICATION	Signal transduction inhibitor, Bcr-Abl inhibitor
CATEGORY	Targeted agent	DRUG MANUFACTURER	ARIAD Pharmaceuticals

MECHANISM OF ACTION
- Potent inhibitor of the non-mutant Bcr-Abl tyrosine kinase.
- In contrast to other Bcr-Abl inhibitors, ponatinib has inhibitory effects against all known Bcr-Abl mutations, including the T315I gatekeeper mutation. Ponatinib was specifically designed to bind and inhibit these mutant forms.
- Inhibits other tyrosine kinases, some of which are involved in tumor growth and tumor angiogenesis, including VEGFR, PDGFR, FGFR, FLT3, TIE-2, Src family kinases, Kit, RET, and EPH.

MECHANISM OF RESISTANCE
- Development of compound mutations in the Bcr-Abl kinase domain.
- Amplification of the anti-apoptotic BCL2 gene.
- Development of T315L and I315M mutations in the Bcr-Abl kinase domain.

ABSORPTION
Absorbed following oral administration at varying levels of bioavailability based on pH levels, with higher gastric pH levels leading to lower oral bioavailability. Peak plasma concentrations are achieved at 6 hours, and steady-state drug levels are achieved at 28 days. Food does not affect oral absorption.

DISTRIBUTION
Extensive plasma proteins binding of >99%.

METABOLISM
Metabolized in the liver primarily by CYP3A4 microsomal enzymes. CYP2C8, CYP2D6, and CYP3A5 liver microsomal enzymes are also involved. Approximately 87% and 5% of an administered dose is eliminated in feces and urine, respectively. The mean terminal elimination half-life is 24 hours.

INDICATIONS
1. FDA-approved for adult patients with chronic-, accelerated-, or blast-phase CML for whom no other TKI is indicated.
2. FDA-approved for adult patients with Ph+ ALL for whom no other TKI is indicated.
3. FDA-approved for adult patients with T315I chronic-, accelerated-, or blast-phase CML or T315I Ph+ ALL.

DOSAGE RANGE
1. Recommended dose is 45 mg PO once daily with or without food.
2. Recommended dose is 30 mg PO once daily if given concurrently with strong CYP3A inhibitors.

DRUG INTERACTION 1
Phenytoin and other drugs that stimulate liver microsomal CYP3A4 enzymes, including carbamazepine, rifampin, phenobarbital, and St. John's Wort—These drugs increase the metabolism of ponatinib, resulting in its inactivation and lower effective drug levels.

DRUG INTERACTION 2
Drugs that inhibit liver microsomal CYP3A4 enzymes, including ketoconazole, voriconazole, posaconazole, itraconazole, erythromycin, and clarithromycin—These drugs decrease the metabolism of ponatinib, resulting in increased drug levels and potentially increased toxicity.

DRUG INTERACTION 3
Warfarin—Patients on warfarin should be closely monitored for alterations in their clotting parameters (PT and INR) and/or bleeding, as ponatinib inhibits the metabolism of warfarin by the liver P450 system. Dose of warfarin may require careful adjustment in the presence of ponatinib therapy.

DRUG INTERACTION 4

Proton pump inhibitors and H2-blockers may reduce the plasma drug concentrations of ponatinib by reducing oral bioavailability.

SPECIAL CONSIDERATIONS

1. Patients should be closely monitored for an increased risk of arterial thromboembolic events, such as cardiovascular, cerebrovascular, and peripheral vascular thrombosis, including fatal myocardial infarction and stroke. This represents a black-box warning.
2. Closely monitor hepatic function prior to and at least monthly thereafter, as hepatotoxicity, liver failure, and death have been reported in patients treated with ponatinib. This represents a black-box warning.
3. Severe bleeding can occur, and caution should be taken in patients with thrombocytopenia or in those on anticoagulation.
4. Therapy should be interrupted in patients undergoing major surgical procedures.
5. Can result in the development of gastrointestinal perforation and fistula formation.
6. Monitor CBC every 2 weeks during the first 3 months, then monthly thereafter.
7. Closely monitor blood pressure, especially in patients with underlying hypertension, as ponatinib can worsen hypertension.
8. Tumor lysis syndrome has been reported. Monitor uric acid levels, and consider allopurinol and adequate hydration.
9. Monitor patients for fluid retention that can manifest as peripheral edema, pericardial effusion, pleural effusion, pulmonary edema, or ascites.
10. Avoid grapefruit, grapefruit juice, Seville oranges, starfruit, pomelos, and St. John's Wort while on therapy.
11. Avoid PPIs and H2-blockers, as they can reduce the oral bioavailability and subsequent efficacy of ponatinib.
12. May cause fetal harm. Women of reproductive potential should use effective contraception during treatment and for 3 weeks after the last dose. Breastfeeding should be avoided while on therapy and for 6 days following the last dose.

TOXICITY 1

Arterial thromboembolic events, such as myocardial infarction and stroke. Serious arterial thrombosis occurs in up to 10% of patients.

TOXICITY 2

Hepatotoxicity with elevation in SGOT/SGPT in 60% of patients. Liver failure and death are rare events.

TOXICITY 3

Pancreatitis.

TOXICITY 4
Hypertension.

TOXICITY 5
Cardiac arrhythmias in the form of complete heart block, sick sinus syndrome, atrial fibrillation, and sinus bradycardia.

TOXICITY 6
Fluid retention manifesting as peripheral edema, pericardial effusion, pleural effusion, pulmonary edema, or ascites.

TOXICITY 7
Bleeding complications, usually associated with severe thrombocytopenia.

TOXICITY 8
Myelosuppression, with neutropenia, thrombocytopenia, and anemia.

TOXICITY 9
Tumor lysis syndrome occurs rarely, in less than 1%.

TOXICITY 10
Gastrointestinal perforation, fistula formation, and wound-healing complications.

TOXICITY 11
Skin toxicity, including skin rash and dry skin.

Pralatrexate

TRADE NAME	Folotyn	CLASSIFICATION	Antimetabolite
CATEGORY	Chemotherapy drug	DRUG MANUFACTURER	Allos Therapeutics

MECHANISM OF ACTION

- 10-Deazaaminopterin antifolate analog with activity in the S-phase of the cell cycle.
- Transported selectively into the cell by the reduced folate carrier type 1 (RFC-1) and rationally designed to have greater affinity to this transport protein.
- Requires polyglutamation by the enzyme folylpolyglutamate synthase (FPGS) for its cytotoxic activity.
- Inhibition of DHFR, resulting in depletion of critical reduced folates.
- Inhibition of de novo thymidylate synthesis.
- Inhibition of de novo purine synthesis.
- Incorporation of dUTP into DNA, resulting in inhibition of DNA synthesis and function.

MECHANISM OF RESISTANCE

- Increased expression of the target enzyme DHFR through either gene amplification or increased transcription, translation, and/or post-translational events.
- Reduced binding affinity of drug to DHFR.
- Decreased carrier-mediated transport of drug into cell through decreased expression and/or activity of RFC-1.
- Decreased formation of cytotoxic pralatrexate polyglutamates through either decreased expression of FPGS or increased expression of GGH.

ABSORPTION

Administered only via the IV route.

DISTRIBUTION

Approximately 67% of drug is bound to plasma proteins.

METABOLISM

Significant intracellular metabolism of drug to the polyglutamated species. Metabolism in the liver through as-yet-undefined mechanisms. Principally cleared by renal excretion, with approximately 34% of an administered dose of drug excreted unchanged in urine. Age-related decline in renal function may lead to a reduction in pralatrexate clearance and an increase in plasma exposure. The terminal half-life of pralatrexate is 12–18 hours, with a prolonged intracellular half-life as a result of pralatrexate polyglutamates.

INDICATIONS

FDA-approved for patients with relapsed or refractory peripheral T-cell lymphoma (PTCL).

DOSAGE RANGE

Recommended dose is 30 mg/m^2 IV weekly for 6 weeks in 7-week cycles.

DRUG INTERACTION 1
Aspirin, NSAIDs, penicillins, probenecid, cephalosporins, and trimethoprim/sulfamethoxazole—These drugs inhibit the renal excretion of pralatrexate, leading to enhanced drug effect and toxicity.

DRUG INTERACTION 2
Leucovorin—Leucovorin rescues the toxic effects of pralatrexate and may also impair the antitumor activity. The active form of leucovorin is the L-isomer.

DRUG INTERACTION 3
Thymidine—Thymidine rescues the toxic effects of pralatrexate and may also impair the antitumor activity.

SPECIAL CONSIDERATIONS
1. Closely monitor CBCs on a periodic basis.
2. Use with caution in patients with abnormal renal function. Dose should be reduced in proportion to the creatinine clearance. Important to obtain baseline CrCl and to monitor renal function before each cycle of therapy.
3. Closely monitor liver function while on treatment. Patients who develop evidence of hepatic impairment or hepatic disease may require dose modification.
4. Dietary folate status of the patient may be an important factor in determining risk for toxicity. Patients with insufficient folate intake may be at increased risk for toxicity. Evaluation of serum homocysteine and methylmalonic acid may be helpful.
5. All patients should receive supplementation with folic acid and vitamin B12 to reduce the incidence and severity of adverse reactions. Folic acid 1–1.25 mg PO daily should begin 10 days prior to the first dose of pralatrexate and continue during the full course of therapy, until 30 days after the last dose of pralatrexate. Vitamin B12 1,000 µg IM should begin no more than 10 weeks prior to the first dose of pralatrexate and should be repeated every 8–10 weeks during therapy. Subsequent vitamin B12 injections may be given on the same day as pralatrexate.
6. Pregnancy category D. Breastfeeding should be avoided.

TOXICITY 1
Myelosuppression with thrombocytopenia, neutropenia, and anemia.

TOXICITY 2
GI toxicity with mucositis, nausea/vomiting, diarrhea, and abdominal pain.

TOXICITY 3
Transient elevations in serum transaminases reported in 10%–15% of patients. Clinically asymptomatic in most cases.

TOXICITY 4
Fatigue and asthenia.

TOXICITY 5
Skin rash.

Pralsetinib

TRADE NAME	Gavreto	CLASSIFICATION	Signal transduction inhibitor, RET inhibitor
CATEGORY	Targeted agent	DRUG MANUFACTURER	Blueprint Medicines

MECHANISM OF ACTION
- Small molecule inhibitor of wild-type RET and oncogenic RET fusion and mutations.
- Inhibits VEGFR2 as well as TRKA and TRKC, FLT3, PDGFRB, JAK1 and JAK2, and FGFR1, albeit at much higher concentrations than for RET.
- RET fusion-positive NSCLC (1%–2%), papillary thyroid cancer (10%–20%), and RET-mutant medullary thyroid cancer (40%–50% sporadic, >90% hereditary) make up the largest fraction of RET-altered tumors.

MECHANISM OF RESISTANCE
- RET solvent front mutations, including G810R, G810S, and G810C.
- RET hinge mutations, Y806C and Y806N, and β2 strand mutations, V738A.
- Emergence of RET V804M gatekeeper mutation.
- RET-independent mechanisms such as acquired MET or KRAS gene amplification.

ABSORPTION
Rapidly absorbed, with a median time to peak drug levels of 2–4 hours after oral ingestion. Steady-state drug levels are achieved in approximately 3–5 days. Food with high-fat content increases C_{max} and AUC.

DISTRIBUTION
Extensive binding (97%) to plasma proteins.

METABOLISM
Metabolized in the liver primarily by CYP3A4 microsomal enzymes and to a lesser extent by CYP2D6 and CYP1A2. After an administered dose of drug, nearly 73% is eliminated in feces (66% as parent drug) and 6% is eliminated in urine (4.82% as parent drug). The terminal half-life of the drug is approximately 16 hours.

INDICATIONS
1. FDA-approved for adult patients with metastatic RET fusion-positive NSCLC.
2. FDA-approved for adult and pediatric patients 12 years and older with advanced or metastatic RET fusion-positive thyroid cancer who require systemic therapy and who are radioactive iodine-refractory.

DOSAGE RANGE
Recommended dose is 400 mg PO once daily on an empty stomach.

DRUG INTERACTION 1
Drugs such as ketoconazole, itraconazole, erythromycin, clarithromycin, atazanavir, indinavir, nefazodone, nelfinavir, ritonavir, saquinavir, telithromycin, and voriconazole may decrease the metabolism of pralsetinib, resulting in increased drug levels and potentially increased toxicity.

DRUG INTERACTION 2
Drugs that are combined P-gp and strong CYP3A inhibitors, such as itraconazole, may lead to increased drug levels and potentially increased toxicity.

DRUG INTERACTION 3
Phenytoin and other drugs that stimulate the liver microsomal CYP3A4 enzymes, including carbamazepine, rifampin, phenobarbital, and St. John's Wort—These drugs may increase the metabolism of pralsetinib, resulting in lower effective drug levels and potentially reduced clinical activity.

SPECIAL CONSIDERATIONS
1. Should be taken on an empty stomach with no food intake for at least 2 hours before and at least 1 hour after ingestion.
2. Dose reduction is not required in the setting of mild to moderate hepatic impairment. Has not been studied in the setting of moderate and severe hepatic impairment.
3. Dose reduction is not required in the setting of mild and moderate renal impairment. Has not been studied in patients with severe renal impairment or in those with end-stage renal disease.
4. Monitor for pulmonary symptoms as pneumonitis as well as potentially severe, life-threatening, and even fatal interstitial lung disease can occur.

5. Monitor LFTs at baseline and every 2 weeks during the first 3 months of therapy, then once a month or as clinically indicated.
6. Monitor blood pressure while on therapy, starting at one week after initiation and then at least on a monthly basis or as clinically indicated.
7. Monitor for tumor lysis syndrome, especially in patients with medullary thyroid cancer with rapidly growing tumors, high tumor burden, renal dysfunction, or dehydration.
8. Monitor for bleeding complications.
9. Should be held for at least 5 days prior to elective surgery given the risk of impaired wound healing. Should not be administered for at least 2 weeks following major surgery and until there is evidence of adequate wound healing.
10. May cause fetal harm when administered to a pregnant woman. Females of reproductive potential should use effective contraception during drug therapy and for at least 2 weeks after the final dose. Breastfeeding should be avoided.

TOXICITY 1
Hypertension.

TOXICITY 2
Hepatotoxicity.

TOXICITY 3
Interstitial lung disease and pneumonitis.

TOXICITY 4
Bleeding complications.

TOXICITY 5
Tumor lysis syndrome.

TOXICITY 6
Impaired wound healing.

TOXICITY 7
Fatigue, asthenia, and anorexia.

TOXICITY 8
Musculoskeletal pain.

TOXICITY 9
GI side effects with constipation, diarrhea, dry mouth, mild nausea.

Procarbazine

$$CH_3NHNHCH_2 \longrightarrow \overset{\overset{O}{\|}}{C}NHC\overset{CH_3}{\underset{CH_3}{H}}$$

TRADE NAME	Matulane, N-methylhydrazine	CLASSIFICATION	Nonclassic alkylating agent
CATEGORY	Chemotherapy drug	DRUG MANUFACTURER	Roche

MECHANISM OF ACTION

- Hydrazine analog that acts as an alkylating agent. Weak monoamine oxidase (MAO) inhibitor and a relative of the MAO inhibitor 1-methyl-2-benzylhydrazine.
- Requires metabolic activation for cytotoxicity. Occurs spontaneously through a non-enzymatic process and/or by an enzymatic reaction mediated by the liver cytochrome P450 system.
- While the precise mechanism of cytotoxicity is unclear, this drug inhibits DNA, RNA, and protein synthesis.
- Cell cycle–nonspecific drug.

MECHANISM OF RESISTANCE

- Enhanced DNA repair secondary to increased expression of AGAT.
- Enhanced DNA repair secondary to AGAT-independent mechanisms.

ABSORPTION

Rapid and complete absorption from the GI tract, reaching peak plasma levels within 1 hour.

DISTRIBUTION

Rapidly and extensively metabolized by the liver cytochrome P450 microsomal system. Procarbazine metabolites cross the blood-brain barrier, and peak CSF levels of drug occur within 30–90 minutes after drug administration.

METABOLISM

Metabolized to active and inactive metabolites by two main pathways, chemical breakdown in aqueous solution and liver microsomal P450 system. Possible formation of free radical intermediates. About 70% of procarbazine is excreted in urine within 24 hours. Less than 5%–10% of the drug is eliminated in an unchanged form. The elimination half-life is short, being less than 1 hour after oral administration.

INDICATIONS
1. Hodgkin's lymphoma.
2. Non-Hodgkin's lymphoma.
3. Brain tumors adjuvant and/or advanced disease.
4. Cutaneous T-cell lymphoma (CTCL).

DOSAGE RANGE
1. Hodgkin's lymphoma: 100 mg/m^2 PO daily for 14 days, as part of MOPP regimen.
2. Brain tumors: 60 mg/m^2 PO daily for 14 days, as part of PCV regimen.

DRUG INTERACTION 1
Alcohol- or tyramine-containing foods—Concurrent use with procarbazine can result in nausea, vomiting, increased CNS depression, hypertensive crisis, visual disturbances, and headache.

DRUG INTERACTION 2
Antihistamines, CNS depressants—Concurrent use of procarbazine with antihistamines can result in CNS and/or respiratory depression.

DRUG INTERACTION 3
Levodopa, meperidine—Concurrent use of procarbazine with levodopa or meperidine results in hypertension.

DRUG INTERACTION 4
Tricyclic antidepressants—Concurrent use of procarbazine with sympathomimetics and tricyclic antidepressants may result in CNS excitation; hypertension; tremors; palpitations; and, in severe cases, hypertensive crisis and/or angina.

DRUG INTERACTION 5
Antidiabetic agents—Concurrent use of procarbazine with antidiabetic agents such as sulfonylurea compounds and insulin may potentiate hypoglycemic effect.

SPECIAL CONSIDERATIONS
1. Monitor CBC while on therapy.
2. Prophylactic use of antiemetics 30 minutes before drug administration to reduce the risk of nausea and vomiting. Incidence and severity of nausea usually decrease with continued therapy.
3. Important to review patient's list of concurrent medications, as procarbazine has several potential drug–drug interactions.
4. Instruct patients to avoid ingestion of alcohol while on procarbazine. May result in disulfiram (Antabuse)-like effect.
5. Instruct patients about specific types of food to avoid during drug therapy (e.g., dark beer, wine, cheese, bananas, yogurt, and pickled and smoked foods).
6. Pregnancy category D. Breastfeeding should be avoided.

TOXICITY 1

Myelosuppression is dose-limiting. Thrombocytopenia is most pronounced, with nadir in 4 weeks and return to normal in 4–6 weeks. Neutropenia usually occurs after thrombocytopenia. Patients with G6PD deficiency may present with hemolytic anemia while on procarbazine therapy.

TOXICITY 2

Nausea and vomiting usually develop in the first days of therapy and improve with continued therapy. Diarrhea may also be observed.

TOXICITY 3

Flu-like syndrome in the form of fever, chills, sweating, myalgias, and arthralgias. Usually occurs with initial therapy.

TOXICITY 4

CNS toxicity in the form of paresthesias, neuropathies, ataxia, lethargy, headache, confusion, and/or seizures.

TOXICITY 5

Hypersensitivity reaction with pruritus, urticaria, maculopapular skin rash, flushing, eosinophilia, and pulmonary infiltrates. Skin rash responds to steroid therapy, and drug treatment may be continued. However, procarbazine-induced interstitial pneumonitis usually requires discontinuation of therapy.

TOXICITY 6

Amenorrhea and azoospermia.

TOXICITY 7

Immunosuppressive activity with increased risk of infections.

TOXICITY 8

Increased risk of secondary malignancies in the form of AML.

Q

Quazartinib

TRADE NAME	Vanflyta, AC220	**CLASSIFICATION**	Signal transduction inhibitor, FLT3 inhibitor
CATEGORY	Targeted agent	**DRUG MANUFACTURER**	Daiichi Sankyo

MECHANISM OF ACTION
- Highly potent, selective, second-generation type 2 FMS-like tyrosine kinase 3 (FLT3) internal tandem duplication (ITD) inhibitor.
- FLT3 ITD mutations present in about 25% of patients with newly diagnosed AML.
- FLT3 ITD mutations associated with more aggressive clinical disease and worse overall prognosis.

MECHANISM OF RESISTANCE
- Mutations in FLT3-ITD, including D835Y, and the F691L gatekeeper mutation.
- Mutations in the RAS/MAPK signaling pathway, including NRAS, KRAS, and BRAF.
- Activation of AXL-1 and PIM1.
- Induction of autophagy signaling network.
- Metabolic reprogramming in the bone marrow microenvironment with dependence on aurora kinase B.

ABSORPTION
Oral bioavailability of 71%, and time to peak drug levels is approximately 4 hours after ingestion. Food with high-fat content does not alter oral absorption.

DISTRIBUTION
Extensive binding (99%) of drug to plasma proteins, mainly serum albumin. Steady-state drug levels are achieved in approximately 15 days.

METABOLISM

Metabolized in the liver primarily by CYP3A4 and CYP3A5 microsomal enzymes. The main metabolite is AC886, which has potent antitumor activity. Approximately 76% of an administered dose is eliminated in feces and 16% is eliminated in urine. The terminal half-lives of quizartinib and AC886 are approximately 81 hours, and 136 hours, respectively.

INDICATIONS

FDA-approved in combination with standard cytarabine and anthracycline induction and cytarabine consolidation and as maintenance monotherapy following consolidation chemotherapy for adult patients with newly diagnosed AML that is FLT3 internal tandem duplication (ITD)-positive as detected by an FDA-approved test.

DOSAGE RANGE

Induction: recommended dose is 35.4 mg PO once daily starting on day 8 for 2 weeks in each cycle (days 8 to 21).

Consolidation: recommended dose is 35.4 mg PO once daily starting on day 6 for 2 weeks in each cycle (days 6 to 19).

Maintenance: recommended dose is 26.5 mg PO once daily on days 1 through 14 of the first cycle if QTc is <450 ms.

Dose should be increased to 53 mg PO once daily on day 15 of the first cycle if QTc is <450 msec.

Continue with the 26.5 mg daily dose if QTc>500 msec was observed during induction or consolidation.

Maintenance therapy should be given once daily with no break between cycles for up to 36 28-day cycles.

DRUG INTERACTION 1

Drugs such as ketoconazole, itraconazole, erythromycin, clarithromycin, atazanavir, indinavir, nefazodone, nelfinavir, ritonavir, saquinavir, telithromycin, and voriconazole may decrease the quazartinib metabolism, resulting in increased drug levels and potentially increased toxicity.

DRUG INTERACTION 2

Drugs such as rifampin, phenytoin, phenobarbital, carbamazepine, and St. John's Wort may increase quazartinib metabolism, resulting in lower effective drug levels.

DRUG INTERACTION 3

Drugs such as antifungal azoles, ondansetron, granisetron, azithromycin, pentamidine, doxycycline, moxifloxacin, prochorperazine, and tacrolimus are associated with QTc interval prolongation and may further increase the QTc interval with quazartinib therapy.

SPECIAL CONSIDERATIONS

1. Dose adjustment is not required for patients with mild or moderate hepatic impairment. Has not been studied in patients with severe hepatic impairment.
2. Dose adjustment is not required for patients with mild or moderate renal impairment (CrCl 30–89 mL/min). Has not been studied in patients with severe renal impairment or in those on hemodialysis.
3. Dose of quazartinib should be reduced when used with strong CYP3A4 inhibitors, as they may increase drug exposure.
4. Monitor ECGs at baseline and then once weekly, as quazartinib therapy can prolong the QTc interval. This is a black-box warning. Avoid the concomitant use of drugs that prolong the QT interval.
5. Monitor electrolyte status and correct any abnormalities, such as hypokalemia and hypomagnesemia.
6. May cause fetal harm. Females of reproductive potential should use effective contraception during drug therapy and for at least 7 months after the final dose. Breastfeeding should be avoided. Females should not breastfeed while on therapy and for 1 month after the last dose.

TOXICITY 1

QTc prolongation, Torsades de Pointes, and in very rare cases, cardiac arrest.

TOXICITY 2

Myelosuppression with neutropenia.

TOXICITY 3

Anorexia and fatigue.

Ramucirumab

TRADE NAME	Cyramza, IMC-1121B	CLASSIFICATION	Monoclonal antibody, anti-VEGFR antibody
CATEGORY	Targeted agent, anti-angiogenesis agent	DRUG MANUFACTURER	Eli Lilly

MECHANISM OF ACTION
- Recombinant fully human IgG1 monoclonal antibody directed against the vascular endothelial growth factor receptor 2 (VEGFR-2) and prevents binding of VEGF-A, VEGF-C, and VEGF-D ligands to their target receptor VEGFR-2.
- VEGFR-2 is the main VEGF-associated receptor that mediates tumor angiogenesis.
- Binds with high affinity to VEGFR-2 (50 pM) and results in inhibition of VEGFR-mediated signaling, which leads to reduced endothelial cell permeability, migration, and proliferation.
- Precise mechanism of action remains unknown.
- Inhibits formation of new blood vessels in primary tumor and metastatic tumors.
- Inhibits tumor blood vessel permeability and reduces interstitial tumoral pressures, and in so doing, may enhance blood flow delivery within tumor.

MECHANISM OF RESISTANCE
- Activation and/or upregulation of alternative pro-angiogenic factor ligands, such as bFGF and HGF.
- Recruitment of bone marrow–derived cells, which circumvents the requirement of VEGF signaling and restores neovascularization and tumor angiogenesis.

DISTRIBUTION
Distribution in the body is not well characterized. The estimated time to reach steady-state levels is approximately 28 days.

METABOLISM
Metabolism of ramucirumab has not been extensively characterized. The mean drug clearance is similar for patients with gastric cancer, NSCLC, and mCRC, and the mean terminal half-life is 14 days.

INDICATIONS
1. Advanced metastatic colorectal cancer—FDA-approved for use in combination with FOLFIRI chemotherapy with disease progression on or after prior therapy with FOLFOX/XELOX plus bevacizumab.

2. Advanced metastatic gastric or gastro-esophageal junction adenocarcinoma—FDA-approved for use as monotherapy or in combination with paclitaxel with disease progression on or after fluoropyrimidine or platinum-containing chemotherapy.
3. Metastatic NSCLC—FDA-approved in combination with docetaxel for metastatic NSCLC in patients with disease progression on or after platinum-based chemotherapy.
4. Metastatic NSCLC—FDA-approved in combination with erlotinib for first-line treatment of NSCLC with EGFR exon 19 deletions or exon 21 (L858R) mutations.
5. Hepatocellular cancer—FDA-approved for HCC with alfa-fetoprotein levels >400 ng/mL and following previous treatment with sorafenib.

DOSAGE RANGE

1. mCRC: recommended dose is 8 mg/kg IV every 2 weeks in combination with FOLFIRI.
2. Advanced gastric or gastro-esophageal junction adenocarcinoma: recommended dose is 8 mg/kg IV every 2 weeks as monotherapy or in combination with paclitaxel.
3. NSCLC: recommended dose is 10 mg/kg IV every 3 weeks in combination with docetaxel.
4. EGFR mutant NSCLC: recommended dose is 10 mg/kg IV every 2 weeks in combination with erlotinib 150 mg PO q day.
5. HCC: recommended dose is 8 mg/kg IV every 2 weeks.

DRUG INTERACTIONS

None well characterized to date.

SPECIAL CONSIDERATIONS

1. Serious, sometimes fatal arterial thromboembolic events, including myocardial infarction, cardiac arrest, cerebrovascular accident, and cerebral ischemia, may occur. Permanently discontinue ramucirumab in patients who experience a severe arterial thromboembolic event.
2. Patients should be warned of the potential for increased risk of hemorrhage and gastrointestinal hemorrhage, including severe and sometimes fatal hemorrhagic events. Patients with gastric cancer receiving NSAIDs were excluded from studies. As a result, the risk of gastric hemorrhage in patients with gastric tumors receiving NSAIDs is unknown.
3. Ramucirumab is associated with an increased incidence of severe hypertension. Use with caution in patients with uncontrolled hypertension. Closely monitor blood pressure every 2 weeks or more frequently as indicated during treatment. Should be permanently discontinued in patients who develop hypertensive crisis.
4. Closely monitor for infusion-related symptoms. May need to treat with diphenhydramine and acetaminophen.

5. Potentially fatal gastrointestinal perforation can occur. Should be permanently discontinued in patients who experience a gastrointestinal perforation.

6. Impaired wound healing can occur with antibodies inhibiting the VEGF signaling pathway, and ramucirumab has the potential to adversely affect wound healing. Should be discontinued in patients with impaired wound healing and withheld prior to surgery. Resume following surgery based on clinical judgment of adequate wound healing. If a patient develops wound-healing complications during therapy, discontinue until the wound is fully healed.

7. Clinical deterioration, as manifested by new-onset or worsening encephalopathy, ascites, or hepatorenal syndrome, has been reported in patients with Child-Pugh Class B or C cirrhosis who received single-agent ramucirumab.

8. Should be used with caution in patients with renal disease. Severe proteinuria, including nephrotic syndrome, has been reported. Should be withheld for urine protein levels that are >2 g over 24 hours and reinitiated at a reduced dose once the urine protein level returns to <2 g over 24 hours. Permanently discontinue if urine protein levels >3 g over 24 hours or in the setting of nephrotic syndrome.

9. Closely monitor thyroid function.

10. No dose adjustments are required in patients with renal impairment.

11. No dose adjustments are required in patients with mild or moderate hepatic impairment. Use with caution in patients with severe hepatic impairment, as increased toxicity may be observed.

12. Pregnancy category B.

TOXICITY 1
Hypertension occurs in up to 20%–30% of patients, with grade 3 hypertension observed in 8%–15% of patients. Usually well controlled with oral anti-hypertensive medication.

TOXICITY 2
Bleeding complications with epistaxis and GI hemorrhage, including severe and sometimes fatal hemorrhagic events.

TOXICITY 3
Fatigue and headache.

TOXICITY 4
Nausea/vomiting, anorexia, abdominal pain, and diarrhea.

TOXICITY 5
GI perforations and wound-healing complications.

TOXICITY 6
Proteinuria with nephrotic syndrome.

TOXICITY 7

Infusion-related symptoms with fever, chills, urticaria, flushing, fatigue, headache, bronchospasm, dyspnea, angioedema, and hypotension. Relatively uncommon (<5%).

TOXICITY 8

Increased risk of arterial thromboembolic events, including myocardial infarction, angina, and stroke. There is also an increased incidence of venous thromboembolic events.

TOXICITY 9

Hypothyroidism.

TOXICITY 10

RPLS occurs rarely (<0.1%), and presents with headache, seizure, lethargy, confusion, blindness, and other visual disturbances.

Regorafenib

TRADE NAME	Stivarga, BAY 73-4506	CLASSIFICATION	Signal transduction inhibitor, TKI
CATEGORY	Targeted agent	DRUG MANUFACTURER	Bayer, Onyx

MECHANISM OF ACTION

- Small-molecule inhibitor of multiple membrane-bound and intracellular kinases involved in oncogenesis, tumor angiogenesis, and maintenance of the tumor microenvironment.
- Inhibits tyrosine kinases associated with vascular endothelial growth factor receptors (VEGFR-1, VEGFR-2, VEGFR-3), platelet-derived growth factor receptors (PDGFR-α, PDGFR-β), and Tie-2.
- Inhibits oncogenic kinases such as c-Kit, RET, RAF-1, and BRAF.
- Inhibits tyrosine kinases associated with fibroblast growth factor receptors (FGFR-1, FGFR-2), DDR2, Trk2A, Eph2A, SAPK2, PTK5, and Abl.

MECHANISM OF RESISTANCE
- Activation of Akt signaling.
- Activation of Notch-1 signaling.
- Increased expression and activity of the multidrug resistant–associated transporter protein 2 (MRP2).
- Mutations in the KRAS gene.
- Defects in PUMA-mediated apoptosis.

ABSORPTION
Rapidly absorbed after an oral dose. Peak plasma levels are reached at a median time of 4 hours. The mean relative bioavailability of tablets compared to oral solution is 69%–83%. Food with a high-fat content increases oral bioavailability of parent drug by 48%.

DISTRIBUTION
Highly bound (99.5%) to human plasma proteins.

METABOLISM
Metabolized in the liver primarily by CYP3A4 and UGT1A9. The main circulating metabolites are M-2 (N-oxide) and M-5 (N-oxide and N-desmethyl), both of which have similar biological activity as parent drug. Approximately 71% of an administered drug is excreted in the feces, with 47% in parent form and 24% as metabolites, and 19% is eliminated in the urine. The terminal half-life of regorafenib is 28 hours, while the terminal half-lives of the M-2 and M-5 metabolites are approximately 25 and 51 hours, respectively.

INDICATIONS
1. FDA-approved for metastatic CRC following treatment with fluoropyrimidine-, oxaliplatin-, and irinotecan-based chemotherapy; an anti-VEGF therapy; and an anti-EGFR therapy if RAS wild-type.
2. FDA-approved for locally advanced, unresectable, or metastatic GIST previously treated with imatinib and sunitinib.
3. FDA-approved for hepatocellular cancer (HCC) following prior therapy with sorafenib.

DOSAGE RANGE
1. Recommended dose is 160 mg PO once daily after a low-fat meal for the first 21 days of a 28-day cycle.
2. Re-DOS strategy is to start at 80 mg/day with weekly escalation in 40-mg increments up to 160 mg/day if no significant drug-related adverse events.
3. Intermittent dosing schedule of 160 mg PO once daily for 1 week on and 1 week off.

DRUG INTERACTION 1

Strong inhibitors of CYP3A4 such as ketoconazole, itraconazole, clarithromycin, nefazodone, telithromycin, and voriconazole decrease regorafenib metabolism, resulting in increased drug levels and potentially increased toxicity.

DRUG INTERACTION 2

Drugs such as rifampin, phenytoin, phenobarbital, carbamazepine, and St. John's Wort increase regorafenib metabolism, resulting in its inactivation and potentially lower effective drug levels.

DRUG INTERACTION 3

Concomitant use of regorafenib, a UGT1A1 inhibitor, and irinotecan, a UGT1A1 substrate, may result in increased exposure of irinotecan and the active SN-38 metabolite, potentially leading to increased toxicity.

SPECIAL CONSIDERATIONS

1. Regorafenib should be taken at the same time each day with a low-fat breakfast that contains less than 600 calories and 30% fat.
2. Dose adjustment is not required in patients with pre-existing mild or moderate hepatic disease; however, regorafenib has not been studied in patients with severe hepatic disease, and use in this population is not recommended.
3. Dose adjustments are not required in patients with renal dysfunction. Has not been studied in patients on dialysis.
4. Regorafenib should be held for > grade 2/3 hand-foot skin reaction, symptomatic grade 2 hypertension, and any NCI CTCAE v3.0 grade 3/4 toxicity.
5. Patients should be warned of the risk of liver toxicity, which represents a black-box warning. LFTs need to be closely monitored while on therapy.
6. Regorafenib should be stopped permanently if a reduced dose of 80 mg is not tolerated, SGOT/SGPT >20 × ULN, SGOT/SGPT >3 × ULN with serum bilirubin >2 × ULN, recurrence of SGOT/SGPT >5 × ULN with dose reduction to 120 mg, and for any grade 4 side effects.
7. Dose of regorafenib can be reduced to 120 mg and 80 mg, respectively, based on specific conditions, which are outlined in the package insert.
8. Dose-escalation strategy starting initially at 80 mg/day and then weekly escalation in 40-mg increments up to 160 mg/day if no significant side effects are observed. This dosing strategy has been shown to reduce the incidence of side effects and maintain clinical activity.
9. Use with caution when administered with agents that are metabolized and/or eliminated by the UGT1A1 pathway, such as irinotecan, as regorafenib is an inhibitor of UGT1A1.
10. Patients receiving regorafenib along with oral warfarin anticoagulant therapy should have their coagulation parameters (PT and INR) monitored frequently, as elevations in INR and bleeding events have been observed.
11. Closely monitor blood pressure while on therapy, especially during the first 6 weeks of therapy, and treat as needed with standard oral antihypertensive medication.

12. Closely monitor LFTs at least every 2 weeks during the first 2 months of therapy and monthly thereafter.
13. Skin toxicities, including rash and hand-foot reaction, should be managed early in the course of therapy with topical treatments for symptomatic relief, temporary interruption, dose reduction, and/or discontinuation. Topical corticosteroids, such as 0.05% clobetasol, should be used for grades 2 and 3 skin toxicities. Sun exposure should be avoided, and periodic dermatologic evaluation is recommended.
14. Regorafenib should be interrupted in patients undergoing major surgical procedures.
15. Avoid Seville oranges, starfruit, pomelos, grapefruit, and grapefruit juice while on regorafenib therapy.
16. May cause fetal harm. Women of reproductive potential should use effective contraception while on therapy and for 2 months after the last dose. Males should use effective contraception for 2 months after the last dose. Breastfeeding should be avoided while on therapy and for 2 weeks after the last dose.

TOXICITY 1
Hypertension occurs in nearly 30% of patients. Usually occurs within 6 weeks of starting therapy and is well controlled with oral antihypertensive medications. Hypertensive crisis has been reported rarely.

TOXICITY 2
Skin toxicity in the form of hand-foot syndrome and skin rash occur in up to 45% and 26%, respectively. Usually appears within the first cycle of drug treatment.

TOXICITY 3
Bleeding complications occur in approximately 20% of patients.

TOXICITY 4
Diarrhea and nausea are the most common GI side effects.

TOXICITY 5
Fatigue and asthenia.

TOXICITY 6
Hepatotoxicity with elevations in SGOT/SGPT and serum bilirubin. Severe drug-induced liver injury resulting in death has been reported rarely.

TOXICITY 7
GI perforation and GI fistula occur rarely.

TOXICITY 8
Myocardial ischemia and/or infarction occur in about 1% of patients.

TOXICITY 9
CNS toxicity in the form of RPLS.

Relatlimab

TRADE NAME	Opdualag	**CLASSIFICATION**	Monoclonal antibody, LAG3 inhibitor, PD-1 inhibitor
CATEGORY	Immune checkpoint inhibitor, immunotherapy	**DRUG MANUFACTURER**	Bristol-Myers Squibb

MECHANISM OF ACTION
- Relatlimab is a humanized IgG4 antibody that binds to the lymphocyte activation gene-3 (LAG-3) receptor expressed on T cells, which then blocks the interaction between LAG-3 receptor and its ligands, including FGL1 and MHCII.
- Blockade of the LAG-3 pathway-mediated immune checkpoint overcomes immune escape mechanisms and enhances T-cell immune response, leading to T-cell activation and proliferation.
- Works best in combination with an anti-PD1 antibody, nivolumab, leading to enhanced T-cell activation.

MECHANISM OF RESISTANCE
- Increased expression and/or activity of other immune checkpoint pathways (e.g., TIGIT, TIM3).
- Increased expression of other immune escape mechanisms.
- Increased infiltration of immune suppressive populations within the tumor microenvironment, which include Tregs, myeloid-derived suppressor cells (MDSCs), and M2 macrophages.
- Release of various cytokines, chemokines, and metabolites within the tumor microenvironment, including CSF-1, tryptophan metabolites, TGF-β, and adenosine.

ABSORPTION
Administered only via the IV route.

DISTRIBUTION
Distribution in body is not well characterized. Steady-state levels are achieved by 16 weeks.

METABOLISM
Metabolism of relatlimab has not been extensively characterized. The terminal half-life is on the order of 26.5 days, similar to nivolumab.

INDICATIONS
FDA-approved for adult and pediatric patients 12 years of age or older with unresectable or metastatic melanoma.

DOSAGE RANGE
Recommended dose is nivolumab 480 mg IV and relatlimab 160 mg IV every 4 weeks.

DRUG INTERACTIONS
None well characterized to date.

SPECIAL CONSIDERATIONS
1. Relatlimab can result in significant immune-mediated adverse reactions due to T-cell activation and proliferation. These immune-mediated reactions may involve any organ system, with the most common reactions being pneumonitis, hepatitis, colitis, hypophysitis, pancreatitis, neurological disorders, and adrenal and thyroid dysfunction.
2. Relatlimab should be withheld for any of the following:
   - Grade 2 pneumonitis
   - Grades 2 or 3 colitis
   - SGOT/SGPT $> 3\times$ ULN and up to $5 \times$ ULN or total bilirubin $> 1.5 \times$ ULN and up to $3 \times$ ULN
   - Symptomatic hypophysitis, adrenal insufficiency, hypothyroidism, hyperthyroidism, or grades 3 or 4 hyperglycemia
   - Grade 2 ocular inflammatory toxicity
   - Grades 2 or 3 pancreatitis or grades 3 or 4 increases in serum amylase or lipase levels
   - Grades 3 or 4 infection
   - Grade 2 infusion-related reactions
   - Grade 3 skin rash
3. Relatlimab should be permanently discontinued for any of the following:
   - Grades 3 or 4 pneumonitis
   - SGOT/SGPT $> 8 \times$ ULN or total bilirubin $> 3 \times$ ULN
   - Grade 4 diarrhea or colitis
   - Grade 4 hypophysitis
   - Myasthenic syndrome/myasthenia gravis, Guillain-Barré syndrome, or meningoencephalitis (all grades)
   - Grades 3 or 4 ocular inflammatory toxicity
   - Grade 4 or any grade of recurrent pancreatitis
   - Grades 3 or 4 infusion-related reactions
   - Grade 4 skin rash
4. Monitor for symptoms and signs of infection.
5. Monitor thyroid and adrenal function prior to and during therapy.
6. Dose modification is not needed for patients with mild or moderate renal dysfunction. Has not been studied in patients with severe renal dysfunction.
7. Dose modification is not needed for patients with mild or moderate hepatic dysfunction. Has not been studied in patients with severe hepatic dysfunction.
8. May cause fetal harm. Advise females of potential of increased risk to a fetus and to use effective contraception during treatment and for at least 5 months after the last dose of drug.

TOXICITY 1
Infusion-related reactions.

TOXICITY 2
Colitis with diarrhea and abdominal pain.

TOXICITY 3
Pneumonitis with dyspnea and cough.

TOXICITY 4
Nausea/vomiting.

TOXICITY 5
Hepatotoxicity with elevations in SGOT/SGPT, alkaline phosphatase, and serum bilirubin.

TOXICITY 6
Endocrinopathies, including hypophysitis, thyroid disorders, adrenal insufficiency, and diabetes.

TOXICITY 7
Neurologic toxicity with neuropathy, myositis, and myasthenia gravis, Guillain-Barré syndrome, or meningoencephalitis.

TOXICITY 8
Musculoskeletal symptoms with arthralgias, oligoarthritis, polyarthritis, tenosynovitis, polymyalgia rheumatica, and myalgias.

TOXICITY 9
Cardiac toxicity with myocarditis, pericarditis, and vasculitis.

TOXICITY 10
Ocular toxicities in the form of uveitis, iritis, conjunctivitis, blepharitis, or episcleritis.

TOXICITY 11
Nephritis and renal dysfunction.

Relugolix

TRADE NAME	Orgovyx	**CLASSIFICATION**	LHRH receptor antagonist
CATEGORY	Hormonal agent	**DRUG MANUFACTURER**	Myovant Sciences

MECHANISM OF ACTION
- First oral non-peptide GnRH receptor antagonist that binds to pituitary GnRH receptors, which then leads to reduced release of LH and FSH, followed by lowered testosterone levels.

ABSORPTION
Oral bioavailability is approximately 60%. No significant effect of food on oral absorption. Steady-state levels reached within 7 days.

DISTRIBUTION
Moderate binding to plasma proteins (68%–71%).

METABOLISM
Metabolism occurs mainly in the liver by CYP3A4 and to a lesser extent by CYP2C8. The drug is primarily eliminated via the hepatobiliary route in feces (83%) with only a small amount eliminated in urine (4.4%). Only 2.2% of an administered dose is eliminated in the parent form. The elimination half-life is 25 hours.

INDICATIONS
Advanced prostate cancer.

DOSAGE RANGE
Loading dose of 360 mg PO on first day of treatment followed by 120 mg PO every day.

DRUG INTERACTIONS

Relugolix is a substrate for P-glycoprotein, so caution should be used in the presence of P-gp inhibitors, such as erythromycin and verapamil, and P-gp inducers, such as rifampin.

SPECIAL CONSIDERATIONS

1. Serum testosterone levels decrease to castrate levels within 3–4 days after initiation of therapy.
2. Results in sustained castration rates that are superior to that of leuprolide.
3. Significantly lower risk of cardiovascular events when compared to leuprolide.

TOXICITY 1

Hot flashes occur in about 50% of patients

TOXICITY 2

Fatigue.

TOXICITY 3

GI side effects with mild diarrhea and constipation.

TOXICITY 4

Cardiovascular events with MI and stroke.

TOXICITY 5

Musculoskeletal pain.

Retifanlimab

TRADE NAME	Zynyz, INCMGA00012	CLASSIFICATION	Anti-PD-1 antibody
CATEGORY	Immunotherapy, immune checkpoint inhibitor	DRUG MANUFACTURER	Incyte

MECHANISM OF ACTION

- Humanized IgG4 antibody that binds to the PD-1 receptor, which is expressed on T cells, and inhibits the interaction between the PD-L1 and PD-L2 ligands and the PD-1 receptor.
- Blockade of the PD-1 pathway-mediated immune checkpoint enhances T-cell immune response, leading to T-cell activation and proliferation.
- May also re-activate B-cell and NK function.

MECHANISM OF RESISTANCE

- Increased expression and/or activity of other immune checkpoint pathways (e.g., TIGIT, TIM3, and LAG3).
- Increased expression of other immune escape mechanisms.
- Increased infiltration of immune suppressive populations within the tumor microenvironment, which include Tregs, myeloid-derived suppressor cells (MDSCs), and M2 macrophages.
- Release of various cytokines, chemokines, and metabolites within the tumor microenvironment, including CSF-1, tryptophan metabolites, TGF-β, and adenosine.

DISTRIBUTION

Distribution in body has not been well characterized. Steady-state levels are achieved by about 6 months.

METABOLISM

Metabolism has not been extensively characterized. The terminal half-life is on the order of 19-20 days.

INDICATIONS

FDA-approved for adult patients with metastatic or recurrent locally advanced Merkel cell cancer. Approved under accelerated approval based on tumor response rate and duration of response.

DOSAGE

Recommended dose is 500 mg IV every 4 weeks.

DRUG INTERACTIONS

None well characterized to date.

SPECIAL CONSIDERATIONS

1. Associated with significant immune-mediated adverse reactions due to T-cell activation and proliferation. These immune-mediated reactions may involve any organ system, with the most common reactions being pneumonitis, colitis, hepatitis, hypophysitis, nephritis, and thyroid dysfunction.
2. Should be withheld for any of the following:
   - Grade 2 pneumonitis
   - Grade 2 or 3 colitis
   - SGOT/SGPT >3 × ULN and up to 8 × ULN or total bilirubin >1.5 × ULN and up to 3 × ULN
   - Grade 2 nephritis with renal dysfunction
   - Grade 3 or 4 endocrinopathies
   - Any other severe or grade 3 treatment-related toxicity
3. Should be permanently discontinued for any of the following:
   - Any life-threatening toxicity
   - Grade 3 or 4 pneumonitis
   - SGOT/SGPT >8 × ULN or total bilirubin >3 × ULN

- Grade 3 or 4 infusion-related reactions
- Grade 4 nephritis
- Any severe or grade 3 toxicity that recurs
- Inability to reduce steroid dose to 10 mg or less of prednisone or equivalent per day within 12 weeks
4. Monitor thyroid function prior to and during therapy.
5. Monitor patients for infusion-related reactions. May need to premedicate with an antipyretic and/or an antihistamine for patients who have previously experienced an infusion reaction.
6. Monitor patients for evidence of transplant-related complications, such as GVHD or hepatic veno-occlusive disease.
7. Dose modification is not needed for patients with mild or moderate renal dysfunction. Has not been studied in patients with severe renal dysfunction or end-stage renal disease.
8. Dose modification is not needed for patients with mild hepatic dysfunction. Has not been studied in patients with moderate or severe hepatic dysfunction.
9. Females should be advised of the potential risk to a fetus and should use effective contraception during treatment and for 4 months after the last dose. Breastfeeding should be avoided while on therapy and for 4 months after the last dose.

TOXICITY 1
Infusion-related reactions.

TOXICITY 2
Colitis with diarrhea and abdominal pain.

TOXICITY 3
Pneumonitis with dyspnea and cough.

TOXICITY 4
Hepatotoxicity with elevations in SGOT/SGPT, alkaline phosphatase, and serum bilirubin.

TOXICITY 5
GI side effects with nausea/vomiting and dry mouth. Pancreatitis can be observed.

TOXICITY 6
Fatigue, anorexia, and asthenia.

TOXICITY 7
Neurologic toxicity with neuropathy, myositis, and myasthenia gravis.

TOXICITY 8
Renal toxicity with nephritis.

TOXICITY 9
Musculoskeletal symptoms presenting with myalgias, arthralgias, oligo or polyarthritis, tenosynovitis, and polymyalgia rheumatica.

TOXICITY 10
Endocrinopathies, including hypogonadism, hypopituitarism, thyroid disorders, adrenal insufficiency, and diabetes.

TOXICITY 11
Maculopapular skin rash, erythema, dermatitis, and pruritus.

Ribociclib

TRADE NAME	Kisqali, LEE-011	CLASSIFICATION	Signal transduction inhibitor, CDK inhibitor
CATEGORY	Targeted agent	DRUG MANUFACTURER	Novartis

MECHANISM OF ACTION
- Inhibitor of cyclin-dependent kinase (CDK) 4 and 6.
- Inhibition of CDK 4/6 leads to inhibition of cell proliferation and growth by blocking progression of cells from G1 to the S-phase of the cell cycle.
- Decreased retinoblastoma protein phosphorylation (pRb), resulting in reduced E2F expression and signaling.

MECHANISM OF RESISTANCE
- Acquired CDK6 amplification, resulting in increased CDK6 expression.
- Increased expression of CDK2.
- Loss of pRb expression.
- Overexpression of cyclins A and E.
- FGFR1 gene amplification.
- Increased expression of 3-phosphoinositide-dependent protein kinase 1 (PDK1) with activation of AKT pathway and other AGC kinases.

ABSORPTION
Oral bioavailability is on the order of 46%. Peak plasma drug levels are achieved within 1–4 hours. Food does not appear to alter the rate and extent of drug absorption.

DISTRIBUTION
Moderate binding (70%) to plasma proteins with extensive tissue distribution. Steady-state drug levels are achieved within 8 days following repeat daily dosing.

METABOLISM
Extensively metabolized in the liver, primarily by CYP3A4 microsomal enzymes, with oxidation reactions being most important. The main metabolites are M13, M4, and M1. Nearly 70% of drug is eliminated via the hepatobiliary route in feces and only 23% in urine, with the majority of drug in metabolite form. Only 17% and 12% of parent drug is eliminated in feces and urine, respectively. The elimination half-life of the parent drug is 32 hours.

INDICATIONS
FDA-approved in combination with an aromatase inhibitor as initial endocrine-based therapy in postmenopausal women with hormone receptor (HR)–positive, HER2-negative advanced or metastatic breast cancer.

DOSAGE RANGE
Recommended dose is 600 mg PO daily for 21 days followed by 7 days off. Each cycle is 28 days. Can be taken with or without food.

DRUG INTERACTION 1
Drugs that stimulate liver microsomal CYP3A4 enzymes, including phenytoin, carbamazepine, rifampin, phenobarbital, and St. John's Wort—These drugs may increase ribociclib metabolism, resulting in lower drug levels and potentially reduced clinical activity.

DRUG INTERACTION 2
Drugs that inhibit liver microsomal CYP3A4 enzymes, including ketoconazole, itraconazole, erythromycin, and clarithromycin—These drugs may reduce ribociclib metabolism, resulting in increased drug levels and potentially increased toxicity.

DRUG INTERACTION 3
Drugs known to prolong QT interval—Avoid the concomitant use of drugs known to prolong the QT interval, such as anti-arrhythmic medications.

SPECIAL CONSIDERATIONS
1. Dose reduction is not required in the setting of mild hepatic impairment. Use with caution in patients with moderate or severe hepatic impairment, as ribociclib has not been studied in these settings.

2. Dose reduction is not required in the setting of mild or moderate renal impairment. Use with caution in patients with severe renal impairment, as ribociclib has not been studied in this setting.
3. Closely monitor CBC and platelet count every 2 weeks during the first 2 months of therapy and at monthly intervals thereafter.
4. Monitor ECGs and electrolyte status at baseline and while on therapy, as ribociclib therapy can result in QT interval prolongation.
5. Monitor LFTs at baseline and every 2 weeks for the first 2 cycles and at the start of each subsequent 4 cycles.
6. Pregnancy category D.

TOXICITY 1
Myelosuppression with neutropenia, anemia, and thrombocytopenia.

TOXICITY 2
Fatigue, anorexia, and asthenia.

TOXICITY 3
Increased risk of infections, with URI and UTI being most common.

TOXICITY 4
Nausea/vomiting, abdominal pain, and diarrhea.

TOXICITY 5
Hepatotoxicity with elevations in SGOT/SGPT and serum bilirubin.

TOXICITY 6
QT prolongation.

Ripretinib

TRADE NAME	Qinlock, DCC-2618	CLASSIFICATION	Signal transduction inhibitor, PDGFR-α and KIT inhibitor
CATEGORY	Targeted agent	DRUG MANUFACTURER	Deciphera

MECHANISM OF ACTION
- Novel type II inhibitor of KIT and platelet-derived growth factor receptor α (PDGFRA) activating and drug-resistant mutations.
- "Switch-control" kinase inhibitor that forces the activation loop into an inactive conformation.
- Inhibitor of all tested KIT and PDGFRA mutants and inhibits a wide range of KIT mutants in drug-resistant GIST.
- Inhibits other kinases, such as PDGFRB, TIE2, VEGFR2, and BRAF.

MECHANISM OF RESISTANCE
None well characterized to date.

ABSORPTION
Rapidly absorbed, with a median time to peak drug levels of 4 hours after oral ingestion for ripretinib and 15.6 hours for its main metabolite, DP-5439. Steady-state drug levels are achieved in 14 days for both ripretinib and DP-5439. Food with high fat content does not alter C_{max} or AUC.

DISTRIBUTION
Extensive binding (99.8%) of parent drug and DP-5439 metabolite to plasma proteins, including albumin and α-1 acid glycoprotein.

METABOLISM
Ripretinib and its main metabolite DP-5439 are metabolized in the liver primarily by CYP3A4 microsomal enzymes and to a lesser extent by CYP2C8 and CYP2D6. After an administered dose of ripretinib, 34% of parent drug and 6% of DP-5439 are eliminated in feces. Only 0.02% of ripretinib and 0.1% of DP-5439 are eliminated in urine. The terminal half-lives of ripretinib and DP-5439 are 14.8 and 17.8 hours, respectively.

INDICATIONS
FDA-approved for advanced GIST following prior treatment with >3 kinase inhibitors, including imatinib.

DOSAGE RANGE
Recommended dose is 150 mg PO once daily and can be taken with or without food.

DRUG INTERACTION 1
Drugs such as ketoconazole, itraconazole, erythromycin, clarithromycin, atazanavir, indinavir, nefazodone, nelfinavir, ritonavir, saquinavir, telithromycin, and voriconazole may decrease the rate of metabolism of ripretinib, resulting in increased drug levels and potentially increased toxicity.

DRUG INTERACTION 2
Phenytoin and other drugs that stimulate the liver microsomal CYP3A4 enzymes, including carbamazepine, rifampin, phenobarbital, and St. John's Wort—These drugs may increase the metabolism of ripretinib, resulting in lower effective drug levels.

SPECIAL CONSIDERATIONS

1. Dose reduction is not required in the setting of mild to moderate hepatic impairment. Has not been studied in the setting of severe hepatic impairment.
2. Dose reduction is not required in the setting of mild to moderate renal impairment. Has not been studied in patients with severe renal impairment or in those with end-stage renal disease.
3. Careful skin exams should be performed at baseline and routinely while on therapy and to closely monitor for new skin lesions.
4. Patients with a history of hypertension should have their blood pressure under good control before initiation of therapy. Monitor blood pressure while on therapy and may need to initiate or adjust antihypertensive medication as needed.
5. Monitor LV ejection fraction with MUGA or echocardiogram at baseline and periodically during treatment.
6. Ripretinib should be held for at least 1 week prior to elective surgery given the risk of impaired wound healing. Should not be administered for at least 2 weeks following major surgery and until there is evidence of adequate wound healing.
7. May cause fetal harm when administered to a pregnant woman. Females of reproductive potential should use effective contraception during drug therapy and for at least one week after the final dose. Breastfeeding should be avoided while on therapy and for at least one week after the final dose.

TOXICITY 1
Alopecia.

TOXICITY 2
Fatigue, asthenia, and anorexia.

TOXICITY 3
Nausea/vomiting, diarrhea, and abdominal pain.

TOXICITY 4
Myalgias and arthralgias.

TOXICITY 5
Hand-foot syndrome.

TOXICITY 6
Elevations in serum lipase.

TOXICITY 7
Hypertension.

TOXICITY 8
Cardiac dysfunction with cardiac failure, diastolic dysfunction, and ventricular hypertrophy.

TOXICITY 9
Hypophosphatemia.

TOXICITY 10
New primary cutaneous malignancies, including cutaneous squamous cell cancer, keratoacanthoma, and melanoma.

Rituximab

TRADE NAME	Rituxan	CLASSIFICATION	Anti-CD20 antibody
CATEGORY	Biologic response modifier agent, targeted agent	DRUG MANUFACTURER	Biogen-IDEC and Genentech

MECHANISM OF ACTION
- Chimeric anti-CD20 antibody consisting of human IgG1-κ constant regions and variable regions from the murine monoclonal anti-CD20 antibody.
- Targets the CD20 antigen, a 35-kDa cell-surface, non-glycosylated phosphoprotein expressed during early pre–B-cell development until the plasma cell stage. Binding of antibodies to CD20 results in inhibition of CD20-mediated signaling that leads to inhibition of cell activation and cell cycle progression.
- CD20 is expressed on more than 90% of all B-cell non-Hodgkin's lymphomas and leukemias.
- CD20 is not expressed on early pre–B cells, plasma cells, normal bone marrow stem cells, antigen-presenting dendritic reticulum cells, or other normal tissues.
- Chimeric antibody mediates complement-dependent cell lysis (CDCL) in the presence of human complement and antibody-dependent cellular cytotoxicity (ADCC) with human effector cells.

ABSORPTION
Administered only via the IV route.

DISTRIBUTION

Peak and trough levels of rituximab correlate inversely with the number of circulating CD20-positive B cells.

METABOLISM

Antibody can be detected in peripheral blood up to 3–6 months after completion of therapy. Elimination pathway has not been well characterized, although antibody-coated cells are reported to undergo elimination via Fc-receptor binding and phagocytosis by the reticuloendothelial system.

INDICATIONS

1. FDA-approved in adult patients for relapsed and/or refractory low-grade or follicular, CD20+, B-cell non-Hodgkin's lymphoma as a single agent.
2. FDA-approved in adult patients for previously untreated low-grade or follicular, CD20+, B-cell non-Hodgkin's lymphoma in combination with first-line chemotherapy and in patients achieving a complete or partial response to rituximab therapy in combination with chemotherapy, as single-agent maintenance therapy.
3. FDA-approved in adult patients for non-progressing (including stable disease) low-grade CD20-positive, B-cell non-Hodgkin's lymphoma as a single agent after CVP chemotherapy.
4. FDA-approved in adult patients for previously untreated diffuse large B-cell, CD20+, non-Hodgkin's lymphoma in combination with CHOP or other anthracycline-based chemotherapy regimens.
5. FDA-approved in adult patients in combination with fludarabine and cyclophosphamide for treatment of previously untreated and previously treated patients with CD20-positive CLL.
6. FDA-approved in pediatric patients aged 6 months or older for previously untreated diffuse large B-cell, Burkitt lymphoma, Burkitt-like lymphoma, or mature B-cell acute leukemia in combination with chemotherapy r.

DOSAGE RANGE

1. NHL: Recommended dose for relapsed or refractory low-grade or follicular NHL is 375 mg/m^2 IV on a weekly schedule for 4 or 8 weeks.
2. NHL: Recommended dose for retreatment of relapsed or refractory low-grade or follicular NHL is 375 mg/m^2 IV on a weekly schedule for 4 weeks.
3. NHL: Recommended dose for previously untreated low-grade or follicular NHL is 375 mg/m^2 IV on day 1 of each cycle of chemotherapy for up to 8 doses. For maintenance therapy, rituximab should be started 8 weeks following completion of rituximab plus chemotherapy and administered as a single agent every 8 weeks for up to 12 doses.
4. NHL: Recommended dose for non-progressing low-grade or follicular NHL after first-line CVP chemotherapy is 375 mg/m^2 IV on a weekly schedule for 4 weeks at 6-month intervals up to a maximum of 16 doses.

5. NHL: Recommended dose for diffuse large B-cell NHL is 375 mg/m^2 IV on day 1 of each cycle of chemotherapy for up to 8 doses.

6. CLL: Recommended dose is 375 mg/m^2 on the day prior to initiation of FC chemotherapy of the first cycle and then 500 mg/m^2 on day 1 of cycles 2–6, with each cycle administered every 28 days.

DRUG INTERACTIONS

None well characterized to date.

SPECIAL CONSIDERATIONS

1. Contraindicated in patients with known type 1 hypersensitivity or anaphylactic reactions to murine proteins or product components.

2. Patients should be premedicated with acetaminophen and diphenhydramine to reduce the incidence of infusion-related reactions.

3. Infusion should be started at an initial rate of 50 mg/hour. If infusion reaction is not observed during the first hour, the infusion rate can be escalated by increments of 50 mg/hour every 30 minutes to a maximum of 400 mg/hour. If the first treatment is well tolerated, the starting infusion rate for the second and subsequent infusions can be administered at 100 mg/hour with 100-mg/hour increments at 30-minute intervals up to 400 mg/hour. Rituximab should **NOT** be given by IV push.

4. Monitor for infusion-related events, which usually occur 30–120 minutes after the start of the first infusion. Infusion should be immediately stopped if signs or symptoms of an allergic reaction are observed. Immediate institution of diphenhydramine, acetaminophen, corticosteroids, IV fluids, and/or vasopressors may be necessary. In most instances, the infusion can be restarted at a reduced rate (50%) once symptoms have completely resolved. Resuscitation equipment should be readily available at bedside.

5. Infusion-related deaths within 24 hours have been reported. Usually occur with the first infusion. Other risk factors include female gender, patients with pre-existing pulmonary disease, and patients with CLL or mantle cell lymphoma.

6. Monitor for tumor lysis syndrome, especially in patients with high numbers of circulating cells (>25,000/mm^3) or high tumor burden. In this setting, the first dose of rituximab can be split into two doses, with 50% of the total dose to be given on days 1 and 2.

7. Use with caution in patients with pre-existing heart disease, including arrhythmias and angina, as there is an increased risk of cardiac toxicity. The development of cardiac arrhythmias requires cardiac monitoring with subsequent infusion of drug. Patients should be monitored during the infusion and in the immediate post-transfusion period.

8. Monitor for the development of skin reactions. Patients experiencing severe skin reactions should not receive further therapy, and skin biopsies may be required to guide future treatment.

9. Pregnancy category C. Breastfeeding should be avoided.

TOXICITY 1

Infusion-related symptoms, including fever, chills, urticaria, flushing, fatigue, headache, bronchospasm, rhinitis, dyspnea, angioedema, nausea, and/or hypotension. Usually occur within 30 minutes to 2 hours after the start of the first infusion, and they usually resolve upon slowing or interrupting the infusion and with supportive care. Incidence decreases with subsequent infusion.

TOXICITY 2

Tumor lysis syndrome. Characterized by hyperkalemia, hyperuricemia, hyperphosphatemia, hypocalcemia, and renal insufficiency. Usually occurs within the first 12–24 hours of treatment. Risk is increased in patients with high numbers of circulating malignant cells (>25,000/mm^3) and/or high tumor burden with bulky lymph nodes.

TOXICITY 3

Skin reactions, including pemphigus, Stevens-Johnson syndrome, lichenoid dermatitis, and toxic epidermal neurolysis. Usual onset ranges from 1 to 13 weeks following drug treatment.

TOXICITY 4

Arrhythmias and chest pain, usually during drug infusion. Increased risk in patients with pre-existing cardiac disease.

TOXICITY 5

Myelosuppression is rarely observed.

TOXICITY 6

Nausea and vomiting. Generally mild.

Rituximab-abbs

TRADE NAME	Truxima, biosimilar to rituximab	CLASSIFICATION	Anti-CD20 antibody
CATEGORY	Biologic response modifier agent, targeted agent	DRUG MANUFACTURER	Celltrion, Teva

INDICATIONS

1. FDA-approved for relapsed and/or refractory low-grade or follicular, CD20+, B-cell non-Hodgkin's lymphoma as a single agent.

R

2. FDA-approved for previously untreated low-grade or follicular, CD20+, B-cell non-Hodgkin's lymphoma in combination with first-line chemotherapy and as single-agent maintenance therapy in patients achieving a complete or partial response to rituximab therapy in combination with chemotherapy.
3. FDA-approved for non-progressing (including stable disease) low-grade CD20-positive, B-cell non-Hodgkin's lymphoma as a single agent after CVP chemotherapy.

Rituximab and human hyaluronidase

TRADE NAME	Rituxan Hycela	CLASSIFICATION	Anti-CD20 antibody
CATEGORY	Biologic response modifier agent, targeted agent	DRUG MANUFACTURER	Biogen and Genentech/ Roche

MECHANISM OF ACTION
- Combination of rituximab, a chimeric anti-CD20 antibody consisting of human IgG1-κ constant regions and variable regions from the murine monoclonal anti-CD20 antibody, and recombinant human hyaluronidase (rHuPh20), an endoglycosidase.
- Hyaluronidase has a local and reversible effect by increasing the permeability of the subcutaneous tissue by depolymerizing hyaluronan.
- Targets the CD20 antigen, a 35-kDa cell-surface, non-glycosylated phosphoprotein expressed during early pre–B-cell development until the plasma cell stage. Binding of antibodies to CD20 results in inhibition of CD20-mediated signaling that leads to inhibition of cell activation and cell cycle progression.
- CD20 is expressed on more than 90% of all B-cell non-Hodgkin's lymphomas and leukemias.
- CD20 is not expressed on early pre–B cells, plasma cells, normal bone marrow stem cells, antigen-presenting dendritic reticulum cells, or other normal tissues.
- Chimeric antibody mediates complement-dependent cell lysis (CDCL) in the presence of human complement and antibody-dependent cellular cytotoxicity (ADCC) with human effector cells.

ABSORPTION
Administered via the SC route.

DISTRIBUTION

Peak and trough levels of rituximab correlate inversely with the number of circulating CD20-positive B cells.

METABOLISM

The pharmacokinetics of SC rituximab are similar to IV rituximab with similar pharmacodynamic effects.

INDICATIONS

1. FDA-approved for relapsed and/or refractory low-grade or follicular, CD20+, B-cell non-Hodgkin's lymphoma as a single agent.
2. FDA-approved for previously untreated low-grade or follicular, CD20+, B-cell non-Hodgkin's lymphoma in combination with first-line chemotherapy and as single-agent maintenance therapy in patients achieving a complete or partial response to rituximab therapy in combination with chemotherapy.
3. FDA-approved for non-progressing (including stable disease) low-grade CD20-positive, B-cell non-Hodgkin's lymphoma as a single agent after CVP chemotherapy.
4. FDA-approved for previously untreated diffuse large B-cell, CD20+, non-Hodgkin's lymphoma in combination with CHOP or other anthracycline-based chemotherapy regimens.
5. FDA-approved in combination with fludarabine and cyclophosphamide for the treatment of previously untreated and previously treated patients with CD20-positive CLL.

DOSAGE RANGE

1. All patients must receive at least one full dose of rituximab by IV infusion before receiving SC rituximab.
2. NHL: Recommended dose for follicular NHL and diffuse large B-cell lymphoma is 1,400 mg/23,400 units (1,400 mg rituximab and 23,400 units hyaluronidase human) SC.
3. CLL: Recommended dose is 1,600 mg/26,800 units (1,600 mg rituximab and 26,800 units hyaluronidase human) SC.

DRUG INTERACTIONS

None well characterized to date.

SPECIAL CONSIDERATIONS

1. Patients should receive at least one full dose of IV rituximab before starting treatment with the SC formulation.
2. Patients should be premedicated with acetaminophen and diphenhydramine to reduce the incidence of infusion-related reactions. Premedication with a steroid should also be considered.
3. Closely monitor patients for at least 15 minutes after administration of SC rituximab.

4. Monitor for infusion-related events, which usually occur 30–120 minutes after the start of the first infusion. Infusion should be immediately stopped if signs or symptoms of an allergic reaction are observed. Immediate institution of diphenhydramine, acetaminophen, corticosteroids, IV fluids, and/or vasopressors may be necessary. In most instances, the infusion can be restarted at a reduced rate (50%) once symptoms have completely resolved. Resuscitation equipment should be readily available at bedside.

5. Infusion-related deaths within 24 hours have been reported with IV rituximab. Other risk factors include female gender, patients with pre-existing pulmonary disease, and patients with CLL or mantle cell lymphoma.

6. Monitor for tumor lysis syndrome, especially in patients with high numbers of circulating cells ($>25,000/mm^3$) or high tumor burden. In this setting, the first dose of rituximab can be split into two doses, with 50% of the total dose to be given on days 1 and 2.

7. Use with caution in patients with pre-existing heart disease, including arrhythmias and angina, as there is an increased risk of cardiac toxicity. The development of cardiac arrhythmias requires cardiac monitoring with subsequent infusion of drug. Patients should be monitored during the infusion and in the immediate post-transfusion period.

8. Monitor for infections, as serious bacterial, fungal, and new or reactivated viral infections can occur during or following completion of rituximab therapy. SC rituximab therapy should be terminated for serious infections, with initiation of appropriate anti-infective therapy.

9. Monitor for the development of skin reactions. Patients experiencing severe skin reactions should not receive further therapy, and skin biopsies may be required to guide future treatment.

10. Rituximab and hyaluronidase is **NOT** indicated for the treatment of non-cancer conditions.

11. Pregnancy category C. Breastfeeding should be avoided.

TOXICITY 1

Infusion-related symptoms with IV rituximab, including fever, chills, urticaria, flushing, fatigue, headache, bronchospasm, rhinitis, dyspnea, angioedema, nausea, and/or hypotension. Usually occur within 30 minutes to 2 hours after the start of the IV infusion. Usually resolve upon slowing or interrupting the infusion and with supportive care. Incidence decreases with subsequent infusion.

TOXICITY 2

Tumor lysis syndrome. Characterized by hyperkalemia, hyperuricemia, hyperphosphatemia, hypocalcemia, and renal insufficiency. Usually occurs within the first 12–24 hours of treatment. Risk is increased in patients with high numbers of circulating malignant cells ($>25,000/mm^3$) and/or high tumor burden with bulky lymph nodes.

TOXICITY 3

Infections, including bacterial and fungal infections. There is also an increased risk of new or reactivated viral infections, such as CMV, HSV, parvovirus B19, varicella zoster virus, West Nile virus, and hepatitis B and C.

TOXICITY 4

Skin rash and erythema with various skin disorders, including pemphigus, Stevens-Johnson syndrome, lichenoid dermatitis, and toxic epidermal neurolysis.

TOXICITY 5

Arrhythmias and chest pain, usually occurring during drug infusion. Increased risk in patients with pre-existing cardiac disease.

TOXICITY 6

Abdominal pain and bowel obstruction and perforation, which can be fatal in some cases.

TOXICITY 7

Progressive multifocal leukoencephalopathy (PML).

Rituximab-pvvr

TRADE NAME	Ruxience, biosimilar to rituximab	**CLASSIFICATION**	Anti-CD20 antibody
CATEGORY	Biologic response modifier agent, targeted agent	**DRUG MANUFACTURER**	Ruxience, Pfizer

INDICATIONS

1. FDA-approved as monotherapy for relapsed and/or refractory low-grade or follicular, CD20+, B-cell non-Hodgkin's lymphoma.
2. FDA-approved in combination with chemotherapy for previously untreated low-grade or follicular, CD20+, B-cell non-Hodgkin's lymphoma in combination with first-line chemotherapy and as single-agent maintenance therapy in patients achieving a complete or partial response to rituximab therapy.
3. FDA-approved as monotherapy for non-progressing (including stable disease) low-grade CD20-positive, B-cell non-Hodgkin's lymphoma after CVP chemotherapy.
4. FDA-approved in combination with CHOP or other anthracycline-based chemotherapy regimens for previously untreated diffuse large B-cell, CD20+, non-Hodgkin's lymphoma.

5. FDA-approved in combination with fludarabine and cyclophosphamide for the treatment of previously untreated and previously treated patients with CD20-positive CLL.
6. NHL: Recommended dose for diffuse large B-cell NHL is 375 mg/m^2 IV on day 1 of each cycle of chemotherapy for up to 8 doses.
7. CLL: Recommended dose is 375 mg/m^2 on the day prior to initiation of FC chemotherapy of the first cycle and then 500 mg/m^2 on day 1 of cycles 2–6, with each cycle administered every 28 days.

Romidepsin

TRADE NAME	Istodax, Depsipeptide	CLASSIFICATION	Histone deacetylase (HDAC) inhibitor
CATEGORY	Targeted agent	DRUG MANUFACTURER	Celgene

MECHANISM OF ACTION
- Bicyclic peptide isolated from *Chromobacterium violaceum*.
- Potent inhibitor of histone deacetylases HDAC1 and HDAC2.
- Inhibition of HDAC activity leads to accumulation of acetyl groups on the histone lysine residues, resulting in chromatin remodeling and open chromatin structure. Induction of cell-cycle arrest in G1- and G2/M-phases and/or apoptosis may then occur.
- Modulator of transcription of genes and cellular gene expression.
- Precise mechanism(s) by which romidepsin exerts its antitumor activity has not been fully characterized.

MECHANISM OF RESISTANCE
None well characterized to date.

ABSORPTION
Administered only via the IV route.

DISTRIBUTION
Significant binding (90%–95%) to plasma proteins.

METABOLISM

Extensive metabolism by CYP3A4, with minor contribution from CYP3A5, CYP1A1, CYP2B6, and CYP2C19. Elimination is mainly via metabolism. The terminal half-life of the parent drug is approximately 3–3.5 hours.

INDICATIONS

FDA-approved for the treatment of patients with CTCL who have received at least one prior systemic therapy.

DOSAGE RANGE

Recommended dose is 14 mg/m^2 on days 1, 8, and 15 of a 28-day cycle.

DRUG INTERACTIONS

1. Warfarin—Patients receiving warfarin should be closely monitored for alterations in their clotting parameters (PT and INR) and/or bleeding, as prolongation of PT and INR has been observed with concomitant use of romidepsin. The dose of warfarin may require careful adjustment in the presence of romidepsin therapy.
2. Phenytoin and other drugs that stimulate liver microsomal CYP3A4 enzymes, including carbamazepine, rifampin, phenobarbital, and St. John's Wort—These drugs may increase romidepsin metabolism, resulting in its inactivation and reduced drug levels.
3. Drugs that inhibit liver microsomal CYP3A4 enzymes, including ketoconazole, itraconazole, voriconazole, atazanavir, indinavir, ritonavir, erythromycin, and clarithromycin—These drugs may decrease romidepsin metabolism, resulting in increased drug levels and potentially increased toxicity.
4. P-glycoprotein inhibitors—Romidepsin is a substrate for the efflux transport protein P-glycoprotein. Caution should be used when romidepsin is given concomitantly with drugs that inhibit P-glycoprotein, as increased drug levels of romidepsin may be observed.

SPECIAL CONSIDERATIONS

1. Dose reduction is not required in patients with mild hepatic impairment. The dose should be reduced to 7 mg/m^2 in patients with moderate hepatic impairment and to 5 mg/m^2 in patients with severe hepatic impairment.
2. Dose reduction is not required in patient with mild to severe renal impairment. Has not been studied in patients with end-stage renal disease.
3. Closely monitor CBC and platelet count while on therapy.
4. Monitor ECG with QT measurement at baseline and periodically during therapy, as QTc prolongation has been observed. Use with caution in patients at risk of developing QT prolongation, including hypokalemia, hypomagnesemia, and congenital long QT syndrome, and in patients taking antiarrhythmic medications or any other products that may cause QT prolongation.
5. May cause fetal harm. Females of reproductive potential should use effective contraception during treatment and for at least 1 month after the last dose. Breastfeeding should be avoided while on therapy and for at least 1 week after the last dose.

TOXICITY 1
Nausea and vomiting are the most common GI toxicities.

TOXICITY 2
Myelosuppression with neutropenia, thrombocytopenia, and anemia.

TOXICITY 3
Fatigue and anorexia.

TOXICITY 4
Infections involving skin, upper respiratory tract, pulmonary system, GI system, and urinary tract.

TOXICITY 5
ECG changes consisting of T-wave flattening, ST segment depression, and rare cases of QTc prolongation. These ECG changes are usually not associated with functional cardiac toxicity.

Rucaparib

TRADE NAME	Rubraca	CLASSIFICATION	Signal transduction inhibitor, PARP inhibitor
CATEGORY	Targeted agent	DRUG MANUFACTURER	Clovis

MECHANISM OF ACTION
- Small-molecule inhibitor of poly (ADP-ribose) polymerase (PARP) enzymes, including PARP1, PARP2, and PARP3.
- Inhibition of PARP enzymatic activity, with increased formation of PARP-DNA complexes, results in cell death.
- Enhanced antitumor activity in tumors that are BRCA1- and BRCA2-deficient and in tumors with deficiencies in other DNA repair genes.

MECHANISM OF RESISTANCE

- Increased expression of the P-glycoprotein drug efflux transporter protein.
- Reduced expression of p53-binding protein 1 (53BP1), which is a critical component of DNA double-strand break (DSB) signaling and repair in mammalian cells.
- Reversion mutations in BRCA1 or BRCA2 that result in restoration of BRCA function.
- Loss of REV7 expression and function leads to restoration of homologous recombination, resulting in PARP resistance.
- Reduced expression of PARP enzymes.
- Increased stabilization of replication forks.

ABSORPTION

Oral bioavailability is approximately 40%. Peak plasma concentrations achieved at about 2 hours after administration. Food with high fat content can slow the rate of absorption but does not alter systemic drug exposure.

DISTRIBUTION

Moderate binding of rucaparib to plasma proteins (70%). Steady-state blood levels are achieved in about 15 days with daily dosing.

METABOLISM

Metabolized in the liver primarily by CYP2D6 microsomal enzymes and to a lesser extent by CYP3A4 and CYP1A2 enzymes. A large fraction of an administered dose of drug is metabolized by oxidation reactions, with several of the metabolites undergoing subsequent glucuronide or sulfate conjugation. Nearly 90% of drug is recovered, with 42% in feces and 44% in urine, with the majority of drug being in metabolite form. The terminal half-life is on the order of 17–19 hours.

INDICATIONS

1. FDA-approved for maintenance treatment of recurrent epithelial ovarian, fallopian tube, or primary peritoneal cancer in complete or partial remission to platinum-based chemotherapy.
2. FDA-approved for treatment of metastatic castration-resistant prostate cancer (mCRPC) that harbors deleterious BRCA mutations (germline and/or somatic) who have been previously treated with androgen receptor-directed therapy and taxane-based chemotherapy. Approved under accelerated approval based on objective response rate and duration of response.

DOSAGE RANGE

Recommended dose for ovarian cancer and prostate cancer is 600 mg PO bid with or without food.

DRUG INTERACTIONS
None well characterized to date.

SPECIAL CONSIDERATIONS
1. Dose adjustment is not required for patients with mild hepatic impairment. Has not been studied in patients with moderate or severe hepatic impairment, and there are no formal recommendations for dosing in these settings.
2. No dose modification is needed in patients with mild or moderate renal impairment (CrCl 30–89 mL/min). Has not been studied in patients with severe renal impairment or in those on dialysis, and there are no formal recommendations for dosing in these settings.
3. Closely monitor CBCs at baseline and monthly intervals. For prolonged hematologic toxicities, interrupt therapy, and monitor CBCs on a weekly basis until recovery. If blood counts have not recovered within 4 weeks, bone marrow analysis and peripheral blood for cytogenetics should be performed to rule out the possibility of MDS/AML.
4. May cause fetal harm. Females of reproductive potential should be warned of the potential risk to a fetus and to use effective contraception.

TOXICITY 1
Myelosuppression with anemia, thrombocytopenia, and neutropenia.

TOXICITY 2
Fatigue, anorexia, and asthenia.

TOXICITY 3
GI side effects in the form of nausea/vomiting, abdominal pain, diarrhea, and constipation.

TOXICITY 4
Elevations in serums transaminases (SGOT/SGPT) and serum cholesterol.

TOXICITY 5
Arthralgias, myalgias, and back pain.

TOXICITY 6
MDS and AML.

Sacituzumab govitecan

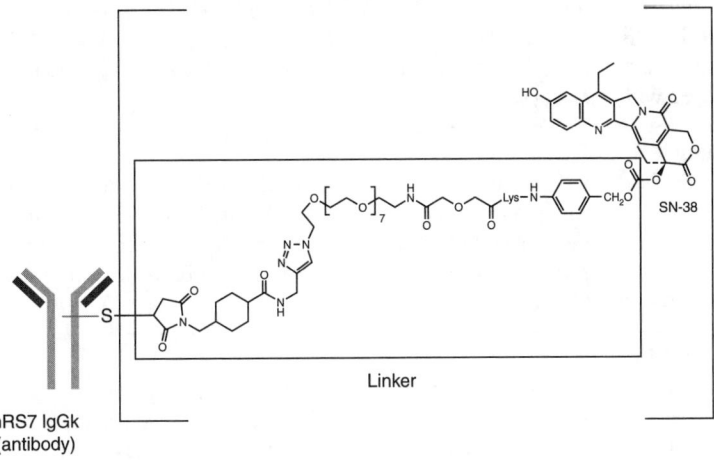

hRS7 IgGk
(antibody)

Linker

SN-38

TRADE NAME	Trodelvy, IMMU-132	**CLASSIFICATION**	Antibody-drug conjugate (ADC)
CATEGORY	Biologic response modifier agent, chemotherapy drug	**DRUG MANUFACTURER**	Immunomedics

MECHANISM OF ACTION

- Antibody-drug conjugate (ADC) made up of the humanized monoclonal antibody, sacituzumab hRS7 IgG1κ, directed against Trop-2 conjugated to govitecan (SN-38,) a topo I inhibitor. Approximately 7–8 molecules of SN-38 are conjugated to each antibody molecule.
- Upon binding to Trop-2, sacituzumab govitecan is rapidly internalized into lysosomes, and SN-38 is then released in the cell to target and inhibit the topo I protein. Inhibition of topo I leads to double-stranded DNA breaks and eventual cell death.
- Trop-2 is a 46-kDa transmembrane calcium signal protein that works through the ERK/MAPK and cyclin D1 signaling pathways to stimulate cell growth and proliferation, invasion, cell survival, and tumorigenesis.
- Trop-2 is overexpressed in many epithelial solid tumors, including breast cancer, and its expression is detected in more than 85% of triple-negative breast cancer.

MECHANISM OF RESISTANCE

None well characterized to date.

ABSORPTION
Administered only via the IV route.

DISTRIBUTION
Moderate binding (77%) of drug to plasma proteins. Steady-state drug levels are achieved within 21 days.

METABOLISM
No formal metabolism studies have been done with sacituzumab govitecan, but the antibody is expected to undergo catabolism to small peptides and amino acids. SN-38 is metabolized by UGT1A1 in the liver. The median terminal half-life of sacituzumab govitecan is 16 hours, and the terminal half-life of free SN-38 is approximately 18 hours.

INDICATIONS
1. FDA-approved for patients with metastatic triple-negative breast cancer who have received at least 2 prior therapies for metastatic disease.
2. FDA-approved for patients with unresectable, locally advanced or metastatic, hormone receptor-(HR) positive, HER2-negative breast cancer who have received endocrine-based therapy and at least 2 additional systemic therapies in the metastatic setting.
3. FDA-approved for patients with locally advanced or metastatic urothelial cancer who previously received a platinum-containing chemotherapy regimen and either PD-1 or PD-L1 inhibitor. Approved under accelerated approval based on tumor response rate and duration of response.

DOSAGE RANGE
Recommended dose for TNBC; HR-positive, HER2-negative breast cancer; and urothelial cancer is 10 mg/kg IV on days 1 and 8 of a 21-day schedule.

DRUG INTERACTION 1
UGT1A1 inhibitors—Concomitant use of sacituzumab govitecan with inhibitors of UGT1A1 may result in increased drug levels of SN-38 and potentially increased toxicity.

DRUG INTERACTION 2
UGT1A1 inducers—Concomitant use of sacituzumab govitecan with inducers of UGT1A1 may result in reduced drug levels of SN-38 and potentially reduced clinical activity.

SPECIAL CONSIDERATIONS
1. Sacituzumab govitecan should be administered as an IV infusion and **NOT** as an IV push or bolus. The first infusion should be administered over 3 hours and patients observed during the infusion and for at least 30 min after the infusion is completed. For all subsequent infusions, the drug can be given over 1–2 hours if the prior infusion was well tolerated.

2. Patients should be premedicated with antipyretics, H1 and H2 blockers prior to infusion, and steroids may be used for patients who previously experienced infusion reactions.
3. Closely monitor CBCs as severe neutropenia may occur. G-CSF should be considered to prevent neutropenic episodes. This is a black-box warning.
4. Treatment can be complicated by a syndrome of "early diarrhea," which is a cholinergic response to SN-38 and consists of diarrhea, diaphoresis, and abdominal cramping during the infusion or within 24 hours of drug administration. The recommended treatment is atropine (0.25–1.0 mg) administered IV unless clinically contraindicated. The routine use of atropine for prophylaxis is not recommended. However, atropine prophylaxis should be administered if a cholinergic event has been experienced with prior treatment.
5. Instruct patients about the possibility of late diarrhea (starting after 24 hours of drug administration), which can lead to serious dehydration and/or electrolyte imbalances if not managed promptly. This side effect is thought to be due to a direct irritation of the gastrointestinal mucosa by SN-38, although other as-yet-unidentified mechanisms may be involved. Loperamide should be taken immediately after the first loose bowel movement. The recommended dose is 4 mg PO as a loading dose, followed by 2 mg every 2 hours around the clock (4 mg every 4 hours during the night). Loperamide can be discontinued once the patient is diarrhea-free for 12 hours. If diarrhea should continue without improvement in the first 24 hours, an oral fluoroquinolone should be added. Hospitalization with IV antibiotics and IV hydration should be considered with continued diarrhea. This is a black-box warning.
6. Dose reduction is not recommended for patients with mild hepatic dysfunction. Sacituzumab govitecan has not been studied in patients with moderate or severe hepatic dysfunction, and use should be avoided in these settings.
7. Has not been studied in patients with renal impairment or with end-stage renal disease.
8. Patients with the UGT1A1 7/7 (UGT1A1*28) genotype may be at increased risk for developing myelosuppression and other side effects, such as diarrhea. Approximately 10% of the North American population is homozygous for this genotype.
9. May cause fetal harm when given to a pregnant woman. Females of reproductive potential should use effective contraception during treatment and for at least 2 months after the last dose. Males with female partners of reproductive potential should use effective contraception while on treatment and for at least 4 months after the last dose. Breastfeeding should be avoided.

TOXICITY 1
Myelosuppression with neutropenia is most commonly observed. Severe or life-threatening neutropenia can occur.

TOXICITY 2

Diarrhea with two different forms: early and late. Early form occurs during the infusion or within 24 hours of drug treatment and is characterized by flushing, diaphoresis, abdominal pain, and diarrhea. Late-form diarrhea occurs after 24 hours, typically at 3–10 days after treatment, can be severe and prolonged, and can lead to dehydration and electrolyte imbalance. Up to 60% of patients may experience some aspect of diarrhea, although only about 10% of patients will experience grade 3/4 diarrhea. Anorexia, nausea, and vomiting are usually mild and dose-related.

TOXICITY 3

Hypersensitivity infusion reactions.

TOXICITY 4

Nausea and vomiting.

TOXICITY 5

Fatigue and anorexia.

TOXICITY 6

Alopecia.

Selinexor

TRADE NAME	Xpovio, KPT-330	CLASSIFICATION	Nuclear export inhibitor, exportin 1 (XPO) inhibitor
CATEGORY	Targeted agent	DRUG MANUFACTURER	Karyopharm

MECHANISM OF ACTION

- Inhibits nuclear export of tumor suppressor proteins, growth regulators, and mRNAs of various oncogenic proteins by blocking exportin 1 (XPO1).

- Leads to accumulation and functional activation of tumor suppressor proteins in the nucleus and prevents the translation of oncoprotein mRNAs with reductions in several key oncoproteins, such as c-myc and cyclin D1. These effects lead to selective induction of apoptosis in tumor cells and largely spares normal cells.
- XPO1 is overexpressed in multiple myeloma and other cancers.

MECHANISM OF RESISTANCE
None well characterized to date.

ABSORPTION
Median time to peak drug levels is 4 hours, and there is no food effect on oral absorption.

DISTRIBUTION
Approximately 95% of drug is bound to plasma proteins.

METABOLISM
Metabolized in the liver primarily by CYP3A4, multiple UGTs, and glutathione-S-transferase microsomal enzymes. Elimination is nearly equal with excretion in feces (41%) and urine (48%), with only <10% eliminated as unchanged parent drug. The terminal half-life of selinexor is approximately 6–8 hours.

INDICATIONS
1. FDA-approved in combination with dexamethasone for adult patients with relapsed or refractory multiple myeloma who have received at least 4 prior therapies and whose disease is refractory to at least 2 proteasome inhibitors, at least 2 immunomodulatory agents, and an anti-CD38 monoclonal antibody.
2. FDA-approved in combination with bortezomib and dexamethasone for adult patients with multiple myeloma who have received at least 1 prior therapy.
3. FDA-approved for adult patients with relapsed or refractory diffuse large B cell (DLBCL), including DLBCL arising from follicular lymphoma, after at least 2 lines of systemic therapy. Approved under accelerated approval based on overall response rate.

DOSAGE RANGE
1. Multiple myeloma: 80 mg PO on days 1 and 3 of each week in combination with dexamethasone.
2. Multiple myeloma in combination with bortezomib and dexamethasone: 100 mg PO once weekly in combination with bortezomib and dexamethasone.
3. Diffuse large B-cell lymphoma: 60 mg PO on days 1 and 3 of each week for a 4-week cycle.

DRUG INTERACTIONS
None well characterized to date.

SPECIAL CONSIDERATIONS

1. Dose adjustment is not needed for patients with mild hepatic dysfunction. Has not been studied in setting of moderate or severe hepatic dysfunction.
2. Dose adjustment is not needed for patients with mild, moderate, or severe renal dysfunction. Has not been studied in setting of end-stage renal disease or in patients on hemodialysis.
3. Monitor CBCs at baseline, during treatment, and as clinically indicated.
4. Monitor serum sodium levels at baseline, during treatment, and as clinically indicated.
5. Patients on selinexor therapy should avoid other drugs that may cause CNS effects such as dizziness or confusion.
6. May cause fetal harm when administered to a pregnant woman. Females of reproductive potential should use an effective non-hormonal method of contraception during drug therapy and for at least 1 week after the final dose. Breastfeeding should be avoided.

TOXICITY 1
Myelosuppression with thrombocytopenia, anemia, and neutropenia.

TOXICITY 2
Fatigue and anorexia.

TOXICITY 3
Hyponatremia.

TOXICITY 4
Nausea/vomiting, diarrhea, constipation, dry mouth, and dysgeusia.

TOXICITY 5
CNS effects with dizziness, mental status changes, confusion, and blurred vision.

Selpercatinib

TRADE NAME	Retevmo	**CLASSIFICATION**	Signal transduction inhibitor, RET inhibitor
CATEGORY	Targeted agent	**DRUG MANUFACTURER**	Eli Lilly and Loxo

MECHANISM OF ACTION
- Small molecule inhibitor of wild-type RET and multiple mutant RET isoforms.
- Inhibits VEGFR1 and VEGFR3 as well as FGFR1, FGFR2, and FGFR3, albeit at much higher concentrations than for RET.
- RET fusion-positive NSCLC (1%–2%) and RET-mutant medullary thyroid cancer (60% sporadic, >90% hereditary) make up the largest fraction of RET-altered tumors.

MECHANISM OF RESISTANCE
- Development of RET solvent front mutations, including G810R, G810S, and G810C.
- Emergence of RET V804M gatekeeper mutation.

ABSORPTION
Rapidly absorbed, with a median time to peak drug levels of 2 hours after oral ingestion. Oral bioavailability is 73%. Steady-state drug levels are achieved in approximately 7 days. Food does not affect drug absorption.

DISTRIBUTION
Extensive binding (96%) to plasma proteins.

METABOLISM
Metabolized in the liver primarily by CYP3A4 microsomal enzymes. After an administered dose of drug, nearly 70% is eliminated via the hepatobiliary route in feces (14% as parent drug) and 24% is eliminated in urine (12% as parent drug). The terminal half-life of the drug is 32 hours.

INDICATIONS

1. FDA-approved for adult patients with locally advanced or metastatic RET fusion-positive NSCLC.
2. FDA-approved for adult and pediatric patients 12 years and older with advanced or metastatic RET-mutant medullary thyroid cancer (MTC) who require systemic therapy.
3. FDA-approved for adult and pediatric patients 12 years and older with advanced or metastatic RET fusion-positive thyroid cancer who require systemic therapy and who are radioactive iodine-refractory.
4. FDA-approved for adult patients with locally advanced or metastatic solid tumors with RET fusion and disease progression on or following prior systematic treatment or who have no satisfactory alternative treatment options.

DOSAGE RANGE

Recommended dose is based on weight.
<50 kg: 120 mg PO daily
>50 kg: 160 mg PO daily

DRUG INTERACTION 1

Drugs such as ketoconazole, itraconazole, erythromycin, clarithromycin, atazanavir, indinavir, nefazodone, nelfinavir, ritonavir, saquinavir, telithromycin, and voriconazole may decrease the rate of metabolism of selpercatinib, resulting in increased drug levels and potentially increased toxicity.

DRUG INTERACTION 2

Phenytoin and other drugs that stimulate the liver microsomal CYP3A4 enzymes, including carbamazepine, rifampin, phenobarbital, and St. John's Wort—These drugs may increase the metabolism of selpercatinib, resulting in lower effective drug levels and potentially reduced clinical activity.

SPECIAL CONSIDERATIONS

1. Dose reduction is not required in the setting of mild and moderate hepatic impairment. Dose reduction is recommended in the setting of severe hepatic impairment, as defined by total bilirubin >3–10 × ULN with any SGOT. If the current dose is 120 mg or 160 mg bid, the dose should be reduced to 80 mg bid.
2. Dose reduction is not required in the setting of mild and moderate renal impairment. Has not been studied in patients with severe renal impairment or in those with end-stage renal disease.
3. Avoid concomitant use with PPIs, H2 receptor blockers, or locally acting antacids. If this can not be avoided, selpercatininb should be taken 2 hours before or 2 hours after antacid or H2 blocker and taken with food when co-administered with a PPI.

4. Monitor LFTs at baseline and every 2 weeks during the first 3 months of therapy, then once a month or as clinically indicated.
5. Monitor blood pressure while on therapy, starting at 1 week after initiation and then at least on a monthly basis or as clinically indicated.
6. Monitor QT interval and electrolyte status periodically as the drug can cause QT interval prolongation.
7. Patients should be warned about the potential risk of hypersensitivity reactions. If such reactions occur, the drug should be stopped, and steroids initiated at a dose of 1 mg/kg. If there are recurrent episodes of hypersensitivity reactions, the drug should be permanently discontinued.
8. Should be held for at least 1 week prior to elective surgery given the risk of impaired wound healing. The drug should not be administered for at least 2 weeks following major surgery and until there is evidence of adequate wound healing.
9. May cause fetal harm when administered to a pregnant woman. Females of reproductive potential should use effective contraception during drug therapy and for at least 1 week after the final dose. Breastfeeding should be avoided.

TOXICITY 1
Hypertension.

TOXICITY 2
Hepatotoxicity.

TOXICITY 3
Hypersensitivity reactions with fever, skin rash, and arthralgias.

TOXICITY 4
QTc interval prolongation.

TOXICITY 5
Hemorrhagic events, including cerebral hemorrhage, tracheostomy site hemorrhage, and hemoptysis.

TOXICITY 6
Impaired wound healing.

TOXICITY 7
GI side effects with dry mouth, nausea/vomiting, diarrhea, and abdominal pain.

Sipuleucel-T

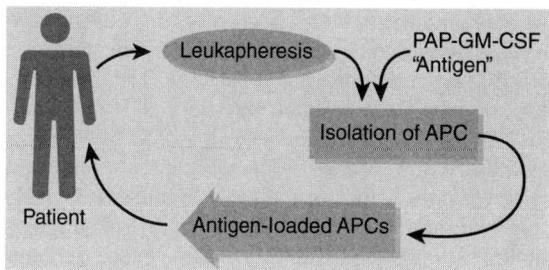

TRADE NAME	Provenge, APC8015	**CLASSIFICATION**	Vaccine
CATEGORY	Immunotherapy, cell therapy	**DRUG MANUFACTURER**	Dendreon

MECHANISM OF ACTION
- Sipuleucel-T is an autologous vaccine prepared using a patient's own peripheral blood mononuclear cells.
- Stimulates T-cell immunity to prostatic acid phosphatase (PAP), an antigen expressed in the majority of prostate cancer but not in non-prostate tissue.
- Composed of autologous antigen-presenting cells (APCs) cultured ex vivo with a fusion protein, termed PA2024, which is made up of PAP linked to GM-CSF. PA2024 provides efficient loading and processing of antigen by APCs.
- Activated APCs trigger autologous immune reaction against PAP-expressing prostate cancer cells.

MECHANISM OF RESISTANCE
- Down-regulation of the cell surface expression of PAP.
- Increased tumor load, rendering vaccine therapy ineffective.
- Activation of the PD-1 immune checkpoint pathway, with increased expression of the PD-1 receptor, which is present on the surface of activated T cells, resulting in inhibition of the immune response.

ABSORPTION
Administered only via the IV route.

INDICATIONS

FDA-approved for the treatment of asymptomatic or minimally symptomatic metastatic, castrate-resistant (hormone-refractory) prostate cancer.

DOSAGE RANGE

1. Sipuleucel-T is for autologous use only.
2. Recommended course is three doses infused over 60 minutes at 2-week intervals.
3. Each dose contains a minimum of 50 million autologous CD54+ cells activated with PAP-GM-CSF in a sealed, patient-specific infusion bag.

DRUG INTERACTIONS

None well characterized to date.

SPECIAL CONSIDERATIONS

1. Patients should be premedicated 30 minutes prior to administration with acetaminophen 1,000 mg PO and diphenhydramine 50 mg PO to reduce the incidence of acute infusion reactions.
2. Monitor for infusion-related events, which typically occur within 1 day of infusion and are more severe following the second infusion.
3. Use with caution in patients with underlying cardiac or pulmonary disease.
4. Universal precautions need to be employed, as sipuleucel-T is not routinely tested for transmissible infectious diseases.
5. The concomitant use of chemotherapy and immunosuppressive medications should be avoided, as they have the potential to reduce the efficacy and/or alter the toxicity of sipuleucel-T.
6. No pregnancy category has been assigned.

TOXICITY 1

Acute infusion reactions in the form of chills, fever, fatigue, and headache. In more severe cases, patients present with dyspnea, cough, hypoxia, and bronchospasm.

TOXICITY 2

Arthralgias, myalgias, muscle cramps/spasms, and bone pain.

TOXICITY 3

Mild nausea, vomiting, constipation, diarrhea, and anorexia.

Sonidegib

TRADE NAME	Odomzo, LDE225	**CLASSIFICATION**	Signal transduction inhibitor, hedgehog inhibitor
CATEGORY	Targeted agent	**DRUG MANUFACTURER**	Novartis

MECHANISM OF ACTION
- Small molecule inhibitor of the hedgehog pathway.
- Binds to and inhibits smoothened, a transmembrane protein that is involved in hedgehog signaling.

MECHANISM OF RESISTANCE
- Increased expression of MAPK signaling.
- Activation/induction of alternative cellular signaling pathways, such as c-Met, FGFR, EGFR, and PI3K/Akt.
- Reactivation of Ras/Raf signaling via mutations in KRAS, NRAS, and BRAF.
- Cross-resistance between sonidegib and vismodegib.

ABSORPTION
Oral bioavailability is low at about 10%. Median time to peak drug levels (T_{max}) is 2–4 hours. Food with high-fat content can significantly increase AUC drug exposure.

DISTRIBUTION
Extensive binding (97%) of sonidegib to plasma proteins.

METABOLISM
Metabolism occurs mainly in the liver by CYP3A microsomal enzymes. The main route of elimination of parent drug and its metabolites is via the hepatobiliary route, with excretion in feces (70%), with renal elimination accounting for 30% of an administered dose. The elimination half-life of sonidegib is approximately 28 days.

INDICATIONS
FDA-approved for patients with locally advanced basal cell cancer that has recurred following surgery or radiation therapy or in those who are not candidates for surgery and/or radiation.

DOSAGE RANGE

Recommended dose is 200 mg PO once daily on an empty stomach, at least 1 hour before or 2 hours after a meal.

DRUG INTERACTION 1

Phenytoin and other drugs that stimulate the liver microsomal CYP3A4 enzymes, including carbamazepine, rifampin, phenobarbital, and St. John's Wort—These drugs may increase the metabolism of sonidegib, resulting in its inactivation and lower effective drug levels.

DRUG INTERACTION 2

Drugs that inhibit the liver microsomal CYP3A4 enzymes, including ketoconazole, itraconazole, erythromycin, and clarithromycin—These drugs may decrease the metabolism of sonidegib, resulting in increased drug levels and potentially increased toxicity.

SPECIAL CONSIDERATIONS

1. Sonidegib should be taken on an empty stomach at least 1 hour before or 2 hours after a meal.
2. Dose reduction is not required in patients with mild, moderate, or severe hepatic impairment.
3. Dose reduction is not required in patients with mild or moderate renal impairment. However, the drug has not been studied in the setting of severe renal impairment or end-stage renal disease.
4. Patients should be advised not to donate blood or blood products while on sonidegib and for at least 20 months after the last drug dose.
5. The pregnancy status of female patients must be verified prior to the start of vismodegib therapy given the risk of embryo-fetal death and/or severe birth defects. This is a black-box warning.
6. Female and male patients of reproductive potential should be counseled on pregnancy prevention and planning. Female patients should be advised on the need for contraception and for at least 20 months after the last dose. Male patients should be advised of the potential risk of drug exposure through semen and to use condoms with a pregnant partner or a female partner of reproductive potential during treatment with sonidegib and for at least 8 months after the last dose. This is a black-box warning.
7. In contrast to vismodegib, proton pump inhibitors can be used while on sonidegib therapy.
8. Closely monitor serum creatine kinase (CK) and creatinine levels at baseline and periodically while on sonidegib therapy, as musculoskeletal adverse reactions, including rhabdomyolysis, have been reported.
9. Patients should be advised to report any new unexplained muscle pain, tenderness, or weakness that occurs during treatment or that persists after sonidegib therapy has been stopped.
10. Pregnancy category X. Breastfeeding should be avoided.

TOXICITY 1

Embryo-fetal deaths and/or severe birth defects.

TOXICITY 2

Musculoskeletal side effects, which include muscle spasms, musculoskeletal pain, myalgia, muscle tenderness, or weakness. Rhabdomyolysis is a rare event.

TOXICITY 3

Elevations in serum CK.

TOXICITY 4

Decreased appetite, weight loss, fatigue, and asthenia.

TOXICITY 5

Change in taste and/or loss of taste.

TOXICITY 6

Alopecia.

TOXICITY 7

Nausea/vomiting, constipation, and diarrhea.

TOXICITY 8

Hepatotoxicity with elevations in SGOT/SGPT.

TOXICITY 9

Elevations in serum lipase and amylase.

Sorafenib

TRADE NAME	Nexavar, BAY 43-9006	CLASSIFICATION	Signal transduction inhibitor, TKI
CATEGORY	Targeted agent, anti-angiogenesis agent	DRUG MANUFACTURER	Bayer and Onyx

MECHANISM OF ACTION
- Inhibits multiple receptor tyrosine kinases (RTKs), some of which are involved in tumor growth, tumor angiogenesis, and metastasis.
- Inhibitor of c-Raf and wild-type and mutant B-Raf.
- Targets vascular endothelial growth factor receptors, VEGF-R2 and VEGF-R3, and platelet-derived growth factor receptor-β (PDGFR-β), and, in so doing, inhibits angiogenesis.

MECHANISM OF RESISTANCE
- Activation of angiogenic switch, with increased expression of alternative pro-angiogenic pathways.
- Increased pericyte coverage to tumor vessels, with increased expression of VEGF and other pro-angiogenic factors.
- Recruitment of pro-angiogenic inflammatory cells from bone marrow, such as tumor-associated macrophages, monocytes, and myeloid-derived suppressor cells (MDSCs).

ABSORPTION
Rapidly absorbed after an oral dose, with peak plasma levels achieved within 2 to 7 hours. Oral administration should be without food at least 1 hour before or 2 hours after eating, as food with a high-fat content reduces oral bioavailability by up to 29%.

DISTRIBUTION
Extensive binding (99%) to plasma proteins. Steady-state drug concentrations are reached in 7 days.

METABOLISM
Metabolized in the liver, primarily by CYP3A4 microsomal enzymes and by glucuronidation mediated by UGT1A9. Parent drug accounts for 70%–85% at steady state, while the pyridine-N-oxide metabolite, which has similar biological activity to sorafenib, accounts for 9%–16%. Elimination is via the hepatobiliary route, with excretion in feces (~77%). Renal elimination of the glucuronidated metabolites accounts for nearly 20% of an administered dose. The terminal half-life of sorafenib is approximately 25–48 hours.

INDICATIONS
1. FDA-approved for the treatment of advanced renal cell cancer.
2. FDA-approved for the treatment of unresectable hepatocellular cancer (HCC).

DOSAGE RANGE
Recommended dose is 400 mg PO bid. Dose may need to be reduced in Asian patients, as they appear to experience increased toxicity to sorafenib.

DRUG INTERACTION 1

Drugs such as ketoconazole and other CYP3A4 inhibitors may decrease the rate of metabolism of sorafenib. However, one study with ketoconazole administered at a dose of 400 mg once daily for 7 days did not alter the mean AUC of a single oral dose of sorafenib 50 mg in healthy volunteers.

DRUG INTERACTION 2

Drugs such as rifampin, phenytoin, phenobarbital, carbamazepine, and St. John's Wort increase the rate of metabolism of sorafenib, resulting in its inactivation and potentially lower effective drug levels.

SPECIAL CONSIDERATIONS

1. Sorafenib should be taken without food at least 1 hour before or 2 hours after a meal.
2. No dose adjustment is necessary in patients with mild or moderatae liver dysfunction. However, sorafenib has not been studied in patients with severe (Child-Pugh Class C) liver dysfunction, and caution should be used in this setting.
3. No dose adjustments are necessary in patients with mild or moderate renal dysfunction. Has not been studied in patients with severe renal dysfunction or in those undergoing dialysis.
4. Use with caution when administering sorafenib with agents that are metabolized and/or eliminated by the UGT1A1 pathway, such as irinotecan, as sorafenib is an inhibitor of UGT1A1.
5. Patients receiving sorafenib along with oral warfarin anticoagulant therapy should have their coagulation parameters (PT and INR) monitored frequently, as elevations in INR and bleeding events have been observed.
6. Closely monitor blood pressure while on therapy, especially during the first 6 weeks of therapy, and treat as needed with standard oral antihypertensive medication.
7. Skin toxicities, including rash and hand-foot reaction, should be managed early in the course of therapy with topical treatments for symptomatic relief, temporary interruption, dose reduction, and/or discontinuation. Sun exposure should be avoided, and periodic dermatologic evaluation is recommended.
8. Sorafenib therapy should be interrupted in patients undergoing major surgical procedures.
9. Avoid Seville oranges, starfruit, pomelos, grapefruit, and grapefruit juice while on sorafenib therapy.
10. Pregnancy category D. Breastfeeding should be avoided.

TOXICITY 1

Hypertension usually occurs within 6 weeks of starting therapy and is usually well controlled with oral antihypertensive medication.

TOXICITY 2

Skin rash. Hand-foot skin reaction occurs in up to 30%. Rare cases of actinic keratoses and cutaneous squamous cell cancer have been reported.

TOXICITY 3
Bleeding complications with epistaxis most commonly observed.

TOXICITY 4
Wound-healing complications.

TOXICITY 5
Constitutional side effects with fatigue and asthenia.

TOXICITY 6
Diarrhea and nausea are the most common GI side effects.

TOXICITY 7
Hypophosphatemia occurs in up to 45% of patients but is usually clinically asymptomatic.

Sotorasib

TRADE NAME	Lumakras, AMG510	**CLASSIFICATION**	Signal transduction inhibitor, KRAS G12C inhibitor
CATEGORY	Targeted agent	**DRUG MANUFACTURER**	Amgen

MECHANISM OF ACTION
- Selective and irreversible small molecule inhibitor of KRAS G12C mutation.
- Forms a covalent bond with the unique cysteine of the KRAS G12C protein, which locks the protein in an inactive GDP-bound state that prevents downstream signaling without affecting wild-type KRAS.
- KRAS G12C mutation present in 13% of NSCLC and 1%–3% of CRC and other solid tumors.
- Results in a pro-inflammatory tumor microenvironment that drives antitumor immunity.

MECHANISM OF RESISTANCE

- Acquired mutations in KRAS at codons 12, 13, 61, 68, 95, and 96.
- Amplification of the KRAS G12C allele.
- Polyclonal RAS-MAPK reactivation with activation/induction of downstream cellular signaling pathways, such as RAS/RAF, PI3K/AKT, and MAPK.
- MET amplification.
- Transformation to squamous cell histology.

ABSORPTION

Median time to peak drug levels is 1 hour, and steady-state drug levels are reached in 22 days. Food with high-fat content increases AUC by about 25%.

DISTRIBUTION

Fairly extensive protein binding (89%).

METABOLISM

Metabolized mainly by non-enzymatic conjugation and oxidative metabolism by liver CYP3A4 microsomal enzymes. Elimination of drug is mainly via the hepatobiliary route in feces (75%), the majority of which (53%) is in parent form. Renal clearance of parent drug and metabolites account for only about 6% of an administered dose. The half-life is on the order of 5.5 hours.

INDICATIONS

FDA-approved for the treatment of KRAS G12C-mutated locally advanced or metastatic non–small cell lung cancer (NSCLC). Approved under accelerated approval based on overall response rate and duration of response.

DOSAGE RANGE

Recommended dose is 960 mg PO daily with or without food.

DRUG INTERACTION 1

Drugs such as ketoconazole, itraconazole, erythromycin, clarithromycin, atazanavir, indinavir, nefazodone, nelfinavir, ritonavir, saquinavir, telithromycin, and voriconazole may decrease sotorasib metabolism, resulting in increased drug levels and potentially increased toxicity.

DRUG INTERACTION 2

Phenytoin and other drugs that stimulate the liver microsomal CYP3A4 enzymes, including carbamazepine, rifampin, phenobarbital, and St. John's Wort—These drugs may increase sotorasib metabolism, resulting in lower effective drug levels and potentially reduced activity.

DRUG INTERACTION 3

Certain P-gp substrates—Avoid concomitant use of sotorasib with certain P-gp substrates, such as digoxin, verapamil, diltiazem, dabigatran, and fexofenadine.

DRUG INTERACTION 4

Avoid concomitant use of gastric acid-reducing agents, such as proton pump inhibitors, H2 blockers, and antacids as they may reduce oral bioavailability of sotorasib.

SPECIAL CONSIDERATIONS

1. Dose reduction is not required in setting of mild hepatic impairment. Has not been studied in the setting of moderate or severe hepatic impairment.
2. Dose reduction is not required in setting of mild or moderate renal impairment. Has not been studied in the setting of severe renal impairment or end-stage renal disease.
3. Monitor LFTs every 3 weeks for the first 3 months of treatment and then once monthly as indicated.
4. Monitor patients for pulmonary symptoms. Therapy should be held in patients presenting with new or progressive pulmonary symptoms and should be permanently stopped if treatment-related pneumonitis or interstitial lung disease (ILD) is confirmed.
5. If treatment with a gastric acid-reducing agent can not be avoided, use a local antacid and take sotorasib 4 hours before or 10 hours after ingestion of the local antacid.
6. There is no currently available data on the risk of sotorasib in pregnant women. Breastfeeding should be avoided while on treatment and for 1 week after the final dose.

TOXICITY 1

GI side effects with diarrhea and nausea/vomiting.

TOXICITY 2

Pulmonary toxicity with increased cough, dyspnea, and pulmonary infiltrates. Interstitial lung disease (ILD) and pneumonitis are the more serious events.

TOXICITY 3

Hepatotoxicity with elevations in SGOT/SGPT and serum bilirubin.

TOXICITY 4

Fatigue and diarrhea.

TOXICITY 5

Arthralgias and musculoskeletal pain.

Streptozocin

TRADE NAME	Streptozotocin, Zanosar	CLASSIFICATION	Alkylating agent
CATEGORY	Chemotherapy drug	DRUG MANUFACTURER	Teva

MECHANISM OF ACTION
- Cell cycle–nonspecific nitrosourea analog.
- Formation of intrastrand cross-links of DNA, resulting in inhibition of DNA synthesis and function.
- Selectively targets pancreatic β cells, possibly due to the presence of a glucose moiety on the compound.
- In contrast to other nitrosourea analogs, no effect on RNA or protein synthesis.

MECHANISM OF RESISTANCE
- Decreased cellular uptake of drug.
- Increased intracellular thiol content due to glutathione and/or glutathione-related enzymes.
- Enhanced activity of DNA repair enzymes.

ABSORPTION
Administered only via the IV route.

DISTRIBUTION
Rapidly cleared from plasma, with an elimination half-life of 35 minutes. Drug concentrates in the liver and kidney, reaching concentrations equivalent to those in plasma. Drug metabolites cross the blood-brain barrier and enter the CSF. Selectively concentrates in pancreatic β cells, presumably due to the glucose moiety on the molecule.

METABOLISM
Metabolized primarily by the liver to active metabolites. The elimination half-life of the drug is short, being less than 1 hour. About 60%–70% of drug is excreted in urine, 20% in unchanged form. Less than 1% of drug is eliminated in stool.

INDICATIONS

1. Pancreatic islet cell cancer.
2. Carcinoid tumors.

DOSAGE RANGE

1. Weekly schedule: 1,000–1,500 mg/m^2 IV weekly for 6 weeks, followed by 4 weeks of observation.
2. Daily schedule: 500 mg/m^2 IV for 5 days every 6 weeks.

DRUG INTERACTION 1

Steroids—Concurrent use of steroids and streptozocin may result in severe hyperglycemia.

DRUG INTERACTION 2

Phenytoin—Phenytoin antagonizes the antitumor effect of streptozocin.

DRUG INTERACTION 3

Nephrotoxic drugs—Avoid concurrent use of streptozocin with nephrotoxic agents, as renal toxicity may be enhanced.

SPECIAL CONSIDERATIONS

1. Use with caution in patients with abnormal renal function. Dose reduction is recommended in this setting, as nephrotoxicity is dose-limiting and can be severe and/or fatal. Baseline CrCl should be obtained, as well as monitoring of renal function before each cycle of therapy. Hydration with 1–2 liters of fluid is recommended to prevent nephrotoxicity.
2. Monitor CBC while on therapy.
3. Avoid the use of other nephrotoxic agents in combination with streptozocin.
4. Carefully administer drug to minimize and/or avoid burning, pain, and extravasation.
5. Pregnancy category D. Breastfeeding should be avoided.

TOXICITY 1

Renal toxicity is dose-limiting. Occurs in 40%–60% of patients and presents with proteinuria and azotemia. May also present as glucosuria, hypophosphatemia, and nephrogenic diabetes insipidus. Permanent renal damage can occur in rare cases.

TOXICITY 2

Nausea and vomiting occur in 90% of patients. More frequently observed with the daily dosage schedule and in some cases can be severe.

TOXICITY 3

Myelosuppression is usually mild, with nadir occurring at 3–4 weeks.

TOXICITY 4
Pain and/or burning at the injection site.

TOXICITY 5
Altered glucose metabolism, resulting in either hypoglycemia or hyperglycemia.

TOXICITY 6
Mild and transient increases in SGOT/SGPT, alkaline phosphatase, and bilirubin. Usual onset is within 2–3 weeks of starting therapy.

Sunitinib

TRADE NAME	Sutent, SU11248	CLASSIFICATION	Signal transduction inhibitor, TKI
CATEGORY	Targeted agent	DRUG MANUFACTURER	Pfizer

MECHANISM OF ACTION
- Inhibits multiple RTKs, some of which are involved in tumor growth, tumor angiogenesis, and metastasis.
- Potent inhibitor of platelet-derived growth factor receptors (PDGFR-α and PDGFR-β), vascular endothelial growth factor receptors (VEGFR-1, VEGFR-2, and VEGFR-3), stem cell factor receptor (Kit), Fms-like tyrosine kinase-3 (Flt3), colony-stimulating factor receptor type 1 (CSF-1R), and glial cell-line derived neurotrophic factor receptor (RET).

MECHANISM OF RESISTANCE
- Increased expression of PDGFR-α, PDGFR-β, VEGFR-1, VEGFR-2, VEGFR-3, c-Kit, CSF-1R, and RET.
- Mutations in RTKs leading to reduce binding affinity to drug.
- Induction of kinome reprogramming with induction of multiple kinases, including FAK, SCR, MET, FGFR2, EGFR, IGF-1R, and ERBB2.
- Epigenetic modifications with increased expression of EZH2.

- Enhanced stability of MCL-1 protein and activation of mTOR signaling.
- Activation of angiogenic switch, with increased expression of alternative pro-angiogenic pathways.
- Increased pericyte coverage to tumor vessels, with increased expression of VEGF and other pro-angiogenic factors.
- Recruitment of pro-angiogenic inflammatory cells from bone marrow, such as tumor-associated macrophages, monocytes, and myeloid-derived suppressor cells (MDSCs).
- Increased degradation and/or metabolism of the drug through as-yet ill-defined mechanisms.

ABSORPTION
Oral bioavailability is nearly 100%, and food does not affect oral absorption.

DISTRIBUTION
Extensive binding (90%–95%) of sunitinib and its primary metabolite to plasma proteins. Peak plasma levels are achieved 6–12 hours after ingestion. Steady-state drug concentrations of sunitinib and its primary active metabolite are reached in 10–14 days.

METABOLISM
Metabolized in the liver primarily by CYP3A4 microsomal enzymes to produce its primary active metabolite, which is further metabolized by CYP3A4. The primary active metabolite comprises 23%–37% of the total exposure. Elimination is via the hepatobiliary route, with excretion in feces (~60%). Renal elimination accounts for only16% of an administered dose. The terminal half-lives of sunitinib and its primary active metabolite are approximately 40–60 hours and 80–110 hours, respectively. With repeated daily administration, sunitinib accumulates 3- to 4-fold, while the primary metabolite accumulates 7- to 10-fold.

INDICATIONS
1. FDA-approved for GIST after disease progression on or intolerance to imatinib.
2. FDA-approved for advanced renal cell cancer (RCC).
3. FDA-approved for the adjuvant treatment of patients at high risk of recurrent RCC following nephrectomy.
4. FDA-approved for progressive, well-differentiated PNET in patients with unresectable locally advanced or metastatic disease.

DOSAGE RANGE
1. GIST and RCC: 50 mg/day PO for 4 weeks, followed by 2 weeks off.
2. GIST and RCC: An alternative schedule is 50 mg/day PO for 2 weeks, followed by 1 week off.
3. Adjuvant therapy of RCC: 50 mg/day PO for 4 weeks followed by 2 weeks off for nine 6-week cycles.
4. PNET: 37.5 mg/day PO continuously.
5. RCC: Alternative schedule is 37.5 mg/day PO continuously for first- and second-line treatment

DRUG INTERACTION 1

Drugs such as ketoconazole, itraconazole, erythromycin, clarithromycin, atazanavir, indinavir, nefazodone, nelfinavir, ritonavir, saquinavir, telithromycin, and voriconazole decrease the rate of sunitinib metabolism, resulting in increased drug levels and potentially increased toxicity.

DRUG INTERACTION 2

Drugs such as rifampin, phenytoin, phenobarbital, carbamazepine, and St. John's Wort increase sunitinib metabolism of, resulting in its inactivation and reduced drug levels.

SPECIAL CONSIDERATIONS

1. Baseline and periodic evaluations of LVEF should be performed while on sunitinib therapy.
2. Use with caution in patients with underlying cardiac disease, especially those who presented with cardiac events within 12 months prior to initiation of sunitinib, such as MI (including severe/unstable angina), coronary/peripheral artery bypass graft, and CHF.
3. In the presence of clinical manifestations of CHF, discontinuation of sunitinib is recommended. The dose of sunitinib should be interrupted and/or reduced in patients without clinical evidence of CHF but with an ejection fraction <50% and >20% below pretreatment baseline.
4. Closely monitor blood pressure while on therapy and treat as needed with standard oral antihypertensive medication. In cases of severe hypertension, temporary suspension of sunitinib is recommended until hypertension is controlled.
5. Closely monitor LFTs at baseline and during each cycle of therapy. Treatment should be interrupted for >grade 3 hepatotoxicity and should be stopped if there is no improvement in LFTs and/or there is evidence of liver failure.
6. No dose adjustment is necessary in patients with mild or moderate (Child-Pugh Class A and B) liver dysfunction. Has not been studied in patients with severe (Child-Pugh Class C) liver disease, and caution should be used in this setting.
7. No dose adjustments are necessary in patients with mild, moderate, or severe renal dysfunction and in patients undergoing dialysis.
8. Monitor for adrenal insufficiency in patients who experience increased stress such as surgery, trauma, or severe infection.
9. Closely monitor thyroid function tests and TSH at 2- to 3-month intervals, as sunitinib treatment results in hypothyroidism. The incidence of hypothyroidism is increased with prolonged duration of therapy.
10. Avoid Seville oranges, starfruit, pomelos, grapefruit, and grapefruit products while on sunitinib therapy.
11. Pregnancy category D. Breastfeeding should be avoided.

TOXICITY 1

Hypertension occurs in up to 30% of patients. Usually occurs within 3–4 weeks of starting therapy and is usually well controlled with oral antihypertensive medication.

TOXICITY 2

Yellowish discoloration of the skin occurs in approximately 30% of patients. Skin rash, dryness, thickness, and/or cracking of skin. Depigmentation of hair and/or skin may also occur.

TOXICITY 3

Bleeding complications with epistaxis most commonly observed.

TOXICITY 4

Hepatotoxicity with elevated LFTs and serum bilirubin. In severe cases, liver failure or death can occur.

TOXICITY 5

Constitutional side effects with fatigue and asthenia, which may be significant in some patients.

TOXICITY 6

Diarrhea, stomatitis, altered taste, and abdominal pain are the most common GI side effects. Pancreatitis has been reported rarely with elevations in serum lipase and amylase.

TOXICITY 7

Increased risk of left ventricular dysfunction, which in some cases results in CHF.

TOXICITY 8

Adrenal insufficiency and hypothyroidism.

TOXICITY 9

TTP, HUS, and thrombotic microangiopathy.

TOXICITY 10

Tumor lysis syndrome is a rare event that usually occurs in the setting of high tumor burden.

Tafasitamab-cxix

TRADE NAME	Monjuvi, XmAb5574	**CLASSIFICATION**	Monoclonal antibody, anti-CD19 antibody
CATEGORY	Targeted agent	**DRUG MANUFACTURER**	MorphoSys AG

MECHANISM OF ACTION
- Fc-modified, humanized anti-CD19 monoclonal antibody directed against the CD19 antigen.
- CD19 is broadly expressed in B-cell malignancies and enhances B-cell receptor signaling and tumor cell proliferation.
- Modified Fc region engineered with the introduction of two amino acids within the Fc region to increase affinity for the activating Fcγreceptor CD16A (FCγRIIIa) on immune cells. This engineered antibody can then mediate immunologic-mediated functions, including ADCC and ADCP.

MECHANISM OF RESISTANCE
None well characterized to date.

ABSORPTION
Administered only via the IV route.

DISTRIBUTION
Total distribution is 9.3 L.

METABOLISM
Metabolism has not been extensively characterized. Terminal half-life is on the order of 17 days.

INDICATIONS
FDA-approved for the treatment of relapsed or refractory DLBCL not otherwise specified, including DLBCL arising from low grade lymphoma, and who are not eligible for autologous stem cell transplant (ASCT).

DOSAGE RANGE
Recommended dose is 12 mg/kg IV according to the following schedule:
  Cycle 1: days 1, 4, 8, 15, and 22 of a 28-day cycle
  Cycles 2 and 3: days 1, 8, 15, and 22 of each 28-day cycle
  Cycle 4 and beyond: days 1 and 15 of each 28-day cycle

DRUG INTERACTIONS
No formal drug interactions have been characterized to date.

SPECIAL CONSIDERATIONS

1. Monitor for infusion-related reactions, which are most frequently seen with the first infusion. The majority of the infusion reactions occur during cycles 1 or 2. Premedication with an antihistamine (diphenhydramine), an antipyretic (acetaminophen), and a steroid (dexamethasone or methylprednisolone) to be administered 30 minutes to 2 hours before tafasitamab infusion can prevent and/or reduce the severity of the infusion reaction.
2. Monitor for signs and symptoms of infection.
3. Monitor CBC prior to each cycle and periodically while on therapy. Patients may need G-CSF for support.
4. Embryo-fetal toxicity. Females of reproductive potential should use effective contraception during drug therapy and for 3 months after the final dose. Breastfeeding should be avoided.

TOXICITY 1
Myelosuppression with neutropenia, thrombocytopenia, and anemia.

TOXICITY 2
Infusion-related symptoms with fever, chills, rash, urticaria, flushing, dyspnea, and hypertension.

TOXICITY 3
Infections with URIs, UTIs, bronchitis, nasopharyngitis, and pneumonia.

TOXICITY 4
Diarrhea, abdominal pain, and nausea/vomiting.

TOXICITY 5
Fatigue and anorexia.

TOXICITY 6
Skin rash and pruritus.

Tagraxofusp-erzs

TRADE NAME	Elzonris, SL-401	**CLASSIFICATION**	Immunotoxin, cytotoxin
CATEGORY	Targeted agent, biologic agent	**DRUG MANUFACTURER**	Stemline Therapeutics

MECHANISM OF ACTION
- Recombinant fusion protein composed of human interleukin-3 (IL-3) fused to a truncated diptheria toxin payload.

- Binds to the alpha chain of IL-3 receptors (CD123) and internalized with subsequent release of the cytotoxic diptheria toxin payload. This then catalyzes ADP ribosylation of elongation factor 2, leading to inhibition of protein synthesis and cell death.
- CD123 receptor is overexpressed in blastic plasmacytoid dendritic cell neoplasm (BPDCN) as well as other hematologic cancers when compared to normal cells.

ABSORPTION
Administered only via the IV route.

DISTRIBUTION
Mean steady-state volume of distribution is 5.1 L.

METABOLISM
Metabolism has not been well characterized. Short terminal half-life of 0.7 hours.

INDICATIONS
FDA-approved for the treatment of adult and pediatric patients 2 years and older with blastic plasmacytoid dendritic cell neoplasm.

DOSAGE RANGE
Recommended dose is 12 mcg/kg once daily on days 1–5 of a 21-day schedule.

DRUG INTERACTION
None well characterized to date.

SPECIAL CONSIDERATIONS
1. Prior to initiation of therapy, ensure that patients have adequate cardiac function and that serum albumin is >3.2 g/dL. Monitor serum albumin levels prior to each dose of therapy, and monitor for signs and symptoms of capillary leak syndrome. This is a black-box warning.
2. Monitor for hypersensitivity reactions. Premedicate patients with H1 antagonist, H2 antagonist, and acetaminophen at 60 minutes prior to each infusion.
3. First treatment cycle should be administered in the inpatient setting. All subsequent cycles may be given in the inpatient or outpatient settings. Patients should be monitored for a minimum of 4 hours following each infusion.
4. Monitor liver function tests and serum bilirubin while on therapy.
5. Dose reduction is not required in patients with mild or moderate hepatic dysfunction. Has not been studied in setting of severe hepatic dysfunction.
6. Dose reduction is not required in patients with mild or moderate renal dysfunction. Has not been studied in setting of severe renal dysfunction or end-stage renal disease.

7. May cause fetal harm. Women should be advised to use effective contraception during treatment and for 1 week after the last dose of treatment. Breastfeeding should be avoided while on therapy and for 1 week after the last dose.

TOXICITY 1
Capillary leak syndrome (CLS) with weight gain, peripheral edema, pulmonary edema, hypotension, and hemodynamic instability.

TOXICITY 2
Hypersensitivity reactions.

TOXICITY 3
Hepatotoxicity with elevation in LFTs and serum bilirubin.

TOXICITY 4
Hypoalbuminemia.

TOXICITY 6
Fatigue and anorexia.

Talazoparib

TRADE NAME	Talzenna	CLASSIFICATION	Signal transduction inhibitor, PARP inhibitor
CATEGORY	Targeted agent	DRUG MANUFACTURER	BioMarin and Pfizer

MECHANISM OF ACTION
- Small-molecule inhibitor of poly (ADP-ribose) polymerase (PARP) enzymes, including PARP1 and PARP2.
- More potent inhibitor of PARP1 when compared to other PARP inhibitors, including olaparib, rucaparib, and veliparib.
- Inhibition of PARP enzymatic activity, with increased formation of PARP-DNA complexes, results in cell death.

- Enhanced antitumor activity in tumors that are BRCA1- and BRCA2-deficient and in tumors with defects in other DNA repair genes.
- Exhibits enhanced antitumor activity when combined with other DNA damaging agents, such as temozolomide, SN-38, or platinum analogs.

MECHANISM OF RESISTANCE
- Increased expression of the P-glycoprotein drug efflux transporter protein.
- Reduced expression of p53-binding protein 1 (53BP1), which is a critical component of DNA double-strand break (DSB) signaling and repair in mammalian cells.
- Reversion mutations in BRCA1 or BRCA2 that result in restoration of BRCA function.
- Loss of REV7 expression and function leads to restoration of homologous recombination, resulting in PARP resistance.

ABSORPTION
Good oral bioavailability. Peak plasma concentrations are achieved in about 1–2 hours after administration. Food does not alter oral absorption.

DISTRIBUTION
Moderate binding of talazoparib to plasma proteins (74%). Steady-state blood levels are achieved in 2–3 weeks with daily dosing.

METABOLISM
Undergoes minimal metabolism in the liver, which is in contrast to other PARP inhibitors. The main metabolic pathways include cysteine conjugation, dehydrogenation, glucuronide conjugation, and mono-oxidation. Nearly 70% of an administered dose of drug is recovered in urine, and nearly 20% is recovered in feces, with more than 50% of drug eliminated in urine in the parent form. The terminal half-life is on the order of 90 hours.

INDICATIONS
1. FDA-approved for treatment of deleterious or suspected deleterious germline BRCA-mutated, HER2-negative, locally advanced or metastatic breast cancer, as detected by an FDA-approved diagnostic assay.
2. FDA-approved in combination with enzalutamide for homologous recombination repair (HRR) gene-mutated metastatic castration-resistant prostate cancer.

DOSAGE RANGE
1. Breast cancer: 1 mg PO daily with or without food.
2. Prostate cancer: 0.5 mg PO daily with enzalutamide. Patients should also receive a GnRH analog concurrently or should have undergone bilateral orchiectomy.

DRUG INTERACTIONS

P-gp inhibitors—Co-administration with P-gp inhibitors may increase talazoparib drug exposure.

SPECIAL CONSIDERATIONS

1. Dose adjustment is not required for patients with mild hepatic impairment. Has not been studied in patients with moderate or severe hepatic impairment, and there are no formal recommendations for dosing in these settings.
2. No dose modification is needed in patients with mild renal impairment (CrCl 60–89 mL/min). The dose of drug should be reduced to 0.75 mg PO once daily in the setting of moderate renal impairment (CrCl 30–59 mL/min). Has not been studied in patients with severe renal impairment or in those on dialysis, and there are no formal recommendations for dosing in these settings.
3. The dose of talazoparib should be reduced to 0.75 mg PO once daily when co-administered with certain P-gp inhibitors (amiodarone, carvedilol, clarithromycin, itraconazole, and verapamil).
4. Closely monitor CBCs at baseline and at monthly intervals. For prolonged hematologic toxicities, interrupt therapy, and monitor CBCs on a weekly basis until recovery. If blood counts have not recovered within 4 weeks, bone marrow analysis and peripheral blood for cytogenetics should be performed to rule out the possibility of MDS/AML.
5. Talazoparib may cause fetal harm. Women of reproductive potential should be warned of the potential risk to a fetus and need to use effective contraception during treatment and for at least 7 months following the last dose of drug.

TOXICITY 1

Myelosuppression with anemia, thrombocytopenia, and neutropenia. Anemia is most commonly observed with >grade 3 anemia in nearly 40% of patients.

TOXICITY 2

Fatigue, anorexia, and asthenia.

TOXICITY 3

GI side effects in the form of nausea/vomiting and diarrhea.

TOXICITY 4

Elevations in serum transaminases (SGOT/SGPT) and alkaline phosphatase.

TOXICITY 5

MDS and AML.

Talimogene Laherparepvec

TRADE NAME	Imlygic, T-vec	**CLASSIFICATION**	Oncolytic virus
CATEGORY	Biologic response modifier agent, immunotherapy	**DRUG MANUFACTURER**	Amgen

MECHANISM OF ACTION

- Talimogene laherparepvec (T-vec) is a first-in-class oncolytic virus based on a modified herpes simplex virus (HSV) type 1 that selectively replicates in and lyses tumor cells.
- T-vec is modified through deletion of two non-essential viral genes, which reduces viral pathogenicity and enhances tumor-selective replication.
- T-vec is further modified with insertion and expression of the gene encoding human granulocyte macrophage colony-stimulating factor (GM-CSF). This results in local production of GM-CSF that then recruits and activates antigen-presenting dendritic cells with subsequent induction of tumor-specific T-cell responses.
- A local antitumor immune response is generated through the combined effects of release of tumor-derived antigens and GM-CSF production. There also appears to be generation of a systemic immune response that acts at non-injected sites, a phenomenon known as an abscopal effect.
- Clinical studies have shown an association between clinical response and presence of interferon-γ-producing MART-1-specific CD8+ T cells and reduction in CD4+ FoxP3+ regulatory T cells, which are consistent with induction of host antitumor immunity.

MECHANISM OF RESISTANCE
None well characterized to date.

ABSORPTION
Administered only via the intratumoral route.

DISTRIBUTION
Distribution in the body has not been well characterized.

METABOLISM
Metabolism of T-vec has not been well characterized.

INDICATIONS
FDA-approved for the local treatment of unresectable cutaneous, subcutaneous, and nodal lesions in patients with recurrent melanoma following initial surgery.

DOSAGE RANGE

1. Initial dose: 10^6 PFU per mL solution
2. Second dose to be administered 3 weeks after initial treatment: 10^8 PFU per mL solution
3. All subsequent doses: 10^8 PFU per mL solution to be administered 2 weeks after the second treatment
4. The following guidelines are used to determine the volume of T-vec to be injected (lesion size is based on longest dimension; when lesions are clustered together, they are to be injected as a single lesion):
   - If the lesion size is >5 cm, inject up to 4 mL.
   - If the lesion size is >2.5 cm to 5 cm, inject up to 2 mL.
   - If the lesion size is >1.5 cm to 2.5 cm, inject up to 1 mL.
   - If the lesion size is >0.5 cm to 1.5 cm, inject up to 0.5 mL.
   - If the lesion size is ≤0.5 cm, inject up to 0.1 mL.

DRUG INTERACTION

Acyclovir or other antiviral agents may reduce the clinical efficacy of T-vec.

SPECIAL CONSIDERATIONS

1. T-vec should be administered by intralesional injection into cutaneous, subcutaneous, and/or nodal lesions that are visible, palpable, or detectable by ultrasound. Please see package insert for complete details regarding how the intralesional injection should be performed.
2. Accidental exposure may lead to transmission of T-vec and herpetic infection. If accidental exposure occurs, exposed individuals should clean the affected areas thoroughly. If signs or symptoms of herpetic infection develop, the exposed individuals must contact their healthcare provider for appropriate treatment.
3. Healthcare providers who are immunocompromised or pregnant should not prepare or administer T-vec. They should not come into direct contact with injection sites, dressings, or body fluids of treated patients.
4. T-vec should **NOT** be administered to immunocompromised patients, including those with a history of leukemia, lymphoma, AIDS or other clinical manifestations of infections with human immunodeficiency viruses, and those on immunosuppressive therapy.
5. T-vec should **NOT** be administered to pregnant patients.
6. No formal recommendations for dosing in the setting of hepatic or renal impairment, as studies have not been conducted in these clinical settings.
7. No clinical data on the potential effect of T-vec on pregnant women, and no information on its impact on breastfeeding. There are no clinical studies to evaluate the effect of T-vec on fertility.

TOXICITY 1

Generalized symptoms, including fatigue, low-grade fever, chills, and myalgias, are most commonly observed.

TOXICITY 2
Herpetic infections with cold sores and herpetic keratitis. Disseminated herpes infection may occur in immunocompromised patients.

TOXICITY 3
Injection-site complications, including pain, erythema, and pruritus at the injection site; necrosis; tumor tissue ulceration; and cellulitis.

TOXICITY 4
Immune-mediated events, including glomerulonephritis, pneumonitis, vasculitis, vitiligo, and psoriasis.

TOXICITY 5
Influenza-like illness.

TOXICITY 6
GI side effects with nausea/vomiting, diarrhea, and constipation.

Talquetamab

TRADE NAME	Talvey, JNJ-64407564	**CLASSIFICATION**	Bispecific antibody
CATEGORY	Biologic response modifier agent, immunotherapy	**DRUG MANUFACTURER**	Janssen

MECHANISM OF ACTION
- Bispecific T-cell engaging (BiTE) humanized IgG4 antibody that binds to G protein-coupled receptor, family C, group 5 member D (GPRC5D) expressed on multiple myeloma cells and CD3 expressed on the surface of T cells.
- This BiTE causes cytotoxic T cells to be physically linked to malignant GPRC5D-positive plasma cells and triggers the signaling cascade, leading to upregulation of cell adhesion molecules, production of cytolytic proteins, release of inflammatory cytokines, and proliferation of T cells, ultimately resulting in lysis of malignant plasma cells.
- GPRC5D expression is enriched on the surface of multiple myeloma cells and is associated with markers of high-risk myeloma.
- Only low level expression of GPRC5D in normal tissues.

ABSORPTION

Administered via the SC route. Mean bioavailability is approximately 59% when administered SC. Time to reach maximal concentrations occurs at 3.7 days after the first dose and 3.6 days after the 17th treatment dose.

DISTRIBUTION

Following SC administration, steady-state levels are achieved 16 weeks after the treatment dose.

METABOLISM

Talquetamab is expected to be broken down into small peptides and amino acids. The terminal half-life is approximately 8.4 hours.

INDICATION

FDA-approved for the treatment of adult patients with relapsed or refractory multiple myeloma following at least 4 prior lines of therapy, including a proteasome inhibitor, an immunomodulatory agent, and an anti-CD38 monoclonal antibody.

DOSAGE RANGE

1. Administered as SC injection according to the step-up dosing schedule in cycle 1 as outlined.
2. Cycle 1, Day 1 – 0.01 mg/kg; Cycle 1, Day 4 – 0.06 mg/kg; Cycle 1, Day 7 – 0.4 mg/kg
3. 0.4 mg/kg SC weekly thereafter

DRUG INTERACTION

None well characterized to date.

SPECIAL CONSIDERATIONS

1. Patients should be premedicated one to three hours prior to each step-up dose and first treatment dose to reduce the risk of CRS with 16 mg dexamethasone (oral or IV), H1 receptor antagonist (oral or IV diphenhydramine), and an antipyretic (oral or IV acetaminophen).
2. Monitor for CRS. This is a black-box warning.
3. Monitor for neurologic toxicity, especially for the immune effector cell-associated neurotoxicity syndrome (ICANS). This is a black-box warning.
4. Monitor for signs and symptoms of infection. Patients should be given PJP prophylaxis prior to starting on therapy.
5. Monitor CBCs closely while on therapy.
6. Monitor for signs and symptoms of oral toxicity
7. Dose reduction is not required in patients with mild or moderate hepatic dysfunction. Has not been studied in setting of severe hepatic dysfunction.

8. Dose reduction is not required in patients with mild or moderate renal dysfunction. Has not been studied in setting of severe renal dysfunction or end-stage renal disease.

9. May cause fetal harm. Women should be advised to use effective contraception during treatment and for 3 months after the last dose of treatment. Breastfeeding should be avoided while on therapy and for 3 months after the last dose.

TOXICITY 1
Cytokine release syndrome (CRS) with fever, chills, hypotension, tachycardia, hypoxia, and headache.

TOXICITY 2
Myelosuppression with neutropenia, thrombocytopenia, and anemia.

TOXICITY 3
Neurological toxicities with headache, motor dysfunction, sensory neuropathy, and encephalopathy. ICANS can present with confusional state and dysgraphia.

TOXICITY 4
Injection site reactions.

TOXICITY 5
Increased risk of viral, bacterial, fungal, and opportunistic infections. Can cause severe or fatal infections.

TOXICITY 6
Oral toxicities with dysgeusia, dry mouth, dysphagia, and stomatitis.

TOXICITY 7
Skin reactions with rash, maculo-papular rash, and erythema.

TOXICITY 8
Hepatotoxicity with elevations in LFTs and serum bilirubin.

TOXICITY 9
Fatigue, anorexia, weight loss.

Tamoxifen

TRADE NAME	Nolvadex	**CLASSIFICATION**	Antiestrogen
CATEGORY	Hormonal agent	**DRUG MANUFACTURER**	AstraZeneca

MECHANISM OF ACTION
- Nonsteroidal antiestrogen with weak estrogen agonist effects.
- Competes with estrogen for binding to ERs. Binding of tamoxifen to ER leads to ER dimerization. The tamoxifen-bound ER dimer is transported to the nucleus, where it binds to DNA sequences referred to as ER elements. This interaction results in inhibition of critical transcriptional processes and signal transduction pathways that are required for cellular growth and proliferation.
- Cell cycle–specific agent that blocks cells in the mid-G1-phase of the cell cycle. Effect may be mediated by cyclin D.
- Stimulates the secretion of transforming growth factor-β (TGF-β), which then acts to inhibit the expression and/or activity of TGF-α and IGF-1, two genes that are involved in cell growth and proliferation.

MECHANISM OF RESISTANCE
- Decreased expression of ER.
- Mutations in ER, leading to decreased binding affinity to tamoxifen.
- Overexpression of several key growth factor receptors, such as EGFR, HER2/neu, IGF-1R, or TGF-β, that counteract the inhibitory effects of tamoxifen.
- Presence of ESR1 mutations.

ABSORPTION
Rapidly and completely absorbed in the GI tract. Peak plasma levels are achieved within 4–6 hours after oral administration.

DISTRIBUTION
Distributes to most body tissues, especially in those expressing estrogen receptors. Present in very low concentrations in CSF. Nearly all of the drug is bound to plasma proteins.

METABOLISM

Extensively metabolized by liver cytochrome P450 enzymes after oral administration. The main metabolite, N-desmethyl tamoxifen, has biologic activity similar to that of the parent drug. Both tamoxifen and its metabolites are excreted primarily (75%) in feces, with minimal clearance in urine. The terminal half-lives of tamoxifen and its metabolites are relatively long, approaching 7–14 days.

INDICATIONS

1. Adjuvant therapy in axillary node–negative breast cancer following surgical resection.
2. Adjuvant therapy in axillary node–positive breast cancer in postmenopausal women following surgical resection.
3. Adjuvant therapy in women with ductal carcinoma in situ (DCIS) after surgical resection and radiation therapy.
4. Metastatic breast cancer in women and men.
5. Approved as a chemopreventive agent for women at high risk for breast cancer. "High-risk" women are defined as women >35 years and with a 5-year predicted risk of breast cancer ≥1.67%, according to the Gail model.
6. Endometrial cancer.

DOSAGE RANGE

Recommended dose for breast cancer patients is 20 mg PO every day.

DRUG INTERACTION 1

Warfarin—Tamoxifen can inhibit metabolism of warfarin by the liver P450 system, leading to increased anticoagulant effect. Coagulation parameters, including PT and INR, must be closely monitored, and dose adjustments may be required.

DRUG INTERACTION 2

Drugs activated by liver P450 system—Tamoxifen and its metabolites are potent inhibitors of hepatic P450 enzymes and may inhibit the metabolic activation of drugs utilizing this pathway, including cyclophosphamide.

DRUG INTERACTION 3

Drugs metabolized by liver P450 system—Tamoxifen and its metabolites are potent inhibitors of hepatic P450 enzymes and may inhibit the metabolism of various drugs, including erythromycin, calcium channel blockers, and cyclosporine.

DRUG INTERACTION 4

Antidepressants that act as selective serotonin reuptake inhibitors (SSRIs) or selective noradrenergic reuptake inhibitors (SNRIs)—Drugs such as paroxetine, fluoxetine, bupropion, duloxetine, and sertraline are inhibitors of CYP2D6, which can interfere and inhibit metabolic activation of tamoxifen, resulting in lower blood levels of the active tamoxifen metabolites.

DRUG INTERACTION 5

Antipsychotics—Drugs such as thioridazine, perphenazine, and pimozide are inhibitors of CYP2D6, which can interfere and inhibit tamoxifen metabolism, resulting in lower blood levels of the active tamoxifen metabolites.

DRUG INTERACTION 6

Drugs such as cimetidine, quinidine, ticlopidine, and terfenadine are inhibitors of CYP2D6, which can interfere and inhibit tamoxifen metabolism, resulting in lower blood levels of the active tamoxifen metabolites.

SPECIAL CONSIDERATIONS

1. Instruct patients to notify physician about menstrual irregularities, abnormal vaginal bleeding, and pelvic pain and/or discomfort while on therapy.
2. Patients should have routine follow-up with a gynecologist, as tamoxifen therapy is associated with an increased risk of endometrial hyperplasia, polyps, and endometrial cancer.
3. Use with caution in patients with abnormal liver function, as there may be an increased risk of drug accumulation, resulting in toxicity.
4. Use with caution in patients with either personal history or family history of thromboembolic disease or hypercoagulable states, as tamoxifen is associated with an increased risk of thromboembolic events. Tamoxifen therapy is associated with antithrombin III deficiency.
5. Initiation of treatment with tamoxifen may induce a transient tumor flare. Tamoxifen should not be given in patients with impending ureteral obstruction, spinal cord compression, or in those with extensive painful bone metastases.
6. Premenopausal patients should be warned about the possibility of developing menopausal symptoms with tamoxifen therapy.
7. Monitor CBC during therapy with tamoxifen, as myelosuppression can occur, albeit rarely.
8. Testing for CYP2D6 is recommended prior to initiation of tamoxifen therapy. Up to 10% of patients are poor metabolizers of tamoxifen based on CYP2D6 alleles, which may result in reduced clinical efficacy.
9. Consider using citalopram, escitalopram, fluvoxamine, mirtazapine, and venlafaxine if an antidepressant is required during treatment with tamoxifen.
10. Avoid the use of medications that inhibit CYP2D6.
11. Pregnancy category D. Breastfeeding should be avoided.

TOXICITY 1

Menopausal symptoms, including hot flashes, nausea, vomiting, vaginal bleeding, and menstrual irregularities. Vaginal discharge and vaginal dryness also observed.

TOXICITY 2

Fluid retention and peripheral edema observed in about 30% of patients.

TOXICITY 3

Tumor flare usually occurs within the first 2 weeks of starting therapy. May observe increased bone pain, urinary retention, back pain with spinal cord compression, and/or hypercalcemia.

TOXICITY 4

Headache, lethargy, and dizziness occur rarely. Visual disturbances, including cataracts, retinopathy, and decreased visual acuity, have been described.

TOXICITY 5

Skin rash, pruritus, hair thinning, and/or partial hair loss.

TOXICITY 6

Myelosuppression is rare, with transient thrombocytopenia and leukopenia. Usually resolves after the first week of treatment.

TOXICITY 7

Thromboembolic complications, including deep vein thrombosis, pulmonary embolism, and superficial phlebitis. Incidence of thromboembolic events may be increased when tamoxifen is given concomitantly with chemotherapy.

TOXICITY 8

Elevations in serum triglycerides.

TOXICITY 9

Increased incidence of endometrial hyperplasia, polyps, and endometrial cancer.

TOXICITY 10

Musculoskeletal symptoms, including carpal tunnel syndrome.

TAS-102

TRADE NAME	Lonsurf	CLASSIFICATION	Antimetabolite
CATEGORY	Chemotherapy drug	DRUG MANUFACTURER	Taiho Oncology

MECHANISM OF ACTION

- Composed of trifluridine, a fluorinated pyrimidine nucleoside analog, and tipiracil, a thymidine phosphorylase inhibitor, at a molar ratio of 1:0.5.
- Presence of tipiracil inhibits trifluridine degradation by thymidine phosphorylase, thereby enhancing trifluridine exposure and subsequent metabolism to the cytotoxic triphosphate metabolite.

- Trifluridine monophosphate inhibits thymidylate synthase, leading to inhibition of thymidylate, a key nucleotide precursor for DNA biosynthesis. The TAS-102 monophosphate metabolite is a much weaker TS inhibitor than the 5-FU metabolite FdUMP.
- Trifluridine triphosphate is incorporated into DNA, resulting in inhibition of DNA synthesis and function.
- Retains activity in 5-FU resistant model systems.
- Appears to have similar clinical activity in KRAS-wt and KRAS-mutant colorectal cancer.

MECHANISM OF RESISTANCE
None well characterized to date.

ABSORPTION
Peak plasma levels of trifluridine are reached in 2 hours. The rate and extent of absorption are reduced by food.

DISTRIBUTION
Trifluridine is mainly bound to serum albumin. Plasma protein binding of tipiracil is less than 10%.

METABOLISM
Trifluridine is primarily eliminated via metabolism by thymidine phosphorylase to form the inactive metabolite 5-trifluoromethyluracil (FTY). No other major metabolites have been identified in plasma or urine. Trifluridine and tipiracil are not metabolized by the liver P450 enzymes. Greater than 90% of an administered dose of drug and its metabolites is cleared in the urine. Following a single dose of TAS-102, the mean 48-hour urinary excretion is 1.5% for unchanged trifluridine, 19.2% for FTY, and 29.3% for unchanged tipiracil. The mean elimination half-life of trifluridine is 2.1 hours and of tipiracil is 2.4 hours.

INDICATIONS
1. FDA-approved for patients with metastatic colorectal cancer as a single agent or in combination with bevacizumab who have been previously treated with fluoropyrimidine-, oxaliplatin-, and irinotecan-based chemotherapy; an anti-VEGF biological therapy; and, if RAS wild-type, an anti-EGFR therapy.
2. FDA-approved for patients with metastatic gastric or GE junction adenocarcinoma previously treated with at least 2 prior lines of chemotherapy that included a fluoropyrimidine; a platinum; either a taxane or irinotecan; and, if appropriate, HER2-targeted therapy.

DOSAGE RANGE
Recommended dose is 35 mg/m^2 PO bid on days 1–5 and 8–12 of a 28-day cycle.

DRUG INTERACTION
None well characterized to date.

SPECIAL CONSIDERATIONS

1. TAS-102 should be taken within 1 hour after completion of morning and evening meals.
2. Use with caution in patients >65 years of age, as the incidence of grade 3/4 myelosuppression is increased in older patients.
3. Closely monitor CBCs prior to and on day 15 of each cycle.
4. TAS-102 should not be initiated until the ANC is >1,500/mm^3, platelets are >75,000/mm^3, and grades 3/4 non-hematologic toxicity has resolved to grades 0 or 1.
5. Within a treatment cycle, TAS-102 should be withheld for any of the following: ANC <500/mm^3, platelets <50,000/mm^3, and grades 3/4 non-hematologic toxicity.
6. No dose adjustment is necessary in patients with mild liver dysfunction. Should not be given to patients with moderate or severe hepatic impairment.
7. No dose adjustment is recommended in patients with mild or moderate renal dysfunction (baseline CrCl, 30–89 mL/min). Has not been studied in patients with severe renal dysfunction (CrCL<30 mL/min) or end-stage renal disease.
8. May consider in patients with the DPD pharmacogenetic syndrome.
9. May cause fetal harm. Females should be advised of the potential risk to a fetus and to use effective contraception. Breastfeeding should be avoided.

TOXICITY 1
Myelosuppression with neutropenia, anemia, and thrombocytopenia.

TOXICITY 2
GI toxicity with diarrhea, abdominal pain, and nausea/vomiting.

TOXICITY 3
Fatigue, asthenia.

TOXICITY 4
Anorexia.

Tazemetostat

TRADE NAME	Tazverik, EPZ-6438	**CLASSIFICATION**	Methyltransferase inhibitor, EZH2 inhibitor
CATEGORY	Targeted agent	**DRUG MANUFACTURER**	Epizyme and Eisai

MECHANISM OF ACTION
- Inhibitor of the Enhancer of zeste homolog 2 (EZH2) methyltransferase and several EZH2 gain of function mutations, including Y646X, A682G, and A692V.
- Inhibits EZH1, albeit at much higher concentrations than for EZH2.
- Aberrant upregulation of EZH2 activity is oncogenic in a wide range of tumors.

MECHANISM OF RESISTANCE
- Emergence of EZH2 mutations that prevent drug binding.
- Activation of the IGF-1R, MEK, and MAPK signaling pathways.

ABSORPTION
Rapidly absorbed with a median time to peak drug levels of 1–2 hours after oral ingestion. Oral bioavailability is relatively modest at only 33%. Steady-state drug levels are achieved in approximately 15 days. Food does not affect drug absorption.

DISTRIBUTION
Extensive binding (96%) to plasma proteins.

METABOLISM
Metabolized in the liver primarily by CYP3A4 microsomal enzymes to form inactive major metabolites M3 and M5. The M5 metabolite undergoes further metabolism by CYP3A4. After an administered dose of drug, nearly 80% is eliminated in feces and 12% is eliminated in urine. The terminal half-life of the drug is 3.1 hours.

INDICATIONS

1. FDA-approved for adult and pediatric patients 16 years and older with metastatic or locally advanced epithelioid sarcoma not eligible for complete resection.
2. FDA-approved for adult patients with relapsed or refractory follicular lymphoma whose tumors are positive for an EZH2 mutation, as detected by an FDA-approved test, and who have received at least 2 prior systemic therapies.
3. FDA-approved for adult patients with relapsed or refractory follicular lymphoma who have no satisfactory alternative treatment options.

DOSAGE RANGE

Recommended dose is 800 mg PO bid and can be taken with or without food.

DRUG INTERACTION 1

Drugs such as ketoconazole, itraconazole, erythromycin, clarithromycin, atazanavir, indinavir, nefazodone, nelfinavir, ritonavir, saquinavir, telithromycin, and voriconazole may decrease the rate of metabolism of tazemetostat, resulting in increased drug levels and potentially increased toxicity.

DRUG INTERACTION 2

Phenytoin and other drugs that stimulate the liver microsomal CYP3A4 enzymes, including carbamazepine, rifampin, phenobarbital, and St. John's Wort—These drugs may increase the metabolism of tazemetostat, resulting in lower effective drug levels.

SPECIAL CONSIDERATIONS

1. Dose reduction is not required in the setting of mild hepatic impairment. Has not been studied in the setting of moderate and severe hepatic impairment.
2. Dose reduction is not required in the setting of renal impairment, including end-stage renal disease.
3. Concomitant use of tazemetostat with moderate or strong CYP3A4 inhibitors should be avoided.
4. Concomitant use of tazemetostat with moderate or strong CYP3A4 inducers should be avoided.
5. Monitor patients for the development of secondary malignancies, including MDS and AML.
6. Can cause fetal harm when administered to a pregnant woman. Females of reproductive potential should use effective contraception during drug therapy and for at least 6 months after the final dose. Breastfeeding should be avoided.

TOXICITY 1

Fatigue, anorexia, and asthenia.

TOXICITY 2

Musculoskeletal pain, myalgias, arthralgias, and bone pain.

TOXICITY 3
Nausea/vomiting, constipation, diarrhea, and abdominal pain.

TOXICITY 4
Anemia and thrombocytopenia.

TOXICITY 5
Hemorrhagic events, including cerebral hemorrhage, tracheostomy site hemorrhage, and hemoptysis.

TOXICITY 6
Impaired wound healing.

TOXICITY 7
GI side effects with dry mouth, nausea/vomiting, diarrhea, and abdominal pain.

TOXICITY 8
Secondary malignancies, including MDS and AML.

Tebentafusp-tebn

TRADE NAME	Kimmtrak, IMC-gp100	**CLASSIFICATION**	Immune mobilizing monoclonal T cell receptor
CATEGORY	Biologic response modifier agent, immunotherapy,	**DRUG MANUFACTURER**	Immunocore

MECHANISM OF ACTION
- First-in-class anti-gp100 immune-mobilizing monoclonal T-cell receptor against cancer (ImmTAC).
- Bispecific gp100 peptide-HLA-A*02:01 directed T-cell receptor (TCR) CD3 T-cell engager.
- Binding to the specific peptide-HLA complexes on the target-cell surface leads to recruitment and activation of polyclonal T cells through CD3, which then results in release of cytolytic proteins and inflammatory cytokines, and proliferation of T cells. These events lead to cell death of melanoma tumor cells.
- gp100 is highly expressed in uveal melanoma, variably in cutaneous melanoma, weakly in normal melanocytes, and only minimally in non-melanocyte tissues.

ABSORPTION
Administered only via the IV route.

DISTRIBUTION
Mean steady-state volume of distribution is 7.56L.

METABOLISM
Tebentafusp is expected to be broken down into small peptides and amino acids. The terminal half-life is approximately 7.5 hours.

INDICATIONS
FDA-approved for the treatment of adult patients with HLA-A*02:01-positive unresectable or metastatic uveal melanoma.

DOSAGE RANGE
1. Administered only as IV injection according to the step-up dosing schedule in cycle 1 as outlined.
2. Cycle 1, Day 1 – 20 µg; Cycle 1, Day 8 – 30 µg; Cycle 1, Day 15 – 68 µg
3. 68 µg IV weekly thereafter

DRUG INTERACTION
None well characterized to date.

SPECIAL CONSIDERATIONS
1. Patients should be premedicated one to three hours prior to each step-up dose and first treatment dose to reduce the risk of CRS with 16 mg dexamethasone (oral or IV), H1 receptor antagonist (oral or IV diphenhydramine), and an antipyretic (oral or IV acetaminophen).
2. Monitor for CRS for at least 16 hours following the first three infusions and then as clinically indicated. This is a black-box warning.
3. Monitor for skin reactions.
4. Monitor liver function tests and serum bilirubin while on therapy
5. Dose reduction is not required in patients with mild hepatic dysfunction. Has not been studied in setting of moderate or severe hepatic dysfunction.
6. Dose reduction is not required in patients with mild or moderate renal dysfunction. Has not been studied in setting of severe renal dysfunction or end-stage renal disease.
7. May cause fetal harm. Women should be advised to use effective contraception during treatment and for 1 week after the last dose of treatment. Breastfeeding should be avoided while on therapy and for 1 week after the last dose.

TOXICITY 1
Cytokine release syndrome (CRS) with fever, chills, hypotension, tachycardia, hypoxia, and headache.

TOXICITY 2
Skin toxicity with rash, pruritus, dry skin, erythema, and cutaneous edema.

TOXICITY 3
Hepatotoxicity with elevation in LFTs and serum bilirubin.

TOXICITY 4
Fatigue.

TOXICITY 5
Mild nausea and vomiting.

Teclistamab-cqyv

TRADE NAME	Tecvalyi, JNJ-64007957	**CLASSIFICATION**	Bispecific antibody
CATEGORY	Biologic response modifier agent, targeted agent	**DRUG MANUFACTURER**	Janssen Pharmaceuticals, Johnson & Johnson

MECHANISM OF ACTION
- Teclistimab is a bispecific antibody that targets both CD3 expressed on the surface of T cells and B-cell maturation antigen (BCMA) expressed on the surface of myeloma cells.
- Mediates T-cell activation and subsequent lysis of BCMA-expressing myeloma cells.

MECHANISM OF RESISTANCE
None well characterized to date.

ABSORPTION
Administered via the SC route with a mean bioavailability of 72%.

DISTRIBUTION
Distribution has not been well characterized.

METABOLISM
Metabolism has not been well characterized. Mean terminal half-life is approximately 18 days.

INDICATIONS

FDA-approved for patients with relapsed or refractory multiple myeloma who have received at least 4 prior lines of therapy, including a proteasome inhibitor, an immunomodulatory agent, and an anti-CD38 monoclonal antibody

DOSAGE RANGE

Step-up dosing schedule: 0.06 mg/kg SC on day 1, 0.3 mg/kg SC on day 4, and then 1.5 mg/kg on day 7.
Recommended dose is 1.5 mg/kg SC on a weekly basis.

DRUG INTERACTION

No known significant interactions have been characterized to date. However, drug treatment may cause release of cytokines, which may suppress activity of CYP3A4 enzymes in liver. This may lead to increased exposure of CYP 3A4 substrates, which may then lead to increased toxicity.

SPECIAL CONSIDERATIONS

1. Administered only via the SC route.
2. Pre-treatment medication with corticosteroid (oral or IV dexamethasone 16 mg), H1-receptor antagonist (oral or IV diphenhydramine 50 mg), and antipyretics (oral or IV acetaminophen 650 mg to 1,000 mg) to be given 1–3 hours before each dose of the step-up schedule and first treatment dose. Pre-treatment medications may be required prior to administration of subsequent doses of teclistimab.
3. Prophylaxis for herpes zoster virus reactivation is recommended.
4. Monitor patients for signs and symptoms of cytokine release syndrome (CRS). Patients should be immediately evaluated for hospitalization at the first sign of CRS. Most events occur after step-up and cycle 1 doses. Median time to onset of CRS is 2 days. This is a black-box warning.
5. Monitor patients for signs and symptoms of neurologic toxicity, including Immune Effector Cell-Associated Neurotoxicity Syndrome (ICANS). This is a black-box warning.
6. Monitor patients for signs and symptoms of infection. Immunoglobulin levels should be monitored while on treatment.
7. Monitor CBC at baseline and during treatment.
8. Monitor LFTS and serum bilirubin at baseline during treatment.
9. Patients should refrain from driving or operating heavy machinery during and for 48 hours after completion of step-up dosing schedule and regular treatment.
10. Teclistimab is only available through a restricted program called the Teclistimab Risk Evaluation and Mitigation Strategy (REMS).
11. No dose adjustments are recommended for patients with mild or moderate renal dysfunction. Has not been studied in the setting of severe renal dysfunction.
12. No dose adjustments are recommended for patients with mild hepatic dysfunction. Has not been studied in the setting of moderate or severe hepatic dysfunction.

13. Embryo-fetal toxicity. May cause fetal harm when administered to a pregnant woman. Females of reproductive potential should use effective contraception during drug therapy and for 5 months after the final dose. Breastfeeding should be avoided.

TOXICITY 1
Myelosuppression with neutropenia, thrombocytopenia, and anemia.

TOXICITY 2
Hypersensitivity reactions.

TOXICITY 3
Cytokine release syndrome (CRS) with fever, hypoxia, chills, hypotension, and sinus tachycardia.

TOXICITY 4
Neurologic toxicity, with ICANS, headache, motor dysfunction, sensory neuropathy, and encephalopathy. Seizures and Guillain-Barré syndrome occur rarely.

TOXICITY 5
Hepatotoxicity with elevations in SGOT/SGPT and serum bilirubin.

TOXICITY 6
Increased risk of infections with URIs, pneumonia, and UTIs. Reactivation of herpes zoster virus can occur.

TOXICITY 7
GI side effects with mild nausea/vomiting, diarrhea, and constipation.

Temozolomide

TRADE NAME	Temodar	CLASSIFICATION	Nonclassic alkylating agent
CATEGORY	Chemotherapy drug	DRUG MANUFACTURER	Merck

MECHANISM OF ACTION

- Imidazotetrazine analog that is structurally and functionally similar to dacarbazine.
- Cell cycle–nonspecific agent.
- Metabolic activation to the reactive compound MTIC is required for antitumor activity.
- Although the precise mechanism of cytotoxicity is unclear, this drug methylates guanine residues in DNA and inhibits DNA, RNA, and protein synthesis. Does not cross-link DNA strands.

MECHANISM OF RESISTANCE

- Increased activity of the DNA repair enzyme O6-methylguanine-DNA methyltransferase (MGMT).
- Defects in mismatch repair (MMR) resulting from mutations in key MMR genes, such as MLH1, MSH2, MSH6, and PMS2.
- Defects in base excision repair (BER).
- Increased expression of tribbles pseudokinase 2 (TRIB2) and mitogen-activated protein kinase kinase kinase 1 (MAP3K1).

ABSORPTION

Rapidly and completely absorbed, with an oral bioavailability approaching 100%. Maximum plasma concentrations are reached within 1 hour after administration. Food reduces the rate and extent of drug absorption.

DISTRIBUTION

Widely distributed in body tissues. Able to cross the blood-brain barrier as a result of its lipophilicity. Levels in brain and CSF are 30%–40% of those achieved in plasma. Relatively weak binding to human plasma proteins.

METABOLISM

Metabolized primarily by non-enzymatic hydrolysis at physiologic pH. Undergoes conversion to the metabolite MTIC, which is further hydrolyzed to AIC, a known intermediate in purine de novo synthesis, and methylhydrazine, the presumed active alkylating species. The liver P450 enzymes play a minor role in the metabolism of temozolomide and MTIC. About 40%–50% of parent drug is excreted in urine within 6 hours of administration, and tubular secretion is the predominant mechanism of renal excretion. The elimination half-life of the drug is 2 hours.

INDICATIONS

1. FDA-approved for refractory anaplastic astrocytoma at first relapse following treatment with a nitrosourea and procarbazine-containing regimen.
2. FDA-approved for newly diagnosed glioblastoma multiforme (GBM) in combination with radiotherapy and then as maintenance treatment.
3. Clinical activity in metastatic melanoma.

DOSAGE RANGE

1. Anaplastic astrocytoma: 150 mg/m^2 PO daily for 5 days every 28 days.
2. Dose is adjusted to nadir neutrophil and platelet counts. If nadir of ANC is acceptable, the dose may be increased to 200 mg/m^2 PO daily for 5 days. If ANC falls below acceptable levels during any cycle, the next dose should be reduced by 50 mg/m^2 PO daily.
3. Newly diagnosed GBM: 75 mg/m^2 PO daily for 42 days along with radiotherapy (60 Gy in 30 fractions). During the maintenance phase, which is started 4 weeks after completion of the combined modality therapy, temozolomide is given on cycle 1 at 150 mg/m^2 PO daily for 5 days followed by 23 days without treatment. For cycles 2–6, the dose of temozolomide may be escalated to 200 mg/m^2 if tolerated.

DRUG INTERACTIONS

None well characterized to date.

SPECIAL CONSIDERATIONS

1. Temozolomide is a moderately emetogenic agent. Aggressive use of antiemetics prior to drug administration is required to decrease the risk of nausea and vomiting.
2. Dose reduction is not recommended in the setting of mild or moderate hepatic dysfunction. Has not been studied in patients with severe hepatic dysfunction.
3. Dose reduction is not recommended in the setting of mild or moderate renal dysfunction. Has not been studied in patients with severe renal dysfunction or in those with end-stage disease.
4. Patients should be warned to avoid sun exposure for several days after drug treatment.
5. Use with caution in elderly patients (age >65), as they are at increased risk for myelosuppression.
6. Patients should be monitored closely for the development of PJP, and those receiving temozolomide and radiotherapy combined modality therapy require PJP prophylaxis.
7. Pregnancy category D. Breastfeeding should be discontinued.

TOXICITY 1

Myelosuppression is dose-limiting. Leukopenia and thrombocytopenia are commonly observed.

TOXICITY 2

Nausea and vomiting. Mild to moderate, usually occurring within 1–3 hours and lasting for up to 12 hours. Aggressive antiemetic therapy strongly recommended.

TOXICITY 3

Headache and fatigue.

TOXICITY 4
Mild elevation in hepatic transaminases.

TOXICITY 5
Photosensitivity.

TOXICITY 6
Teratogenic, mutagenic, and carcinogenic.

Temsirolimus

TRADE NAME	Torisel, CCI-779	CLASSIFICATION	Signal transduction inhibitor, mTOR inhibitor
CATEGORY	Targeted agent	DRUG MANUFACTURER	Pfizer

MECHANISM OF ACTION
- Potent inhibitor of the mammalian target of rapamycin (mTOR) kinase, which is a key component of cellular signaling pathways involved in the growth and proliferation of tumor cells.
- Inhibition of mTOR signaling results in cell cycle arrest, induction of apoptosis, and inhibition of angiogenesis.

MECHANISM OF RESISTANCE
- Activation of PI3K/AKT signaling.
- Activation of signal transduction pathways via TORC2.
- Alterations in integrin $\alpha5$ and $\beta3$ expression.
- Increased expression of integrin $\alpha7$ (ITGA7).

ABSORPTION
Administered only via the IV route.

DISTRIBUTION
Widely distributed in tissues. Steady-state drug concentrations are reached in 7–8 days.

METABOLISM
Metabolism in the liver primarily by CYP3A4 microsomal enzymes. The main metabolite is sirolimus, which is a potent inhibitor of mTOR signaling, with the other metabolites accounting for <10% of all metabolites measured. Elimination is mainly hepatic with excretion in feces. Renal elimination of parent drug and its metabolites account for only 5% of an administered dose. The terminal half-life of the parent drug is 17 hours, while that of sirolimus is 55 hours.

INDICATIONS
FDA-approved for advanced renal cell cancer.

DOSAGE RANGE
Recommended dose is 25 mg IV administered on a weekly schedule.

DRUG INTERACTION 1
Phenytoin and other drugs that stimulate liver microsomal CYP3A4 enzymes, including carbamazepine, rifampin, phenobarbital, and St. John's Wort—These drugs may increase the rate of metabolism of temsirolimus, resulting in its inactivation and lower effective drug levels.

DRUG INTERACTION 2
Drugs that inhibit liver microsomal CYP3A4 enzymes, including ketoconazole, itraconazole, erythromycin, and clarithromycin—These drugs may decrease the rate of metabolism of temsirolimus, resulting in increased drug levels and potentially increased toxicity.

SPECIAL CONSIDERATIONS
- Use with caution in patients with mild hepatic impairment, and dose reduction to 15 IV/week is recommended. Should not be given to patients with bilirubin >1.5 × ULN.
- Dose reduction is not recommended in patients with renal impairment. However, the drug has not been studied in patients on hemodialysis.
- Patients should be premedicated with an H1-antagonist antihistamine (diphenhydramine 25–50 mg IV) 30 minutes before the start of therapy to reduce the incidence of hypersensitivity reactions.
- Closely monitor serum glucose levels in all patients, especially those with diabetes mellitus.
- Closely monitor patients for new or progressive pulmonary symptoms, including cough, dyspnea, and fever. Temsirolimus therapy should be interrupted pending further diagnostic evaluation.

- Patients are at increased risk for developing opportunistic infections while on temsirolimus given its potential immunosuppressive effects.
- Closely monitor serum triglyceride and cholesterol levels while on therapy.
- Patients should be advised to report the development of fever, abdominal pain, and/or bloody stools, as temsirolimus may cause bowel perforation on rare occasions.
- Closely monitor renal function during therapy, as temsirolimus can cause progressive and severe renal failure, especially in patients with pre-existing renal impairment.
- Use with caution after surgical procedures, as temsirolimus can impair the process of wound healing.
- Avoid grapefruit juice and other grapefruit products while on temsirolimus.
- Avoid the use of live vaccines and/or close contact with those who have received live vaccines while on temsirolimus.
- Pregnancy category D. Breastfeeding should be avoided.

TOXICITY 1
Asthenia and fatigue.

TOXICITY 2
Pruritus, dry skin, with mainly a pustular, acneiform skin rash.

TOXICITY 3
Nausea/vomiting, mucositis, and anorexia. On rare occasions, bowel perforations can occur and present as fever, abdominal pain, and bloody stools.

TOXICITY 4
Hyperlipidemia with increased serum triglycerides and/or cholesterol in up to 90% of patients.

TOXICITY 5
Hyperglycemia in up to 80%–90% of patients.

TOXICITY 6
Allergic hypersensitivity reactions occur in 10% of patients.

TOXICITY 7
Pulmonary toxicity in the form of ILD manifested by increased cough, dyspnea, fever, and pulmonary infiltrates. Observed in less than 1% of patients and more frequent in patients with underlying pulmonary disease.

TOXICITY 8
Renal toxicity with elevation in serum creatinine and rare cases of renal failure.

TOXICITY 9
Peripheral edema.

Tepotinib

TRADE NAME	Tepmetko	**CLASSIFICATION**	Signal transduction inhibitor, MET inhibitor
CATEGORY	Targeted agent	**DRUG MANUFACTURER**	EMD Serono

MECHANISM OF ACTION
- Selective small molecule inhibitor of mesenchymal-epithelial transition (MET) tyrosine kinase, including the mutant variant produced by exon 14 skipping (METex14).
- Leads to downstream inhibition of key signaling pathways involved in proliferation, motility, migration, and invasion.
- MET is a receptor tyrosine kinase overexpressed or mutated in several tumor types, including NSCLC (3%–4%).

MECHANISM OF RESISTANCE
- Activation of several RTKs, including EGFR, ErbB2, ErbB3, FGFR2, FGFR3, AXL, RET, and M-CSFR.
- Increased expression of Src homology 2 domain-containing phosphatase 2 (SHP2).
- Gene amplification of PIK3CA resulting in increased expression of PIK3CA.
- Increased signaling mediated by MAPK pathway.

ABSORPTION
High oral bioavailability of about 72% with low inter-individual variability. Median time to peak drug levels of 8 hours after oral ingestion. Food with high fat, high calorie content increases C_{max} and AUC.

DISTRIBUTION
Large volume of distribution with extensive binding (98%) to plasma proteins.

METABOLISM
Metabolized in the liver primarily by CYP3A4 and CYP2C8 microsomal enzymes. Two major metabolites have been identified, M506 and M668. Only the M506 metabolite is detected in plasma. After an administered dose of drug, 85% is eliminated in feces (45% as parent drug), and 14% is eliminated in urine (7% as parent drug). The terminal half-life of the drug is 6.5 hours.

INDICATIONS
FDA-approved for adult patients with metastatic NSCLC with a MET exon 14 skipping alterations.

DOSAGE RANGE
Recommended dose is 450 mg PO once daily with food.

DRUG INTERACTION 1
Drugs such as ketoconazole, itraconazole, erythromycin, clarithromycin, atazanavir, indinavir, nefazodone, nelfinavir, ritonavir, saquinavir, telithromycin, and voriconazole may decrease the rate of metabolism of tepotinib, resulting in increased drug levels and potentially increased toxicity.

DRUG INTERACTION 2
Phenytoin and other drugs that stimulate the liver microsomal CYP3A4 enzymes, including carbamazepine, rifampin, phenobarbital, and St. John's Wort—These drugs may increase the metabolism of tepotinib, resulting in lower effective drug levels and potentially reduced activity.

DRUG INTERACTION 3
Certain P-gp substrates–Tepotinib is a P-gp inhibitor, so concomitant use of tepotinib may increase the concentration of certain P-gp substrates, such as digoxin, verapamil, diltiazem, dabigatran, and fexofenadine.

SPECIAL CONSIDERATIONS
1. Dose reduction is not recommended in the setting of mild or moderate hepatic impairment. Has not been studied in the setting of severe hepatic impairment.
2. Dose reduction is not recommended in the setting of mild or moderate renal impairment. Has not been studied in the setting of severe renal impairment or end-stage renal disease.
3. Monitor patients for new pulmonary symptoms as tepotinib can cause interstitial lung disease and pneumonitis.
4. Monitor LFTs at baseline and every 2 weeks during the first 3 months of therapy, then once a month or as clinically indicated.
5. Embryo-fetal toxicity. Females of reproductive potential should use effective contraception during drug therapy and for at least 1 week after the final dose. Breastfeeding should be avoided.

TOXICITY 1
Interstitial lung disease and pneumonitis, which, in rare cases, can be fatal.

TOXICITY 2
Hepatotoxicity with elevations in SGOT/SGPT and serum bilirubin.

TOXICITY 3
Peripheral edema.

TOXICITY 4
GI toxicities with nausea/vomiting, diarrhea, constipation, and abdominal pain.

TOXICITY 5
Fatigue, asthenia, and anorexia.

TOXICITY 6
Musculoskeletal pain.

Thalidomide

TRADE NAME	Thalomid	CLASSIFICATION	Immunomodulatory agent, anti-angiogenic agent
CATEGORY	Unclassified therapeutic agent, biologic response modifier agent	DRUG MANUFACTURER	Celgene

MECHANISM OF ACTION
- Mechanism of action has not been fully characterized.
- Inhibition of TNF-α synthesis and down-modulation of selected cell-surface adhesion molecules.
- May exert an anti-angiogenic effect through inhibition of bFGF and VEGF as well as through as-yet-undefined mechanisms.

MECHANISM OF RESISTANCE
None well characterized to date.

ABSORPTION
Oral bioavailability of thalidomide is not known due to poor aqueous solubility. Slowly absorbed from the GI tract, with peak plasma levels reached 3–6 hours after oral administration.

DISTRIBUTION
Extent of binding to plasma proteins is not known. Remains unclear whether thalidomide is present in the ejaculate of males.

METABOLISM
Non-enzymatic hydrolysis appears to be the principal mechanism of thalidomide breakdown. However, the exact metabolic pathway(s) has not been fully characterized. The precise route of drug excretion is not well defined.

INDICATIONS
1. FDA-approved in combination with dexamethasone for newly diagnosed multiple myeloma.
2. FDA-approved for cutaneous manifestations of erythema nodosum leprosum (ENL).
3. Clinical activity in MDS and in a broad range of solid tumors.

DOSAGE RANGE
No standard dose recommendations for use in cancer patients have been established. When used in combination with chemotherapy, doses are typically titrated up to 400 mg PO daily and given as a single bedtime dose. As a single agent, doses have been in the range of 100–1,200 mg daily.

DRUG INTERACTION 1
Barbiturates, chlorpromazine, and reserpine—Sedative effect of thalidomide is enhanced with concurrent use of these medications.

DRUG INTERACTION 2
Alcohol—Sedative effect of thalidomide is enhanced with concurrent use of alcohol.

SPECIAL CONSIDERATIONS
1. Pregnancy category X. Severe fetal malformations can occur if even one capsule is taken by a pregnant woman. All women should have a baseline β-human chorionic gonadotropin before starting therapy with thalidomide. All women of childbearing potential should practice two forms of birth control throughout treatment with thalidomide: one highly effective (intrauterine device, hormonal contraception, partner's vasectomy) and one additional barrier method (latex condom, diaphragm, cervical cap). It is strongly recommended that these precautionary measures begin 4 weeks before initiation of therapy, continue while on therapy, and continue for at least 4 weeks after therapy is discontinued.
2. Breastfeeding while on therapy should be avoided given the potential for serious adverse reactions from thalidomide in nursing infants. It remains unknown whether thalidomide is excreted in human milk.
3. Men taking thalidomide must use latex condoms for every sexual encounter with a woman of childbearing potential, since thalidomide may be present in semen.

4. Patients with AIDS should have their HIV mRNA levels monitored after the first and third months after treatment initiation with thalidomide, then every 3 months thereafter, as HIV mRNA levels may be increased while on thalidomide.
5. Instruct patients to avoid operating heavy machinery or driving a car while on thalidomide, as the drug can cause drowsiness.
6. Patients who develop a skin rash during therapy with thalidomide should have prompt medical evaluation. Serious skin reactions, including Stevens-Johnson syndrome, which may be fatal, have been reported.
7. Associated with an increased risk of thromboembolic complications, including DVT and PE, and prophylaxis with low-molecular-weight heparin, warfarin, or aspirin can help to prevent and/or reduce the incidence.

TOXICITY 1
Teratogenic effect is most serious toxicity. Severe birth defects or death to an unborn fetus. Manifested as absent or defective limbs, hypoplasia or absence of bones, facial palsy, absent or small ears, absent or shrunken eyes, congenital heart defects, and GI and renal abnormalities.

TOXICITY 2
General neurologic-related events with fatigue, orthostatic hypotension, and dizziness. Specific peripheral neuropathy in the form of numbness, tingling, and pain in the feet or hands does not appear to be dose- or duration-related. Prior exposure to neurotoxic agents increases the risk of neurotoxicity.

TOXICITY 3
Constipation is most common GI toxicity.

TOXICITY 4
No direct myelosuppressive effects. Certain patient populations (ENL and HIV) have reported a higher incidence of abnormalities in blood counts.

TOXICITY 5
Skin toxicity with maculopapular skin rash, urticaria, and dry skin. Serious dermatologic reactions, including Stevens-Johnson syndrome, have been reported. Patients who develop a skin rash during therapy with thalidomide should discontinue therapy. Therapy can be restarted with caution if the rash was not exfoliative, purpuric, or bullous or otherwise suggestive of a serious skin condition.

TOXICITY 6
Daytime sedation or fatigue following an evening dose often associated with larger initial doses.

TOXICITY 7
Increased risk of thromboembolic complications, including DVT and PE.

Thioguanine

TRADE NAME	6-Thioguanine, 6-TG	CLASSIFICATION	Antimetabolite, purine analog
CATEGORY	Chemotherapy drug	DRUG MANUFACTURER	GlaxoSmithKline

MECHANISM OF ACTION
- Cell cycle–specific purine analog with activity in the S-phase.
- Parent drug is inactive. Requires intracellular phosphorylation by the enzyme HGPRT to the cytotoxic monophosphate form, which is then eventually metabolized to the triphosphate metabolite form.
- Monophosphate metabolite inhibits de novo purine synthesis by inhibiting PRPP amidotransferase.
- Incorporation of thiopurine triphosphate nucleotides into DNA, resulting in inhibition of DNA synthesis and function.
- Incorporation of thiopurine triphosphate nucleotides into RNA, resulting in alterations in RNA processing and/or translation.

MECHANISM OF RESISTANCE
- Decreased expression of the activating enzyme HGPRT.
- Increased expression of the catabolic enzyme alkaline phosphatase or the conjugating enzyme TPMT.
- Decreased cellular transport of drug.
- Decreased expression of mismatch repair enzymes (e.g., hMLH1, hMSH2).
- Cross-resistance between thioguanine and mercaptopurine.

ABSORPTION
Oral absorption of drug is incomplete and variable. Only 30% of an oral dose is absorbed. Peak plasma levels are reached in 2–4 hours after ingestion.

DISTRIBUTION
Distributes widely into the RNA and DNA of peripheral blood and bone marrow cells. Crosses the placenta but does not appear to cross the blood-brain barrier.

METABOLISM
Metabolized in the liver by the processes of deamination and methylation. Main pathway of inactivation is catalyzed by guanine deaminase (guanase). In contrast to 6-mercaptopurine, metabolism of thioguanine does not involve xanthine oxidase. Metabolites are eliminated in both feces and urine. Plasma half-life is on the order of 80–90 minutes.

INDICATIONS
1. Acute myelogenous leukemia.
2. Acute lymphoblastic leukemia.
3. Chronic myelogenous leukemia.

DOSAGE RANGE
1. Induction: 100 mg/m^2 PO every 12 hours on days 1–5, usually in combination with cytarabine.
2. Maintenance: 100 mg/m^2 PO every 12 hours on days 1–5, every 4 weeks, usually in combination with other agents.
3. Single-agent: 1–3 mg/kg PO daily.

DRUG INTERACTIONS
None well characterized to date.

SPECIAL CONSIDERATIONS
1. Dose of drug does not need to be reduced in patients with abnormal liver and/or renal function.
2. In contrast to 6-mercaptopurine, dose of drug does not need to be reduced in the presence of concomitant allopurinol therapy.
3. Administer on an empty stomach to facilitate absorption.
4. Use with caution in the presence of other hepatotoxic drugs, as the risk of thioguanine-associated hepatotoxicity is increased.
5. Pregnancy category D. Breastfeeding should be avoided.

TOXICITY 1
Myelosuppression is dose-limiting. Neutropenia tends to precede thrombocytopenia, with nadir at 10–14 days and recovery by day 21.

TOXICITY 2
Nausea and vomiting. Dose-related, usually mild.

TOXICITY 3
Mucositis and diarrhea. May be severe, requiring dose reduction.

TOXICITY 4
Hepatotoxicity in the form of elevated serum bilirubin and transaminases. Veno-occlusive disease has been reported rarely.

TOXICITY 5
Immunosuppression with increased risk of bacterial, fungal, and parasitic infections.

TOXICITY 6
Transient renal toxicity.

TOXICITY 7
Mutagenic, teratogenic, and carcinogenic.

Thiotepa

$$\triangleright N - \overset{\overset{\displaystyle S}{\|}}{\underset{\underset{\displaystyle N}{|}}{P}} - N \triangleleft$$

TRADE NAME	Thioplex	**CLASSIFICATION**	Alkylating agent
CATEGORY	Chemotherapy drug	**DRUG MANUFACTURER**	Ben Venue Labs

MECHANISM OF ACTION
- Ethylenimine analog chemically related to nitrogen mustard.
- Functions as an alkylating agent by alkylating the N-7 position of guanine.
- Cell cycle–nonspecific agent.
- Inhibits DNA, RNA, and protein synthesis.

MECHANISM OF RESISTANCE
- Decreased uptake of drug into cell.
- Increased activity of DNA repair enzymes.
- Increased expression of sulfhydryl proteins, including glutathione and glutathione-related proteins.

ABSORPTION
Mainly administered by the IV route. Can also be given by the intravesical route where the absorption from the bladder is variable, ranging from 10%–100% of an administered dose. Incomplete and erratic absorption via the oral route.

DISTRIBUTION
Widely distributed throughout the body. About 40% of drug is bound to plasma proteins.

METABOLISM
Extensively metabolized by the liver microsomal P450 system to both active and inactive metabolites. About 60% of a dose is eliminated in urine within 24–72 hours, with only a small amount excreted as parent drug. Elimination half-life is on the order of 2–3 hours.

INDICATIONS
1. Breast cancer.
2. Ovarian cancer.
3. Superficial transitional cell cancer of the bladder.
4. Hodgkin's and non-Hodgkin's lymphoma.
5. High-dose transplant setting for breast and ovarian cancer.

DOSAGE RANGE

1. Usual dose is 10–20 mg/m^2 IV given every 3–4 weeks.
2. High-dose transplant setting: Doses range from 180 to 1,100 mg/m^2 IV.
3. Intravesical instillation: Dose for bladder instillation is 60 mg administered in 60 mL sterile water weekly for up to 4 weeks.

DRUG INTERACTIONS

Myelosuppressive agents—Bone marrow toxicity of thiotepa is enhanced when combined with other myelosuppressive anticancer agents.

SPECIAL CONSIDERATIONS

1. Monitor CBC while on therapy, as thiotepa is highly toxic to the bone marrow.
2. Use with caution in regimens including other myelosuppressive agents, as the risk of bone marrow toxicity is significantly increased.
3. Resuscitation equipment and medications should be available during administration of drug, as there is a risk of hypersensitivity reaction.
4. Monitor CBC after intravesical administration of drug into the bladder, as severe bone marrow depression can arise from systemically absorbed drug.
5. Caution patients about the risk of skin changes such as rash, urticaria, bronzing, flaking, and desquamation that can occur following high-dose therapy. Topical skin care should be initiated promptly.
6. Pregnancy category D. Breastfeeding should be avoided.

TOXICITY 1

Myelosuppression is dose-limiting. Leukopenia nadir at 7–10 days, with recovery by day 21. Platelet count nadir occurs at day 21, with usual recovery by days 28–35.

TOXICITY 2

Nausea and vomiting. Dose-dependent. Usual onset is 6–12 hours after treatment.

TOXICITY 3

Mucositis may be dose-limiting with high-dose therapy.

TOXICITY 4

Allergic reaction in the form of skin rash, hives, and rarely bronchospasm.

TOXICITY 5

Chemical and/or hemorrhagic cystitis. Occurs rarely following intravesical treatment.

TOXICITY 6
Skin changes with rash and bronzing of skin, erythema, flaking, and desquamation developing after high-dose therapy.

TOXICITY 7
Teratogenic, mutagenic, and carcinogenic. Increased risk of secondary malignancies, usually AML. Breast cancer and NSCLC have also been reported.

Tisagenlecleucel

TRADE NAME	Kymriah, CTL019, Tisa-cel	**CLASSIFICATION**	CAR T-cell therapy
CATEGORY	Cellular therapy, immunotherapy	**DRUG MANUFACTURER**	Novartis

MECHANISM OF ACTION
- CD19-directed genetically modified autologous T-cell immunotherapy that binds to CD19-expressing target cells.
- Prepared from the patient's own peripheral blood mononuclear cells that are enriched for T cells and then genetically modified ex vivo by lentiviral transduction to express a chimeric antigen receptor (CAR) made up of a murine anti-CD19 single-chain variable fragment linked to CD3-zeta domain to provide a T-cell activation signal and a 4-1BB (CD137) domain to provide a co-stimulatory signal. The anti-CD19 CAR T cells are expanded ex vivo and infused back into the patient, where they target CR19-expressing cells.
- Lymphocyte depletion conditioning regimen with cyclophosphamide and fludarabine leads to increased systemic levels of IL-15 and other pro-inflammatory cytokines and chemokines that enhance CAR T-cell activity.
- The conditioning regimen may also decrease immunosuppressive regulatory T cells, activate antigen-presenting cells, and induce pro-inflammatory tumor cell damage.

MECHANISM OF RESISTANCE
- Selection of alternatively spliced CD19 isoforms that lack the CD19 epitope recognized by the CAR T cells.
- Antigen loss or modulation.
- Insufficient reactivity against tumors cells with low antigen density.
- Emergence of an antigen-negative clone.
- Lineage switch from lymphoid to myeloid leukemia phenotype.

ABSORPTION
Administered only via the IV route.

DISTRIBUTION
Distributed in peripheral blood and bone marrow. Peak levels of anti-CD19 CAR T cells are observed at 9–10 days after infusion.

METABOLISM
Metabolism of tisagenlecleucel has not been well characterized.

INDICATIONS
1. FDA-approved for patients up to 25 years of age with B-cell precursor acute lymphoblastic leukemia (ALL) that is refractory or in second or later relapses.
2. FDA-approved for relapsed or refractory large B-cell lymphoma after two or more lines of systemic therapy, including diffuse large B-cell lymphoma (DLBCL), high-grade B-cell lymphoma, and DLBCL arising from follicular lymphoma.
3. FDA-approved for relapsed or refractory follicular lymphomas after 2 or more lines of systemic therapy. Approved under accelerated approval based on response rate and duration of response.
4. Tisagenlecleucel is **NOT** approved for patients with primary CNS lymphoma.

DOSAGE RANGE
- For pediatric and young adult patients with B-cell ALL, a lymphodepleting chemotherapy regimen of cyclophosphamide 500 mg/m^2 IV daily for 2 days and fludarabine 30 mg/m^2 IV daily for 4 days should be administered. Tisagenlecleucel should then be infused 2–14 days after completion of the lymphodepleting regimen.
- For adult patients with DLBCL, a lymphodepleting chemotherapy regimen of cyclophosphamide 250 mg/m^2 IV daily for 3 days and fludarabine 25 mg/m^2 IV daily for 3 days should be administered. Tisagenlecleucel should then be infused 2–11 days after completion of the lymphodepleting regimen.
- For adult patients with DLBCL, a lymphodepleting regimen may be omitted if a patient's WBC count is less than 1,000 within 1 week of CAR T-cell infusion.
- Patients should be premedicated with acetaminophen 650 mg PO and diphenhydramine 12.5 mg IV 1 hour before infusion of tisagenlecleucel.
- For pediatric and young adult patients with B-cell ALL, dosing of tisagenlecleucel is based on patient weight at the time of leukapheresis.
- Patients <50 kg: administer 0.2–5.0 × 10^6 CAR-positive viable T cells per kg body weight.
- Patients >50 kg: administer 0.1–2.5 × 10^8 CAR-positive viable T cells.
- For adult patients with DLBCL, administer 0.6–6.0 × 10^8 CAR-positive viable T cells.

DRUG INTERACTIONS
None characterized to date.

SPECIAL CONSIDERATIONS
1. Available only through a restricted program under a Risk Evaluation and Mitigation Strategy (REMS).
2. Monitor for hypersensitivity infusion reactions. Patients should be premedicated with acetaminophen 650 mg PO and diphenhydramine 12.5 mg IV at 1 hour prior to CAR T-cell infusion. Prophylactic use of systemic corticosteroids should be avoided, as they may interfere with the clinical activity of tisagenlecleucel.
3. Monitor patients at least daily for 7 days following infusion for signs and symptoms of cytokine release syndrome (CRS), which may be fatal or life-threatening in some cases. The median time to onset is 3 days, and the median duration is 8 days. Patients need to be monitored for up to 4 weeks after infusion. Please see package insert for guidelines regarding the appropriate management for CRS. This is a black-box warning.
4. Monitor for signs and symptoms of neurologic toxicities, which may be fatal or life-threatening in some cases. These neurologic events usually occur within 8 weeks after infusion, and severe neurologic events occur more frequently in patients who experience more severe CRS. This is a black-box warning.
5. Monitor for signs and symptoms of infection.
6. Monitor CBCs periodically after infusion.
7. Immunoglobulin levels should be monitored after treatment with tisagenlecleucel. Infection precautions, antibiotic prophylaxis, and immunoglobulin replacement may need to be instituted.
8. Patients should be advised not to drive and not to engage in operating heavy or potentially dangerous machinery for at least 8 weeks after receiving tisagenlecleucel.
9. Patients will require life-long monitoring for secondary malignancies.
10. Pregnancy category D. Breastfeeding should be avoided.

TOXICITY 1
Hypersensitivity infusion reactions.

TOXICITY 2
CRS with fever, hypotension, tachycardia, chills, and hypoxia. More serious events include cardiac arrhythmias (both atrial and ventricular), decreased cardiac ejection fraction, cardiac arrest, capillary leak syndrome, hepatotoxicity, renal failure, and prolongation of coagulation parameters PT and PTT.

TOXICITY 3
Neurologic toxicity, which includes headache, delirium, encephalopathy, tremors, somnolence, dizziness, aphasia, imbalance and gait instability, and seizures.

TOXICITY 4

Myelosuppression with thrombocytopenia and neutropenia, which can be prolonged for several weeks after infusion.

TOXICITY 5

Fever, fatigue, and anorexia.

TOXICITY 6

Infections, with unspecific pathogen, bacterial, and viral infections most common.

TOXICITY 7

Hypogammaglobulinemia.

TOXICITY 8

Hepatitis B reactivation.

TOXICITY 9

Secondary malignancies.

Tisotumab vedotin-tftv

TRADE NAME	Tivdak	CLASSIFICATION	Antibody-drug conjugate
CATEGORY	Biologic response modifier agent, chemotherapy drug	DRUG MANUFACTURER	Seagen and Genmab A/S

MECHANISM OF ACTION

- Antibody-drug conjugate made up of the fully human monoclonal antibody, tisotumab, directed against tissue factor, conjugated to the microtubule-disrupting agent monomethyl auristatin E (MMAE).
- Upon binding to tissue factor, tisotumab vedotin is rapidly internalized, and MMAE is then released inside the cell via proteolytic cleavage.
- Tissue factor is expressed in several cancers, including cervical cancer, NSCLC, endometrial cancer, prostate cancer, ovarian cancer, esophageal cancer, and bladder cancer.
- Tissue factor contributes to tumor progression by using tissue factor procoagulant activity and protease-activated receptor-2 (PAR-2) signaling.
- MMAE is a microtubule-disrupting agent that disrupts the microtubule network of actively dividing cells leading to cell cycle arrest and apoptosis.
- May also mediate antibody-dependent cellular phagocytosis and antibody-dependent cellular cytotoxicity.

MECHANISM OF RESISTANCE

None well characterized to date.

ABSORPTION

Administered only via the IV route.

DISTRIBUTION

Moderate binding (68%-82%) of drug to plasma proteins. Steady-state drug levels are achieved within 21 days.

METABOLISM

Tisotumab vedotin is expected to undergo catabolism to small peptides, amino acids, unconjugated MMAE, and unconjugated MMAE-related catabolites. The elimination of tisotumab vedotin has not been well characterized. The median terminal half-life of tisotumab vedotin and unconjugated MMAE is 4 days and 2.56 days, respectively.

INDICATIONS

FDA-approved for patients with recurrent or metastatic cervical cancer with disease progression on or after chemotherapy.

DOSAGE RANGE

Recommended dose is 2 mg/kg IV (up to a maximum of 200 mg) on day 1 of a 21-day schedule.

DRUG INTERACTION

None well characterized to date.

SPECIAL CONSIDERATIONS

1. Patients should have an eye exam that includes visual acuity and slit lamp exam at baseline, prior to each dose, and as clinically indicated.
2. Topical corticosteroid eye drops should be administered in each eye prior to each infusion. Eye drops need to be continued in each eye for 72 hours after infusion.
3. Topical ocular vasoconstrictor drops should be administered in each eye prior to each infusion. Cooling eye pads are to be used during drug infusion.
4. Topical lubricating eye drops should be administered for the duration of therapy and for 30 days after the last dose of drug.
5. Patients should be advised to avoid wearing contact lenses for the entire duration of therapy.
6. Monitor patients for signs and symptoms of neurologic changes.
7. Monitor patients for signs and symptoms of hemorrhage.
8. Monitor patients for new respiratory symptoms, such as cough and dyspnea.
9. May cause fetal harm when given to a pregnant woman. Females of reproductive potential should use effective contraception during treatment and for at least 2 months after the last dose. Breastfeeding should be avoided. Males with female partners of reproductive potential should use effective contraception while on treatment and for at least 4 months after the last dose.

TOXICITY 1
Ocular toxicity with conjunctival reactions, dry eye, corneal reactions, keratitis, and blepharitis. Visual acuity changes may also occur.

TOXICITY 2
Neurologic toxicity with peripheral neuropathy, motor neuropathy, muscular weakness, and rarely demyelinating peripheral polyneuropathy.

TOXICITY 3
Hemorrhage with epistaxis, hematuria, and vaginal bleeding.

TOXICITY 4
Pneumonitis.

TOXICITY 5
Fatigue and anorexia.

TOXICITY 6
Mild nausea and vomiting

Tivozanib

TRADE NAME	Fotivda, AV-951	**CLASSIFICATION**	Signal transduction inhibitor, TKI
CATEGORY	Targeted agent	**DRUG MANUFACTURER**	AVEO

MECHANISM OF ACTION
- Potent and selective inhibitor of VEGFR-1, VEGFR-2, VEGFR-3. More potent than other small molecule VEGR inhibitors, including sunitinib, sorafenib, and pazopanib.
- Inhibits platelet-derived growth factor receptor (PDGFR)-α and c-Kit, but with at least one order of magnitude less potency than VEGFR inhibition.

MECHANISM OF RESISTANCE
- Increased expression of VEGFR-1, VEGFR-2, VEGFR-3, PDGFR, and c-Kit.
- Mutations in target VEGFRs, resulting in alterations in drug-binding affinity.
- Activation of angiogenic switch, with increased expression of alternative pro-angiogenic pathways.
- Increased pericyte coverage to tumor vessels, with increased expression of VEGF and other pro-angiogenic factors.
- Recruitment of pro-angiogenic inflammatory cells from bone marrow, such as tumor-associated macrophages, monocytes, and myeloid-derived suppressor cells (MDSCs).

ABSORPTION
Good oral absorption with median time to peak concentrations of 10 hours. Steady-state drug levels are achieved in 14 days. Food does not appear to affect oral absorption.

DISTRIBUTION
Extensive binding (>99%) of tivozanib to plasma proteins, mainly albumin.

METABOLISM
Undergoes metabolism in the liver primarily by CYP3A4 microsomal enzymes. Elimination is mainly via the hepatobiliary route with excretion in feces, nearly 80%, with renal elimination accounting for about 12% of the administered dose. The mean terminal half-life is 4.5–5 hours.

INDICATIONS
FDA-approved for relapsed or refractory advanced renal cell carcinoma following 2 or more prior systemic therapies.

DOSAGE RANGE
Recommended dose is 1.34 mg PO once daily with or without food for 21 days on a 28-day cycle.

DRUG INTERACTIONS
Concomitant administration of strong CYP3A4 inducers such as phenytoin, carbamazepine, rifampin, phenobarbital, and St. John's Wort increases the rate of metabolism of tivozanib, resulting in its inactivation and reduced effective drug levels.

SPECIAL CONSIDERATIONS
1. Monitor blood pressure while on therapy. Blood pressure should be well controlled prior to initiation of tivozanib.
2. Monitor patients for bleeding complications, especially in those who are at increased risk or who have a prior history of bleeding issues.
3. Use with caution in patients with cardiovascular and cerebrovascular disease, especially those with prior MI, angina, stroke, and TIA.
4. Closely monitor thyroid function tests, as tivozanib therapy results in hypothyroidism.
5. Baseline and periodic urinalysis during treatment is recommended, and tivozanib should be discontinued in the setting of grade 4 proteinuria.
6. Avoid Seville oranges, starfruit, pomelos, grapefruit, and grapefruit products while on tivozanib therapy, as they can inhibit CYP3A4 activity, resulting in increased drug levels.
7. Patients are at increased risk for developing allergic-type reaction that is in response to the tartrazine dye that is contained in the drug capsule.
8. Dose reduction is not recommended for patients with mild hepatic impairment. Dose of drug should be reduced to 0.89 mg in setting of moderate hepatic impairment. Has not been studied in the setting of severe hepatic impairment.
9. Dose reduction is not recommended for patients with mild to severe renal impairment.
10. Embryo-fetal toxicity. May cause fetal harm. Females of reproductive potential should use effective contraception during drug therapy and for at least 1 month after the final dose. Breastfeeding should be avoided.

TOXICITY 1
Hypertension occurs in up to 45% of patients, with about 24% grade 3/4 events.

TOXICITY 2
Diarrhea, nausea/vomiting, and mucositis are the most common GI side effects.

TOXICITY 3
Fatigue, asthenia, and anorexia.

TOXICITY 4
Bleeding complications with hematuria, epistaxis, and hemoptysis.

TOXICITY 5
Increased risk of arterial thromboembolic events, including MI, angina, TIA, and stroke as well as increased risk of venous-thromboembolic events.

TOXICITY 6
Proteinuria.

TOXICITY 7
Hypothyroidism.

TOXICITY 8
Rare cases of cardiac failure.

TOXICITY 9
RPLS presenting with seizures, headaches, visual disturbances, confusion, or altered mental status.

Topotecan

TRADE NAME	Hycamtin	CLASSIFICATION	Topoisomerase I inhibitor
CATEGORY	Chemotherapy drug	DRUG MANUFACTURER	GlaxoSmithKline

MECHANISM OF ACTION
- Semisynthetic derivative of camptothecin, an alkaloid extract from the *Camptotheca acuminata* tree.

- Inhibits topoisomerase I function. Binds to and stabilizes the topoisomerase I-DNA complex and prevents the religation of DNA after it has been cleaved by topoisomerase I. The collision between this stable cleavable complex and the advancing replication fork results in double-strand DNA breaks and cellular death.
- Antitumor activity requires the presence of topoisomerase I and ongoing DNA synthesis.

MECHANISM OF RESISTANCE
- Decreased expression of topoisomerase I.
- Mutations in topoisomerase I enzyme, with reduced binding affinity to drug.
- Increased expression of the multidrug-resistant phenotype, with overexpression of P170 glycoprotein. Results in enhanced efflux of drug and decreased intracellular accumulation of drug.
- Decreased accumulation of drug into cells through non–multidrug-resistance-related mechanisms.

ABSORPTION
Rapidly absorbed with peak plasma concentrations occurring between 1 and 2 hours following oral administration. Oral bioavailability is about 40%, and topotecan can be given without regard to food.

DISTRIBUTION
Widely distributed in body tissues. Binding to plasma proteins is on the order of 10%–35%. Levels of drug in the CSF are only 30% of those in plasma. Peak drug levels are achieved within 1 hour after drug administration.

METABOLISM
Rapid conversion of topotecan in plasma and in aqueous solution from the lactone closed ring form to the carboxylate acid open form. At acidic pH, topotecan is mainly in the lactone ring, while at physiologic and basic pH, the carboxylate form predominates. Only about 20%–30% of a given dose is present as the active lactone metabolite at 1 hour after drug administration. The major route of elimination of topotecan is renal excretion, accounting for 40%–68% of drug clearance. Metabolism in the liver appears to be minimal and is mediated by the liver microsomal P450 system. The elimination half-life is approximately 3 hours.

INDICATIONS
1. Ovarian cancer—FDA-approved in patients with advanced ovarian cancer who failed platinum-based chemotherapy.
2. SCLC—FDA-approved in patients with sensitive disease who progressed on first-line chemotherapy.
3. Cervical cancer—FDA-approved in combination with cisplatin for the treatment of stage IV-B, recurrent, or persistent carcinoma of the cervix that is not amenable to curative treatment with surgery and/or radiation therapy.

DOSAGE RANGE

1. IV: Recommended dose is 1.5 mg/m^2/day IV for 5 consecutive days given every 21 days.
2. Oral: Recommended dose is 2.3 mg/m^2/day for 5 consecutive days given every 21 days.

DRUG INTERACTION

None well characterized.

SPECIAL CONSIDERATIONS

1. Dose reduction is not recommended in patients with mild or moderate renal impairment. Dose should be reduced to 0.75 5 mg/m^2/day IV for 5 consecutive days given every 21 days in the setting of severe renal impairment. Baseline CrCl should be obtained, as well as periodic monitoring of renal function while on therapy.
2. Dose reduction is not recommended in the setting of hepatic impairment.
3. Monitor CBC on a weekly basis.
4. Carefully monitor administration of drug, as it is a mild vesicant. The infusion site should be carefully monitored for extravasation, in which case flushing with sterile water, elevation of the extremity, and local application of ice are recommended. In severe cases, a plastic surgeon should be consulted.
5. If granulocyte nadir count is low, begin G-CSF 24 hours after the completion of topotecan therapy.
6. Pregnancy category D. Breastfeeding should be avoided.

TOXICITY 1

Myelosuppression is dose-limiting, with neutropenia being most commonly observed. Nadir typically occurs at days 7–10, with full recovery by days 21–28.

TOXICITY 2

Nausea and vomiting. Mild-to-moderate and dose-related. Occurs in 60%–80% of patients. Diarrhea with abdominal pain also observed.

TOXICITY 3

Headache, fever, malaise, arthralgias, and myalgias.

TOXICITY 4

Microscopic hematuria. Seen in 10% of patients.

TOXICITY 5

Alopecia.

TOXICITY 6

Transient elevation in serum transaminases, alkaline phosphatase, and bilirubin.

Toremifene

TRADE NAME	Fareston	CLASSIFICATION	Antiestrogen
CATEGORY	Hormonal agent	DRUG MANUFACTURER	Orion and GTx

MECHANISM OF ACTION
- Synthetic analog of tamoxifen.
- Nonsteroidal antiestrogen that directly binds to estrogen receptors on breast cancer cells. Affinity for estrogen receptor is 4- to 5-fold higher than tamoxifen. Blocks downstream intracellular signal transduction pathways, leading to inhibition of cell growth and induction of apoptosis.

MECHANISM OF RESISTANCE
Cross-resistance between toremifene, tamoxifen, and other antiestrogen agents.

ABSORPTION
Well absorbed after oral administration. Food does not interfere with oral absorption.

DISTRIBUTION
Widely distributed to body tissues. Extensive (>99%) binding to plasma proteins, mainly albumin. Steady-state plasma concentrations are reached in 4–6 weeks.

METABOLISM
Extensive metabolism in the liver by the cytochrome P450 system. Major metabolites, N-demethyltoremifene and 4-hydroxytoremifene, have long terminal half-lives of 4–6 days secondary to enterohepatic recirculation. Parent drug and metabolites are excreted mainly in bile and feces. Minimal excretion in urine.

INDICATIONS
Metastatic breast cancer in postmenopausal women with ER+ tumors or in cases where ER status is not known. Not recommended in ER– tumors.

DOSAGE RANGE

Recommended dose is 60 mg PO daily until disease progression.

DRUG INTERACTION 1

Thiazide diuretics—Decrease renal clearance of calcium and increase the risk of hypercalcemia associated with toremifene.

DRUG INTERACTION 2

Warfarin—Toremifene inhibits liver P450 metabolism of warfarin, resulting in an increased anticoagulant effect. Coagulation parameters, PT and INR, should be closely monitored, and dose adjustments made accordingly.

DRUG INTERACTION 3

Phenobarbital, carbamazepine, phenytoin—Liver P450 metabolism of toremifene may be enhanced by phenobarbital, carbamazepine, and phenytoin, resulting in reduced blood levels and reduced clinical efficacy.

DRUG INTERACTION 4

Ketoconazole and erythromycin—Liver P450 metabolism of toremifene may be inhibited by ketoconazole and erythromycin, resulting in elevated blood levels and enhanced clinical efficacy.

SPECIAL CONSIDERATIONS

1. Patients with a prior history of thromboembolic events must be carefully monitored while on therapy, as toremifene is thrombogenic.
2. Use with caution in the setting of brain and/or vertebral body metastases, as tumor flare with bone and/or muscular pain, erythema, and transient increase in tumor volume can occur upon initiation of therapy.
3. Monitor CBC, LFTs, and serum calcium on a regular basis.
4. Contraindicated in patients with a prior history of endometrial hyperplasia. Increased risk of endometrial cancer associated with therapy. Onset of vaginal bleeding during therapy requires immediate gynecologic evaluation.
5. Baseline and biannual eye exams are recommended, as toremifene can lead to cataract formation.
6. Pregnancy category D. Breastfeeding should be avoided. Not known whether toremifene is excreted in breast milk.

TOXICITY 1

Hot flashes, sweating, menstrual irregularity, milk production in breast, and vaginal discharge and bleeding are commonly observed.

TOXICITY 2

Transient tumor flare manifested by bone and/or tumor pain.

TOXICITY 3

Ocular toxicity with cataract formation and xerophthalmia.

TOXICITY 4
Nausea, vomiting, and anorexia.

TOXICITY 5
Myelosuppression is usually mild.

TOXICITY 6
Rare skin toxicity in the form of rash, alopecia, and peripheral edema.

Tositumomab

TRADE NAME	Bexxar	CLASSIFICATION	Monoclonal antibody, anti-CD20 antibody
CATEGORY	Biologic response modifier agent, targeted agent	DRUG MANUFACTURER	Corixa and GlaxoSmithKline

MECHANISM OF ACTION
- Radioimmunotherapeutic monoclonal antibody-based regimen composed of the tositumomab monoclonal antibody and the radiolabeled monoclonal antibody I-131 tositumomab, a radio-iodinated derivative of tositumomab that has been covalently linked to I-131.
- The antibody moiety is tositumomab, which targets the CD20 antigen, a 35-kDa cell-surface, non-glycosylated phosphoprotein expressed during early pre–B-cell development until the plasma cell stage. Binding of the antibody to CD20 induces a transmembrane signal that blocks cell activation and cell cycle progression.
- CD20 is expressed on more than 90% of all B-cell non-Hodgkin's lymphomas and leukemias. CD20 is not expressed on early pre–B cells, plasma cells, normal bone marrow stem cells, antigen-presenting dendritic reticulum cells, or other normal tissues.
- Ionizing radiation from the I-131 radioisotope results in cell death.

ABSORPTION
Administered only via the IV route.

DISTRIBUTION
Higher clearance, shorter terminal half-life, and larger volumes of distribution observed in patients with higher tumor burden, splenomegaly, and/or bone marrow involvement.

METABOLISM
Elimination of I-131 occurs by decay and excretion in the urine. Total body clearance is 67% of an administered dose, and nearly 100% of drug clearance is accounted for in the urine.

INDICATIONS
Relapsed and/or refractory CD20-positive, follicular non-Hodgkin's lymphoma with and without transformation—disease is refractory to rituximab therapy and has relapsed following chemotherapy.

DOSAGE RANGE
Treatment schema is as follows: Day 0, begin Lugol's solution or oral potassium iodide solution. Day 1, dosimetric dose: 450 mg unlabeled tositumomab, followed by 5 mCi of I-131 tositumomab (35 mg). Measurement of whole body counts and calculation of therapeutic dose. Day 7 up to day 14, therapeutic dose: 450 mg unlabeled tositumomab, followed by calculated therapeutic dose of I-131 tositumomab to deliver 75 cGy. Days 8–21, continue Lugol's solution or oral potassium iodide solution.

DRUG INTERACTIONS
None well characterized to date.

SPECIAL CONSIDERATIONS
1. Contraindicated in patients with known type I hypersensitivity or known hypersensitivity to any component of the Bexxar therapeutic regimen.
2. TSH levels should be monitored before treatment and on an annual basis thereafter.
3. Before receiving the dosimetric dose of I-131, patients must receive at least 3 doses of SSKI, 3 doses of Lugol's solution, or 1 dose of 130 mg potassium iodide (at least 24 hours prior to the dosimetric dose).
4. Should be administered only by physicians and healthcare professionals who are qualified and experienced in the safe use and handling of radioisotopes.
5. Patients should be premedicated with acetaminophen and diphenhydramine before each administration of tositumomab in the dosimetric and therapeutic steps to reduce the incidence of infusion-related reactions.
6. The same IV tubing set and filter must be used throughout the dosimetric and therapeutic step, as a change in filter can result in loss of effective drug delivery.
7. Monitor for infusion-related events, which usually occur during or within 48 hours of infusion. Infusion rate should be reduced by 50% for mild to moderate allergic reaction and immediately stopped for a severe reaction. Immediate institution of diphenhydramine, acetaminophen, corticosteroids, IV fluids, and/or vasopressors may be necessary. In the setting of a severe reaction, the infusion can be restarted at a reduced rate (50%) once symptoms have completely resolved. Resuscitation equipment should be readily available at bedside.

8. Tositumomab therapy should not be given to patients with >25% involvement of the bone marrow by lymphoma and/or impaired bone marrow reserve or to patients with platelet count <100,000/mm^3 or neutrophil count <1,500/mm^3.
9. CBCs and platelet counts should be monitored weekly following tositumomab therapy for up to 10–12 weeks after therapy.
10. Should be given only as a single-course treatment.
11. May have direct toxic effects on the male and female reproductive organs, and effective contraception should be used during therapy and for up to 12 months following the completion of therapy.
12. Pregnancy category X. Contraindicated in women who are pregnant.
13. Breastfeeding should be discontinued immediately prior to starting therapy.

TOXICITY 1
Infusion-related symptoms, including fever, chills, urticaria, flushing, fatigue, headache, bronchospasm, rhinitis, dyspnea, angioedema, nausea, and/or hypotension. Usually resolve upon slowing and/or interrupting the infusion and with supportive care.

TOXICITY 2
Myelosuppression with neutropenia, thrombocytopenia, and anemia. The time to nadir is typically 4–7 weeks, and the duration of cytopenias is 30 days. Severe cytopenias may persist beyond 12 weeks after therapy in 5%–7% of patients.

TOXICITY 3
Mild asthenia and fatigue occur in up to 40% of patients.

TOXICITY 4
Infections with majority of infection events being of viral origin and relatively minor. Up to 10% of patients experience more serious infections that require hospitalization.

TOXICITY 5
Mild nausea and vomiting.

TOXICITY 6
Hypothyroidism.

TOXICITY 7
Secondary malignancies occur in about 2%–3% of patients. AML and MDS have been reported, with a cumulative incidence of 1.4% at 2 years and 4.8% at 4 years following therapy.

TOXICITY 8
Development of human anti-mouse antibody responses (HAMAs). Rare event in less than 1%–2% of patients.

Trabectedin

TRADE NAME	Yondelis	CLASSIFICATION	Alkylating agent
CATEGORY	Chemotherapy drug	DRUG MANUFACTURER	Janssen/Johnson & Johnson

MECHANISM OF ACTION

- Tetrahydroisoquinoline alkylating agent that binds to the N2 position of guanine residues in the minor groove of DNA, leading to formation of DNA adducts and to bending of the DNA helix toward the major groove.
- DNA adduct formation results in single- and double-strand breaks and inhibition of DNA synthesis and function.
- Induces cell cycle arrest and cell death that is not dependent on p53.
- Antitumor activity may also relate to effects on the tumor microenvironment.
- Has potent immunomodulatory effects, with cytotoxic effects against monocytes and tumor-associated macrophages.
- Inhibits production of pro-inflammatory and pro-angiogenic mediators in the tumor microenvironment.
- Cell cycle nonspecific. Active in all phases of the cell cycle.

MECHANISM OF RESISTANCE

- Multidrug-resistant phenotype with increased expression of P170 glycoprotein.
- Increased expression of ABCB1 transport protein.
- Increased expression of IGF-1R and insulin receptor substrate-1.
- Increased expression and activity of zinc finger proteins, including ZNF93 and ZNF43.

ABSORPTION

Administered only via the IV route.

DISTRIBUTION

Mean steady-state volume of distribution exceeds 5,000 L. Based on in vitro testing, about 97% of drug bound to plasma proteins.

METABOLISM

Rapidly and extensively metabolized by CYP3A liver microsomal enzymes. There is negligible unchanged drug in feces and urine following drug administration. Elimination is mainly hepatic, with excretion in feces (~58%), with renal elimination accounting for only 6% of an administered dose. The terminal elimination half-life is approximately 175 hours.

INDICATIONS

FDA-approved for the treatment of unresectable or metastatic liposarcoma or leiomyosarcoma following a prior anthracycline-containing regimen.

DOSAGE RANGE

Recommended dose is 1.5 mg/m^2 as a 24-hour infusion every 3 weeks. The drug should be administered through a central venous line.

DRUG INTERACTION 1

Drugs such as ketoconazole, itraconazole, erythromycin, clarithromycin, atazanavir, indinavir, nefazodone, nelfinavir, ritonavir, saquinavir, telithromycin, and voriconazole may decrease the rate of metabolism of trabectedin, resulting in increased drug levels and potentially increased toxicity.

DRUG INTERACTION 2

Drugs such as rifampin, phenytoin, phenobarbital, carbamazepine, and St. John's Wort may increase the rate of metabolism of trabectedin, resulting in its inactivation and lower effective drug levels.

SPECIAL CONSIDERATIONS

1. Use with caution in patients with hepatic dysfunction. Dose reduction is recommended in patients with moderate hepatic dysfunction, and a dose of 0.9 mg/m^2 should be administered. Trabectedin should not be given in the setting of severe hepatic dysfunction.
2. Dose reduction is not recommended in patients with mild or moderate renal dysfunction. Has not been studied in patients with severe renal dysfunction and end-stage renal disease.
3. Closely monitor CBCs on a periodic basis, with a focus on the ANC.
4. Trabectedin should be held for >grade 2 neutropenia.
5. Closely monitor CPK levels prior to each cycle of therapy, as rhabdomyolysis and musculoskeletal toxicity can occur.
6. LFTs should be monitored, as hepatotoxicity, including hepatic failure, is associated with trabectedin.
7. Baseline and periodic evaluation of LVEF by echocardiogram of MUGA. Trabectedin should be held for LVEF below the lower limit of normal and permanently discontinued for symptomatic cardiomyopathy or persistent LV dysfunction that does not return to the lower limit of normal within 3 weeks.

8. Trabectedin must be administered through a central line, as drug extravasation can cause tissue necrosis.
9. Pregnancy category D. Breastfeeding should be avoided.

TOXICITY 1
Myelosuppression with neutropenia. Severe and fatal neutropenic sepsis may occur.

TOXICITY 2
Rhabdomyolysis and musculoskeletal toxicity.

TOXICITY 3
Hepatotoxicity with elevations in SGOT/SGPT, bilirubin, and alkaline phosphatase.

TOXICITY 4
Cardiac toxicity with reduction in LVEF, diastolic dysfunction, CHF, and cardiac failure.

TOXICITY 5
GI toxicity with nausea/vomiting, constipation, and diarrhea.

TOXICITY 6
Fatigue and anorexia.

Trametinib

TRADE NAME	Mekinist	CLASSIFICATION	Signal transduction inhibitor, MEK inhibitor
CATEGORY	Targeted agent	DRUG MANUFACTURER	Novartis

MECHANISM OF ACTION

- Reversible inhibitor of mitogen-activated extracellular signal-regulated kinase 1 (MEK1) and kinase 2 (MEK2) activity.
- Results in inhibition of downstream regulators of the extracellular signal-regulated kinase (ERK) pathway, leading to inhibition of cellular proliferation.
- Inhibits growth of BRAF-V600 mutation–positive melanoma.

MECHANISM OF RESISTANCE

- Increased expression and/or activation of the PI3K/AKT pathway.
- Reactivation of the MAPK signaling pathway.
- Emergence of MEK2 mutations.
- Presence of NRAS mutations.
- Increased expression and/or activation of the HER2-neu pathway.

ABSORPTION

Oral bioavailability is on the order of 70%. Peak plasma drug concentrations are achieved in 1.5 hours after oral ingestion. Food with a high fat content reduces C_{max}, T_{max}, and AUC.

DISTRIBUTION

Extensive binding (97.4%) of trametinib to plasma proteins.

METABOLISM

Metabolized mainly via deacetylation alone or with mono-oxygenation or in combination with glucuronidation biotransformation pathways in the liver. The process of deacetylation is mediated by hydrolytic enzymes, such as carboxylesterases or amidases. Elimination is hepatic, with excretion in feces (>80%), with renal elimination accounting for <20% of an administered dose. The median terminal half-life of trametinib is approximately 4–5 days.

INDICATIONS

1. FDA-approved as a single agent or in combination with dabrafenib for unresectable or metastatic melanoma with BRAF-V600E or V600K mutation as determined by an FDA-approved diagnostic test.
2. FDA-approved in combination with dabrafenib for the adjuvant treatment of early-stage melanoma with involvement of lymph nodes following complete surgical resection and with BRAF-V600E or BRAF-V600K mutation as determined by an FDA-approved diagnostic test.
3. FDA-approved in combination with dabrafenib for metastatic NSCLC with BRAF-V600E mutation as determined by an FDA-approved diagnostic test.
4. FDA-approved in combination with dabrafenib for locally advanced or metastatic anaplastic thyroid cancer (ATC) with BRAF-V600E mutation and no appropriate locoregional treatment options.
5. FDA-approved in combination with dabrafenib for adult and pediatric patients 6 years of age and older with unresectable or metastatic solid tumors with BRAF-V600E mutation who have progressed following prior treatment and who have no satisfactory alternative treatment options.

Approved under accelerated approval based on overall response rate and duration of response.

6. FDA-approved for pediatric patients 1 year of age and older with low-grade glioma with a BRAF V600E mutation who require systemic therapy.

DOSAGE RANGE

1. Recommended dose for adult patients as a single agent or in combination with dabrafenib is 2 mg PO daily. Should be taken at least 1 hour before or at least 2 hours after a meal.
2. Recommended dose for tablets or oral solution in pediatric patients is based on body weight as outlined in the package insert.

DRUG INTERACTIONS

None well characterized to date.

SPECIAL CONSIDERATIONS

1. Baseline and periodic evaluations of LVEF should be performed while on therapy. Approximately 10% of patients will develop cardiomyopathy at a median time of 63 days. Treatment should be held if the absolute LVEF drops by 10% from pretreatment baseline. Therapy should be permanently stopped for symptomatic cardiomyopathy or persistent, asymptomatic LVEF dysfunction that does not resolve within 4 weeks.
2. Patients should be warned about the possibility of visual disturbances.
3. Careful eye exams should be done at baseline and with any new visual changes to rule out the possibility of retinal detachments or retinal vein occlusion.
4. Monitor patients for pulmonary symptoms. Therapy should be held in patients presenting with new or progressive pulmonary symptoms and should be terminated in patients diagnosed with treatment-related pneumonitis or ILD.
5. Monitor patients for serious skin toxicity and secondary infections, with the median time to onset of 15 days. The median time to resolution of skin toxicity is 48 days.
6. BRAF testing using an FDA-approved diagnostic test to confirm the presence of the BRAF-V600E or BRAF-V600K mutation is required for determining which patients should receive trametinib therapy.
7. Dose adjustment is not recommended for patients with mild hepatic dysfunction. However, caution should be used in patients with moderate or severe hepatic dysfunction.
8. Dose adjustment is not recommended for patients with mild or moderate renal dysfunction. Use with caution in patients with severe renal dysfunction.
9. May cause fetal harm. Women of reproductive potential should use effective contraception during treatment and for 4 months after the last dose. Breastfeeding should be avoided during treatment and for 4 months after the last dose.

TOXICITY 1
Cardiac toxicity in the form of cardiomyopathy.

TOXICITY 2
Ophthalmologic side effects, including retinal detachment and retinal vein occlusion.

TOXICITY 3
Pulmonary toxicity with ILD presenting as cough, dyspnea, hypoxia, pleural effusion, or infiltrates. Observed rarely in about 2% of patients.

TOXICITY 4
Skin toxicity with rash, dermatitis, acneiform rash, hand-foot syndrome, erythema, pruritus, and paronychia. Severe skin toxicity observed in 12% of patients.

TOXICITY 5
Diarrhea, mucositis, and abdominal pain are the most common GI side effects.

TOXICITY 6
Hypertension.

TOXICITY 7
Lymphedema.

Trastuzumab

TRADE NAME	Herceptin, Anti-HER2-antibody	CLASSIFICATION	Signal transduction inhibitor, anti-HER2 antibody
CATEGORY	Biologic response modifier agent, targeted agent	DRUG MANUFACTURER	Genentech/ Roche

MECHANISM OF ACTION
- Recombinant humanized monoclonal antibody directed against the extracellular domain (IV) of the HER2 growth factor receptor. This receptor is overexpressed in several human cancers, including 25%–30% of breast cancers and up to 20% of gastric cancers.
- Precise mechanism(s) of action remains unknown.
- Inhibits HER2 intracellular signaling pathways.

- Immunologic mechanisms may also be involved in antitumor activity, which include recruitment of antibody-dependent cellular cytotoxicity (ADCC) and/or complement-mediated cell lysis.

MECHANISM OF RESISTANCE
- Mutations in the HER2 growth factor receptor, leading to reduced binding affinity to trastuzumab.
- Reactivation of HER signaling through acquisition of the HER2 L755S mutation.
- Decreased expression of HER2.
- Expression of P95HER2, a constitutively active, truncated form of the HER2 receptor.
- Increased expression of HER3.
- Activation/induction of alternative cellular signaling pathways, such as the PI3K/AKT, IGF-1 receptor, and/or the c-Met receptor.

DISTRIBUTION
Distribution in body has not been well characterized.

METABOLISM
Metabolism of trastuzumab has not been extensively characterized. Half-life is on the order of 6 days with a weekly schedule and 16 days with the every-3-week schedule.

INDICATIONS
1. Metastatic breast cancer—First-line therapy in combination with paclitaxel. Patient's tumor must express HER2 protein to be treated with this monoclonal antibody.
2. Metastatic breast cancer—Second- and third-line therapy as a single agent in patients whose tumors overexpress the HER2 protein.
3. Early-stage breast cancer—FDA-approved for the adjuvant therapy of node-positive, HER2-overexpressing breast cancer as part of a treatment regimen containing doxorubicin, cyclophosphamide, and either paclitaxel or docetaxel.
4. Metastatic gastric and gastroesophageal junction adenocarcinoma—FDA-approved in combination with cisplatin and capecitabine or 5-FU for the treatment of patients with HER2-overexpressing metastatic gastric or gastroesophageal junction adenocarcinoma who have not received prior treatment for metastatic disease.

DOSAGE RANGE
1. Recommended loading dose of 4 mg/kg IV administered over 90 minutes, followed by maintenance dose of 2 mg/kg IV on a weekly basis. One week following the last weekly dose of trastuzumab, administer trastuzumab at 6 mg/kg as an intravenous infusion over 30–90 minutes every 3 weeks.

2. Alternative schedule is to give a loading dose of 8 mg/kg IV administered over 30–90 minutes, followed by maintenance dose of 6 mg/kg IV every 3 weeks.

DRUG INTERACTIONS

Anthracyclines, taxanes—Increased risk of cardiac toxicity when trastuzumab is used in combination with anthracyclines and/or taxanes.

SPECIAL CONSIDERATIONS

1. Caution should be used in treating patients with pre-existing cardiac dysfunction. Careful baseline assessment of cardiac function (LVEF) before treatment and frequent monitoring (every 3 months) of cardiac function while on therapy. Trastuzumab should be held for >16% absolute decrease in LVEF from a normal baseline value. Trastuzumab therapy should be stopped immediately in patients who develop clinically significant congestive heart failure. When trastuzumab is used in the adjuvant setting, cardiac function should be assessed every 6 months for at least 2 years following the completion of therapy.
2. Carefully monitor for infusion reactions, which typically occur during or within 24 hours of drug administration. Administer initial loading dose over 90 minutes, and then observe patient for 1 hour following completion of the loading dose. May need to treat with diphenhydramine and acetaminophen. Rarely, in severe cases, may need to treat with IV fluids and/or pressors.
3. Maintenance doses are administered over 30 minutes if loading dose was well tolerated without fever and chills. However, if fever and chills were experienced with the loading dose, maintenance doses should be administered over 90 minutes.
4. Pregnancy category D.

TOXICITY 1

Infusion-related symptoms with fever, chills, urticaria, flushing, fatigue, headache, bronchospasm, dyspnea, angioedema, and hypotension. Occur in 40%–50% of patients. Usually mild to moderate in severity and observed most commonly with administration of the first infusion.

TOXICITY 2

Mild GI toxicity in the form of nausea/vomiting and diarrhea.

TOXICITY 3

Cardiac toxicity in the form of dyspnea, peripheral edema, and reduced left ventricular function. Significantly increased risk when used in combination with an anthracycline-based regimen. In most instances, cardiac dysfunction is readily reversible.

TOXICITY 4

Myelosuppression. Increased risk and severity when trastuzumab is administered with chemotherapy.

TOXICITY 5

Generalized pain, asthenia, and headache.

TOXICITY 6

Pulmonary toxicity in the form of increased cough, dyspnea, rhinitis, sinusitis, pulmonary infiltrates, and/or pleural effusions.

Trastuzumab-pkrb

TRADE NAME	Herzuma, biosimilar to trastuzumab	CLASSIFICATION	Signal transduction inhibitor, amti-HER2 antibody
CATEGORY	Targeted agent	DRUG MANUFACTURER	Teva

INDICATIONS

1. Metastatic breast cancer—First-line therapy in combination with paclitaxel. Patient's tumor must express HER2 protein to be treated with this monoclonal antibody.
2. Metastatic breast cancer—Second- and third-line therapy as a single agent in patients whose tumors overexpress the HER2 protein.
3. Early-stage breast cancer—FDA-approved for the adjuvant therapy of node-positive, HER2-overexpressing breast cancer as part of a treatment regimen containing doxorubicin, cyclophosphamide, and either paclitaxel or docetaxel.
4. Metastatic gastric and gastroesophageal junction adenocarcinoma—FDA-approved in combination with cisplatin and capecitabine or 5-FU for the treatment of patients with HER2-overexpressing metastatic gastric or gastroesophageal junction adenocarcinoma who have not received prior treatment for metastatic disease.

Trastuzumab deruxtecan

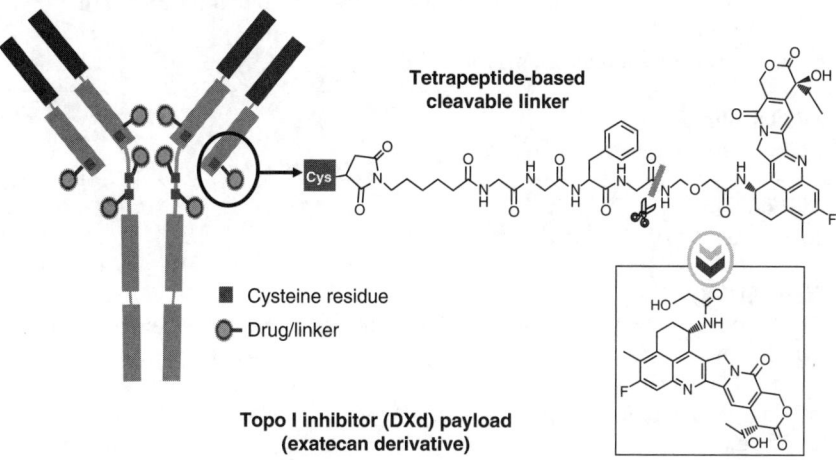

Humanized anti-HER2 IgG1
mAb with same AA
sequence as trastuzumab

Tetrapeptide-based
cleavable linker

Cys

■ Cysteine residue
●– Drug/linker

Topo I inhibitor (DXd) payload
(exatecan derivative)

TRADE NAME	Enhertu, DS-8201	CLASSIFICATION	Antibody-drug conjugate
CATEGORY	Biologic response modifier agent/ chemotherapy drug	DRUG MANUFACTURER	Daiichi Sankyo and AstraZeneca

MECHANISM OF ACTION
- HER2-targeted antibody-drug conjugate made up of a humanized anti-HER2 IgG1 antibody and the topoisomerase I (topo I) inhibitor DXd.
- Upon binding to the HER2 receptor, trastuzumab deruxtecan undergoes receptor-mediated internalization and lysosomal degradation, leading to intracellular release of the DXd molecule.
- Binding of DXd to topo I leads to inhibition of DNA synthesis and function, which leads to DNA damage and apoptotic cell death. DXd is a 10-fold more potent topo I inhibitor than SN38, the active metabolite of irinotecan.
- Inhibits HER2 downstream signaling pathways.
- Immunologic-mediated mechanisms, such as antibody-dependent cell-mediated cytotoxicity (ADCC), may also be involved in antitumor activity.
- Activity of trastuzumab deruxtecan is dependent on HER2 expression and not on HER2 gene amplification.
- Higher drug-to-antibody ratio than ado-trastuzumab emtansine.

MECHANISM OF RESISTANCE

- Reduced expression of HER2 receptor.
- Poor internalization of the antibody-drug conjugate.
- Impaired lysosomal proteolytic activity leading to reduced intracellular levels of the DXd molecule.
- Defective intracellular and endosomal trafficking of the HER2-DXd complex.
- Increased expression of p95HER2.

ABSORPTION

Administered only via the IV route.

DISTRIBUTION

Extensive binding (97%) to plasma proteins.

METABOLISM

The trastuzumab antibody is expected to be broken down into small peptides and amino acids. DXd is metabolized by the liver CYP3A4 microsomal enzymes. The median elimination half-life of trastuzumab deruxtecan is approximately 5.7 days, and the median apparent elimination half-life of DXd is on the order of 5.8 days.

INDICATIONS

1. FDA-approved for patients with unresectable or metastatic HER2-positive breast cancer who have received a prior anti-HER2-based regimens in either the metastatic setting or in the neoadjuvant or adjuvant setting and have developed disease recurrence during or within 6 months of completing therapy.
2. FDA-approved for patients with unresectable or metastatic HER2-low breast cancer (IHC 1+ or IHC 2+/ISH-) who have received a prior chemotherapy in the metastatic setting or or developed disease recurrence during or within 6 months of completing adjuvant chemotherapy.
3. FDA-approved for patients with locally advanced or metastatic HER2-positive gastric or gastro-esophageal junction adenocarcinoma who have received a prior trastuzumab-containing regimen.
4. FDA-approved for patients with unresectable or metastatic NSCLC whose tumors have activating HER2 mutations. Approved under accelerated approval based on objective response rate and duration of response.
5. Clinical activity in mCRC.

DOSAGE RANGE

1. Recommended dose for breast cancer and NSCLC is 5.4 mg/kg IV every 3 weeks.
2. Recommended dose for gastric cancer is 6.4 mg/kg IV every 3 weeks.

DRUG INTERACTIONS

None well characterized to date.

SPECIAL CONSIDERATIONS

1. Trastuzumab deruxtecan can **NOT** be substituted for or with trastuzumab or ado-trastuzumab emtansine.
2. Baseline and periodic evaluations of left ventricular ejection fraction (LVEF) should be performed while on therapy. Treatment should be permanently stopped if the LVEF drops <40% or absolute reduction from pre-treatment baseline is >20%. Treatment should also be permanently stopped in patients who develop symptomatic congestive heart failure.
3. Carefully monitor for infusion-related reactions, especially during the first infusion.
4. Monitor patients for pulmonary symptoms. Therapy should be held in patients presenting with new or progressive pulmonary symptoms and should be permanently stopped in patients with grade 2 or higher treatment-related pneumonitis or interstitial lung disease (ILD). This is a black-box warning.
5. Closely monitor CBC on a periodic basis.
6. HER2 testing using an FDA-approved diagnostic test to confirm the presence of HER2 protein overexpression is required for determining which patients should receive trastuzumab deruxtecan.
7. No dose adjustment is recommended for patients with mild or moderate hepatic dysfunction. Use with caution in patients with severe hepatic dysfunction as the drug has not been studied in this setting.
8. No dose adjustment is recommended for patients with mild or moderate renal dysfunction. Use with caution in patients with severe renal dysfunction, as there is only very limited information about the drug in this setting.
9. May cause embryo-fetal harm. Patients should be educated on the need for effective contraception. Females of reproductive potential should use effective contraception during treatment and for 7 months after the last dose. Males with female partners should use effective contraception during treatment and for 4 months after the last dose. Breastfeeding should be avoided while on therapy and for 7 months after the last dose.

TOXICITY 1

Pulmonary toxicity presenting as cough, dyspnea, fever, and infiltrates. Severe interstitial lung disease, including pneumonitis can occur in up to 9% of patients.

TOXICITY 2

Infusion-related reactions.

TOXICITY 3

Cardiac toxicity with cardiomyopathy.

TOXICITY 4
Myelosuppression with neutropenia and anemia.

TOXICITY 5
Asthenia, fatigue, and anorexia.

TOXICITY 6
Mild nausea and vomiting, constipation, and diarrhea.

Tremelimumab-actl

TRADE NAME	Imjudo	**CLASSIFICATION**	Monoclonal antibody, anti-CTLA4 antibody
CATEGORY	Immunotherapy, immune checkpoint inhibitor	**DRUG MANUFACTURER**	AstraZeneca

MECHANISM OF ACTION
- Binds to cytotoxic T-lymphocyte-associated antigen 4 (CTLA-4), which is expressed on the surface of activated CD4 and CD8 T lymphocytes, resulting in inhibition of the interaction between CTLA-4 and its target ligands CD80 and CD86.
- Blockade of CTLA-4 enhances T-cell immune responses, including T-cell activation and proliferation.

MECHANISM OF RESISTANCE
- Increased expression and/or activity of other immune checkpoint pathways (e.g., TIGIT, TIM3, and LAG3).
- Increased expression of other immune escape mechanisms.
- Increased infiltration of immune suppressive populations within the tumor microenvironment, which include Tregs, myeloid-derived suppressor cells (MDSCs), and M2 macrophages.
- Release of various cytokines, chemokines, and metabolites within the tumor microenvironment, including CSF-1, tryptophan metabolites, TGF-β, and adenosine.

ABSORPTION
Administered only via the IV route.

DISTRIBUTION
Steady-state concentrations are generally reached by approximately 12 weeks.

METABOLISM
Metabolism has not been extensively characterized. The terminal half-life is on the order of 17–18 days.

INDICATIONS
1. FDA-approved in combination with durvalumab for adult patients with unresectable hepatocellular cancer (HCC).
2. FDA-approved in combination with durvalumab and platinum-based chemotherapy for adult patients with metastatic NSCLC with no EGFR mutation or ALK-genomic tumor alteration.

DOSAGE RANGE
1. HCC: Weight >30 kg–recommended dose is 300 mg IV as a single dose in combination with durvalumab 1,500 mg at cycle 1/day 1 followed by durvalumab as a single agent every 4 weeks.
   Weight<30 kg–recommended dose is 4 mg/kg IV as a single dose in combination with durvalumab 20 mg/kg at cycle 1/day 1 followed by durvalumab as a single agent every 4 weeks.
2. NSCLC: Weight >30 kg–recommended dose is 75 mg IV every 3 weeks in combination with durvalumab 1,500 mg and platinum-based chemotherapy for 4 cycles, followed by durvalumab 1,500 mg IV as a single agent with histology-based pemetrexed therapy every 4 weeks, and a fifth dose of tremelimumab 75 mg in combination with durvalumab dose 6 at week 16.
   Weight<30 kg–recommended dose is 1 mg/kg IV every 3 weeks in combination with durvalumab 20 mg/kg and platinum-based chemotherapy for 4 cycles, followed by durvalumab 20 mg/kg IV as a single agent with histology-based pemetrexed therapy every 4 weeks, and a fifth dose of tremelimumab 1 mg/kg in combination with durvalumab dose 6 at week 16.

DRUG INTERACTIONS
None well characterized to date.

SPECIAL CONSIDERATIONS
1. Monitor patients for infusion reactions. Infusions should be interrupted, slowed, or permanently discontinued based on the severity of the reaction.
2. Tremelimumab can result in severe and fatal immune-mediated adverse reactions due to T-cell activation and proliferation. These immune-mediated reactions may involve any organ system, with the most common reactions being enterocolitis, hepatitis, dermatitis, neuropathy, and endocrinopathy. They typically occur during treatment, although some of these reactions may occur weeks to months after completion of therapy.

3. Tremelimumab should be permanently discontinued for any of the following:
   - Grade 3/4 colitis
   - Grade 3/4 pneumonitis
   - Any grade intestinal perforation
   - SGOT/SGPT >8 × ULN or total bilirubin >3 × ULN
   - Stevens-Johnson syndrome, toxic epidermal necrolysis, or rash complicated by full-thickness dermal ulceration or necrotic, bullous, or hemorrhagic manifestations
   - Grade 3/4 neurological toxicities
   - Grade 4 nephritis with renal dysfunction
4. Tremelimumab should be withheld for any moderate immune-mediated adverse reaction or for symptomatic endocrinopathy.
5. Monitor thyroid function tests at the start of treatment and before each dose.
6. Advise females of potential of increased risk to a fetus. Females of reproductive potential should use effective contraception during treatment and for 3 months after the last dose. Breastfeeding should be avoided while on therapy and for 3 months after the last dose.

TOXICITY 1
Fatigue and anorexia.

TOXICITY 2
Infusion-related reactions.

TOXICITY 3
Immune-mediated enterocolitis presenting as diarrhea, abdominal pain, fever, and ileus.

TOXICITY 4
Immune-mediated hepatotoxicity that can range from moderate to severe life-threatening hepatotoxicity.

TOXICITY 5
Immune-mediated dermatitis with rash and pruritis. Severe, life-threatening dermatitis in the form of Stevens-Johnson syndrome; toxic epidermal necrolysis; full-thickness dermal ulceration; or necrotic, bullous, or hemorrhagic skin lesions occurs rarely.

TOXICITY 6
Endocrinopathies with hypophysitis, adrenal insufficiency, hypopituitarism, hypogonadism, hyperthyroidism or hypothyroidism, and diabetes.

TOXICITY 7
Neurotoxicity with motor weakness, sensory alterations, myositis, myasthenia gravis, and Guillain-Barré–like syndromes.

TOXICITY 8
Cardiac toxicity with myocarditis, pericarditis, and vasculitis.

TOXICITY 9
Ocular toxicities in the form of uveitis, iritis, conjunctivitis, blepharitis, or episcleritis.

TOXICITY 10
Other immune-mediated adverse reactions, temporal arteritis, polymyalgia rheumatica, vasculitis, and arthritis.

Tretinoin

TRADE NAME	All-trans-retinoic acid, ATRA, Vesanoid	CLASSIFICATION	Retinoid
CATEGORY	Differentiating agent	DRUG MANUFACTURER	Roche

MECHANISM OF ACTION
- Precise mechanism of action has not been fully elucidated.
- Induces differentiation of acute promyelocytic cells to normal myelocyte cells, thereby decreasing cellular proliferation.
- Upon entry into cells, tretinoin binds to the cytoplasmic protein, cellular retinoic acid binding protein (CRABP). The retinoid CRABP complex is transported to the nucleus, where it binds to retinoid-dependent receptors known as RAR and/or RXR. This process affects the transcription and subsequent expression of various target cellular genes involved in growth, proliferation, and differentiation.
- Effects on the immune system may also contribute to antitumor activity.
- Induces apoptosis through as-yet-undetermined mechanisms.

MECHANISM OF RESISTANCE
- Alteration in drug metabolism by the liver P450 system. Tretinoin induces the activity of cytochrome P450 enzymes, which are responsible for its oxidative metabolism. Plasma concentrations decrease to about one-third of their day 1 values after 1 week of continuous therapy.
- Increased expression of CRABP, which acts to sequester tretinoin within the cell, preventing its subsequent delivery to the nucleus.

ABSORPTION

Well absorbed by the GI tract, reaching peak plasma concentration between 1 and 2 hours after oral administration.

DISTRIBUTION

Binds extensively (>95%) to plasma proteins, mainly to albumin. The apparent volume of distribution has not been determined.

METABOLISM

Undergoes oxidative metabolism by the liver cytochrome P450 system. Several metabolites have been identified, including 13-cis retinoic acid, 4-oxo trans-retinoic acid, 4-oxo cis-retinoic acid, and 4-oxo trans-retinoic acid glucuronide. Excreted in urine (63%) and in feces (31%). The terminal elimination half-life is approximately 40–120 minutes.

INDICATIONS

Acute promyelocytic leukemia (APL)—Induction of remission in patients with APL characterized by the t(15;17) translocation and/or the presence of the PML/RAR-α gene following progression and/or relapse with anthracycline-based chemotherapy or for whom anthracycline-based chemotherapy is contraindicated.

DOSAGE RANGE

Recommended dose is 45 mg/m^2/day PO divided in two daily doses for a minimum of 45 days and a maximum of 90 days.

DRUG INTERACTION 1

Drugs metabolized by liver P450 system—Tretinoin is metabolized by liver P450 enzymes. Caution should be exercised when using drugs that induce this enzyme system, such as rifampin and phenobarbital, and drugs that inhibit this system, including ketoconazole, cimetidine, erythromycin, verapamil, diltiazem, and cyclosporine.

DRUG INTERACTION 2

Vitamin A supplements—Use of vitamin A supplements may increase toxicity of tretinoin.

SPECIAL CONSIDERATIONS

1. Contraindicated in patients with known hypersensitivity to retinoids.
2. Monitor for new-onset fever, respiratory symptoms, and leukocytosis, as 25% of patients develop the retinoic acid syndrome. Tretinoin should be stopped immediately, and high-dose dexamethasone, 10 mg IV q 12 hours, should be given for 3 days or until resolution of symptoms. In most cases, therapy can be resumed once the syndrome has completely resolved. Usually occurs during the first month of treatment.
3. Use with caution in patients with pre-existing hypertriglyceridemia and in those with diabetes mellitus, obesity, and/or predisposition to excessive alcohol intake. Serum triglyceride and cholesterol levels should be closely monitored.

4. Monitor CBC, coagulation profile, and LFTs on a frequent basis during therapy.
5. Oral absorption of tretinoin may be increased when taken with food.
6. No formal recommendations for dosing in the presence of hepatic or renal impairment, as the drug has not been studied in these settings.
7. Pregnancy category D. Breastfeeding should be avoided.

TOXICITY 1

Vitamin A toxicity is nearly universal. Most common side effects are headache, usually occurring in the first week of therapy with improvement thereafter, and fever, dryness of the skin and mucous membranes, skin rash, peripheral edema, mucositis, pruritus, and conjunctivitis.

TOXICITY 2

Retinoic acid syndrome. Occurs in 25% of patients and can be dose-limiting. Characterized by fever, leukocytosis, dyspnea, weight gain, diffuse pulmonary infiltrates on chest X-ray, and pleural and/or pericardial effusions. More commonly observed with WBC >10,000/mm^3. Usually observed during the first month of therapy but may follow the initial drug dose.

TOXICITY 3

Flushing, hypotension, hypertension, phlebitis, and congestive heart failure. Cardiac ischemia, myocardial infarction, stroke, myocarditis, pericarditis, and pulmonary hypertension are rarer events, each being reported in less than 3% of patients.

TOXICITY 4

Increased serum cholesterol and triglyceride levels occur in up to 60% of patients. Usually reversible upon completion of treatment.

TOXICITY 5

CNS toxicity in the form of dizziness, anxiety, paresthesias, depression, confusion, and agitation. Hallucinations, agnosia, aphasia, slow speech, asterixis, cerebellar disorders, convulsion, coma, dysarthria, encephalopathy, facial paralysis, hemiplegia, and hyporeflexia are less often seen.

TOXICITY 6

GI toxicity. Relatively common and manifested by abdominal pain, constipation, diarrhea, and GI bleeding. Elevations in serum transaminases and alkaline phosphatase occur in 50%–60% of patients and usually resolve after completion of therapy.

TOXICITY 7

Alterations in hearing sensation with hearing loss. About 25% of patients describe earache or a fullness in the ears.

TOXICITY 8
Renal dysfunction and dysuria occur rarely.

TOXICITY 9
Pseudotumor cerebri. Benign intracranial hypertension with papilledema, headache, nausea and vomiting, and visual disturbances.

Tucatinib

TRADE NAME	Tukysa	**CLASSIFICATION**	Signal transduction inhibitor, ErB inhibitor
CATEGORY	Targeted agent	**DRUG MANUFACTURER**	Seattle Genetics

MECHANISM OF ACTION
- Potent and selective small-molecule inhibitor of the tyrosine kinase associated with HER2 (ErbB2), resulting in inhibition of ErbB tyrosine kinase phosphorylation and downstream signaling.
- Inhibition of HER2 results in inhibition of critical mitogenic and anti-apoptotic signals involved in proliferation, growth, invasion/metastasis, angiogenesis, and response to chemotherapy and/or radiation therapy.

MECHANISM OF RESISTANCE
- Gatekeeper mutation in HER2-associated tyrosine kinase, T798I, leading to reduced binding affinity to tucatinib.
- Increased activity of CYP3A4 microsomal enzymes.

ABSORPTION
Oral absorption yields peak plasma levels in about 2 hours after ingestion. Food does not affect oral absorption. Time to steady-state drug levels is 4 days.

DISTRIBUTION
Extensive binding (97.1%) to plasma proteins.

METABOLISM

Metabolism in the liver primarily by CYP2C8 microsomal enzymes and to a smaller extent by CYP3A4. Elimination is mainly hepatic, with about 86% of drug excreted in feces. Renal elimination of parent drug and its metabolites accounts for only about 4% of an administered dose. The terminal half-life of the parent drug is 8.5 hours.

INDICATIONS

1. FDA-approved in combination with trastuzumab and capecitabine for advanced unresectable or metastatic HER2-positive breast cancer, including brain metastases, following one or more prior anti-HER2-based regimens in the metastatic setting.
2. FDA-approved in combination with trastuzumab for unresectable or metastatic RAS wild-type, HER2-positive colorectal cancer that has progressed on treatment with fluoropyrimidine-, oxaliplatin-, and irinotecan-based chemotherapy.

DOSAGE RANGE

Recommended dose is 300 mg PO bid.

DRUG INTERACTION 1

Phenytoin and other drugs that stimulate the liver microsomal CYP3A4 enzymes, including carbamazepine, rifampin, phenobarbital, and St. John's Wort—These drugs may increase the rate of metabolism of tucatinib, resulting in its inactivation and lower effective drug levels.

DRUG INTERACTION 2

Drugs that inhibit the liver microsomal CYP3A4 enzymes, including ketoconazole, itraconazole, erythromycin, and clarithromycin—These drugs may decrease the rate of metabolism of tucatinib, resulting in increased drug levels and potentially increased toxicity.

DRUG INTERACTION 3

Moderate CYP2C8 inducers—These drugs may increase the rate of metabolism of tucatinib, resulting in its inactivation and lower effective drug levels.

DRUG INTERACTION 4

Strong CYP2C8 inhibitors—These drugs may reduce the rate of metabolism of tucatinib, resulting in increased drug levels and potentially increased toxicity.

SPECIAL CONSIDERATIONS

1. Dose reduction is not recommended in patients with mild or moderate hepatic impairment (Child-Pugh Class A or B). Dose should be reduced to 200 mg bid in patients with severe hepatic impairment (Child-Pugh Class C).
2. Dose reduction is not recommended in patients with mild to moderate renal impairment. Should not be used in patients with severe renal impairment as the drug has not been studied in this setting.

3. Avoid concomitant use of moderate CYP2C8 inducers and strong CYP2C8 inhibitors.

4. Closely monitor patients for diarrhea, as severe diarrhea may develop while on therapy. Anti-diarrheal prophylaxis with loperamide is recommended during the first 2 cycles of therapy and should be initiated with the first dose.

5. Important to aggressively manage diarrhea with additional anti-diarrheals, fluids, and close monitoring of electrolyte status. Therapy should be held in patients experiencing severe and/or persistent diarrhea.

6. Specific dose modifications are recommended in the setting of diarrhea. Please see package insert for specific details.

7. Specific dose modifications are in place for drug-induced hepatotoxicity. Please see package insert for specific details.

8. Avoid Seville oranges, starfruit, pomelos, and grapefruit products while on therapy.

9. Closely monitor liver function tests every 3 weeks during therapy and as clinically indicated.

10. Embryo-fetal toxicity. May cause fetal harm. Females of reproductive potential should use effective contraception during treatment and for 1 week after the last dose. Breastfeeding should be avoided while on treatment and for 1 week after the last dose.

TOXICITY 1

Diarrhea is the most common dose-limiting toxicity. Mild nausea/vomiting, abdominal pain, and dyspepsia may also occur.

TOXICITY 2

Hepatotoxicity with elevations in transaminases (SGOT, SGPT) and serum bilirubin.

TOXICITY 3

Fatigue and anorexia.

TOXICITY 4

Muscle weakness, arthralgias, and musculoskeletal symptoms.

TOXICITY 5

Maculopapular skin rash, dry skin, and pruritus.

Umbralisib

TRADE NAME	Ukoniq	**CLASSIFICATION**		Signal transduction inhibitor, PI3K and casein kinase inhibitor
CATEGORY	Targeted agent	**DRUG MANUFACTURER**		TG Therapeutics

MECHANISM OF ACTION

- First-in-class dual inhibitor of PI3K-δ and casein kinase 1ϵ (CK1ϵ).
- Expression of the PI3K-δ isoform is restricted to cells of hematopoietic origin and plays a central role in B-cell development. Expressed in normal and malignant B cells.
- Exhibits greater selectivity for PI3K-δ over the α-, β-, and γ-isoforms.
- CK1ϵ is involved in protein translation of key oncogenes, such as MYC, BCL-2, and CCND1, and in the development of lymphoid malignancies.

MECHANISM OF RESISTANCE

- Activation of alternative pathways, including MAPK, ER, HER2, AXL, PIM-1, and FOXO transcription factors.
- Signaling via other PI3K isoforms.
- Activation of downstream effectors in PI3K pathway, such as AKT and mTOR.
- Loss of PTEN expression.

ABSORPTION

Peak plasma drug levels are achieved in about 4 hours after ingestion. Food with high fat and high calorie content increases oral absorption.

DISTRIBUTION
Extensive binding (>99%) to plasma proteins. Steady-state drug levels are reached in approximately 3 days.

METABOLISM
Metabolism by CYP3A4, CYP2C9, and CYP1A2. Elimination is mainly via the hepatobiliary route, with 81% of an administered dose eliminated in feces. Renal elimination accounts for only 3% of an administered dose. Approximately 17% and <1% of an administered dose is eliminated in feces and urine, respectively, in the parent form. The terminal half-life is 91 hours.

INDICATIONS
1. FDA-approved for relapsed or refractory marginal zone lymphoma (MZL) following at least one prior anti-CD20-based regimen.
2. FDA-approved for relapsed or refractory follicular lymphoma (FL) following at least 3 prior lines of systemic therapy.
3. These two indications are under accelerated approval based on overall response rate.

DOSAGE RANGE
Recommended dose is 800 mg PO once daily with food.

DRUG INTERACTIONS
No significant drug interactions have been identified to date.

SPECIAL CONSIDERATIONS
1. Dose reduction is not required in setting of mild hepatic impairment (Child-Pugh Class A). Has not been studied in the setting of moderate or severe hepatic impairment.
2. Dose reduction is not required in setting of mild or moderate renal impairment. Has not been studied in setting of severe renal impairment, or end-stage renal disease, or in patients on dialysis.
3. Monitor for signs and symptoms of infection.
4. Monitor CBC at least every 2 weeks for the first 2 months of therapy.
5. Monitor LFTs at baseline and periodically while on therapy.
6. Patients should be educated on the signs and symptoms of skin reactions.
7. Patients should start on anti-diarrheal medication, increase oral fluid intake, and notify their physician if diarrhea should occur while on therapy.
8. Patients may experience an allergic reaction that results from the tartrazine dye in the drug capsule. Most frequently seen in patients with aspirin hypersensitivity.
9. May cause fetal harm when administered to a pregnant woman. Women of reproductive potential should use effective contraception during drug therapy and for at least 1 month after the final dose. Breastfeeding should be avoided.

TOXICITY 1
Diarrhea or non-infectious colitis.

TOXICITY 2
Myelosuppression with neutropenia, anemia, and thrombocytopenia.

TOXICITY 3
Nausea and vomiting.

TOXICITY 4
Fatigue and anorexia.

TOXICITY 5
Infections with URIs, pneumonia, and opportunistic infections, including PJP.

TOXICITY 6
Hepatotoxicity with increases in SGOT/SGPT and serum bilirubin.

TOXICITY 7
Skin reactions, including maculopapular rash, erythema, pruritus, and exfoliative rash.

TOXICITY 8
Allergic reactions occur rarely.

Vandetanib

TRADE NAME	Caprelsa	CLASSIFICATION	Signal transduction inhibitor, TKI
CATEGORY	Targeted agent	DRUG MANUFACTURER	AstraZeneca

MECHANISM OF ACTION
- Small molecule inhibitor of tyrosine kinases associated with the EGFR family, VEGFR, rearranged during transfection (RET), protein tyrosine kinase 6 (BRK), Tie-2, EPH receptors, and Src family members.
- Inhibition of these receptor tyrosine kinases results in inhibition of critical signaling pathways involved in proliferation, growth, invasion/metastasis, and angiogenesis.

MECHANISM OF RESISTANCE
- Increased expression of target receptor tyrosine kinases (RTKs), such as EGFR and VEGFR.
- Alterations in binding affinity of the drug to RTKs resulting from mutations in the tyrosine kinase domain (e.g., EGFR T790M mutation).
- Activation/induction of alternative cellular signaling pathways, such as IGF-1R and c-Met.

ABSORPTION
Oral absorption is slow, with peak plasma concentrations achieved at a median of 6 hours, and is unaffected by food.

DISTRIBUTION
Binds to human serum albumin and α1-acid glycoprotein on the order of 90%. With daily dosing, steady-state blood levels are achieved in about 28 days.

METABOLISM
Following oral administration, parent vandetanib and metabolites, including N-oxide vandetanib and N-desmethyl vandetanib, are detected in plasma, urine, and feces. A glucuronide conjugate is observed as a minor metabolite. N-desmethyl vandetanib is primarily produced by CYP3A4 and vandetanib N-oxide by flavin-containing monooxygenase enzymes FMO1 and FMO3.

Approximately 70% is recovered, with 45% in feces and 25% in urine. The terminal half-life is prolonged on the order of >100 hours.

INDICATIONS
FDA-approved for symptomatic or progressive medullary thyroid cancer with unresectable locally advanced or metastatic disease.

DOSAGE RANGE
Recommended dose is 300 mg PO daily and may be taken with or without food.

DRUG INTERACTIONS
1. Drugs that stimulate liver microsomal CYP3A4 enzymes, including phenytoin, carbamazepine, rifampin, phenobarbital, and St. John's Wort—These drugs may increase vandetanib metabolism, resulting in its inactivation and lower effective drug levels.
2. Drugs that inhibit liver microsomal CYP3A4 enzymes, including ketoconazole, itraconazole, erythromycin, and clarithromycin—These drugs may reduce vandetanib metabolism, resulting in increased drug levels and potentially increased toxicity.
3. Drugs that are associated with QT prolongation—Certain phenothiazines (chlorpromazine, mesoridazine, and thioridazine), antiarrhythmic drugs (including, but not limited to, amiodarone, disopyramide, procainamide, sotalol, dofetilide, quinidine) and other drugs that may prolong the QT interval (including but not limited to chloroquine, clarithromycin, erythromycin, dolasetron, granisetron, haloperidol, methadone, moxifloxacin, and pimozide), pentamidine, posaconazole, saquinavir, sparfloxacin, terfenadine, and troleandomycin.

SPECIAL CONSIDERATIONS
1. Vandetanib is only available through a restricted distribution program. This program is designed to inform healthcare providers about the potential serious risks of QT prolongation, Torsades de Pointes, and sudden death from vandetanib.
2. Contraindicated in patients with the congenital long QT syndrome.
3. Closely monitor ECG with QTc measurements at baseline and periodically during therapy, as QTc prolongation has been observed. Use with caution in patients with CHF, bradyarrhythmias, concomitant use of drugs that prolong QT interval, and electrolyte abnormalities (hypokalemia and hypomagnesemia). This represents a black-box warning.
4. In the event of corrected QTc (QTc) interval >500 msec, vandetanib needs to be held until QTc returns to <450 msec, at which time a reduced dose should be administered.
5. Not recommended for patients with moderate (Child-Pugh Class B) or severe (Child-Pugh Class C) hepatic impairment.
6. Use with caution in patients with moderate or severe (CrCl <30 mL/min) renal impairment, and in this setting, the starting dose should be reduced to 200 mg.
7. Vandetanib tablets should not be crushed. When vandetanib tablets cannot be taken whole, they can be dispensed in a glass containing

2 ounces of non-carbonated water and stirred for approximately 10 minutes until the tablet is dispersed.

8. Closely monitor thyroid function tests, as increases in the dose of thyroid replacement therapy may be required while on vandetanib. Thyroid-stimulating hormone (TSH) levels should be obtained at baseline, at 2–4 weeks and 8–12 weeks after starting treatment, and every 3 months thereafter.

9. Closely monitor BP while on therapy. Use with caution in patients with uncontrolled hypertension. Should be discontinued in patients who develop hypertensive crisis. Blood pressure is usually well controlled with oral antihypertensive medication.

10. Patients with recent history of hemoptysis of ≥½ teaspoon of red blood should not receive vandetanib. Discontinue vandetanib in patients who develop severe hemorrhage.

11. Vandetanib treatment can result in RPLS, as manifested by headache, seizure, lethargy, confusion, blindness, and other visual side effects, as well as other neurologic disturbances. Brain MRI is helpful in confirming the diagnosis.

12. Pregnancy category D. Breastfeeding should be avoided.

TOXICITY 1
Mild to moderate skin reactions with rash, acne, dry skin, dermatitis, pruritis, and other skin reactions (including photosensitivity reactions and palmar-plantar erythrodysesthesia syndrome). Rare cases of severe skin reactions (including Stevens-Johnson syndrome) resulting in deaths have been reported.

TOXICITY 2
Diarrhea and nausea/vomiting.

TOXICITY 3
Fatigue.

TOXICITY 4
Hypertension. In rare cases, heart failure has been observed.

TOXICITY 5
Bleeding complications.

TOXICITY 6
QT prolongation and Torsades de Pointes.

TOXICITY 7
ILD or pneumonitis.

TOXICITY 8
RPLS with seizures, headache, visual disturbances, confusion, or altered mental function.

Vemurafenib

TRADE NAME	Zelboraf, PLX4032	**CLASSIFICATION**	Signal transduction inhibitor, BRAF inhibitor
CATEGORY	Targeted agent	**DRUG MANUFACTURER**	Genentech-Roche

MECHANISM OF ACTION
- Inhibits mutant forms of BRAF serine-threonine kinase, including BRAF-V600E, which results in constitutive activation of MAPK signaling.
- Does not inhibit wild-type BRAF or other Raf kinases, including ARAF and CRAF.

MECHANISM OF RESISTANCE
- Presence of NRAS mutations.
- Presence of MEK1 and MEK2 mutations, leading to increased expression of MAPK signaling.
- Mutations in MAP2K1, which encodes the MEK1 kinase, and MAP2K2 gene, which encodes the MEK2 kinase. These mutations lead to activation of MAPK signaling downstream of RAF.
- Activation/induction of alternative cellular signaling pathways, such as c-Met, FGFR, EGFR, and PI3K/Akt.
- Reactivation of Ras/Raf signaling via mutations in KRAS, NRAS, and BRAF.
- Increased expression of BRAF through gene amplification.
- Loss of tumor suppressor genes stromal antigen 2 (STAG2) and STAG3.

ABSORPTION
Oral bioavailability is on the order of 58%. Food with high fat content increases systemic exposure to drug without altering the mean terminal half-life.

DISTRIBUTION
Extensive binding (>99%) of vemurafenib to plasma proteins. Steady-state drug levels are reached in 15–22 days following initiation of therapy.

METABOLISM
Metabolized in the liver primarily by CYP3A4 microsomal enzymes to produce its primary active metabolite, which is further metabolized by CYP3A4. Elimination is via the hepatobiliary route with excretion in feces (~94%). Renal elimination is minor accounting for only approximately 1% of an administered dose. The terminal half-life of vemurafenib is approximately 57 hours.

INDICATIONS
1. FDA-approved for unresectable or metastatic melanoma with BRAF-V600E mutation as determined by an FDA-approved test.
2. Not recommended for wild-type BRAF melanoma.
3. FDA-approved for Erdheim-Chester disease (ECD) with BRAF-V600 mutation.

DOSAGE RANGE
Recommended dose is 960 mg PO bid.

DRUG INTERACTION 1
Drugs such as ketoconazole, itraconazole, erythromycin, clarithromycin, atazanavir, indinavir, nefazodone, nelfinavir, ritonavir, saquinavir, telithromycin, and voriconazole may decrease the rate of metabolism of vemurafenib, resulting in increased drug levels and potentially increased toxicity.

DRUG INTERACTION 2
Drugs such as rifampin, phenytoin, phenobarbital, carbamazepine, and St. John's Wort may increase the rate of metabolism of vemurafenib, resulting in its inactivation and lower effective drug levels.

SPECIAL CONSIDERATIONS
1. Baseline and periodic evaluations of ECG and electrolyte status should be performed while on therapy. ECGs should be done at day 15, monthly during the first 3 months of therapy, and every 3 months thereafter. If the QTc >500 msec, therapy should be interrupted. Use with caution in patients at risk of developing QT prolongation, including hypokalemia, hypomagnesemia, and congenital long QT syndrome, and in patients taking antiarrhythmic medications or any other drugs that may cause QT prolongation.
2. Closely monitor LFTs and serum bilirubin.
3. Careful skin exams should be done at baseline and every 2 months while on therapy, given the increased incidence of cutaneous squamous cell cancers.

4. Monitor for severe dermatologic reactions, such as Stevens-Johnson syndrome and toxic epidermal necrolysis. Therapy should be terminated in patients who experience these skin reactions.
5. Patients should be cautioned to avoid sun exposure while on therapy.
6. Monitor patients for eye reactions, including uveitis, iritis, and retinal vein occlusion.
7. BRAF testing using an FDA-approved test to confirm the presence of the BRAF-V600E mutation is required for determining which patients should receive vemurafenib therapy.
8. No dose adjustment is needed for patients with mild or moderate hepatic and/or renal dysfunction. However, caution should be used in patients with severe hepatic and/or renal dysfunction.
9. Pregnancy category D. Breastfeeding should be avoided.

TOXICITY 1
Cutaneous squamous cell cancers and keratoacanthomas occur in up to 25% of patients. Usually occur within 7–8 weeks of starting therapy.

TOXICITY 2
Skin reactions, including Stevens-Johnson syndrome and toxic epidermal necrolysis, have been reported.

TOXICITY 3
Cardiac toxicity with QTc prolongation.

TOXICITY 4
Elevations in serum bilirubin and SGOT/SGPT.

TOXICITY 5
Photosensitivity.

TOXICITY 6
Ophthalmologic side effects, including uveitis, iritis, photophobia, and retinal vein occlusion.

TOXICITY 7
Fatigue.

Venetoclax

TRADE NAME	Venclexta	CLASSIFICATION	Signal transduction inhibitor, BCL-2 inhibitor
CATEGORY	Targeted agent	DRUG MANUFACTURER	AbbVie, Genentech/ Roche

MECHANISM OF ACTION
- Selective small-molecule inhibitor of BCL-2, an important anti-apoptotic protein.
- Activity in tumor cells that overexpress BCL-2, such as CLL.
- Restores the process of apoptosis by binding directly to the BCL-2 protein, displacing pro-apoptotic proteins, such as BIM, which then triggers mitochondrial outer membrane permeabilization and subsequent activation of caspases.

MECHANISM OF RESISTANCE
- Increased expression of MCL1 and BCL-X_L.
- Mutations in the BCL2 gene with Phe104Ile and Gly101Val as two common resistant mutations with reduced binding affinity to the drug.
- Mutations in CREBBP, KMT2C/D, and EZH2.
- Mutations in IDH1 and FLT3.
- Mutations in SMARCA4.
- Increased degradation and/or metabolism of drug.

ABSORPTION
Rapidly absorbed after an oral dose, with peak plasma levels achieved within 5–8 hours. Oral bioavailability on the order of 40%–60%. Food with a high fat content reduces oral bioavailability by up to 15%.

DISTRIBUTION
Highly bound (>99%) to plasma proteins. Steady-state drug concentrations are reached in 15 days.

METABOLISM
Metabolized in the liver primarily by CYP3A4 and CYP3A5 microsomal enzymes. The major metabolite is M27, which also has BCL-2 inhibitory activity. Elimination is hepatic, with excretion in feces (>99.9%), with renal elimination only accounting for <0.1% of an administered dose. Unchanged parent drug represents approximately 21% of an administered dose in feces. The terminal half-life of venetoclax is approximately 26 hours.

INDICATIONS
1. FDA-approved for CLL or small lymphocytic lymphoma (SLL).
2. FDA-approved in combination with azacitidine, decitabine, or low-dose cytarabine for newly diagnosed AML in adults who are >75 years of age or who have comorbidities that preclude use of intensive induction chemotherapy.

DOSAGE RANGE
1. CLL/SLL: Initial therapy starting at 20 mg PO once daily for 7 days following by a weekly ramp-up schedule over 5 weeks to the final recommended dose of 400 mg PO once daily.
2. AML: On day 1, start at 100 mg, increase to 200 mg on day 2, and then to 400 mg on day 3. On day 4, use 400 mg in combination with azacitidine or decitabine and 600 mg in combination with low-dose cytarabine.

DRUG INTERACTION 1
Drugs such as ketoconazole, itraconazole, erythromycin, clarithromycin, atazanavir, indinavir, nefazodone, nelfinavir, ritonavir, saquinavir, telithromycin, and voriconazole may decrease the rate of metabolism of venetoclax, resulting in increased drug levels and potentially increased toxicity. The dose of venetoclax should be reduced by at least 50% if a moderate CYP3A4 inhibitor is used.

DRUG INTERACTION 2
Drugs such as rifampin, phenytoin, phenobarbital, carbamazepine, and St. John's Wort may increase the rate of metabolism of venetoclax, resulting in its inactivation and lower effective drug levels.

DRUG INTERACTION 3
Drugs such as amiodarone, azithromycin, captopril, carvedilol, cyclosporine, felodipine, quinidine, ranolazine, and ticagrelor, which are P-glycoprotein inhibitors, may decrease the rate of metabolism of venetoclax, resulting in increased drug levels and potentially increased toxicity. The dose of venetoclax should be reduced by at least 50% if a P-glycoprotein inhibitor is used.

DRUG INTERACTION 4
Warfarin—Patients receiving warfarin should be closely monitored for alterations in their clotting parameters (PT and INR) and/or bleeding, as venetoclax may inhibit the metabolism of warfarin by the liver P450 system. Dose of warfarin may require careful adjustment in the presence of venetoclax therapy.

SPECIAL CONSIDERATIONS
1. Use with caution in patients with hepatic dysfunction. Dose reduction is not recommended in patients with mild or moderate hepatic dysfunction, although there may be an increased risk of toxicity in patients with moderate hepatic dysfunction. Has not been studied in severe hepatic dysfunction.
2. Dose reduction is not recommended for patients with mild or moderate renal dysfunction. Has not been studied in patients with severe renal dysfunction or in those on dialysis.
3. Closely monitor CBC, and consider using growth factors to support neutrophil count.
4. All patients should be closely monitored for the possibility of tumor lysis syndrome (TLS), with an increased risk in patients with high tumor burden and/or high peripheral white blood cell count. TLS can occur within 6–8 hours following the first dose of venetoclax. Patients with reduced renal function (CrCl <80 mL/min) should be monitored more frequently and require more intense prophylaxis to reduce the risk of TLS.
5. Closely monitor serum chemistries, such as potassium, phosphate, BUN/creatinine, and uric acid, for evidence of tumor lysis syndrome.
6. Patients receiving venetoclax along with oral warfarin anticoagulant therapy should have their coagulation parameters (PT and INR) monitored frequently, as elevations in INR and bleeding events have been observed.
7. Oral bioavailability is not affected by gastric acid–reducing agents, such as proton pump inhibitors, H2-receptor antagonists, and antacids.
8. Venetoclax tablets should be taken with a meal and water and swallowed whole and not chewed, crushed, or broken prior to ingestion.
9. CLL patients without a 17p deletion at the initial time of diagnosis should be re-tested at the time of disease relapse, as acquisition of 17p deletion may occur.
10. Avoid Seville oranges, starfruit, pomelos, grapefruit, and grapefruit juice while on venetoclax therapy.
11. Live attenuated vaccines should not be administered prior to, during, or after venetoclax therapy.
12. Pregnancy category D. Breastfeeding should be avoided.

TOXICITY 1
Tumor lysis syndrome, especially in the setting of high tumor burden and high peripheral white blood cell count.

TOXICITY 2
Myelosuppression with neutropenia, anemia, and thrombocytopenia.

TOXICITY 3
GI toxicity with diarrhea, nausea/vomiting, abdominal pain, and reduced appetite.

TOXICITY 4
Fatigue, asthenia, and anorexia.

TOXICITY 5
Pulmonary toxicity with cough, URI, sinusitis, and dyspnea.

TOXICITY 6
Infections, including pneumonia, herpes simplex, urinary tract infections, viral infections, and influenza-like illness.

Vinblastine

TRADE NAME	Velban, VBL	CLASSIFICATION	Vinca alkaloid, anti-microtubule agent
CATEGORY	Chemotherapy drug	DRUG MANUFACTURER	Eli Lilly

MECHANISM OF ACTION
- Plant alkaloid extracted from the periwinkle plant *Catharanthus roseus*.
- Cell cycle–specific with activity in the mitosis (M) phase.
- Inhibits tubulin polymerization, disrupting formation of microtubule assembly during mitosis. This results in an arrest in cell division, ultimately leading to cell death.
- May also inhibit DNA, RNA, and protein synthesis.

MECHANISM OF RESISTANCE
- Overexpression of the P170 glycoprotein encoded by the multidrug-resistant gene, resulting in enhanced efflux of drug and decreased intracellular drug accumulation. Cross-resistance may be observed with other natural products, such as taxanes, epipodophyllotoxins, anthracyclines, and actinomycin-D.
- Mutations in α- and β-tubulin proteins, with decreased binding affinity to vinblastine.

ABSORPTION
Administered only via the IV route.

DISTRIBUTION
Widely and rapidly distributed into most body tissues. Binds extensively to platelets, RBCs, and WBCs within 30 minutes of administration. Poor penetration into the CSF.

METABOLISM
Metabolized in the liver by the cytochrome P450 microsomal system. Small quantities of at least one metabolite, desacetyl vinblastine, may be as active as the parent drug. Majority of vinblastine is excreted in metabolite form via the hepatobiliary system. Only about 10% of the parent drug is excreted in feces. Approximately 14% of the drug is eliminated by the kidneys. Plasma terminal half-life of about 25 hours.

INDICATIONS
1. Hodgkin's and non-Hodgkin's lymphoma.
2. Testicular cancer.
3. Breast cancer.
4. Kaposi's sarcoma.
5. Renal cell carcinoma.

DOSAGE RANGE
1. Hodgkin's lymphoma: 6 mg/m^2 IV on days 1 and 15, as part of the ABVD regimen.
2. Testicular cancer: 0.15 mg/kg IV on days 1 and 2, as part of the PVB regimen.

DRUG INTERACTION 1
Drugs metabolized by liver P450 system—Vinblastine should be used cautiously in patients receiving medications that inhibit drug metabolism via the hepatic cytochrome P450 system, including calcium channel blockers, cimetidine, cyclosporine, erythromycin, metoclopramide, and ketoconazole.

DRUG INTERACTION 2
Phenytoin—Vinblastine reduces blood levels of phenytoin through either reduced absorption of phenytoin or an increase in the rate of its metabolism and elimination.

DRUG INTERACTION 3
Bleomycin—Risk of Raynaud's syndrome may be increased with the combination of vinblastine and bleomycin.

SPECIAL CONSIDERATIONS
1. Use with caution in patients with abnormal liver function, as toxicity of vinblastine may be significantly enhanced. Dose reduction is recommended in this setting.

2. Vinblastine should be infused as a rapid push in a free-flowing IV line to avoid extravasation. If extravasation occurs, the infusion should be discontinued immediately. Flushing with sterile water, elevation of the involved extremity, and local application of ice are recommended. In severe cases, a plastic surgeon should be consulted.
3. Patients should be warned about the risk of constipation upon starting therapy, and a bowel regimen including a high-fiber diet and a stool softener should be initiated.
4. Observe for hypersensitivity reactions, especially when the drug is administered in association with mitomycin-C.
5. Contamination of the eye may lead to severe irritation and even corneal ulceration. If accidental contamination occurs, the eyes should be immediately and thoroughly washed.
6. Pregnancy category D. Breastfeeding should be avoided.

TOXICITY 1
Myelosuppression is dose-limiting, with neutropenia being most commonly observed. Thrombocytopenia and anemia are less common.

TOXICITY 2
GI side effects with mucositis and nausea/vomiting.

TOXICITY 3
Alopecia is common, usually mild, and reversible.

TOXICITY 4
Hypertension is most common cardiovascular side effect. Occurs as a consequence of autonomic dysfunction.

TOXICITY 5
Neurotoxicity occurs much less frequently than with vincristine. Presents with the same manifestations as seen with vincristine: peripheral neuropathy and autonomic nervous system dysfunction (orthostatic hypotension, paralytic ileus, and urinary retention). Cranial nerve paralysis, ataxia, cortical blindness, seizures, and coma may occur but less commonly.

TOXICITY 6
Vesicant. Extravasation may cause local skin damage.

TOXICITY 7
Syndrome of inappropriate antidiuretic hormone secretion (SIADH).

TOXICITY 8
Headache and depression.

TOXICITY 9
Vascular events, such as stroke, MI, and Raynaud's syndrome.

V

Vincristine

TRADE NAME	Oncovin, VCR	CLASSIFICATION	Vinca alkaloid, anti-microtubule agent
CATEGORY	Chemotherapy drug	DRUG MANUFACTURER	Eli Lilly

MECHANISM OF ACTION

- Plant alkaloid derived from the periwinkle plant *Catharanthus roseus*.
- Cell cycle specific with activity in the mitosis (M) phase.
- Inhibits tubulin polymerization, disrupting formation of microtubule assembly during mitosis. This results in an arrest in cell division, ultimately leading to cell death.
- May also inhibit DNA, RNA, and protein synthesis.

MECHANISM OF RESISTANCE

- Overexpression of the P170 glycoprotein encoded by the multidrug-resistant gene, resulting in enhanced efflux of drug and decreased intracellular drug accumulation. Cross-resistance may be observed with other natural products, such as taxanes, epipodophyllotoxins, anthracyclines, and actinomycin-D.
- Mutations in α- and β-tubulin proteins, with decreased affinity to vincristine.

ABSORPTION

Administered only via the IV route.

DISTRIBUTION

Widely and rapidly distributed into body tissues within 30 minutes of administration. Poor penetration across the blood-brain barrier and into the CSF.

METABOLISM

Metabolized in the liver by the cytochrome P450 microsomal system. The majority of vincristine (80%) is excreted via the hepatobiliary route in bile and feces. Only 15%–20% of the drug is recovered in urine. Terminal half-life is long, on the order of 85 hours.

INDICATIONS

1. Acute lymphoblastic leukemia.
2. Hodgkin's and non-Hodgkin's lymphoma.
3. Multiple myeloma.
4. Rhabdomyosarcoma.
5. Neuroblastoma.
6. Ewing's sarcoma.
7. Wilms' tumor.
8. Chronic leukemias.
9. Thyroid cancer.
10. Brain tumors.
11. Trophoblastic neoplasms.

DOSAGE RANGE

1. Doses usually vary between 0.5 and 1.4 mg/m^2. The total individual dose should be capped at 2 mg to prevent the development of neurotoxicity.
2. Continuous infusion: 0.4 mg/day IV continuous infusion for 4 days, as part of the VAD regimen for multiple myeloma.

DRUG INTERACTION 1

Drugs metabolized by liver P450 system—Vincristine should be used with caution in patients receiving medications that inhibit drug metabolism via the hepatic cytochrome P450 system.

DRUG INTERACTION 2

Phenytoin—Vincristine reduces the blood levels of phenytoin and its subsequent efficacy through either reduced absorption of phenytoin or an increase in the rate of its metabolism and/or elimination.

DRUG INTERACTION 3

Digoxin—Vincristine reduces the blood levels of digoxin, resulting in decreased efficacy.

DRUG INTERACTION 4

Cisplatin and paclitaxel—Concurrent administration of vincristine with other neurotoxic agents such as cisplatin and paclitaxel may increase the risk and severity of neurotoxicity.

DRUG INTERACTION 5

L-asparaginase—When used in combination with L-asparaginase, vincristine should be administered 12–24 hours before, as L-asparaginase inhibits vincristine clearance.

DRUG INTERACTION 6

Methotrexate—Vincristine increases the cellular uptake of methotrexate, resulting in enhanced antitumor activity and toxicity.

DRUG INTERACTION 7

Filgrastim—Concurrent use of vincristine with filgrastim may result in severe atypical neuropathy.

SPECIAL CONSIDERATIONS

1. Use with caution in patients with abnormal liver function, as increased toxicity may be observed. Dose reduction is recommended in this setting.
2. Vincristine should be infused as a rapid push over 1 minute in a side port of a free-flowing IV line to avoid extravasation. If extravasation occurs, the infusion should be discontinued immediately. Application of ice to the area of leakage along with elevation of involved extremity may minimize discomfort and the possibility of cellulitis. In severe cases, a plastic surgeon should be consulted.
3. Contamination of the eye may lead to severe irritation and even corneal ulceration. If accidental contamination occurs, the eye should be washed immediately and thoroughly.
4. Patients should be warned about the risk of constipation upon starting therapy, and a bowel regimen including stool softeners and high-fiber diet should be initiated. Patients should be advised to seek medical attention if persistent nausea, vomiting, and abdominal pain develop after beginning therapy.
5. Careful baseline neurologic evaluation should be performed before starting therapy and at the start of each cycle. The onset of severe signs and/or symptoms of neurotoxicity warrants immediate discontinuation of the drug. Avoid the simultaneous use of drugs associated with neurologic toxicity. Risk factors for neurotoxicity include elderly patients and those with pre-existing neuropathies and/or neuromuscular disorders.
6. Pregnancy category D. Breastfeeding should be avoided.

TOXICITY 1

Neurotoxicity is most common dose-limiting toxicity. Clinical manifestations include peripheral neuropathy (paresthesias, paralysis, and loss of deep tendon reflexes), autonomic nervous system dysfunction (orthostasis, sphincter problems, and paralytic ileus), cranial nerve palsies, ataxia, cortical blindness, seizures, and coma. Bone, back, limb, jaw, and parotid gland pain may also occur.

TOXICITY 2
GI side effects with nausea/vomiting, constipation, and abdominal pain. Paralytic ileus and abdominal obstruction occur rarely.

TOXICITY 3
Alopecia, skin rash, and fever.

TOXICITY 4
Vesicant. Extravasation may cause local tissue injury, inflammation, and necrosis.

TOXICITY 5
Myelosuppression. Generally mild and much less significant than with vinblastine.

TOXICITY 6
SIADH.

TOXICITY 7
Hypersensitivity reactions.

Vinorelbine

TRADE NAME	Navelbine, NVB	**CLASSIFICATION**	Vinca alkaloid, anti-microtubule agent
CATEGORY	Chemotherapy drug	**DRUG MANUFACTURER**	Sagent

MECHANISM OF ACTION
- Semisynthetic alkaloid derived from vinblastine.
- Cell cycle specific with activity in mitosis (M) phase.

- Inhibits tubulin polymerization, disrupting formation of microtubule assembly during mitosis. This results in an arrest in cell division, ultimately leading to cell death.
- Relatively high specificity for mitotic microtubules, with lower affinity for axonal microtubules.
- May also inhibit DNA, RNA, and protein synthesis.

MECHANISM OF RESISTANCE

- Overexpression of the P170 glycoprotein encoded by the multidrug-resistant gene, resulting in enhanced efflux of drug and decreased intracellular drug accumulation. Cross-resistance may be observed with other natural products, such as taxanes, epipodophyllotoxins, anthracyclines, and actinomycin-D.
- Mutations in α- and β-tubulin proteins, with decreased binding affinity to vinorelbine.

ABSORPTION

Administered only via the IV route.

DISTRIBUTION

Widely and rapidly distributed into most body tissues, with a large apparent volume of distribution (>30 L/kg). Extensive binding to plasma proteins (about 80%).

METABOLISM

Metabolized in the liver by the cytochrome P450 microsomal system. Small quantities of at least one metabolite, desacetyl vinorelbine, have antitumor activity similar to that of parent drug. Majority of vinorelbine excreted in feces via the hepatobiliary system (50%). About 15%–20% of the drug is eliminated by the kidneys. Prolonged terminal half-life of 27–43 hours secondary to relatively slow efflux of drug from peripheral tissues.

INDICATIONS

1. NSCLC.
2. Breast cancer.
3. Ovarian cancer.

DOSAGE RANGE

Recommended dose is 30 mg/m^2 IV on a weekly schedule either as a single agent or in combination with cisplatin.

DRUG INTERACTION 1

Drugs metabolized by the liver P450 system—Vinorelbine should be used cautiously in patients receiving medications that inhibit drug metabolism via the hepatic cytochrome P450 system.

DRUG INTERACTION 2

Phenytoin—Vinorelbine reduces blood levels of phenytoin through either reduced absorption of phenytoin or an increase in the rate of its metabolism and elimination.

DRUG INTERACTION 3

Cisplatin—Risk of myelosuppression increases when vinorelbine is used in combination with cisplatin.

DRUG INTERACTION 4

Mitomycin-C—Increased risk of acute allergic reactions when vinorelbine is used in combination with mitomycin-C.

SPECIAL CONSIDERATIONS

1. Use with caution in patients with abnormal liver function, as toxicity of vinorelbine may be enhanced. Dose reduction is recommended in this setting.
2. Use with caution in patients previously treated with chemotherapy and/or radiation therapy, as their bone marrow reserve may be compromised.
3. Vinorelbine should be infused as a rapid push in a free-flowing IV line to avoid extravasation. If extravasation occurs, the infusion should be discontinued immediately. Flushing with sterile water, elevation of the extremity, and local application of ice are recommended. In severe cases, a plastic surgeon should be consulted.
4. Contamination of the eye may lead to severe irritation and even corneal ulceration. If accidental contamination occurs, the eye should be immediately and thoroughly washed.
5. Pregnancy category D. Breastfeeding should be avoided.

TOXICITY 1

Myelosuppression is dose-limiting, and neutropenia is most commonly observed. Nadirs occur by day 7, with recovery by day 14. Thrombocytopenia and anemia are less common.

TOXICITY 2

Nausea and vomiting. Usually moderate and occur within first 24 hours after treatment.

TOXICITY 3

GI toxicities in the form of constipation (35%), diarrhea (17%), stomatitis (<20%), and anorexia (<20%).

TOXICITY 4

Transient elevation in LFTs, including SGOT and bilirubin. Usually clinically asymptomatic.

TOXICITY 5
Vesicant. Extravasation may cause local tissue injury and inflammation.

TOXICITY 6
Neurotoxicity occurs much less frequently than with other vinca alkaloids. Vinorelbine has lower affinity for axonal microtubules than observed with vincristine or vinblastine. Increased risk in patients with pre-existing neuromuscular disease.

TOXICITY 7
Alopecia observed in 10%–15% of patients.

TOXICITY 8
SIADH.

TOXICITY 9
Hypersensitivity and/or allergic reactions presenting as dyspnea and bronchospasm. Incidence is increased when used in combination with mitomycin-C.

TOXICITY 10
Generalized fatigue occurs in 35% of patients, and incidence increases with cumulative doses.

Vismodegib

TRADE NAME	Erivedge	CLASSIFICATION	Signal transduction inhibitor, hedgehog inhibitor
CATEGORY	Targeted agent	DRUG MANUFACTURER	Genentech-Roche

MECHANISM OF ACTION
- Small molecule inhibitor of the hedgehog signaling pathway.
- Binds to and inhibits smoothened, a transmembrane protein that is involved in hedgehog signaling.

MECHANISM OF RESISTANCE
- Increased expression of MAPK signaling.
- Activation/induction of alternative cellular signaling pathways, such as c-Met, FGFR, EGFR, and PI3K/Akt.
- Reactivation of Ras/Raf signaling via mutations in KRAS, NRAS, and BRAF.

ABSORPTION
Oral bioavailability is approximately 32%. Food does not affect oral absorption.

DISTRIBUTION
Extensive binding (>99%) of vismodegib to plasma proteins, including albumin and α1-acid glycoprotein.

METABOLISM
Mainly excreted as unchanged drug. Several minor metabolites are produced in the liver, primarily by CYP3A4, CYP3A5, and CYP2C9 microsomal enzymes. Elimination is via the hepatobiliary route, with excretion in feces (82%), with renal elimination accounting for only 4.4% of an administered dose. The elimination half-life of vismodegib is approximately 4 days.

INDICATIONS
FDA-approved for metastatic basal cell cancer or locally advanced basal cell cancer that has recurred following surgery, or in patients who are not candidates for surgery and/or radiation.

DOSAGE RANGE
Recommended dose is 150 mg PO on a daily basis.

DRUG INTERACTION 1
Proton pump inhibitors, H2-receptor inhibitors, and antacids—Drugs that alter the pH of the upper GI tract may alter vismodegib solubility, thereby reducing drug bioavailability and decreasing systemic drug exposure.

DRUG INTERACTION 2
P-glycoprotein inhibitors (clarithromycin, erythromycin, azithromycin)—Drugs that inhibit P-glycoprotein may increase systemic exposure of vismodegib, resulting in increased toxicity, as vismodegib is a substrate of the P-glycoprotein efflux transport protein.

SPECIAL CONSIDERATIONS
1. Vismodegib may be taken with or without food. Capsules should not be opened or crushed and should be swallowed whole.

2. Safety and efficacy of vismodegib have not been studied in patients with hepatic and/or renal impairment.

3. Patients should be advised not to donate blood or blood products while on vismodegib and for at least 7 months after the last drug dose.

4. The pregnancy status of female patients must be verified prior to the start of vismodegib therapy given the risk of embryo-fetal death and/or severe birth defects. This is a black-box warning.

5. Female and male patients of reproductive potential should be counseled on pregnancy prevention and planning. Female patients should be advised on the need for contraception, while males should be advised of the potential risk of drug exposure through semen. Women who have been exposed to vismodegib during pregnancy, either directly or through seminal fluid, should participate in the pregnancy pharmacovigilance program by contacting the Genentech Adverse Event Line at (888-835-2555).

6. Avoid drugs that alter the pH of the upper GI tract, such as proton pump inhibitors, H2-receptor inhibitors, and antacids, while on vismodegib therapy.

7. Dose reduction is not recommended in the setting of hepatic impairment.

8. Dose reduction is not recommended in the setting of renal impairment.

9. May cause fetal harm. Women of reproductive potential should use effective contraception during therapy and for 24 months after the final dose. Breastfeeding is not recommended while on therapy and for 24 months after the last dose.

TOXICITY 1
Embryo-fetal deaths and/or severe birth defects. This is a black-box warning.

TOXICITY 2
Muscle spasms and arthralgias.

TOXICITY 3
Decreased appetite, fatigue, and weight loss.

TOXICITY 4
Change in taste and/or loss of taste.

TOXICITY 5
Alopecia.

TOXICITY 6
Nausea/vomiting, constipation, and diarrhea.

Vorinostat

TRADE NAME	Zolinza	CLASSIFICATION	Histone deacetylase (HDAC) inhibitor
CATEGORY	Chemotherapy drug	DRUG MANUFACTURER	Merck

MECHANISM OF ACTION
- Potent inhibitor of histone deacetylases HDAC1, HDAC2, HDAC3 (Class I), and HDAC6 (Class II).
- Inhibition of HDAC activity leads to accumulation of acetyl groups on the histone lysine residues, resulting in open chromatin structure and transcriptional activation. Induction of cell cycle arrest and/or apoptosis may then occur.
- The precise mechanism(s) by which vorinostat exerts its antitumor activity has not been fully characterized.

MECHANISM OF RESISTANCE
- Increased expression of target HDACs.
- Mutations in the target HDACs, leading to reduced binding affinity to drug.
- Increased expression/activity of the IGF2/IGF-1R signaling pathway.
- Increased activation of MAPK signaling.
- Reduced expression of the pro-apoptotic protein Bim.

ABSORPTION
Oral bioavailability of 43%. Absorption is not significantly affected with food.

DISTRIBUTION
Significant binding (75%) to plasma proteins and extensive tissue distribution. Peak plasma levels are achieved 4 hours after ingestion.

METABOLISM
Metabolism involves glucuronidation and hydrolysis followed by β-oxidation. In vitro studies suggest minimal biotransformation by the cytochrome P450 system. Elimination is mainly via metabolism, and renal elimination of parent drug accounts for <1% of an administered dose. The terminal half-life of the parent drug is 2 hours.

INDICATIONS
FDA-approved for patients with CTCL who have progressive, persistent, or recurrent disease on or after two systemic therapies.

DOSAGE RANGE
Recommended dose is 400 mg PO daily.

DRUG INTERACTION 1
Warfarin—Patients receiving warfarin should be closely monitored for alterations in their clotting parameters (PT and INR) and/or bleeding, as prolongation of PT and INR has been observed with concomitant use of vorinostat. The dose of warfarin may require careful adjustment in the presence of vorinostat therapy.

DRUG INTERACTION 2
HDAC inhibitors—Severe thrombocytopenia and GI bleeding have been reported when vorinostat and other HDAC inhibitors, such as valproic acid, are used together. CBC and platelet counts should be monitored every 2 weeks for the first 2 months of therapy.

SPECIAL CONSIDERATIONS
1. Use with caution in patients with hepatic impairment. The starting dose should be reduced to 300 mg PO daily in the setting of mild or moderate hepatic impairment (bilirubin 1–3 × ULN or AST > ULN). Has not been studied in patients with severe hepatic impairment (bilirubin > 3 × ULN).
2. Has not been evaluated in setting of renal impairment.
3. Patients should be instructed to drink at least 2 L/day of fluids to maintain hydration.
4. Closely monitor CBC and platelet count every 2 weeks during the first 2 months of therapy and at monthly intervals thereafter.
5. Monitor ECG with QTc measurement at baseline and periodically during therapy, as QTc prolongation has been observed. Use with caution in patients at risk of developing QTc prolongation, including hypokalemia, hypomagnesemia, or congenital long QT syndrome; patients taking anti-arrhythmic medications or any other products that may cause QTc prolongation; and patients taking cumulative high-dose anthracycline therapy.
6. Closely monitor serum glucose levels, especially in diabetic patients, as hyperglycemia may develop while on therapy. Alterations in diet and/or therapy for increased glucose may be necessary.
7. Pregnancy category D. Breastfeeding should be avoided.

TOXICITY 1
Nausea/vomiting and diarrhea are the most common GI toxicities.

TOXICITY 2
Myelosuppression with thrombocytopenia and anemia more common than neutropenia.

TOXICITY 3
Fatigue and anorexia.

TOXICITY 4
Cardiac toxicity with QTc prolongation.

TOXICITY 5
Hyperglycemia.

TOXICITY 6
Increased risk of thromboembolic complications, including DVT and PE.

Zanubrutinib

TRADE NAME	Brukinsa, BGB-3111	CLASSIFICATION	Signal transduction inhibitor, BTK inhibitor
CATEGORY	Targeted agent	DRUG MANUFACTURER	BeiGene and Catalent

MECHANISM OF ACTION
- Potent and selective next generation small molecule inhibitor of Bruton's tyrosine kinase (BTK).
- BTK is a key signaling protein of the B-cell antigen receptor (BCR) and cytokine receptor pathways.
- Greater selectivity for BTK and fewer off-target effects when compared to ibrutinib.

MECHANISM OF RESISTANCE
- Mutations in the Cys481 residue in the BTK active site lead to reduced binding affinity to zanubrutinib.
- Mutations in the gene encoding phospholipase C-γ2 (PLCG2).
- Increased expression of kinases SYK and LYN, which are critical for activation of mutant PLCG2.

ABSORPTION
Rapidly absorbed after oral ingestion, with peak plasma drug levels reached in about 2 hours. Food does not appear to alter oral bioavailability.

DISTRIBUTION
Extensive binding (94%) to plasma proteins. Steady-state drug levels are achieved in approximately 8 days.

METABOLISM
Metabolism in the liver by CYP3A4 microsomal enzymes. Elimination is mainly hepatic (87%), with excretion in feces (38% unchanged). Renal elimination accounts for only 8% of an administered dose (<1% unchanged). Short terminal half-life of the drug on the order of 2–4 hours.

INDICATIONS

1. FDA-approved for adult patients with mantle cell lymphoma (MCL) who have received at least one prior therapy. Approved under accelerated approval based on overall response rate.
2. FDA-approved for adult patients with relapsed or refractory marginal zone lymphoma who have received at least one anti-CD20 regimen.
3. FDA-approved for adult patients with Waldenstrom's macroglobulinemia.
4. FDA-approved for adult patients with CLL or small lymphocytic lymphoma (SLL).

DOSAGE RANGE

Recommended dose is 160 mg PO bid or 320 mg PO once daily. Should be swallowed whole with or without food.

DRUG INTERACTION 1

Phenytoin and other drugs that stimulate the liver microsomal CYP3A4 enzymes, including carbamazepine, rifampin, phenobarbital, and St. John's Wort—These drugs may increase the metabolism of zanubrutinib, resulting in its inactivation and lower effective drug levels.

DRUG INTERACTION 2

Drugs that inhibit the liver microsomal CYP3A4 enzymes, including ketoconazole, itraconazole, erythromycin, and clarithromycin—These drugs may decrease the metabolism of zanubrutinib, resulting in increased drug levels and potentially increased toxicity.

DRUG INTERACTION 3

Proton pump inhibitors—Patients should avoid the use of proton pump inhibitors, as they may reduce oral bioavailability and lead to reduced drug plasma concentrations. If treatment with a gastric acid–reducing agent is required, an antacid or an H2-antagonist should be considered.

SPECIAL CONSIDERATIONS

1. Dose reduction is not required in setting of mild or moderate hepatic impairment (Child-Pugh Class A or B). Dose of zanubrutinib should be reduced to 80 mg PO bid in setting of severe hepatic impairment.
2. Dose reduction is not required in setting of mild or moderate renal impairment. Has not been studied in setting of severe renal impairment, end-stage renal disease, or in patients on dialysis.
3. Zanubrutinib capsules should be swallowed whole with water.
4. Closely monitor CBCs while on therapy.
5. Monitor patients for signs and symptoms of infection. Should consider prophylaxis for herpes simplex virus, PJP, and other infections.
6. Monitor patients for signs and symptoms of bleeding. Concomitant use of antiplatelet or anticoagulant medications may increase the bleeding risk.

7. Patients should be advised to protect against sun exposure.
8. Can cause fetal harm when administered to a pregnant woman. Females of reproductive potential should use effective contraception during drug therapy and for at least 1 week after the final dose. Breastfeeding should be avoided.

TOXICITY 1
Bleeding in the form of purpura, petechiae, ecchymoses, gastrointestinal (GI) bleeding, intracranial bleeds, hemothorax, and hematuria.

TOXICITY 2
Infections with pneumonia being most common. Bacterial, viral, or fungal infections, including herpes simplex virus and PJP. Hepatitis B virus reactivation can occur.

TOXICITY 3
Myelosuppression with neutropenia, thrombocytopenia, and anemia.

TOXICITY 4
Musculoskeletal pain with myalgias, arthralgias, and back pain.

TOXICITY 5
Second primary cancers with skin cancer, basal cell and squamous cell cancers, and other solid tumors.

TOXICITY 6
Fatigue, headache, and myalgias.

TOXICITY 7
Atrial fibrillation/atrial flutter.

Ziv-aflibercept

TRADE NAME	Zaltrap	CLASSIFICATION	Monoclonal antibody, anti-VEGF antibody
CATEGORY	Biologic response modifier agent, targeted agent	DRUG MANUFACTURER	Regeneron/ Sanofi-Aventis

MECHANISM OF ACTION

- Recombinant fusion protein made up of portions of the extracellular domains of human VEGFR-1 and VEGFR-2 fused to the Fc portion of the human IgG1 molecule.
- Functions as a soluble receptor that binds to VEGF-A, VEGF-B, and PlGF. Binds with much higher affinity to VEGF-A than bevacizumab.
- Precise mechanism(s) of action remains unknown.
- Binding of VEGF ligands prevents their subsequent interaction with VEGF receptors on the surface of endothelial cells and tumors, and in so doing, results in inhibition of downstream VEGFR-mediated signaling.
- Inhibits formation of new blood vessels in primary tumor and metastatic tumors.
- Inhibits tumor blood vessel permeability and reduces interstitial tumoral pressures, and, in so doing, may enhance blood flow delivery within tumor.

MECHANISM OF RESISTANCE

- Increased expression/activity of IL6/STAT3 signaling pathway.
- Increased expression of pro-angiogenic factor ligands, such as bFGF and HGF.
- Increased expression of Ang-2.
- Recruitment of bone marrow–derived cells, which circumvents the requirement of VEGF signaling and restores neovascularization and tumor angiogenesis.

DISTRIBUTION

Distribution in body has not been well characterized. The time to reach steady-state levels is on the order of 14 days.

METABOLISM

Metabolism of ziv-aflibercept has not been extensively characterized. The elimination half-life of free ziv-aflibercept is on the order of 6 days, with minimal clearance by the liver or kidneys. Tissue half-life has not been well characterized.

INDICATIONS

Metastatic colorectal cancer—FDA-approved for use in combination with FOLFIRI in patients with mCRC that is resistant to or has progressed following an oxaliplatin-based regimen.

DOSAGE RANGE

1. Recommended dose is 4 mg/kg IV every 2 weeks.
2. Alternative dosing schedule is 6 mg/kg IV every 3 weeks.

DRUG INTERACTION

None well characterized to date.

SPECIAL CONSIDERATIONS

1. Patients should be warned of the increased risk of arterial thromboembolic events, including myocardial infarction and stroke. This is a black-box warning.
2. Patients should be warned of the potential for serious and sometimes fatal bleeding complications, including GI hemorrhage, hemoptysis, hematuria, and post-procedural hemorrhage. This is a black-box warning.
3. Ziv-aflibercept treatment can result in the development of GI perforations and wound dehiscence, which in some cases has resulted in death. These events represent a black-box warning for the drug. Use with caution in patients who have undergone recent surgical and/or invasive procedures.
4. Ziv-aflibercept treatment should be held for at least 4 weeks prior to elective surgery and should not be given for at least 28 days after any surgical and/or invasive intervention and until the surgical wound is completely healed.
5. Ziv-aflibercept treatment can result in fistula formation of both GI and non-GI sites.
6. Use with caution in patients with uncontrolled hypertension, as ziv-aflibercept can result in grade 3 hypertension in about 20% of patients. Should be permanently discontinued in patients who develop hypertensive crisis. In most cases, however, hypertension is well managed with increasing the dose of the antihypertensive medication and/or with the addition of another antihypertensive medication.
7. Monitor older patients for diarrhea and dehydration, as the incidence of diarrhea is increased in patients >65 years of age.
8. Monitor urine for proteinuria by urine dipstick analysis and urinary protein creatinine ratio. A 24-hour urine collection is recommended for patients with a urine dipstick of ≥2+ for protein or a urine protein creatinine (UPCR) greater than 1.
9. Ziv-aflibercept should be terminated in patients who develop nephrotic syndrome (>3 g/24 hours). Therapy should be interrupted for proteinuria >2 g/24 hours and resumed when <2 g/24 hours.
10. Ziv-aflibercept can result in RPLS, which presents with headache, seizure, lethargy, confusion, blindness, and other visual side effects, as well as other neurologic disturbances. Magnetic resonance imaging (MRI) is required to confirm the diagnosis.
11. Closely monitor CBC while on therapy.
12. Pregnancy category C. Breastfeeding should be avoided.

TOXICITY 1

Gastrointestinal perforations and wound-healing complications.

TOXICITY 2

Bleeding complications. Serious, life-threatening intracranial and pulmonary hemorrhage/hemoptysis occur in rare cases.

TOXICITY 3

Increased risk of arterial thromboembolic events, including myocardial infarction, angina, and stroke. There is a slightly increased risk of venous thromboembolic complications, such as DVT and PE.

TOXICITY 4

Hypertension occurs in up to 40% of patients, with grade 3 hypertension observed in 20% of patients. Usually well controlled with oral antihypertensive medication.

TOXICITY 5

Myelosuppression with neutropenia. Febrile neutropenia occurs in about 4% of patients.

TOXICITY 6

GI toxicities in the form of diarrhea and mucositis.

TOXICITY 7

Proteinuria with nephrotic syndrome in up to nearly 10% of patients.

TOXICITY 8

CNS events with dizziness and depression. RPLS is a rare event, and presents with headache, seizure, lethargy, confusion, blindness, and other visual disturbances.

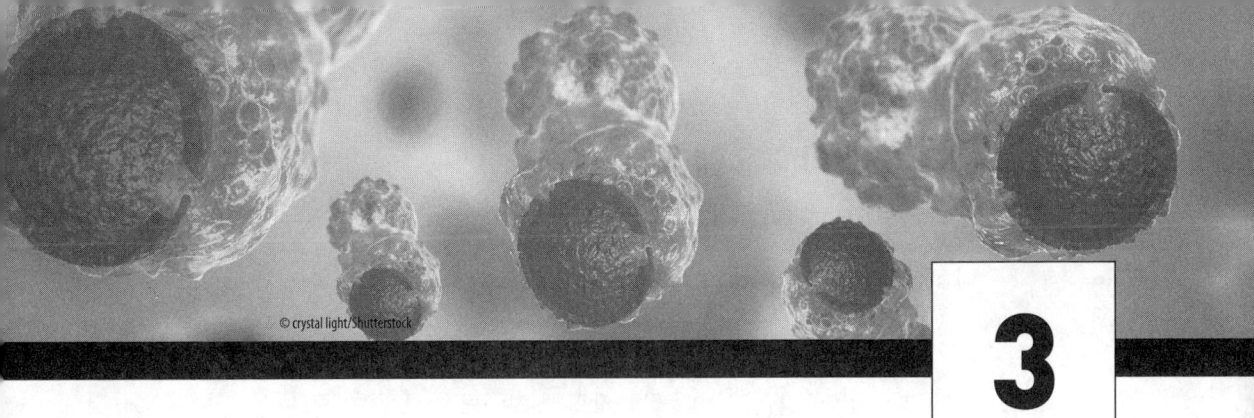

3

Guidelines for Chemotherapy and Dosing Modifications

M. Sitki Copur, Amalia Sofianidi, Laurie J. Harrold, and Edward Chu

Successful administration of chemotherapy relies on several critical patient factors: age; performance status; co-morbid illnesses; prior therapy; and baseline hematologic, hepatic, and renal status. The dose of a given chemotherapeutic agent should be adjusted accordingly to reflect these parameters, as well as any specific drug-induced toxicities that may have been experienced with prior treatment. This chapter outlines performance scales that have been established to determine functional status; reviews methods to calculate creatinine clearance, body surface area, and drug dose; and provides recommendations for dosing in the setting of hepatic and renal dysfunction. General guidelines for dialyzing chemotherapeutic agents in the setting of drug overdose or renal failure are provided. A more detailed review for each individual drug is provided in Chapter 2. The reader is also advised to refer to the published literature for further details regarding recommendations for specific dose modifications for each drug.

Table 3-1. Performance Scales

Karnofsky

(%)	Performance
100	Normal, no evidence of disease
90	Able to carry on normal activity, minor signs or symptoms of disease
80	Normal activity with effort, some signs or symptoms of disease
70	Unable to perform normal activity, cares for self
60	Requires occasional assistance
50	Requires considerable assistance and frequent medical care
40	Disabled, requires special care and assistance
30	Severely disabled, hospitalization may be required
20	Hospitalization necessary for support, very sick
10	Moribund, rapid progression of disease
0	Dead

ECOG

(%)	Performance
0	Asymptomatic, normal activity
1	Fully ambulatory, symptomatic, able to perform activities of daily living
2	Symptomatic, up and about, in bed less than 50% of time
3	Symptomatic, capable of only limited self-care, in bed more than 50% of time
4	Completely disabled, cannot perform any self-care, bedridden 100% of time
5	Dead

Box 3-1. Determination of Creatinine Clearance

- The creatinine clearance is determined by the Cockcroft–Gault formula (Cockcroft DW, Gault MH. *Nephron*. 1976;16(1):31–34), which factors in age, weight, and serum creatinine.

  Males:

  $$\text{Creatinine Clearance (mL/min)} = \frac{\text{weight (kg)} \times (140 - \text{age})}{72 \times \text{serum creatinine (mg/dL)}}$$

  Females:

  $$\text{Creatinine Clearance (mL/min)} = \frac{\text{weight (kg)} \times (140 - \text{age}) \times 0.85}{72 \times \text{serum creatinine (mg/dL)}}$$

- Creatinine clearance can also be determined from a timed urine collection.

  $$\text{Creatinine Clearance (mL/min)} = \frac{\text{urine creatine}}{\text{serum creatine}} \times \frac{\text{urine volume}}{\text{time}}$$

Box 3-2. Determination of Target Area Under the Curve (AUC)

AUC refers to the area under the drug concentration × time curve and provides the best measure of total systemic drug exposure. It is expressed in concentration × units (mg/mL × min).

A formula for quantifying exposure to carboplatin based on dose and renal function was developed by Calvert et al. (Calvert AH, et al. *J Clin Oncol*. 1989;7(11):1748–1756) and is as follows:

$$\text{Carboplatin Dose (mg)} = \text{target AUC (mg/mL} \times \text{min)} \times \{\text{GFR (mL/min)} + 25\}$$

Based on this formula, the total dose is in mg and **NOT** mg/m^2. Target AUC is usually between 4 and 6 mg/mL/min. AUCs >7 are generally associated with increased toxicity with no improvement in clinical activity.

Box 3-3. Determination of Drug Dose

- Drug doses are usually calculated according to body surface area (BSA, mg/m^2).
- BSA is determined by using a nomogram scale or by using a BSA calculator.
- Once the BSA is determined, multiply the BSA by the amount of drug specified in the regimen to give the total dose of drug to be administered.
- Dosing of obese patients remains controversial. Ideal body weight (IBW), as opposed to the actual body weight, may be used to calculate BSA. It is important to refer to an IBW table to determine the IBW based on the individual's actual height. Once the IBW is determined, add one-third of the IBW to the IBW, which is then used to determine the BSA.
- IBW can be calculated from the following formulas: IBW for men (kg): 52.0 kg + 1.9 kg per inch over 5 feet; IBW for women (kg): 49.0 kg + 1.7 kg per inch over 5 feet.[1]
- Full weight–based chemotherapy doses may be used in obese patients, especially when the treatment has curative intent.[2]

1. Peterson CM, Thomas DM, Blackburn GL, Heymsfield SB. Universal equation for estimating ideal body weight and body weight at any BMI [published correction appears in *Am J Clin Nutr.* 2017 Mar;105(3):772]. *Am J Clin Nutr.* 2016;103(5):1197–1203. doi:10.3945/ajcn.115.121178

2. Griggs JJ, Mangu PB, Anderson H, et al. Appropriate chemotherapy dosing for obese adult patients with cancer: American Society of Clinical Oncology clinical practice guideline. *J Clin Oncol.* 2012;30(13):1553–1561. doi:10.1200/JCO.2011.39.9436.

Table 3-2. Calculation of Body Surface Area in Adult Amputees

Body Part	% Surface Area of Amputated Part
Hand and five fingers	3.0
Lower part of arm	4.0
Upper part of arm	6.0
Foot	3.0
Lower part of leg	6.0
Thigh	12.0

BSA (m^2) = BSA – [(BSA) × (%BSA$_{part}$)], where BSA = body surface area, BSA$_{part}$ = body surface area of amputated part.

Reproduced from Colangelo PM, Welch DW, Rich DS, Jeffrey LP. Two methods for estimating body surface area in adult amputees. *Am J Hosp Pharm.* 1984;41(12):2650–2655. doi:10.1093/ajhp/41.12.2650. Reproduced with permission of the American Society of Hospital Pharmacists.

Table 3-3. General Guidelines for Chemotherapy Dosage Based on Hepatic Function

Drug	Recommended Dose Reduction for Hepatic Dysfunction
Abemaciclib	No dose reduction for Child–Pugh Class A and B hepatic dysfunction. Has not been studied in setting of severe hepatic dysfunction.
Acalabrutinib	No dose reduction for Child–Pugh Class A and B hepatic dysfunction. Has not been studied in setting of severe hepatic dysfunction.
Adagrasib	No dose reduction is necessary for mild to severe hepatic dysfunction.
Afatinib	No dose reduction for Child–Pugh Class A and B hepatic dysfunction. Has not been studied in patients with Child–Pugh Class C hepatic dysfunction.
Alectinib	No dose reduction is necessary for mild hepatic dysfunction. Has not been studied in setting of moderate or severe hepatic dysfunction.
Alemtuzumab	N/A
Alpelisib	No dose reduction is necessary for mild, moderate, and severe hepatic dysfunction.
Altretamine	No dose reduction is necessary.
Amifostine	No dose reduction is necessary.
Aminoglutethimide	No dose reduction is necessary.
Amsacrine	Reduce dose by 25% if bilirubin >2.0 mg/dL.
Anastrozole	No formal recommendation for dose reduction.
	Dose reduction may be necessary in patients with hepatic dysfunction.
Apalutamide	No dose reduction for Child–Pugh Class A and B hepatic dysfunction. Has not been studied in setting of severe hepatic dysfunction.
Arsenic trioxide	No dose reduction is necessary.
Asparaginase	No dose reduction is necessary.
Atezolizumab	No dose reduction for mild hepatic dysfunction. Has not been studied in setting of moderate or severe hepatic dysfunction.
Avapritinib	No dose reduction for mild or moderate hepatic dysfunction. Has not been studied in setting of severe hepatic dysfunction.

Table 3-3 (cont.)

Drug	Recommended Dose Reduction for Hepatic Dysfunction
Avelumab	No dose reduction for mild or moderate hepatic dysfunction. Has not been studied in setting of severe hepatic dysfunction (bilirubin >3 × ULN).
Axicabtagene ciloleucel	N/A
Azacitidine	No dose reduction is necessary.
Belinostat	No dose reduction for mild hepatic dysfunction. Has not been studied in setting of moderate or severe hepatic dysfunction.
Bendamustine	Use with caution in patients with mild hepatic dysfunction. Omit in the presence of moderate (SGOT or SGPT 2.5–10 × ULN and total bilirubin >1.5 × ULN) or severe (total bilirubin >3 × ULN) hepatic dysfunction.
Bevacizumab	N/A
Bicalutamide	No formal recommendation for dose reduction. Dose reduction may be necessary when bilirubin >3.0 mg/dL.
Binimetinib	No dose reduction for mild hepatic dysfunction. For patients with moderate or severe hepatic dysfunction, the dose should be reduced to 30 mg PO bid.
Bleomycin	No dose reduction is necessary.
Blinatumomab	N/A
Bosutinib	Reduce dose to 200 mg PO daily in patients with mild, moderate, and severe hepatic dysfunction.
Brigatinib	No dose reduction for mild hepatic dysfunction. Has not been studied in setting of moderate or severe hepatic dysfunction.
Buserelin	No dose reduction is necessary.
Busulfan	No dose reduction is necessary.
Cabazitaxel	No dose reduction for mild hepatic dysfunction. Dose should be reduced to 15 mg/m^2 in patients with moderate hepatic dysfunction. Should not be given in patients with severe hepatic dysfunction (t. bilirubin >3 × ULN.
Cabozantinib	No dose reduction of Cabometyx for mild hepatic dysfunction. Dose of Cabometyx should be reduced to 40 mg PO daily in patients with moderate hepatic dysfunction (Child-Pugh Class B). Dose of Cometriq should be reduced to 80 mg PO daily in patients mild or moderate with hepatic dysfunction. Neither Cabometyx nor Cometriq have been studied in setting of severe hepatic dysfunction (Child-Pugh Class C).

Table 3-3 (cont.)

Drug	Recommended Dose Reduction for Hepatic Dysfunction
Calaspargase pegol-mknl	No dose reduction is necessary.
Capecitabine	No formal recommendation for dose reduction.
	Patients need to be closely monitored in setting of moderate and severe hepatic dysfunction.
Capmatinib	No dose reduction is necessary.
Carboplatin	No dose reduction is necessary.
Carfilzomib	N/A
Carmustine	No dose reduction is necessary.
Cemiplimab-rwlc	No dose reduction for mild hepatic dysfunction. Has not been studied in patients with moderate or severe hepatic dysfunction.
Ceritinib	No dose reduction for mild hepatic dysfunction. Patients need to be closely monitored in setting of moderate and severe hepatic dysfunction, and dose reduction may be necessary.
Cetuximab	No dose reduction is necessary.
Chlorambucil	No dose reduction is necessary.
Cisplatin	No dose reduction is necessary.
Cladribine	No dose reduction is necessary.
Cobimetinib	No dose reduction is necessary.
Copanlisib	No dose reduction for mild hepatic dysfunction. Has not been studied in patients with moderate or severe hepatic dysfunction (total bilirubin $\geq 1.5 \times$ ULN, any AST).
Crizotinib	No dose reduction for mild hepatic dysfunction. Dose should be reduced to 200 mg PO bid in patients with moderate hepatic dysfunction and to 250 PO daily in patients with severe hepatic dysfunction.
Cyclophosphamide	Reduce by 25% if bilirubin 3.0–5.0 mg/dL or SGOT >180 mg/dL.
	Omit if bilirubin >5.0 mg/dL.
Cytarabine	No formal recommendation for dose reduction.
Dabrafenib	No dose reduction is necessary for mild hepatic dysfunction.
	Dose reduction may be necessary with moderate or severe hepatic dysfunction.
Dacarbazine	No dose reduction is necessary.

Table 3-3 (cont.)

Drug	Recommended Dose Reduction for Hepatic Dysfunction
Dacomitinib	No dose reduction for mild or moderate hepatic dysfunction. Has not been studied in setting of severe hepatic dysfunction.
Dactinomycin	Reduce dose by 50% if bilirubin >3.0 mg/dL.
Daratumumab	No dose reduction for mild hepatic dysfunction. Has not been studied in patients with moderate or severe hepatic dysfunction.
Daratumumab and hyaluronidase	No dose reduction for mild hepatic dysfunction. Has not been studied in patients with moderate or severe hepatic dysfunction.
Daunorubicin	Reduce dose by 25% if bilirubin 1.5–3.0 mg/dL. Reduce dose by 50% if bilirubin >3.0 mg/dL. Omit if bilirubin >5.0 mg/dL.
Daunorubicin and cytarabine liposome	No dose reduction for patients with serum bilirubin <3 mg/dL. Has not been studied in patients with serum bilirubin >3 mg/dL, and caution should be used in this setting.
Decitabine	N/A
Decitabine/ Cedazuridine	No dose reduction for mild hepatic dysfunction. Has not been studied in patients with moderate or severe hepatic dysfunction.
Docetaxel	Omit if bilirubin >1.5 mg/dL, SGOT/SGPT >1.5 × ULN and alkaline phosphatase >2.5 × ULN.
Doxorubicin	Reduce dose by 50% if bilirubin 1.5–3.0 mg/dL. Reduce dose by 75% if bilirubin 3.1–5.0 mg/dL. Omit if bilirubin >5.0 mg/dL.
Doxorubicin liposome	Reduce dose by 50% if bilirubin 1.5–3.0 mg/dL. Reduce dose by 75% if bilirubin 3.1–5.0 mg/dL. Omit if bilirubin >5.0 mg/dL.
Durvalumab	No dose reduction for mild hepatic dysfunction. Has not been studied in setting of moderate or severe hepatic dysfunction.
Duvelisib	No dose reduction for mild, moderate, or severe hepatic dysfunction.
Elacestrant	No dose reduction for mild hepatic dysfunction. Dose should be reduced to 258 mg in patients with moderate hepatic dysfunction. Has not been studied in setting of severe hepatic dysfunction.

Table 3-3 (cont.)

Drug	Recommended Dose Reduction for Hepatic Dysfunction
Elotuzumab	No dose reduction for mild hepatic dysfunction. Has not been studied in setting of moderate or severe hepatic dysfunction.
Enasidenib	No dose reduction for mild hepatic dysfunction. Has not been studied in setting of moderate or severe hepatic dysfunction.
Encorafenib	No dose reduction for mild hepatic dysfunction. Has not been studied in setting of moderate or severe hepatic dysfunction.
Enfortumab vedotin	No dose reduction for mild hepatic dysfunction. Has not been studied in setting of moderate or severe hepatic dysfunction.
Entrectinib	No dose reduction for mild hepatic dysfunction. Has not been studied in setting of moderate or severe hepatic dysfunction.
Epcoritamab	No dose reduction for mild hepatic dysfunction. Has not been studied in setting of moderate or severe hepatic dysfunction.
Eribulin	Dose should be reduced to 1.1 mg/m^2 in patients with mild hepatic dysfunction and to 0.7 mg/m^2 in patients with moderate hepatic dysfunction. Has not been studied in setting of severe hepatic dysfunction.
Erlotinib	No formal recommendations for dose reduction. Dose reduction or interruption should be considered in patients with severe hepatic dysfunction and/or in those with a bilirubin >3 × ULN.
Estramustine	No dose reduction is necessary.
Etoposide	Reduce dose by 50% if bilirubin 1.5–3.0 mg/dL or SGOT 60–180 mg/dL. Omit if bilirubin >3 mg/dL or SGOT >180 mg/dL.
Etoposide phosphate	Reduce dose by 50% if bilirubin 1.5–3.0 mg/dL or SGOT 60–180 mg/dL. Omit if bilirubin >3 mg/dL or SGOT >180 mg/dL.
Everolimus	Reduce dose to 5 mg/day in setting of moderate hepatic dysfunction (Child–Pugh Class B). Should not be given in setting of severe hepatic dysfunction (Child–Pugh Class C).
Floxuridine	No dose reduction is necessary.
Fludarabine	No dose reduction is necessary.

Table 3-3 (cont.)

Drug	Recommended Dose Reduction for Hepatic Dysfunction
5–Fluorouracil	No formal recommendation for dose reduction. Should not be given if bilirubin >5.0 mg/dL.
Flutamide	No formal recommendation for dose reduction, but dose reduction should be considered if bilirubin >3.0 mg/dL.
Futibatinib	No dose reduction for mild hepatic dysfunction. Has not been studied in setting of moderate or severe hepatic dysfunction.
Gefitinib	No formal recommendation for dose reduction. Dose reduction or interruption should be considered in patients with moderate or severe hepatic dysfunction.
Gemcitabine	No dose reduction is necessary.
Gemtuzumab	No dose reduction for mild hepatic dysfunction. Has not been studied in setting of moderate or severe hepatic dysfunction, and dose reduction may be required.
Gilteritinib	No dose for mild or moderate hepatic dysfunction. Has not been studied in setting of severe hepatic dysfunction.
Glasdegib	No dose reduction for mild hepatic dysfunction. Has not been studied in setting of moderate or severe hepatic dysfunction.
Goserelin	No dose reduction is necessary.
Hydroxyurea	No dose reduction is necessary.
Ibrutinib	No formal recommendation for dose reduction in presence of hepatic dysfunction, and dose reduction may be required.
Idarubicin	Reduce dose by 25% if bilirubin 1.5–3.0 mg/dL or SGOT 60–180 mg/dL. Reduce dose by 50% if bilirubin 3.0–5.0 or SGOT >180 mg/dL. Omit if bilirubin >5.0 mg/dL.
Ifosfamide	No dose reduction is necessary.
Imatinib	Reduce dose from 400 mg to 300 mg or from 600 mg to 400 mg if bilirubin >1.5 or SGOT >2.5 × ULN. Omit if bilirubin >3 mg/dL or SGOT >5 × ULN.
Infigratinib	Reduce dose to 100 mg PO daily for 21 days with 1-week off for mild hepatic dysfunction. Reduce dose to 75 mg PO daily for 21 days with 1-week off for moderate hepatic dysfunction. Has not been studied in the setting of severe hepatic dysfunction.

Table 3-3 (cont.)

Drug	Recommended Dose Reduction for Hepatic Dysfunction
Inotuzumab	No dose reduction for mild hepatic dysfunction. Has not been studied in setting of moderate or severe hepatic dysfunction.
Interferon–α	No dose reduction is necessary.
Interleukin–2	Omit if signs of hepatic failure (ascites, encephalopathy, jaundice) are observed. Do **NOT** restart sooner than 7 weeks after recovery from severe hepatic dysfunction.
Irinotecan	No formal recommendation for dose reduction in presence of hepatic dysfunction. Dose reduction may be necessary. Patients with UGT1A1*28 genotype should have their dose reduced.
Irinotecan liposome	N/A
Isatuximab	No dose reduction for mild hepatic dysfunction. Has not been studied in setting of moderate or severe hepatic dysfunction.
Isotretinoin	No formal recommendation for dose reduction in presence of mild or moderate hepatic dysfunction. Dose reduction may be necessary.
Ivosidenib	No dose reduction for mild or moderate hepatic dysfunction. Has not been studied in setting of severe hepatic dysfunction.
Ixabepilone	Omit when used in combination with capecitabine if SGOT or SGPT >2.5 × ULN or bilirubin >1 × ULN. When used as monotherapy, reduce dose to 32 mg/m^2 if SGOT or SGPT ≤10 × ULN and bilirubin ≤1.5 × ULN. The dose should be reduced to 20–30 mg/m^2 if SGOT or SGPT ≤10 × ULN and bilirubin >1.5 × ULN to ≤3 × ULN.
Ixazomib	No dose reduction for mild hepatic dysfunction. Dose should be reduced in patients with moderate or severe hepatic dysfunction.
Lapatinib	No formal recommendation for dose reduction for mild or moderate hepatic dysfunction. Reduce dose to 750 mg/day in setting of severe hepatic dysfunction (Child–Pugh Class C).
Larotrectinib	No dose reduction for mild hepatic dysfunction. Dose should be reduced by 50% in setting of moderate and severe hepatic dysfunction.
Lenalidomide	No formal recommendations for dose reduction.

Table 3-3 (cont.)

Drug	Recommended Dose Reduction for Hepatic Dysfunction
Lenvatinib	No dose reduction for mild or moderate hepatic dysfunction. In patients with severe hepatic dysfunction, dose should be reduced to 14 mg PO daily for patients with thyroid cancer and to 10 mg PO daily for patients with renal cell cancer.
Leuprolide	No dose reduction is necessary.
Lomustine	No dose reduction is necessary.
Loncastuximab tesirine	No dose reduction for mild hepatic dysfunction. Has not been studied in setting of moderate or severe hepatic dysfunction.
Lorlatinib	No dose reduction for mild hepatic dysfunction. Has not been studied in patients with moderate or severe hepatic dysfunction.
Lurbinectedin	No dose reduction for mild hepatic dysfunction. Has not been studied in setting of moderate or severe hepatic dysfunction.
Lutetium Lu177 dotatate	No dose reduction for mild or moderate hepatic dysfunction. Has not been studied in patients with severe hepatic dysfunction (total bilirubin $>3 \times$ ULN and any AST).
Margetuximab	No dose reduction for mild hepatic dysfunction. Has not been studied in setting of moderate or severe hepatic dysfunction.
Mechlorethamine	No dose reduction is necessary.
Megestrol acetate	No dose reduction is necessary.
Melphalan	No dose reduction is necessary.
Melphalan flufenamide	No dose reduction for mild hepatic dysfunction. Has not been studied in setting of severe hepatic dysfunction.
6–Mercaptopurine	No dose reduction is necessary.
Methotrexate	Reduce dose by 25% if bilirubin 3.1–5.0 mg/dL or SGOT >180 mg/dL. Should not be given if bilirubin >5.0 mg/dL.
Mitomycin–C	No dose reduction is necessary.
Mitotane	No formal recommendation for dose reduction in presence of hepatic dysfunction. Dose reduction may be necessary.
Mitoxantrone	No formal recommendation for dose reduction in presence of hepatic dysfunction. Dose reduction may be necessary when bilirubin >3.0 mg/dL.

Table 3-3 (cont.)

Drug	Recommended Dose Reduction for Hepatic Dysfunction
Mosunetuzumab	No dose reduction for mild hepatic dysfunction. Has not been studied in setting of moderate to severe hepatic dysfunction.
Moxetumomab pasudotox	No dose reduction for mild, moderate, or severe hepatic dysfunction.
Necitumumab	No dose reduction for mild or moderate hepatic dysfunction. Has not been studied in setting of severe hepatic dysfunction.
Nelarabine	N/A
Neratinib	No dose reduction for mild or moderate hepatic dysfunction. Reduce dose to 80 mg in setting of severe hepatic dysfunction.
Nilutamide	No formal recommendation for dose reduction. Dose reduction may be necessary if bilirubin >3.0 mg/dL.
Niraparib	No dose reduction for mild hepatic dysfunction. Has not been studied in setting of moderate or severe hepatic dysfunction.
Nivolumab	No dose reduction for mild hepatic dysfunction. Has not been studied in setting of moderate or severe hepatic dysfunction.
Obinutuzumab	Has not been studied in setting of hepatic dysfunction.
Ofatumumab	N/A
Olaparib	No dose reduction for mild hepatic dysfunction. Has not been studied in setting of moderate or severe hepatic dysfunction.
Olutasidenib	No dose reduction for mild or moderate hepatic dysfunction. Has not been studied in setting of severe hepatic dysfunction.
Osimertinib	No dose reduction for mild or moderate hepatic dysfunction. Has not been studied in setting of severe hepatic dysfunction.
Oxaliplatin	No dose reduction is necessary.
Paclitaxel	No formal recommendation for dose reduction if bilirubin 1.5–3.0 mg/dL or SGOT 60–180 mg/dL. Should not be given if bilirubin >5.0 mg/dL or SGOT >180 mg/dL.
Palbociclib	No dose reduction for mild hepatic dysfunction. Has not been studied in setting of moderate or severe hepatic dysfunction.
Panitumumab	No dose reduction is necessary.

Table 3-3 (cont.)

Drug	Recommended Dose Reduction for Hepatic Dysfunction
Pazopanib	Reduce dose to 200 mg/day in setting of moderate hepatic dysfunction. No formal guidelines for severe hepatic dysfunction.
Pegasparaginase	No dose reduction is necessary.
Pembrolizumab	No dose reduction for mild hepatic dysfunction. Has not been studied in setting of moderate or severe hepatic dysfunction.
Pemetrexed	No dose reduction is necessary.
Pemigatinib	No dose reduction for mild or moderate hepatic dysfunction. Has not been studied in setting of severe hepatic dysfunction.
Pertuzumab	N/A
Pirtobrunitib	No dose reduction for mild, moderate, or severe hepatic dysfunction.
Polatuzumab vedotin	No dose reduction for mild hepatic dysfunction. Has not been studied in setting of moderate or severe hepatic dysfunction.
Pomalidomide	Should not be given if bilirubin >2.0 mg/dL and SGOT/SGPT >3 × ULN.
Ponatinib	Reduce dose to 30 mg PO daily if SGOT/SGPT >3 × ULN. Should not be given if SGOT/SGPT ≥3 × ULN and bilirubin >2 × ULN and alkaline phosphatase <2 × ULN.
Pralatrexate	N/A
Procarbazine	No formal recommendation for dose reduction in presence of hepatic dysfunction. Dose reduction may be necessary.
Ramucirumab	N/A
Regorafenib	No dose reduction for mild or moderate hepatic dysfunction. Omit in the setting of severe hepatic dysfunction.
Relugolix	No dose reduction for mild or moderate hepatic dysfunction. Has not been studied in setting of severe hepatic dysfunction.
Retifanlimab	No dose reduction for mild hepatic dysfunction. Has not been studied in setting of moderate or severe hepatic dysfunction.
Ribociclib	No dose reduction for mild hepatic dysfunction. Reduce dose to 400 mg in patients with moderate or severe hepatic dysfunction.

Table 3-3 (cont.)

Drug	Recommended Dose Reduction for Hepatic Dysfunction
Ripretinib	No dose reduction for mild or moderate hepatic dysfunction. Has not been studied in setting of severe hepatic dysfunction.
Rituximab	No dose reduction is necessary.
Rituxumab-abbs	No dose reduction is necessary.
Rituximab and human hyaluronidase	N/A
Rucaparib	No dose reduction for mild hepatic dysfunction. Has not been studied in setting of moderate or severe hepatic dysfunction.
Sacituzumab govitecan	No dose reduction for mild hepatic dysfunction. Has not been studied in setting of moderate or severe hepatic dysfunction.
Selinexor	No dose reduction for mild hepatic dysfunction. Has not been studied in setting of moderate or severe hepatic dysfunction.
Selpercatinib	No dose reduction for mild or moderate hepatic dysfunction. Dose should be reduced to 80 mg PO bid in setting of severe hepatic dysfunction.
Sonidegib	No dose reduction is necessary.
Sorafenib	No formal recommendation for dose reduction in presence of hepatic dysfunction.
Streptozocin	No dose reduction is necessary.
Sunitinib	No dose reduction for Child–Pugh Class A or B hepatic dysfunction. Dose reduction may be necessary in patients with Child–Pugh Class C hepatic dysfunction, although there are no formal recommendations.
Talazoparib	No dose reduction for mild hepatic dysfunction. Has not been studied in setting of moderate or severe hepatic dysfunction.
Tamoxifen	No dose reduction is necessary.
Tazemetostat	No dose reduction for mild hepatic dysfunction. Has not been studied in setting of moderate or severe hepatic dysfunction.
Temozolomide	No dose reduction is necessary.
Tepotinib	No dose reduction for mild or moderate hepatic dysfunction. Has not been studied in setting of severe hepatic dysfunction.

Table 3-3 (cont.)

Drug	Recommended Dose Reduction for Hepatic Dysfunction
Thalidomide	N/A
Thioguanine	Should not be given if bilirubin >5.0 mg/dL.
Thiotepa	No formal recommendation for dose reduction.
Tisagenlecleucel	N/A
Tivozanib	No dose reduction for mild hepatic dysfunction. Reduce dose to 0.89 mg PO once daily for 21 days on a 28-day cycle for moderate hepatic dysfunction (total bilirubin >1.5-3 × ULN and any AST). Has not been studied in severe hepatic dysfunction.
Topotecan	No dose reduction is necessary.
Trabectedin	No dose reduction for mild hepatic dysfunction. Dose should be reduced to 0.9 mg/m^2 in setting of moderate hepatic dysfunction (bilirubin ≤1.5–3.0 × ULN and SGOT/SGPT ≤8 × ULN). Should not be administered in setting of severe hepatic dysfunction (bilirubin ≤3.0–10.0 × ULN and any SGOT/SGPT).
Trametinib	No dose reduction for mild hepatic dysfunction. Dose reduction may be necessary in patients with moderate and severe hepatic dysfunction.
Trastuzumab	No dose reduction is necessary.
Trastuzumab deruxtecan	No dose reduction for mild or moderate hepatic dysfunction. Has not been studied in setting of severe hepatic dysfunction.
Tremelimumab	No dose reduction for mild or moderate hepatic dysfunction. Has not been studied in setting of severe hepatic dysfunction.
Tretinoin	Reduce dose to a maximum of 25 mg/m^2 if bilirubin 3.1–5.0 mg/dL or SGOT >180 mg/dL. Should not be given if bilirubin >5.0 mg/dL.
Trifluridine/tipiracil	No dose reduction for mild hepatic dysfunction. Has not been studied in setting of moderate or severe hepatic dysfunction.
Tucatinib	No dose reduction for mild or moderate hepatic dysfunction. Dose should be reduced to 200 mg PO bid in patients with severe hepatic dysfunction.

Table 3-3 (cont.)

Drug	Recommended Dose Reduction for Hepatic Dysfunction
Umbralisib	No dose reduction for mild hepatic dysfunction. Has not been studied in setting of moderate or severe hepatic dysfunction.
Vemurafenib	No dose reduction for mild or moderate hepatic dysfunction. Dose reduction may be required with severe hepatic dysfunction.
Venetoclax	No dose reduction for mild or moderate hepatic dysfunction. Has not been studied in setting of severe hepatic dysfunction.
Vinblastine	No dose reduction if bilirubin <1.5 mg/dL and SGOT <60 mg/dL.
	Reduce by 50% if bilirubin 1.5–3.0 mg/dL and SGOT 60–180 mg/dL.
	Should not be given if bilirubin >3.0 mg/dL or SGOT >180 mg/dL.
Vincristine	No dose reduction if bilirubin <1.5 mg/dL and SGOT <60 mg/dL.
	Reduce by 50% if bilirubin 1.5–3.0 mg/dL and SGOT 60–180 mg/dL.
	Should not be given if bilirubin >3.0 mg/dL or SGOT >180 mg/dL.
Vinorelbine	No dose reduction if bilirubin <2.0 mg/dL.
	Reduce dose by 50% if bilirubin 2.0–3.0 mg/dL.
	Reduce dose by 75% if bilirubin 3.1–5 mg/dL.
	Should not be given if bilirubin >5 mg/dL.
Vorinostat	Reduce dose to 300 mg PO daily in setting of mild or moderate hepatic dysfunction. Has not been studied in setting of severe hepatic dysfunction.
Zanubrutinib	No dose reduction for mild or moderate hepatic dysfunction. Dose should be reduced to 80 mg PO bid in setting of severe hepatic dysfunction.
Ziv-aflibercept	No dose reduction is necessary in patients with mild or moderate hepatic dysfunction. Has not been studied in setting of severe hepatic dysfunction.

N/A—not available

ULN—upper limit of normal

Table 3-4. General Guidelines for Chemotherapy Dosage Based on Renal Function

Drug	Recommended Dose Reduction for Renal Dysfunction
Abemaciclib	No dose reduction for mild or moderate renal dysfunction. Has not been studied in severe renal dysfunction or in end-stage renal disease.
Acalabrutinib	No dose reduction for mild or moderate renal dysfunction. Has not been studied in the setting of end-stage renal disease.
Adagrasib	No dose reduction for mild to severe renal dysfunction. Has not been studied in setting of end-stage renal disease.
Afatinib	No dose reduction for mild renal dysfunction. Dose reduction may be necessary with moderate or severe renal dysfunction.
Alectinib	No dose reduction for mild or moderate renal dysfunction. Has not been studied in severe renal dysfunction or in end-stage renal disease.
Alemtuzumab	N/A
Alpelisib	No dose reduction for mild or moderate renal dysfunction. Has not been studied in severe renal dysfunction or in end-stage renal disease.
Altretamine	N/A
Aminoglutethimide	N/A
Anastrozole	No dose reduction is necessary.
Apalutamide	No dose reduction for mild or moderate renal dysfunction. Has not been studied in severe renal dysfunction or in end-stage renal disease.
Arsenic trioxide	No formal recommendation for dose reduction in the presence of renal dysfunction. Dose reduction may be necessary.
Asparaginase erwinia	N/A
L–Asparaginase	Omit if CrCl <60 mL/min.
Atezolizumab	No dose reduction is necessary.
Avapritinib	No dose reduction for mild and moderate renal dysfunction. Has not been studied in severe renal dysfunction or in end-stage renal disease.

Table 3-4 (cont.)

Drug	Recommended Dose Reduction for Renal Dysfunction
Avelumab	No dose reduction is necessary.
Axicabtagene ciloleucel	N/A
Belantamab mafadotin	No dose reduction for mild or moderate renal dysfunction. Has not been studied in severe renal dysfunction or in end-stage renal disease.
Belinostat	No dose reduction for mild or moderate renal dysfunction. Has not been studied in patients with CrCl <39 mL/min.
Bendamustine	Omit if CrCl <30 mL/min.
Bevacizumab	N/A
Bicalutamide	No dose reduction is necessary.
Binimetinib	No dose reduction for mild, moderate, or severe renal dysfunction.
Bleomycin	No dose reduction if CrCl >50 mL/min. Reduce dose by 25% if CrCl 10–50 mL/min. Reduce dose by 50% if CrCl <10 mL/min.
Blinatumomab	No dose reduction for mild or moderate renal dysfunction. Has not been studied in severe renal dysfunction or in end-stage renal disease.
Bosutinib	No dose reduction for mild or moderate renal dysfunction. Dose should be reduced to 300 mg PO daily in patients with severe renal dysfunction. Has not been studied in end-stage renal disease.
Brigatinib	No dose reduction for mild or moderate renal dysfunction. Has not been studied in severe renal dysfunction or in end-stage renal disease.
Buserelin	N/A
Busulfan	No dose reduction is necessary.
Cabazitaxel	No dose reduction for mild, moderate, or severe renal dysfunction. Has not been studied in end-stage renal disease or in patients on dialysis.
Cabozantinib	No dose reduction for mild or moderate renal dysfunction. Has not been studied in setting of severe renal dysfunction or in end-stage renal disease.
Calaspargase pegol-mknl	No dose reduction is necessary.

Table 3-4 (cont.)

Drug	Recommended Dose Reduction for Renal Dysfunction
Capecitabine	No dose reduction if CrCl >50 mL/min. Reduce dose by 25% if CrCl 30–50 mL/min. Should not be given if CrCl <30 mL/min.
Capmatinib	No dose reduction for mild or moderate renal dysfunction. Has not been studied in severe renal dysfunction or in end-stage renal disease.
Carboplatin	No dose reduction if CrCl >60 mL/min. AUC dose is modified according to CrCl.
Carfilzomib	No dose reduction is necessary.
Carmustine	Should not be given if CrCl <70 mL/min.
Cemiplimab-rwlc	No dose reduction for CrCl >25 mL/min. Has not been studied in patients with end-stage renal disease or in those on hemodialysis.
Ceritinib	N/A
Cetuximab	No dose reduction is necessary.
Chlorambucil	No dose reduction is necessary.
Cisplatin	No dose reduction if CrCl >60 mL/min. Reduce dose by 50% if CrCl 30–60 mL/min. Should not be given if CrCl <30 mL/min.
Cladribine	No dose reduction if CrCl >50 mL/min. Reduce dose by 25% if CrCl 10–50 mL/min. Reduce dose by 50% if CrCl <10 mL/min. No dose reduction if CrCl >60 mL/min.
Clofarabine	No dose reduction if CrCl >60 mL/min. Reduce dose by 50% if CrCl 30–60 mL/min. Use with caution in patients with CrCl <30 mL/min or on hemodialysis.
Cobimetinib	No dose reduction for mild or moderate renal dysfunction. No recommended dose has been established for patients with severe renal dysfunction.
Copanlisib	No dose reduction for mild or moderate renal dysfunction. Has not been studied in severe renal dysfunction, in end-stage renal disease, or in patients on dialysis.

Table 3-4 (cont.)

Drug	Recommended Dose Reduction for Renal Dysfunction
Crizotinib	No dose reduction for mild or moderate renal dysfunction. Dose should be reduced to 250 mg PO daily in patients with severe renal dysfunction not requiring dialysis.
Cyclophosphamide	No dose reduction if CrCl >20 mL/min. Reduce dose by 25% if CrCl 10–20 mL/min. Reduce dose by 50% if CrCl <10 mL/min.
Cytarabine	No formal recommendation for dose reduction in presence of renal dysfunction. Dose reduction may be necessary.
Dacarbazine	No formal recommendation for dose reduction in presence of renal dysfunction. Dose reduction may be necessary.
Dacomitinib	No dose reduction for mild or moderate renal dysfunction. Has not been studied in severe renal dysfunction or in end-stage renal disease.
Dactinomycin	N/A
Daratumumab	No dose reduction is necessary.
Daratumumab and hyaluronidase	No dose reduction is necessary.
Dasatinib	No dose reduction is necessary.
Daunorubicin	Reduce dose by 50% if serum creatinine >3.0 mg/dL.
Daunorubicin and cytarabine liposome	No dose reduction for mild or moderate renal dysfunction. Has not been studied in severe renal dysfunction or in end-stage renal disease.
Decitabine	N/A
Decitabine/ cedazuridine	No dose reduction for mild or moderate renal dysfunction. Has not been studied in severe renal dysfunction or in end-stage renal disease.
Docetaxel	No dose reduction is necessary.
Doxorubicin	No dose reduction is necessary.
Doxorubicin liposome	No dose reduction is necessary.
Durvalumab	No dose reduction for mild or moderate renal dysfunction. Has not been studied in severe renal dysfunction.

Table 3-4 (cont.)

Drug	Recommended Dose Reduction for Renal Dysfunction
Duvelisib	No dose reduction for mild or moderate renal dysfunction. Has not been studied in severe renal dysfunction or in end-stage renal disease.
Elacestrant	No dose reduction for mild or moderate renal dysfunction. Has not been studied in severe renal dysfunction or end-stage renal disease.
Elotuzumab	No dose reduction is necessary.
Enasidenib	No dose reduction if CrCl ≥30 mL/min.
Encorafenib	No dose reduction for mild or moderate renal dysfunction. Has not been studied in severe renal dysfunction or in end-stage renal disease.
Enfortumab vedotin	No dose reduction for mild, moderate, or severe renal dysfunction. Has not been studied in patients with end-stage renal disease or in those on hemodialysis.
Entrectinib	No dose reduction for mild or moderate renal dysfunction. Has not been studied in severe renal dysfunction or in end-stage renal disease.
Epcoritamab	No dose reduction for mild or moderate renal dysfunction. Has not been studied in severe renal dysfunction or in end-stage renal disease.
Eribulin	No dose reduction for mild renal dysfunction. Dose should be reduced to 1.1 mg/m² in setting of moderate or severe renal dysfunction.
Erlotinib	No dose reduction is necessary.
Estramustine	N/A
Etoposide	No dose reduction if CrCl >50 mL/min. Reduce dose by 25% if CrCl 15–50 mL/min. Reduce dose by 50% if CrCl <15 mL/min.
Etoposide phosphate	No dose reduction if CrCl >50 mL/min. Reduce dose by 25% if CrCl 10–50 mL/min. Reduce dose by 50% if CrCl <10 mL/min.
Everolimus	No dose reduction is necessary.
Floxuridine	No dose reduction is necessary.
Fludarabine	No dose reduction if CrCl >70 mL/min. Reduce dose by 20% if CrCl 30–70 mL/min. Should not be given if CrCl <30 mL/min.
5–Fluorouracil	No dose reduction is necessary.

Table 3-4 (cont.)

Drug	Recommended Dose Reduction for Renal Dysfunction
Flutamide	N/A
Futibatinib	No dose reduction for mild or moderate renal dysfunction. Has not been studied in severe renal dysfunction, end-stage renal disease, or in patients on dialysis.
Gefitinib	No dose reduction is necessary.
Gemcitabine	No dose reduction is necessary.
Gemtuzumab	No dose reduction for mild or moderate renal dysfunction. Has not been studied in severe renal dysfunction or in patients on dialysis.
Gilteritinib	No dose reduction for mild or moderate renal dysfunction. Has not been studied in severe renal dysfunction or in patients on dialysis.
Glasdegib	No dose reduction for mild or moderate renal dysfunction. Has not been studied in severe renal dysfunction or in patients on dialysis.
Goserelin	No dose reduction is necessary.
Hydroxyurea	Reduce dose by 50% if CrCl 10–50 mL/min. Reduce dose by 80% if CrCl <10 mL/min.
Ibrutinib	No dose reduction for mild or moderate renal dysfunction. Has not been studied in severe renal dysfunction or in patients on dialysis.
Idarubicin	No dose reduction is necessary.
Idecabtagene vicleucel	N/A
Ifosfamide	No dose reduction if CrCl >60 mL/min. Reduce dose by 20% if CrCl 46–59 mL/min. Reduce dose by 25% if CrCl 31–45 mL/min. Reduce dose by 30% if CrCl <30 mL/min. Use with caution and may omit if CrCl <40 mL/min.
Imatinib	No dose reduction is necessary.
Infigratinib	Dose should be reduced to 100 mg PO daily for 21 days with 1-week off for mild and moderate renal dysfunction (CrCl, 30-89 mL/min). Has not been studied in severe renal impairment or end-stage renal disease.
Inotuzumab	No dose reduction for mild, moderate, or severe renal dysfunction. Has not been studied in end-stage renal disease or in patients on dialysis.

Table 3-4 (cont.)

Drug	Recommended Dose Reduction for Renal Dysfunction
Interferon–α	No dose reduction is necessary.
Interleukin–2	Omit or discontinue if serum creatinine >4.5 mg/dL.
Irinotecan	No dose reduction is necessary.
Irinotecan liposome	No dose reduction for mild or moderate renal dysfunction. Has not been studied in severe renal dysfunction or in end-stage renal disease.
Isatuximab	No dose reduction is necessary.
Isotretinoin	N/A
Ivosidenib	No dose reduction for mild or moderate renal dysfunction. Has not been studied in severe renal dysfunction or in end-stage renal disease.
Ixabepilone	No formal recommendation for dose reduction.
Ixazomib	No dose reduction for mild or moderate renal dysfunction. Dose should be reduced in severe renal dysfunction or in end-stage renal disease.
Lapatinib	No dose reduction is necessary.
Larotrectinib	No dose reduction for mild to severe renal dysfunction.
Lenalidomide	No formal recommendation for dose reduction. In the setting of moderate or severe renal dysfunction, dose reduction may be necessary.
Lenvatinib	No dose reduction for mild or moderate renal dysfunction. In severe renal dysfunction, dose should be reduced to 14 mg PO daily for thyroid cancer and to 10 mg PO daily for renal cell cancer. Has not been studied in end-stage renal disease or in patients on dialysis.
Leuprolide	N/A
Lisocabtagene maraleucel	N/A
Lomustine	Omit if CrCl <60 mL/min.
Loncastuximab tesirine	No dose reduction for mild or moderate renal dysfunction (CrCl, 30–90 mL/min). Has not been studied in severe renal dysfunction, end-stage renal disease, or in patients on dialysis.
Lorlatinib	No dose reduction for mild or moderate renal dysfunction. Dose should reduced to 75 mg PO daily in setting of severe renal dysfunction. Has not been studied in patients on dialysis.

Table 3-4 (cont.)

Drug	Recommended Dose Reduction for Renal Dysfunction
Lurbinectedin	No dose reduction for mild or moderate renal dysfunction. Has not been studied in severe renal dysfunction or in end-stage renal disease.
Lutetium Lu177 dotatate	No dose reduction for mild or moderate renal dysfunction. Has not been studied in severe renal dysfunction or in patients on dialysis.
Margetuximab	No dose reduction for mild or moderate renal dysfunction. Has not been studied in severe renal dysfunction or in end-stage renal disease.
Mechlorethamine	N/A
Megestrol acetate	N/A
Melphalan	No formal recommendation for dose reduction. However, use with caution in the presence of renal dysfunction.
Melphalan flufenamide	No dose reduction for mild renal dysfunction (CrCL, 45–89 mL/min). Has not been studied in moderate to severe renal dysfunction (CrCL, 15–44 mL/min).
6–Mercaptopurine	No formal recommendation for dose reduction in presence of renal dysfunction.
Methotrexate	No dose reduction if CrCl >60 mL/min. Reduce by 50% if CrCl 30–60 mL/min. Should not be given if CrCl <30 mL/min.
Mitomycin–C	No dose reduction if CrCl >60 mL/min. Reduce dose by 25% if CrCl 10–60 mL/min. Reduce dose by 50% if CrCl <10 mL/min.
Mitotane	N/A
Mitoxantrone	No dose reduction is necessary.
Mosunetuzumab	No dose reduction for mild or moderate renal dysfunction. Has not been studied in severe renal dysfunction or end-stage renal disease.
Moxetumomab pasudotox	No dose reduction for mild or moderate renal dysfunction. Has not been studied in severe renal dysfunction, end-stage renal disease, or in patients on dialysis.
Necitumumab	No formal studies have been done in setting of renal dysfunction.
Nelarabine	No formal recommendation for dose reduction. Dose reduction may be necessary in setting of moderate or severe renal dysfunction.

Table 3-4 (cont.)

Drug	Recommended Dose Reduction for Renal Dysfunction
Neratinib	No dose reduction is necessary.
Nilotinib	No dose reduction is necessary.
Nilutamide	No dose reduction is necessary.
Niraparib	No dose reduction for mild or moderate renal dysfunction. Has not been studied in setting of severe renal dysfunction or in patients with end-stage renal disease.
Nivolumab	No dose reduction is necessary.
Obinutuzumab	No dose reduction for mild or moderate dysfunction. Has not been studied in severe renal dysfunction or end-stage renal disease.
Ofatumumab	N/A
Olaparib	No dose reduction for mild renal dysfunction. Dose should be reduced to 300 mg bid in presence of moderate renal dysfunction. Has not been studied in setting of severe renal dysfunction, end-stage renal disease, or in patients on dialysis.
Olutasidenib	No dose reduction for mild or moderate renal dysfunction. Has not been studied in severe renal dysfunction, end-stage renal disease, or in patients on dialysis.
Osimertinib	No dose reduction for mild, moderate, or severe renal dysfunction. Has not been studied in end-stage renal disease.
Oxaliplatin	No dose reduction for CrCl >20 mL/min. Has not been studied in patients with CrCl <20 mL/min.
Paclitaxel	No dose reduction is necessary.
Palbociclib	No dose reduction for mild or moderate renal dysfunction. Has not been studied in severe renal dysfunction or end-stage renal disease.
Panitumumab	No dose reduction is necessary.
Pazopanib	No dose reduction is necessary.
Pegasparaginase	N/A
Pembrolizumab	No dose reduction is necessary.
Pemetrexed	No dose reduction is necessary when CrCl >45 mL/min. Omit if CrCL <45 mL/min.

Table 3-4 (cont.)

Drug	Recommended Dose Reduction for Renal Dysfunction
Pemigatinib	No dose reduction for mild or moderate renal dysfunction. Has not been studied in severe renal dysfunction or end-stage renal disease.
Pertuzumab	No dose reduction for mild or moderate renal dysfunction. Has not been studied in severe renal dysfunction or end-stage renal disease.
Pirtobrunitib	No dose reduction for mild or moderate renal dysfunction. Dose reduced from 200 to 100 mg in patients with severe renal dysfunction.
Polatuzumab vedotin	No dose reduction for mild or moderate renal dysfunction. Has not been studied in severe renal dysfunction or end-stage renal disease.
Pomalidomide	No dose reduction for patients with serum creatinine <3.0 mg/dL. Should not be given if serum creatinine >3.0 mg/dL.
Ponatinib	No dose reduction for mild renal dysfunction. Dose reduction may be necessary in the setting of moderate or severe renal dysfunction.
Pralatrexate	No dose reduction if CrCl >30 mL/min. If CrCl is 15–29 mL/min, reduce dose to 15 mg/m^2. Should not be given if CrCl <15 mL/min.
Pralsetinib	No dose reduction for mild or moderate renal dysfunction. Has not been studied in severe renal dysfunction or end-stage renal disease.
Procarbazine	Omit if CrCl <30 mL/min.
Ramucirumab	N/A
Regorafenib	No dose reduction for mild, moderate, or severe renal dysfunction. Has not been studied in end-stage renal disease or in patients on hemodialysis.
Relugolix	No dose reduction for mild, moderate, or severe renal dysfunction. Has not been studied in setting of end-stage renal disease or in patients on hemodialysis.
Retifanlimab	No dose reduction for mild or moderate renal dysfunction. Has not been studied in severe renal dysfunction or end-stage renal disease.
Ribociclib	N/A
Ripretinib	No dose reduction for mild, moderate, or severe renal dysfunction. Has not been studied in setting of end-stage renal disease or in patients on hemodialysis.

Table 3-4 (cont.)

Drug	Recommended Dose Reduction for Renal Dysfunction
Rituximab	N/A
Rituximab-abbs	N/A
Rituximab and human hyaluronidase	N/A
Rucaparib	No dose reduction for mild or moderate renal dysfunction. Has not been studied in severe renal dysfunction or in end-stage renal disease.
Sacituzumab govitecan	N/A
Selinexor	No dose reduction for mild, moderate, or severe renal dysfunction. Has not been studied in end-stage renal disease or in patients on dialysis.
Selpercatinib	No dose reduction for mild or moderate renal dysfunction. Has not been studied in severe renal dysfunction or end-stage renal disease.
Sonidegib	No dose reduction for mild or moderate renal dysfunction. Has not been studied in severe renal dysfunction or end-stage renal disease.
Sorafenib	No dose reduction if CrCl >40 mL/min. Reduce dose to 200 mg PO bid if CrCl 20–39 mL/min. Dosing has not been well-defined in setting of CrCl <20 mL/min. Has not been studied in patients on dialysis.
Sotorasib	No dose reduction for mild or moderate renal impairment. Has not been studied in severe renal dysfunction or end-stage renal disease.
Streptozocin	No dose reduction if CrCl >60 mL/min. Reduce dose by 25% if CrCl 10–50 mL/min. Reduce dose by 50–75% if CrCl <10 mL/min.
Sunitinib	No dose reduction is necessary.
Talazoparib	No dose reduction for mild renal dysfunction. Dose should be reduced to 0.75 mg PO once daily for moderate renal dysfunction. Has not been studied in severe renal dysfunction, end-stage renal disease, or in patients on dialysis.
Tamoxifen	No dose reduction is necessary.
Tazemetostat	No dose reduction is necessary.

Table 3-4 (cont.)

Drug	Recommended Dose Reduction for Renal Dysfunction
Temozolomide	N/A
Temsirolimus	No dose reduction is necessary.
Tepotinib	No dose reduction for mild or moderate renal dysfunction. Has not been studied in severe renal dysfunction or end-stage renal disease.
Thalidomide	No formal recommendation for dose reduction in presence of renal dysfunction.
Thioguanine	N/A
Thiotepa	No formal recommendation for dose reduction in presence of renal dysfunction.
Tisagenlecleucel	N/A
Tivozanib	No dose reduction for mild to severe renal dysfunction. Has not been studied in end-stage renal disease or in patients on dialysis.
Topotecan	No dose reduction is necessary if CrCl >40 mL/min. Reduce dose to 0.75 mg/m^2/day if CrCl 20–39 mL/min. Should not be given if CrCl <20 mL/min.
Trabectedin	No dose reduction for mild or moderate renal dysfunction. Has not been studied in severe renal dysfunction or in end-stage renal disease.
Trametinib	No dose reduction for mild or moderate renal dysfunction. No formal recommendation for dose reduction in severe renal dysfunction or in end-stage renal disease.
Trastuzumab	N/A
Trastuzumab deruxtecan	No dose reduction for mild or moderate renal dysfunction. Has not been studied in severe renal dysfunction or in end-stage renal disease.
Tremelimumab	No dose reduction for mild or moderate renal dysfunction. Has not been studied in severe renal dysfunction or in end-stage renal disease.
Tretinoin	Give a maximum of 25 mg/m^2 in the presence of renal dysfunction.
Trifluridine/tipiracil	No dose reduction for mild or moderate renal dysfunction. Has not been studied in severe renal dysfunction or in end-stage renal disease.
Tucatinib	No dose reduction for mild or moderate renal dysfunction. Has not been studied in severe renal dysfunction or in end-stage renal disease.

Table 3-4 (cont.)

Drug	Recommended Dose Reduction for Renal Dysfunction
Umbralisib	No dose reduction for mild or moderate renal dysfunction. Has not been studied in severe renal dysfunction or end-stage renal disease.
Vandetanib	No dose reduction for mild renal dysfunction. Dose should be reduced to 200 mg PO daily in moderate to severe renal dysfunction. Has not been studied in end-stage renal disease or in patients on dialysis.
Venetoclax	No dose reduction for mild or moderate renal dysfunction. Has not been studied in severe renal dysfunction or in end-stage renal disease.
Vinblastine	No dose reduction is necessary.
Vincristine	No dose reduction is necessary.
Vinorelbine	No dose reduction is necessary.
Vorinostat	No dose reduction is necessary.
Zanubrutinib	No dose reduction for mild or moderate renal dysfunction. Has not been studied in severe renal dysfunction or in end-stage renal disease.
Ziv-aflibercept	N/A

CrCl—creatinine clearance

N/A—not available

Table 3-5. Guidelines for Dialysis of Chemotherapy Drugs

Drug	Hemodialysis			Peritoneal Dialysis		
	YES	NO	UNKNOWN	YES	NO	UNKNOWN
Afatinib			X			X
Alemtuzumab			X			X
Alpelisib			X			X
Altretamine			X			X
Aminoglutethimide	X					X
Amsacrine			X			X
Anastrozole			X			X
Arsenic trioxide			X			X
Atezolizumab			X			X

Table 3-5 (cont.)

Drug	Hemodialysis			Peritoneal Dialysis		
	YES	NO	UNKNOWN	YES	NO	UNKNOWN
Avapritinib			X			X
Avelumab			X			X
Azacitidine			X			X
Bevacizumab			X			X
Bicalutamide			X			X
Binimetinib			X			X
Bleomycin		X			X	
Bortezomib	X					X
Bosutinib			X			X
Brigatinib			X			X
Buserelin			X			X
Busulfan			X			X
Cabozantinib			X			X
Calapargase pegol-mknl			X			X
Capecitabine			X			X
Capmatinib			X			X
Carboplatin	X				X	
Carfilzomib	X					X
Carmustine		X			X	
Cemiplimab-rwlc			X			X
Ceritinib			X			X
Cetuximab			X			X
Chlorambucil			X			X
Cisplatin	X					X
Cladribine			X			X
Clofarabine			X			X
Cyclophosphamide	X			X		
Cytarabine	X				X	
Dabrafenib			X			X
Dacarbazine			X			X
Dacomitinib			X			X
Dactinomycin			X			X

Table 3-5 (cont.)

Drug	Hemodialysis			Peritoneal Dialysis		
	YES	NO	UNKNOWN	YES	NO	UNKNOWN
Daunorubicin		X				X
Decitabine/Cedazuridine			X			X
Docetaxel		X				X
Doxorubicin		X				X
Doxorubicin liposome			X			X
Duvelisib			X			X
Enasidenib			X			X
Encorafenib			X			X
Enfortumab vedotin			X			X
Epirubicin		X				X
Erdafitinib			X			X
Estramustine			X			X
Etoposide		X			X	
Etoposide phosphate		X				X
Floxuridine		X				X
Fludarabine		X				X
5–Fluorouracil	X					X
Flutamide		X				X
Gemcitabine	X				X	
Gilteritinib			X			X
Glasdegib			X			X
Goserelin			X			X
Hydroxyurea		X				X
Ibrutinib		X				X
Idarubicin		X				X
Ifosfamide	X			X		
Imatinib		X				X
Irinotecan	X					X
Isatuximab		X				X
Isotretinoin		X				X
Ivosidenib			X			X
Ixazomib		X				X

Table 3-5 (cont.)

Drug	Hemodialysis			Peritoneal Dialysis		
	YES	NO	UNKNOWN	YES	NO	UNKNOWN
Lapatinib			X			X
Larotrectinib			X			X
Lenalidomide			X			X
Leuprolide		X				X
Lomustine	X					X
Lorlatinib			X			X
Mechlorethamine			X			X
Megestrol acetate			X			X
Melphalan	X					X
6–Mercaptopurine			X			X
Methotrexate	X			X		
Mitomycin–C			X			X
Mitotane			X			X
Mitoxantrone			X			X
Mogamulizumab-kcpc			X			X
Moxetumomab pasudotox			X			X
Nelarabine			X			X
Nilotinib		X				X
Nilutamide			X			X
Nivolumab			X			X
Ofatumumab			X			X
Oxaliplatin	X					X
Paclitaxel		X			X	
Pazopanib			X			X
Pembrolizumab			X			X
Pemetrexed		X				X
Pemigatinib			X			X
Pentostatin			X			X
Pertuzumab			X			X
Polatuzumab vedotin			X			X
Pomalidomide			X			X
Ponatinib			X		X	

Table 3-5 (cont.)

Drug	Hemodialysis			Peritoneal Dialysis		
	YES	NO	UNKNOWN	YES	NO	UNKNOWN
Pralatrexate			X			X
Procarbazine			X			X
Ramucirumab			X			X
Regorafenib			X			X
Ripretinib			X			X
Rituximab			X			X
Rucaparib			X			X
Selinexor			X			X
Selpercatinib			X			X
Sorafenib		X			X	
Streptozocin			X			X
Sunitinib		X				X
Talazoparib			X			X
Tamoxifen	X					X
Temozolomide			X			X
Temsirolimus			X			X
Thalidomide			X			X
Thioguanine			X			X
Thiotepa			X			X
Topotecan			X			X
Trametinib			X			X
Trastuzumab			X			X
Tucatinib			X			X
Vemurafenib			X			X
Vinblastine		X				X
Vincristine		X				X
Vinorelbine		X				X
Vorinostat			X			X
Zanubrutinib			X			X
Ziv–aflibercept			X			X

Box 3-4. Classification of Teratogenic Potential and Use in Pregnancy for Chemotherapy Agents

Pregnancy Category A. Controlled studies show no risk in pregnancy.

Controlled studies in pregnant women have not shown an increased risk of fetal abnormalities when the drug is administered during pregnancy. The possibility of fetal harm appears remote when the drug is used during pregnancy.

Pregnancy Category B. No evidence of risk in pregnancy.

a. Controlled studies in animals have shown that the drug poses a risk to the fetus. However, studies in pregnant women have failed to show such a risk.

b. Controlled studies in animals do not show evidence of impaired fertility or harm to the fetus. However, similar studies have not been performed in humans. Because animal studies are not entirely predictive of human response, the drug should be used during pregnancy only if clearly needed.

Pregnancy Category C. Risk in pregnancy cannot be ruled out.

Controlled studies either have not been conducted in animals or show that the drug is teratogenic or has an embryocidal effect and/or other adverse effect in animals. However, there are no adequate and well–controlled studies in pregnant women. The drug should be used during pregnancy only if the potential benefit justifies the potential risk to the fetus. The drug can cause fetal harm when administered to a pregnant woman. If the drug is used during pregnancy, or if a patient becomes pregnant while taking this drug, the patient should be informed of the potential hazard to the fetus. However, the potential benefits of treatment may outweigh any potential risk.

Pregnancy Category D. Clear evidence of risk in pregnancy.

The drug can cause fetal harm when administered to a pregnant woman. If the drug is used during pregnancy, or if a patient becomes pregnant while taking this drug, the patient should be informed of the potential hazard to the fetus. However, the potential benefits of treatment may outweigh any potential risk.

Pregnancy Category X. Absolutely contraindicated in pregnancy.

The drug has been shown to cause fetal harm when administered to a pregnant woman. The drug is absolutely contraindicated in women who are or who may become pregnant. If this drug is used during pregnancy or if a patient becomes pregnant while taking this drug, the patient should be informed of the potential hazard to the fetus. In this setting, the potential risk outweighs any potential benefit from treatment.

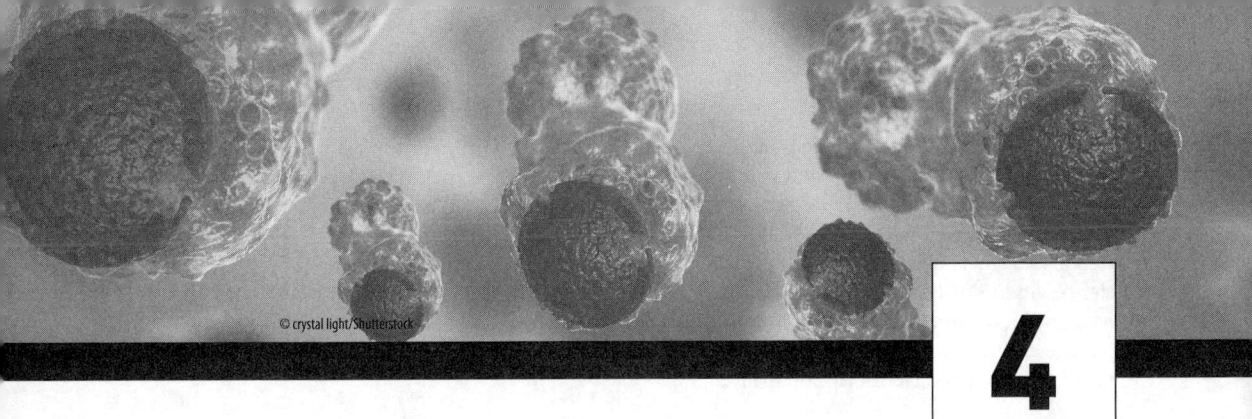
© crystal light/Shutterstock

4

Common Chemotherapy Regimens in Clinical Practice

Chaoyuan Kuang, M. Sitki Copur, Fernand Bteich, Matthew Lee, Laurie J. Harrold, and Edward Chu

This chapter provides some of the common combination regimens and selected single-agent regimens for solid tumors and hematologic malignancies. They are organized alphabetically by the specific cancer type. In each case, the regimens selected are based on the published literature and are used in clinical practice in the medical oncology community. It should be emphasized that not all of the drugs and dosages in the regimens have been officially approved by the Food and Drug Administration (FDA) for the treatment of a particular tumor. As such, the reader should be aware that some of these treatment regimens may not be approved for reimbursement. This chapter should serve as a quick reference for physicians and healthcare providers actively engaged in the practice of cancer treatment and provides several options for treating an individual tumor type. It is not intended to be an all-inclusive review of current treatments, nor is it intended to endorse and/or prioritize any particular combination or single-agent regimen.

It is important to emphasize that the reader should carefully review the original reference for each of the regimens cited to confirm the specific doses and schedules and to check the complete prescribing information contained within the package insert for each agent.

Considerable efforts have been made to ensure the accuracy of the regimens presented. However, it is possible that printing and/or typographical errors may have been made in the preparation of this book. As a result, no liability can be assumed for their use. Moreover, the reader should be reminded that several variations in combination and single-agent regimens exist based on institutional and/or individual experience. Additionally, modifications in dose and schedule may be required according to individual performance status, comorbid illnesses, baseline blood counts, baseline hepatic and/or renal function, development of toxicity, and co-administration of other prescription and non-prescription drugs.

ADRENOCORTICAL CANCER

Combination Regimens

Etoposide + Doxorubicin + Cisplatin + Mitotane

Etoposide:	100 mg/m^2 IV on days 5–7
Doxorubicin:	20 mg/m^2 on days 1 and 8
Cisplatin:	40 mg/m^2 IV on days 1 and 9
Mitotane:	4 g PO daily

Repeat cycle every 21 days [1].

Streptozocin + Mitotane

Streptozocin:	1,000 mg IV on days 1–5 for cycle 1 and 2,000 mg IV on days 1–5 on subsequent cycles
Mitotane:	4 g PO daily

Repeat cycle every 28 days [1].

ANAL CANCER

Combined Modality Therapy

5-Fluorouracil + Mitomycin-C + Radiation Therapy (RTOG/ECOG regimen)

5-Fluorouracil:	1,000 mg/m^2/day IV continuous infusion on days 1–4 and 29–32
Mitomycin-C:	10 mg/m^2 IV (maximum of 20 mg) on days 1 and 29
Radiation therapy:	180 cGy/day, 5 days/week for a total of 5 weeks (total dose, 4,500 cGy)

Chemotherapy is given concurrently with radiation therapy [2].

5-Fluorouracil + Mitomycin-C + Radiation Therapy (EORTC regimen)

5-Fluorouracil:	200 mg/m^2/day IV continuous infusion on days 1–26
Mitomycin-C:	10 mg/m^2 IV on day 1
Radiation therapy:	180 cGy/day, 5 days/week for a total of 4 weeks (total dose, 3,600 cGy)

Chemotherapy is given concurrently with radiation therapy [3]. There is a 2-week break following the completion of this first treatment, after which the second treatment is initiated with concurrent chemotherapy and radiation therapy.

5-Fluorouracil:	200 mg/m^2/day IV continuous infusion on days 1–17
Mitomycin-C:	10 mg/m^2 IV on day 1
Radiation therapy:	Total dose, 2,340 cGy over 17 days

Capecitabine + Mitomycin-C + Radiation Therapy

Capecitabine:	825 mg/m^2 PO bid on Monday–Friday
Mitomycin-C:	10 mg/m^2 IV on days 1 and 29
Radiation therapy:	Total dose, 5,500 cGy over 6 weeks

Chemotherapy is given concurrently with radiation therapy [4].

5-Fluorouracil + Cisplatin + Radiation Therapy

5-Fluorouracil:	1,000 mg/m^2/day IV continuous infusion on days 1–4 of each week of radiation therapy
Cisplatin:	75 mg/m^2 on days 1, 29, 57, and 85 during radiation therapy
Radiation therapy:	Total dose, 4,500 cGy over 5 weeks

Chemotherapy is given concurrently with radiation therapy [5].

XELOX + Radiation Therapy

Capecitabine:	825 mg/m^2 PO bid on Monday–Friday for 6 weeks
Oxaliplatin:	50 mg/m^2 IV on days 1, 8, 22, 29
Radiation Therapy:	180 cGy/day, 5 days/week for a total of 6 weeks

Chemotherapy is given concurrently with radiation therapy [6].

Metastatic Disease

Combination Regimens

5-Fluorouracil + Cisplatin

5-Fluorouracil: 1,000 mg/m^2/day IV continuous infusion on days 1–5

Cisplatin: 100 mg/m^2 IV on day 2

Repeat cycles every 4 weeks [7].

Carboplatin + Paclitaxel

Carboplatin: AUC of 5, IV on day 1

Paclitaxel: 175 mg/m^2 IV on day 1

Repeat cycles every 3 weeks [8].

mFOLFOX6

Oxaliplatin: 85 mg/m^2 IV on day 1

5-Fluorouracil: 400 mg/m^2 IV bolus on day 1, then 2,400 mg/m^2 IV continuous infusion over 46 hours

Leucovorin: 400 mg/m^2 IV on day 1

Repeat cycles every 2 weeks [9].

FOLCIS

Cisplatin: 40 mg/m^2 IV on day 1

5-Fluorouracil: 400 mg/m^2 IV bolus on day 1, then 2,000 mg/m^2 IV continuous infusion over 46 hours

Leucovorin: 400 mg/m^2 IV on day 1

Repeat cycles every 2 weeks [10].

Single-Agent Regimens

Pembrolizumab

Pembrolizumab: 10 mg/kg IV on day 1 or 200 mg IV on day 1

Repeat cycles every 2 weeks if using 10 mg/kg dosing, or every 3 weeks if using 200 mg dosing [11].

Nivolumab

Nivolumab: 480 mg IV on day 1

Repeat cycles every 4 weeks [12].

BASAL CELL CANCER

Single-Agent Regimens

Vismodegib

Vismodegib: 150 mg PO daily

Continue treatment until disease progression [13].

Sonidegib

Sonidegib: 200 mg PO daily

Continue treatment until disease progression [14].

Cemiplimab

Cemiplimab: 350 mg IV on day 1

Repeat cycle every 21 days [15].

BILIARY TRACT CANCER

Adjuvant Therapy

Capecitabine

Capecitabine: $1,250$ mg/m^2 PO bid on days 1–14

Repeat cycles every 21 days for a total of 8 cycles [16].

Locally Advanced Disease

Capecitabine + Gemcitabine + Concurrent RT/Capecitabine

Capecitabine: $1,500$ mg/m^2 PO on days 1–14

Gemcitabine: $1,000$ mg/m^2 IV on days 1 and 8

Repeat cycle every 21 days for 4 cycles [17] followed by

Capecitabine: $1,330$ mg/m^2 PO daily concurrent with

Radiation therapy: 45 Gy to regional lymph nodes; 54 to 59.4 Gy to tumor bed

Metastatic Disease

Combination Regimens

Gemcitabine + Cisplatin + Durvalumab

Gemcitabine: $1,250$ mg/m^2 IV on days 1 and 8

Cisplatin: 25 mg/m^2 on days 1 and 8

Durvalumab: $1,500$ mg IV on day 1

Repeat cycle every 21 days, and treat for up to 8 cycles [18]. After completion of gemcitabine and cisplatin, administer durvalumab monotherapy once every 4 weeks until disease progression or toxicity.

Gemcitabine + Cisplatin

Gemcitabine:	1,250 mg/m^2 IV on days 1 and 8
Cisplatin:	75 mg/m^2 on day 1

Repeat cycle every 21 days [19].

or

Gemcitabine:	1,000 mg/m^2 IV on days 1 and 8
Cisplatin:	25–30 mg/m^2 on days 1 and 8

Repeat cycle every 21 days for 8 cycles [20].

Gemcitabine + Cisplatin + Nab-Paclitaxel

Gemcitabine:	800 mg/m^2 IV on days 1 and 8
Cisplatin:	25 mg/m^2 IV on days 1 and 8
Nab-Paclitaxel:	100 mg/m^2 IV on days 1 and 8

Repeat cycle every 21 days [21].

Gemcitabine + Capecitabine

Gemcitabine:	1,000 mg/m^2 IV on days 1 and 8
Capecitabine:	650 mg/m^2 PO bid on days 1–14

Repeat cycle every 21 days [22].

Gemcitabine + Oxaliplatin

Gemcitabine:	1,000 mg/m^2 IV on day 1
Oxaliplatin:	100 mg/m^2 on day 2

Repeat cycle every 14 days [23].

5-Fluorouracil + Cisplatin

5-Fluorouracil:	400 mg/m^2 IV on day 1, followed by 600 mg/m^2 IV infusion over 22 hours on days 1 and 2
Cisplatin:	50 mg/m^2 IV on day 2

Repeat cycle every 21 days [24].

Oxaliplatin + 5-Fluorouracil + Leucovorin (FOLFOX4)

Oxaliplatin:	85 mg/m^2 IV on day 1
5-Fluorouracil:	400 mg/m^2 IV bolus, followed by 600 mg/m^2 IV continuous infusion for 22 hours on days 1 and 2
Leucovorin:	200 mg/m^2 IV on days 1 and 2 as a 2-hour infusion before 5-fluorouracil

Repeat cycle every 2 weeks [25].

Capecitabine + Cisplatin

Capecitabine: $1{,}250$ mg/m^2 PO bid on days 1–14

Cisplatin: 60 mg/m^2 IV on day 2

Repeat cycle every 21 days [26].

Capecitabine + Oxaliplatin

Capecitabine: $1{,}000$ mg/m^2 PO bid on days 1–14

Oxaliplatin: 130 mg/m^2 IV on day 1

Repeat cycle every 21 days [27].

Gemcitabine + Nab-Paclitaxel

Gemcitabine: $1{,}000$ mg/m^2 IV on days 1, 8, and 15

Nab-Paclitaxel: 125 mg/m^2 IV on days 1, 8, and 15

Repeat cycle every 28 days [28].

Dabrafenib + Trametinib (BRAF:V600E mutation)

Dabrafenib: 150 mg PO bid

Trametinib: 2 mg PO daily

Continue treatment until disease progression [29].

Single-Agent Regimens

Capecitabine

Capecitabine: $1{,}000$ mg/m^2 PO bid on days 1–14

Repeat cycle every 21 days [30]. Dose may be reduced to 825–900 mg/m^2 PO bid on days 1–14.

Pembrolizumab

Pembrolizumab: 200 mg IV on day 1

Repeat cycle every 3 weeks [31]. Used only in the setting of MSI/dMMR and TMB-H tumors.

Gemcitabine

Gemcitabine: $1{,}000$ mg/m^2 IV on days 1 and 8

Repeat cycle every 21 days [32].

Ivosidenib (IDH1 mutation)

Ivosidenib: 500 mg PO daily

Repeat cycle every 28 days [33].

Pemigatinib (FGFR2 fusions or rearrangements)

Pemigatinib: 13.5 mg PO daily for 14 days
Repeat cycle every 21 days [34].

Futibatinib (FGFR2 fusions or rearrangements)

Futibatinib: 20 mg PO daily
Continue until disease progression of toxicity [35].

Infigratinib (FGFR2 fusions or rearrangements)

Infigratinib: 125 mg PO daily for 21 days
Repeat cycle every 28 days [36].

BLADDER CANCER

Adjuvant Therapy

Single-Agent Regimens

Nivolumab

Nivolumab: 240 mg IV day on 1
Repeat cycle every 2 weeks for up to 1 year [37].

Advanced Disease

Combination Regimens

ITP

Ifosfamide: 1,500 mg/m^2 IV on days 1–3
Paclitaxel: 200 mg/m^2 IV over 3 hours on day 1
Cisplatin: 70 mg/m^2 IV on day 1
Repeat cycle every 21 days [38]. G-CSF support is recommended. Regimen can also be administered every 28 days.

Dose-Dense Gemcitabine + Cisplatin

Gemcitabine: 2,500 mg/m^2 IV on day 1
Cisplatin: 35 mg/m^2 IV on days 1 and 2
Repeat cycle every 14 days for up to 6 cycles [39].

Gemcitabine + Cisplatin

Gemcitabine: 1,000 mg/m^2 IV on days 1, 8, and 15
Cisplatin: 75 mg/m^2 IV on day 1
Repeat cycle every 28 days [40].

Gemcitabine + Carboplatin

Gemcitabine: 1,000 mg/m^2 IV on days 1 and 8
Carboplatin: AUC of 4, IV on day 1
Repeat cycle every 21 days up to 6 cycles [41].

Gemcitabine + Paclitaxel

Gemcitabine: 1,000 mg/m^2 IV on days 1, 8, and 15
Paclitaxel: 200 mg/m^2 IV on day 1
Repeat cycle every 21 days [42].
or
Gemcitabine: 2,500 mg/m^2 IV on day 1
Paclitaxel: 150 mg/m^2 IV on day 1
Repeat cycle every 14 days [43].

Gemcitabine + Docetaxel

Gemcitabine: 1,000 mg/m^2 IV on days 1, 8, and 15
Docetaxel: 60 mg/m^2 IV on day 1
Repeat cycle every 28 days [44].

Dose-Dense MVAC

Methotrexate: 30 mg/m^2 IV on days 1, 15, and 22
Vinblastine: 3 mg/m^2 IV on days 2, 15, and 22
Doxorubicin: 30 mg/m^2 IV on day 2
Cisplatin: 70 mg/m^2 IV on day 2
Repeat cycle every 28 days [45].

CMV

Cisplatin: 100 mg/m^2 IV on day 2 (give 12 hours after methotrexate)

Methotrexate: 30 mg/m^2 IV on days 1 and 8
Vinblastine: 4 mg/m^2 IV on days 1 and 8
Repeat cycle every 21 days [46].

MCV

Methotrexate:	30 mg/m^2 IV on days 1, 15, and 22
Carboplatin:	AUC of 4.5, IV on day 1
Vinblastine:	3 mg/m^2 IV on days 1, 15, and 22

Repeat cycle every 28 days [47].

Docetaxel + Cisplatin

Docetaxel:	75 mg/m^2 IV on day 1
Cisplatin:	75 mg/m^2 IV on day 1

Repeat cycle every 21 days up to 6 cycles [48].

Paclitaxel + Carboplatin

Paclitaxel:	225 mg/m^2 IV over 3 hours on day 1
Carboplatin:	AUC of 6, IV on day 1, given 15 minutes after paclitaxel

Repeat cycle every 21 days [49].

CAP

Cyclophosphamide:	400 mg/m^2 IV on day 1
Doxorubicin:	40 mg/m^2 IV on day 1
Cisplatin:	75 mg/m^2 IV on day 2

Repeat cycle every 21 days [50].

5-Fluorouracil + Mitomycin-C + Radiation Therapy

5-Fluorouracil:	500 mg/m^2/day IV continuous infusion on days 1–5 and 16–20 of radiotherapy
Mitomycin-C:	12 mg/m^2 IV on day 1

Radiation therapy 275 cGy/day, 5 days/week for a total of 4 weeks (total dose, 5,500 cGy) or 200 cGy/day for 6.5 weeks (total dose, 6,400 cGy)

Chemotherapy is given concurrently with radiation therapy [51].

Enfortumab vedotin + Pembrolizumab

Enfortumab vedotin:	1.25 mg/kg (up to maximum of 125 mg) IV on days 1, 8, and 15
Pembrolizumab:	200 mg IV on day 1

Repeat cycle every 21 days [52].

Single-Agent Regimens

Gemcitabine

Gemcitabine:	1,200 mg/m^2 IV on days 1, 8, and 15

Repeat cycle every 28 days [53].

Paclitaxel

Paclitaxel: 250 mg/m^2 IV over 24 hours on day 1
Repeat cycle every 21 days [54].
or
Paclitaxel: 80 mg/m^2 IV weekly for 3 weeks
Repeat cycle every 4 weeks [55].

Pemetrexed

Pemetrexed: 500 mg/m^2 IV on day 1
Repeat cycle every 21 days [56]. Folic acid at 350–1,000 μg PO daily beginning 1–2 weeks prior to therapy and vitamin B12 at 1,000 μg IM to start 1–2 weeks prior to first dose of therapy and repeated every 3 cycles.

Atezolizumab

Atezolizumab: 1,200 mg IV on day 1
Repeat cycle every 21 days [57].

Avelumab

Avelumab: 10 mg/kg IV on day 1
Repeat cycle every 14 days [58].

Durvalumab

Durvalumab: 10 mg/kg IV on day 1
Repeat cycle every 14 days [59].

Nivolumab

Nivolumab: 240 mg IV on day 1
Repeat cycle every 14 days [60]. May also administer 480 mg IV on day 1 with cycles repeated every 28 days.

Pembrolizumab

Pembrolizumab: 200 mg IV on day 1
Repeat cycle every 21 days [61]. May also administer 400 mg IV every 6 weeks.

Erdafitinib

Erdafitinib: 8 mg PO daily
Continue treatment until disease progression [62]. Increase dose to 9 mg daily if serum phosphate level <5.5 mg/dL, and there are no ocular disorders or grade ≥2 adverse events.

Enfortumab vedotin-ejfv

Enfortumab vedotin-ejfv:
Repeat cycle every 28 days [63].

1.25 mg/kg IV on days 1, 8, and 15

Sacituzumab govitecan

Sacituzumab govitecan:
Repeat cycle every 28 days [64].

10 mg/kg IV on days 1 and 8

Mitomycin

Mitomycin:

Instill 4 mg/mL via ureteral catheter or nephrostomy tube with total instillation volume not to exceed 15 mL (60 mg)

Instill once weekly for 6 weeks [65]. For patients with a complete response 3 months after initiation of therapy, mitomycin instillations may be administered once a month for a maximum of 11 additional instillations.

Nadofaragene

Nadofaragene:

Instill 75 mL (3×10^{11} viral particles/mL) via ureteral catheter

Instill once every 3 months for up to 12 months [66].

BLASTIC DENDRITIC CELL PLASMACYTOID CANCER

Single-Agent Regimens

Tagraxofusp

Tagraxofusp:
Repeat cycle every 21 days [66a].

12 mcg/kg IV on days 1-5

BRAIN CANCER

Adjuvant Therapy

Combination Regimens

Temozolomide Radiation Therapy

Radiation therapy:

200 cGy/day for 5 days per week for total of 6 weeks

Temozolomide:	75 mg/m^2 PO daily for 6 weeks with radiation therapy. After a 4-week break, 150 mg/m^2 PO on days 1–5

Repeat temozolomide monotherapy every 28 days for up to 6 cycles [67]. If well tolerated, can increase dose to 200 mg/m^2 on subsequent cycles. Patients should be placed on either inhaled pentamidine or trimethoprim/sulfamethoxazole for PCP prophylaxis during the combined-modality regimen.

PCV

Procarbazine:	60 mg/m^2 PO on days 8–21
Lomustine:	130 mg/m^2 PO on day 1
Vincristine:	1.4 mg/m^2 IV on days 8 and 29

Repeat cycle every 8 weeks for 6 cycles [68].

Single-Agent Regimens

Carmustine

Carmustine:	220 mg/m^2 IV on day 1

Repeat cycle every 6–8 weeks for 1 year [69].

or

Carmustine:	75–100 mg/m^2 IV on days 1 and 2

Repeat cycle every 6–8 weeks [69].

Advanced Disease

Combination Regimens

PCV

Procarbazine:	75 mg/m^2 PO on days 8–21
Lomustine:	130 mg/m^2 PO on day 1
Vincristine:	1.4 mg/m^2 IV on days 8 and 29

Repeat cycle every 8 weeks [70].

Irinotecan + Bevacizumab

Irinotecan:	125 mg/m^2 IV on day 1
Bevacizumab:	10 mg/kg IV on day 1

Repeat cycle every 2 weeks for 6 cycles [71].

Temozolomide + Bevacizumab

Temozolomide:	100 mg/m^2 PO on days 1–5 and days 15-19
Bevacizumab:	10 mg/kg IV on days 1 and 15

Repeat cycle every 28 days [72].

Carboplatin + Irinotecan + Bevacizumab

Carboplatin: AUC of 4, IV on day 1
Irinotecan: 340 mg/m^2 IV on days 1 and 14
Bevacizumab: 10 mg/kg IV on days 1 and 14
Repeat cycle every 28 days [73].

Temozolomide + Lomustine

Temozolomide: 100 mg/m^2 PO on days 2–6
Lomustine: 100 mg/m^2 PO on day 1
Repeat cycle every 28 days up to 6 cycles [74].

Single-Agent Regimens
Carmustine

Carmustine: 200 mg/m^2 IV on day 1
Repeat cycle every 6–8 weeks [75].

Procarbazine

Procarbazine: 150 mg/m^2 PO daily divided into
                                                            3 doses

Repeat daily [75].

Temozolomide

Temozolomide: 150 mg/m^2 PO on days 1–5
Repeat cycle every 28 days [76]. If tolerated, can increase dose to 200 mg/m^2.

Irinotecan

Irinotecan: 350 mg/m^2 IV over 90 min on day 1
Repeat cycle every 3 weeks [77].
or
Irinotecan: 125 mg/m^2 IV weekly for 4 weeks
Repeat cycle every 6 weeks [78].

Bevacizumab

Bevacizumab: 15 mg/kg IV on day 1
Repeat cycle every 3 weeks [79].

BREAST CANCER

Neoadjuvant Therapy

Combination Regimens

ACT

Doxorubicin:	60 mg/m^2 IV on day 1
Cyclophosphamide:	600 mg/m^2 IV on day 1
Docetaxel:	100 mg/m^2 IV on day 1

Repeat cycle every 21 days for a total of 4 cycles, followed by surgery [80].

Docetaxel + Carboplatin + Pertuzumab + Trastuzumab

Docetaxel:	75 mg/m^2 IV on day 1
Carboplatin:	AUC 6, IV on day 1
Pertuzumab:	840 mg IV loading dose on day 1 and then 420 mg IV every 3 weeks
Trastuzumab:	8 mg/kg IV loading dose on day 1 and then 6 mg/kg IV every 3 weeks

Repeat cycle every 21 days [81].

Adjuvant Therapy

Combination Regimens: HER2-negative disease

AC

Doxorubicin:	60 mg/m^2 IV on day 1
Cyclophosphamide:	600 mg/m^2 IV on day 1

Repeat cycle every 21 days for a total of 4 cycles [82].

AC→T

Doxorubicin:	60 mg/m^2 IV on day 1
Cyclophosphamide:	600 mg/m^2 IV on day 1

Repeat cycle every 21 days for a total of 4 cycles, followed by

Paclitaxel:	175 mg/m^2 IV on day 1

Repeat cycle every 21 days for a total of 4 cycles [83].

AC→T (weekly)

Doxorubicin:	60 mg/m^2 IV on day 1
Cyclophosphamide:	600 mg/m^2 IV on day 1

Repeat cycle every 21 days for a total of 4 cycles, followed by

Paclitaxel:	80 mg/m^2 IV on day 1

Repeat on a weekly schedule for 12 weeks [84].

AC→Docetaxel

Doxorubicin:	60 mg/m^2 IV on day 1
Cyclophosphamide:	600 mg/m^2 IV on day 1

Repeat cycle every 21 days for a total of 4 cycles, followed by

Paclitaxel:	100 mg/m^2 IV on day 1

Repeat cycle every 21 days for a total of 4 cycles [85].

AC→Docetaxel (weekly)

Doxorubicin:	60 mg/m^2 IV on day 1
Cyclophosphamide:	600 mg/m^2 IV on day 1

Repeat cycle every 21 days for a total of 4 cycles, followed by

Docetaxel:	35 mg/m^2 IV on day

Repeat weekly for a total of 12 weeks [86].

TC

Docetaxel:	75 mg/m^2 IV on day 1
Cyclophosphamide:	600 mg/m^2 IV on day 1

Repeat cycle every 21 days for a total of 4 cycles [87].

TAC

Docetaxel:	75 mg/m^2 IV on day 1
Doxorubicin:	50 mg/m^2 IV on day 1
Cyclophosphamide:	500 mg/m^2 IV on day 1

Repeat cycle every 21 days for a total of 6 cycles [88].

CAF

Cyclophosphamide:	600 mg/m^2 IV on day 1
Doxorubicin:	60 mg/m^2 IV on day 1
5-Fluorouracil:	600 mg/m^2 IV on day 1

Repeat cycle every 28 days for a total of 4 cycles [89].

Epirubicin + CMF

Epirubicin:	100 mg/m^2 IV on day 1

Repeat cycle every 21 days for 4 cycles, followed by

Cyclophosphamide:	600 mg/m^2 IV on day 1
Methotrexate:	40 mg/m^2 IV on day 1
5-Fluorouracil:	600 mg/m^2 IV on day 1

Repeat cycle every 21 days for a total of 4 cycles [90].

FEC

5-Fluorouracil:	500 mg/m^2 IV on day 1
Epirubicin:	100 mg/m^2 IV on day 1
Cyclophosphamide:	500 mg/m^2 IV on day 1

Repeat cycle every 21 days for a total of 6 cycles [91].

FEC→Docetaxel

5-Fluorouracil:	500 mg/m^2 IV on day 1
Epirubicin:	100 mg/m^2 IV on day 1
Cyclophosphamide:	500 mg/m^2 IV on day 1

Repeat cycle every 21 days for a total of 6 cycles [92], followed by

Docetaxel:	100 mg/m^2 IV on day 1

Repeat cycle every 21 days for 3 cycles.

Dose-Dense Combination Regimens: HER2-negative disease

AC→T

Doxorubicin:	60 mg/m^2 IV on day 1
Cyclophosphamide:	600 mg/m^2 IV on day 1

Repeat cycle every 14 days for a total of 4 cycles, followed by

Paclitaxel:	175 mg/m^2 IV on day 1

Repeat cycle every 14 days for a total of 4 cycles [93].
Administer pegfilgrastim 6 mg SC on day 2 of each treatment cycle.

A→T→C

Doxorubicin:	60 mg/m^2 IV on day 1

Repeat cycle every 2 weeks for 4 cycles, followed by

Paclitaxel:	175 mg/m^2 IV on day 1

Repeat cycle every 2 weeks for 4 cycles, followed by

Cyclophosphamide:	600 mg/m^2 IV on day 1

Repeat cycle every 2 weeks for 4 cycles.
Administer filgrastim 5 μg/kg SC on days 3–10 of each treatment cycle [94].

AC→Docetaxel

Doxorubicin:	60 mg/m^2 IV on day 1
Cyclophosphamide:	600 mg/m^2 IV on day 1

Repeat cycle every 14 days for a total of 4 cycles, followed by

Cyclophosphamide:	75 mg/m^2 IV on day 1

Repeat cycle every 14 days for a total of 4 cycles [95].
Administer pegfilgrastim 6 mg SC on day 2 of each treatment cycle.

Docetaxel→AC

Docetaxel:	75 mg/m^2 IV on day 1

Repeat cycle every 14 days for a total of 4 cycles, followed by

Doxorubicin:	60 mg/m^2 IV on day 1
Cyclophosphamide:	600 mg/m^2 IV on day 1

Repeat cycle every 14 days for a total of 4 cycles [95].

Administer pegfilgrastim 6 mg SC on day 2 of each treatment cycle.

Combination Regimens: HER2-positive disease

AC→T + Trastuzumab

Doxorubicin:	60 mg/m^2 IV on day 1
Cyclophosphamide:	600 mg/m^2 IV on day 1

Repeat cycle every 21 days for a total of 4 cycles, followed by

Paclitaxel:	80 mg/m^2 IV over 1 hour on day 1
Trastuzumab:	4 mg/kg IV loading dose, then 2 mg/kg IV weekly

Repeat weekly for 12 weeks, followed by

Trastuzumab:	2 mg/kg IV weekly

Repeat weekly for 40 weeks [96].

AC→T + Trastuzumab (dose-dense)

Doxorubicin:	60 mg/m^2 IV on day 1
Cyclophosphamide:	600 mg/m^2 IV on day 1

Repeat cycle every 14 days for a total of 4 cycles, followed by

Paclitaxel:	175 mg/m^2 IV on day 1

Repeat cycle every 14 days for a total of 4 cycles.

Trastuzumab:	4 mg/kg IV loading dose along with paclitaxel and then 2 mg/kg IV weekly

Trastuzumab is administered for a total of 1 year [97].

TCH

Docetaxel:	75 mg/m^2 IV on day 1
Carboplatin:	AUC of 6, IV on day 1
Trastuzumab:	4 mg/kg IV loading dose and then 2 mg/kg IV weekly

Repeat chemotherapy every 21 days for a total of 6 cycles. At the completion of chemotherapy, trastuzumab is administered at 6 mg/kg IV every 3 weeks for a total of 1 year [98].

DH→FEC

Docetaxel:	100 mg/m^2 IV on day 1
Trastuzumab	4 mg/kg IV loading dose on day 1 and then 2 mg/kg IV weekly

Repeat cycle every 21 days for 3 cycles, followed by

5-Fluorouracil:	600 mg/m^2 IV on day 1
Epirubicin:	60 mg/m^2 IV on day 1
Cyclophosphamide:	600 mg/m^2 IV on day 1

Repeat cycle every 21 days for 3 cycles [99].

Pertuzumab + Trastuzumab + Docetaxel

Docetaxel:	75 mg/m^2 IV on day 1
Trastuzumab:	8 mg/kg IV loading dose on day 1 and then 6 mg/kg IV every 3 weeks
Pertuzumab:	840 mg IV loading dose on day 1 and then 420 mg IV every 3 weeks

Repeat cycle every 21 days [100].

Single-Agent Regimens

Neratinib

Neratinib:	240 mg PO daily

Repeat daily for 1 year in patients following trastuzumab-based adjuvant therapy [101].

Ado-trastuzumab emtansine

Ado-trastuzumab emtansine:	3.6 mg/kg IV on day 1

Repeat cycle every 21 days for a total of 14 cycles [102].

Hormonal Regimens

Tamoxifen

Tamoxifen:	20 mg PO daily

Repeat daily for 5 years in patients with ER+ tumors or ER status unknown [103].

Anastrozole

Anastrozole:	1 mg PO daily

Repeat daily for 5 years in patients with ER+ tumors or ER status unknown [104].

Letrozole

Letrozole:	2.5 mg PO daily

Repeat daily for 5 years in patients with ER+ or PR+ tumors [105].

Tamoxifen + Letrozole [106]

Tamoxifen:	20 mg PO daily for 5 years, followed by
Letrozole:	2.5 mg PO daily for 5 years

Tamoxifen + Exemestane [107]

Tamoxifen:	20 mg PO daily for 2–3 years, followed by
Exemestane:	25 mg PO daily for the remainder of 5 years

Tamoxifen + Goserelin + Zoledronic acid

Tamoxifen:	20 mg PO daily
Goserelin:	3.6 mg SC every 28 days
Zoledronic acid	4 mg IV every 6 months

Continue treatment for a total of 3 years [108].

Anastrozole + Goserelin + Zoledronic acid

Anastrozole:	1 mg PO daily
Gosrelin:	3.6 mg SC every 28 days
Zoledronic acid	4 mg IV every 6 months

Continue treatment for a total of 3 years [108].

Olaparib

Olaparib:	300 mg PO bid daily

Repeat cycle every 24 days and continue treatment for 12 months [109].

Abemaciclib + Tamoxifen

Abemaciclib:	150 mg PO bid for 2 years
Tamoxifen:	20 mg PO daily for 5 years

Continue treatment with abemaciclib for 2 years and with tamoxifen for 5 years [110].

Abemaciclib + Aromatase Inhibitor

Abemaciclib:	150 mg PO bid for 2 years
Aromatase Inhibitor:	PO daily for five years

Continue treatment with abemaciclib for 2 years and with aromatase inhibitor for 5 years [111].

Everolimus + Exemestane [112]

Everolimus:	10 mg PO daily
Exemestane:	25 mg PO daily

Metastatic Disease

Combination Regimens: HER2-negative disease

AC

Doxorubicin:	60 mg/m^2 IV on day 1
Cyclophosphamide:	600 mg/m^2 IV on day 1

Repeat cycle every 21 days [82].

AT

Doxorubicin:	50 mg/m^2 IV on day 1
Paclitaxel:	150 mg/m^2 IV over 24 hours on day 1

Repeat cycle every 21 days [113].

or

Doxorubicin:	60 mg/m^2 IV on day 1

Repeat cycle every 21 days up to a maximum of 8 cycles, followed by

Paclitaxel:	175 mg/m^2 IV on day 1

Repeat cycle every 21 days until disease progression [113].

or

Paclitaxel:	175 mg/m^2 IV on day 1

Repeat cycle every 21 days until disease progression, followed by

Doxorubicin:	60 mg/m^2 IV on day 1

Repeat cycle every 21 days up to a maximum of 8 cycles [113].

CAF

Cyclophosphamide:	600 mg/m^2 IV on day 1
Doxorubicin:	60 mg/m^2 IV on day 1
5-Fluorouracil:	600 mg/m^2 IV on day 1

Repeat cycle every 21 days [89].

CEF

Cyclophosphamide:	75 mg/m^2 PO on days 1–14
Epirubicin:	60 mg/m^2 IV on days 1 and 8
5-Fluorouracil:	500 mg/m^2 IV on days 1 and 8

Repeat cycle every 28 days [114].

CMF

Cyclophosphamide:	600 mg/m^2 IV on day 1
Methotrexate:	40 mg/m^2 IV on day 1
5-Fluorouracil:	600 mg/m^2 IV on day 1

Repeat cycle every 21 days [90].

Capecitabine + Docetaxel (XT)

Capecitabine:	1,250 mg/m^2 PO bid on days 1–14
Docetaxel:	75 mg/m^2 IV on day 1

Repeat cycle every 21 days [115]. May decrease dose of capecitabine to 825–1,000 mg/m^2 PO bid on days 1–14 to reduce the risk of toxicity without compromising clinical efficacy.

Capecitabine + Paclitaxel (XP)

Capecitabine:	825 mg/m^2 PO bid on days 1–14
Paclitaxel:	175 mg/m^2 IV on day 1

Repeat cycle every 21 days [116].

Capecitabine + Navelbine (XN)

Capecitabine:	1,000 mg/m^2 PO bid on days 1–14
Navelbine:	25 mg/m^2 IV on days 1 and 8

Repeat cycle every 21 days [116].

Capecitabine + Ixabepilone (XI)

Capecitabine:	1,000 mg/m^2 PO bid on days 1–14
Ixabepilone:	40 mg/m^2 IV on day 1

Repeat cycle every 21 days [117].

Docetaxel + Doxorubicin

Docetaxel:	75 mg/m^2 IV on day 1
Doxorubicin:	50 mg/m^2 IV on day 1

Repeat cycle every 21 days [118].

Doxorubicin liposome + Docetaxel

Doxorubicin liposome:	30 mg/m^2 on day 1
Docetaxel:	60 mg/m^2 on day 1

Repeat cycle every 21 days [119].

FEC-100

5-Fluorouracil:	500 mg/m^2 IV on day 1
Epirubicin:	100 mg/m^2 IV on day 1
Cyclophosphamide:	500 mg/m^2 IV on day 1

Repeat cycle every 21 days [120].

FEC-75

5-Fluorouracil:	500 mg/m^2 IV on day 1
Epirubicin:	75 mg/m^2 IV on day 1
Cyclophosphamide:	500 mg/m^2 IV on day 1

Repeat cycle every 21 days [121].

FEC-50

5-Fluorouracil:	500 mg/m^2 IV on day 1
Epirubicin:	50 mg/m^2 IV on day 1
Cyclophosphamide:	500 mg/m^2 IV on day 1

Repeat cycle every 21 days [121].

Gemcitabine + Paclitaxel

Gemcitabine:	1,250 mg/m^2 IV on days 1 and 8
Paclitaxel:	175 mg/m^2 IV on day 1

Repeat cycle every 21 days [122].

Carboplatin + Paclitaxel

Carboplatin:	AUC of 6, IV on day 1
Paclitaxel:	200 mg/m^2 IV over 3 hours on day 1

Repeat cycle every 21 days [123].

Carboplatin + Docetaxel

Carboplatin:	AUC of 6, IV day on 1
Docetaxel:	75 mg/m^2 IV on day 1

Repeat cycle every 21 days [124].

Paclitaxel + Bevacizumab

Paclitaxel:	90 mg/m^2 IV on days 1, 8, and 15
Bevacizumab:	10 mg/kg on days 1 and 15

Repeat cycle every 28 days [125].

Atezolizumab + Nab-Paclitaxel

Atezolizumab:	840 mg IV on days 1 and 15
Nab-Paclitaxel:	100 mg/m² IV on days 1, 8, and 15

Repeat cycle every 28 days [126].

Combination Regimens: HER2-positive disease

Pertuzumab + Trastuzumab + Docetaxel

Pertuzumab:	840 mg IV loading dose on day 1 and then 420 mg IV every 3 weeks
Trastuzumab:	8 mg/kg IV loading dose on day 1 and then 6 mg/kg IV every 3 weeks
Docetaxel:	75 mg/m² IV on day 1

Repeat cycle every 21 days [100].

Trastuzumab + Paclitaxel

Trastuzumab:	4 mg/kg IV loading dose and then 2 mg/kg weekly
Paclitaxel:	175 mg/m² IV over 3 hours on day 1

Repeat cycle every 21 days [127].
or

Trastuzumab:	4 mg/kg IV loading dose and then 2 mg/kg weekly
Paclitaxel:	80 mg/m² IV weekly

Repeat cycle every 4 weeks [128].

Trastuzumab + Docetaxel

Trastuzumab:	4 mg/kg IV loading dose and then 2 mg/kg IV on days 8 and 15
Docetaxel:	35 mg/m² IV on days 1, 8, and 15

First cycle is administered weekly for 3 weeks, with 1 week of rest. For subsequent cycles,

Trastuzumab:	2 mg/kg IV weekly
Docetaxel:	35 mg/m² IV weekly

Repeat cycle every 4 weeks [129].

TCH

Carboplatin:	AUC of 6, IV on day 1
Docetaxel:	75 mg/m² IV on day 1
Trastuzumab:	4 mg/kg IV loading dose on day 1 and then 2 mg/kg IV on days 8 and 15, 2 mg/kg IV weekly thereafter

Repeat cycle every 21 days [130].

Gemcitabine + Carboplatin + Trastuzumab

Gemcitabine:	1,500 mg/m^2 IV on day 1
Carboplatin:	AUC of 2.5, IV on day 1
Trastuzumab:	8 mg/kg IV loading dose on day 1 and then 4 mg/kg IV every 2 weeks

Repeat cycle every 2 weeks [131].

Trastuzumab + Navelbine

Trastuzumab:	4 mg/kg IV loading dose and then 2 mg/kg IV weekly
Navelbine:	25 mg/m^2 IV weekly

Repeat on a weekly basis until disease progression [132].

Trastuzumab + Gemcitabine

Trastuzumab:	4 mg/kg IV loading dose and then 2 mg/kg IV weekly
Gemcitabine:	1,200 mg/m^2 IV weekly for 2 weeks

Repeat cycle every 21 days [133].

Trastuzumab + Capecitabine

Trastuzumab:	4 mg/kg IV loading dose and then 2 mg/kg IV weekly
Capecitabine:	1,250 mg/m^2 PO bid on days 1–14

Repeat cycle every 21 days [134].
or

Trastuzumab:	8 mg/kg IV loading dose and then 6 mg/kg IV on day 1 of all subsequent cycles
Capecitabine:	1,250 mg/m^2 PO bid on days 1–14

Repeat cycle every 21 days [135].

Trastuzumab + Lapatinib

Trastuzumab:	4 mg/kg IV loading dose and then 2 mg/kg IV weekly
Lapatinib:	1,000 mg PO daily

Continue until disease progression [136].

Capecitabine + Lapatinib

Capecitabine:	1,000 mg/m^2 PO bid on days 1–14

Lapatinib: 1,250 mg PO daily
Repeat cycle every 21 days [137].

Capecitabine + Neratinib
Capecitabine: 750 mg/m^2 PO bid on days 1–14
Neratinib: 240 mg PO daily
Repeat cycle every 21 days [138].

Tucatinib + Trastuzumab + Capecitabine
Tucatinib: 300 mg PO bid
Trastuzumab: 8 mg/kg IV loading dose followed by
                                            6 mg/kg IV on day 1
Capecitabine: 1,000 mg/m^2 PO bid on days 1–21
Repeat cycle every 21 days [139].

Margetuximab-cmkb + Capecitabine
Margetuximab: 15 mg/kg IV on day 1
Capecitabine: 1,000 mg/m^2 PO bid on days 1–14
Repeat cycle every 21 days [140].

Margetuximab-cmkb + Eribulin
Margetuximab: 15 mg/kg IV on day 1
Eribulin: 1.4 mg/m^2 IV on days 1 and 8
Repeat cycle every 21 days [140].

Margetuximab-cmkb + Vinorelbine
Margetuximab: 15 mg/kg IV on day 1
Vinorelbine: 25 mg/m^2 IV on days 1 and 8
Repeat cycle every 21 days [140].

Margetuximab-cmkb + Gemcitabine
Margetuximab: 15 mg/kg IV on day 1
Gemcitabine: 1,000 mg IV on days 1 and 8
Repeat cycle every 21 days [140].

Combination Regimens: Hormone-Receptor Positive, HER2-Negative Disease
Everolimus + Exemestane [112]
Everolimus: 10 mg PO daily
Exemestane: 25 mg PO daily

Palbociclib + Letrozole

Palbociclib:	125 mg PO daily for 21 days
Letrozole:	2.5 mg PO daily

Repeat cycle every 21 days [141].

Ribociclib + Letrozole

Ribociclib:	600 mg PO daily for 21 days
Letrozole:	2.5 mg PO daily

Repeat cycle every 28 days [142].

Palbociclib + Fulvestrant

Palbociclib:	125 mg PO daily for 21 days
Fulvestrant:	500 mg IM on days 1 and 15 of first cycle and then 500 mg IM on day 1 for all subsequent cycles

Repeat cycle every 28 days [143].

Abemaciclib + Fulvestrant

Abemaciclib:	150 mg PO bid
Fulvestrant:	500 mg IM on days 1 and 15 of first cycle and then 500 mg IM on day 1 for all subsequent cycles

Repeat cycle every 28 days [144].

Alpelisib + Fulvestrant

Alpelisib:	300 mg PO daily
Fulvestrant:	500 mg IM on days 1, 15, and 29 and then once per month

Repeat cycle every 28 days [145].

Abemaciclib + Anastrozole

Abemaciclib:	150 mg PO bid
Anastrozole:	1 mg PO daily

Repeat cycle every 28 days [146].

Abemaciclib + Letrozole

Abemaciclib:	150 mg PO bid
Letrozole:	2.5 mg PO daily

Repeat cycle every 28 days [146].

Single-Agent Regimens: Hormone-Receptor Positive and HER2-Positive Disease

Tamoxifen

Tamoxifen: 20 mg PO daily [147]

Toremifene

Toremifene: 60 mg PO daily [148]

Exemestane

Exemestane: 25 mg PO daily [149]

Anastrozole

Anastrozole: 1 mg PO daily [150]

Letrozole

Letrozole: 2.5 mg PO daily [151]

Fulvestrant

Fulvestrant: 250 mg IM on day 1

Repeat injection every month [152].

or

Fulvestrant: 500 mg IM loading dose on day 1, then 500 mg IM on days 15 and 29

Continue treatment on a monthly basis until disease progression [153].

Elacestrant (ESR1 mutation)

Elacestrant: 345 mg PO daily

Repeat cycle every 28 days until disease progression [154].

Megestrol

Megestrol: 40 mg PO qid [155]

Trastuzumab

Trastuzumab: 4 mg/kg IV loading dose and then 2 mg/kg IV weekly

Repeat cycle weekly for a total of 10 weeks. In the absence of disease progression, continue weekly maintenance dose of 2 mg/kg [156].

or

Trastuzumab: 8 mg/kg IV loading dose, then 6 mg/kg IV every 3 weeks

Continue treatment until disease progression [157].

Margetuximab

Margetuximab: 15 mg/kg IV on day 1
Repeat cycle every 21 days [158].

Trastuzumab and hyaluronidase

Trastuzumab and hyaluronidase: 600 mg trastuzumab SC and
                                                10,000 units hyaluronidase SC
                                                on day 1

Repeat cycle every 21 days [159].

Ado-trastuzumab emtansine

Ado-trastuzumab: 3.6 mg/kg IV on day 1
Repeat cycle every 21 days [160].

Trastuzumab deruxtecan-nxki

Trastuzumab deruxtecan: 5.4 mg/kg IV on day 1
Repeat cycle every 21 days [161].

Capecitabine

Capecitabine: 1,250 mg/m^2 PO bid on days 1–14

Repeat cycle every 21 days [162]. May decrease dose to 850–1,000 mg/m^2 PO bid on days 1–14 to reduce risk of toxicity without compromising clinical efficacy.

Docetaxel

Docetaxel: 100 mg/m^2 IV on day 1
Repeat cycle every 21 days [163].
or
Docetaxel: 35–40 mg/m^2 IV weekly for 6 weeks
Repeat cycle every 8 weeks [164].

Paclitaxel

Paclitaxel: 175 mg/m^2 IV over 3 hours on day 1
Repeat cycle every 21 days [165].
or
Paclitaxel: 80–100 mg/m^2 IV weekly for 3 weeks
Repeat cycle every 4 weeks [166].

Ixabepilone

Ixabepilone: 40 mg/m^2 IV on day 1
Repeat cycle every 21 days [167].

Vinorelbine
Vinorelbine: 30 mg/m^2 IV on day 1
Repeat cycle every 7 days [168].

Doxorubicin
Doxorubicin: 20 mg/m^2 IV on day 1
Repeat cycle every 7 days [169].

Gemcitabine
Gemcitabine: 725 mg/m^2 IV weekly for 3 weeks
Repeat cycle every 28 days [170].

Doxorubicin liposome
Doxorubicin liposome: 40 mg/m^2 IV on day 1
Repeat cycle every 28 days [171].

Abraxane
Abraxane: 260 mg/m^2 IV on day 1
Repeat cycle every 21 days [172].
or
Abraxane: 125 mg/m^2 IV on days 1, 8, and 15
Repeat cycle every 28 days [173].

Eribulin
Eribulin: 1.4 mg/m^2 IV on days 1 and 8
Repeat cycle every 21 days [174].

Olaparib
Olapraib: 300 mg PO bid
Repeat cycle every 28 days [175].

Talazoparib
Talazoparib: 1 mg PO daily
Repeat cycle every 28 days [176].

Sacituzumab govitecan-hziy
Sacituzumab govitecan: 10 mg/kg IV on days 1 and 8
Repeat cycle every 21 days [177].

Single-Agent Regimens: Hormone-Receptor Positive and HER2-Negative Disease

Abemaciclib

Abemaciclib: 150 mg PO bid

Repeat cycle every 28 days [178].

CANCER OF UNKNOWN PRIMARY

Combination Regimens

PCE

Paclitaxel:	200 mg/m^2 IV over 1 hour on day 1
Carboplatin:	AUC of 6, IV on day 1
Etoposide:	50 mg alternating with 100 mg PO on days 1–10

Repeat cycle every 21 days [179].

EP

Etoposide:	100 mg/m^2 IV on days 1–5
Cisplatin:	100 mg/m^2 IV on day 1

Repeat cycle every 21 days [180].

PEB

Cisplatin:	20 mg/m^2 IV on days 1–5
Etoposide:	100 mg/m^2 IV on days 1–5
Bleomycin:	30 units IV on days 1, 8, and 15

Repeat cycle every 21 days [181].

GCP

Gemcitabine:	1,000 mg/m^2 IV on days 1 and 8
Carboplatin:	AUC of 5, IV on day 1
Paclitaxel:	200 mg/m^2 IV on day 1

Repeat cycle every 21 days for 4 cycles [182]. To be followed by paclitaxel at 70 mg/m^2 IV every week for 6 weeks with a 2-week rest. Repeat for a total of 3 cycles.

Gemcitabine + Cisplatin + Paclitaxel

Gemcitabine:	1,000 mg/m^2 IV on days 1 and 8
Cisplatin:	75 mg/m^2 IV on day 1
Paclitaxel:	175 mg/m^2 IV on day 1

Repeat cycle every 21 days [183].

Gemcitabine + Irinotecan

Gemcitabine:	1,000 mg/m^2 IV on days 1 and 8
Irinotecan:	100 mg/m^2 IV on days 1 and 8

Repeat cycle every 21 days [184].

Capecitabine + Oxaliplatin

Capecitabine:	1,000 mg/m^2 PO on days 1–14
Oxaliplatin:	130 mg/m^2 IV on day 1

Repeat cycle every 21 days [185].

Bevacizumab + Erlotinib

Bevacizumab:	10 mg/kg IV on day 1
Erlotinib:	150 mg PO daily

Continue until disease progression [186].

Single-Agent Regimens

Pembrolizumab

Pembrolizumab:	200 mg IV on day 1

Repeat cycle every 3 weeks [187]. May also administer 400 mg IV every 6 weeks.

CARCINOID TUMORS AND NEUROENDOCRINE TUMORS

Combination Regimens

5-Fluorouracil + Streptozocin

5-Fluorouracil:	400 mg/m^2/day IV on days 1–5
Streptozocin:	500 mg/m^2/day IV on days 1–5

Repeat cycle every 6 weeks [188].

Doxorubicin + Streptozocin

Doxorubicin:	50 mg/m^2 IV on days 1 and 22
Streptozocin:	500 mg/m^2/day IV on days 1–5

Repeat cycle every 6 weeks [188].

Cisplatin + Etoposide

Cisplatin:	45 mg/m^2/day IV continuous infusion on days 2 and 3
Etoposide:	130 mg/m^2/day IV continuous infusion on days 1–3

Repeat cycle every 21 days [189].

Everolimus + Octreotide LAR

Everolimus:	10 mg PO daily
Octreotide LAR:	30 mg IM on day 1

Repeat cycle every 28 days [190].

Capecitabine + Temozolomide

Capecitabine:	750 mg/day PO on days 1–14
Temozolomide:	200 mg/m^2/day PO on days 10–14

Repeat cycle every 28 days [191].

Single-Agent Regimens

Octreotide

Octreotide:	150–250 µg SC tid

Continue until disease progression [192].

Lanreotide

Lanreotide:	120 mg SC on day 1

Repeat cycle every 21 days [193].

Sunitinib

Sunitinib:	50 mg PO daily for 4 weeks

Repeat cycle every 6 weeks [194].

Everolimus

Everolimus:	10 mg PO daily

Continue treatment until disease progression [195].

Lutetium Lu 177 dotatate

Lutetium Lu 177 dotatate:	120 mg SC on day 1

Repeat every 8 weeks for a total of 4 doses [196]. Long-acting octreotide 30 mg IM should be administered at 4 to 24 hours after each dose of lutetium Lu 177 dotatate.

CERVICAL CANCER

Combination Regimens

Cisplatin + Radiation Therapy

Radiation therapy:	1.8 to 2 Gy per fraction (total dose, 45 Gy)
Cisplatin:	40 mg/m^2 IV weekly (maximal dose, 70 mg per week)

Cisplatin is given 4 hours before radiation therapy on weeks 1–6 [197].

Paclitaxel + Cisplatin

Paclitaxel.	135 mg/m^2 IV over 24 hours on day 1
Cisplatin:	75 mg/m^2 IV on day 2

Repeat cycle every 21 days [198].

Cisplatin + Topotecan

Cisplatin:	50 mg/m^2 IV on day 1
Topotecan:	0.75 mg/m^2/day IV on days 1–3

Repeat cycle every 21 days [199].

Paclitaxel + Topotecan

Paclitaxel:	175 mg/m^2 IV on day 1
Topotecan:	0.75 mg/m^2 IV on days 1–3

Repeat cycle every 21 days [200].

Paclitaxel + Topotecan + Bevacizumab

Paclitaxel:	175 mg/m^2 IV on day 1
Topotecan:	0.75 mg/m^2/day IV on days 1–3
Bevacizumab:	15 mg/kg IV on day 1

Repeat cycle every 21 days [200].

Cisplatin + Paclitaxel + Bevacizumab

Cisplatin:	50 mg/m^2 IV on day 1
Paclitaxel:	135 or 175 mg/m^2 IV on day 1
Bevacizumab:	15 mg/kg IV on day 1

Repeat cycle every 21 days [201].

BIP

Bleomycin:	30 U IV over 24 hours on day 1
Ifosfamide:	5,000 mg/m^2 IV over 24 hours on day 2

| Mesna: | 6,000 mg/m^2 IV over 36 hours on day 2 |
| Cisplatin: | 50 mg/m^2 IV on day 2 |

Repeat cycle every 21 days [202].

BIC

Bleomycin:	30 U IV on day 1
Ifosfamide:	2,000 mg/m^2 IV on days 1–3
Mesna:	400 mg/m^2 IV, 15 minutes before ifosfamide dose, then 400 mg/m^2 IV at 4 and 8 hours following ifosfamide
Carboplatin:	200 mg/m^2 IV on day 1

Repeat cycle every 21 days [203].

Cisplatin + 5-Fluorouracil

| Cisplatin: | 75 mg/m^2 IV on day 1 |
| 5-Fluorouracil: | 1,000 mg/m^2/day IV continuous infusion on days 2–5 |

Repeat cycle every 21 days [204].

Cisplatin + Vinorelbine

| Cisplatin: | 80 mg/m^2 IV on day 1 |
| Vinorelbine: | 25 mg/m^2 IV on days 1 and 8 |

Repeat cycle every 21 days [205].

Cisplatin + Irinotecan

| Cisplatin: | 60 mg/m^2 IV on day 1 |
| Irinotecan: | 60 mg/m^2 IV on days 1, 8, and 15 |

Repeat cycle every 28 days [206].

Cisplatin + Gemcitabine

| Cisplatin: | 50 mg/m^2 IV on day 1 |
| Gemcitabine: | 1,000 mg/m^2 IV on days 1 and 8 |

Repeat cycle every 21 days for up to 6 cycles [207].
or
| Cisplatin: | 30 mg/m^2 IV on day 1 |
| Gemcitabine: | 800 mg/m^2 IV on days 1 and 8 |

Repeat cycle every 28 days [208].

Carboplatin + Docetaxel

| Carboplatin: | AUC of 6, IV on day 1 |
| Docetaxel: | 60 mg/m^2 IV on day 1 |

Repeat cycle every 21 days [209].

Cisplatin + Pemetrexed

Cisplatin:	50 mg/m^2 IV on day 1
Pemetrexed:	500 mg/m^2 IV on day 1

Repeat cycle every 21 days [210]. Folic acid at 350–1,000 µg PO q day and vitamin B12 at 1,000 µg IM to start 1 week prior to first dose of pemetrexed and repeated every 3 cycles.

Pembrolizumab + Paclitaxel + Cisplatin/Carboplatin + Bevacizumab

Pembrolizumab:	200 mg IV on day 1
Paclitaxel:	175 mg/m^2 IV on day 1
Cisplatin:	50 mg/m^2 IV on day 1
or	
Carboplatin:	AUC of 5 IV on day 1
Bevacizumab:	15 mg/kg IV on day 1

Repeat cycle every 21 days for 6 cycles and/or for 2 cycles beyond complete response [211].

Single-Agent Regimens

Docetaxel

Docetaxel:	100 mg/m^2 IV on day 1

Repeat cycle every 21 days [212].

Paclitaxel

Paclitaxel:	175 mg/m^2 IV over 3 hours on day 1

Repeat cycle every 21 days [213].

Irinotecan

Irinotecan:	125 mg/m^2 IV weekly for 4 weeks

Repeat cycle every 6 weeks [214].

Topotecan

Topotecan:	1.5 mg/m^2/day on days 1–5

Repeat cycle every 21 days [215].

Pemetrexed

Pemetrexed:	500 mg/m^2 IV on day 1

Repeat cycle every 21 days [216]. Folic acid at 350–1,000 µg PO q day and vitamin B12 at 1,000 µg IM to start 1 week prior to first dose of therapy and repeated every 3 cycles.

Gemcitabine

Gemcitabine:	800 mg/m^2 IV on days 1, 8, and 15

Repeat cycle every 28 days [217].

Tisotumab vedotin

Tisotumab vedotin:	2 mg/kg (up to a maximum of 200 mg) IV on day 1

Repeat cycle every 21 days [218].

Pembrolizumab

Pembrolizumab:	200 mg IV on day 1

Repeat cycle every 3 weeks [219]. May also administer 400 mg IV every 6 weeks.

COLORECTAL CANCER

Total Neoadjuvant Therapy for Rectal Cancer (TNT)

Combination Regimens

FOLFOX 6

Oxaliplatin:	85 mg/m^2 IV on day 1
5-Fluorouracil:	400 mg/m^2 IV bolus on day 1, followed by 2,400 mg/m^2 IV continuous infusion over 46 hours on days 1 and 2
Leucovorin:	400 mg/m^2 IV on day 1 as a 2-hour infusion before 5-fluorouracil

Eight cycles of neoadjuvant induction therapy followed by short course or long course chemoradiation with infusional 5-FU or capecitabine [220].

or

CAPOX

Capecitabine:	850 mg/m^2 PO bid on days 1–14
Oxaliplatin:	130 mg/m^2 IV on day 1

Repeat cycle every 21 days.

Administer 5 cycles of neoadjuvant induction chemotherapy followed by short-course or long- course chemoradiation with infusional 5-FU or capecitabine [221].

Single Agent Regimen

Dostarlimab (MSI-H/dMMR)

Dostarlimab:	500 mg IV on day 1

Repeat cycle every 3 weeks for 9 cycles [222]. To be followed by standard radiation therapy (total dose, 5,040 cGy given in 28 fractions) with concurrent administration of capecitabine at standard doses and then total mesorectal excision.

Neoadjuvant Combined Modality Therapy for Rectal Cancer

Combination Regimens

5-Fluorouracil + Radiation Therapy (German AIO regimen)

5-Fluorouracil:	1,000 mg/m²/day IV continuous infusion on days 1–5

Repeat infusional 5-FU on weeks 1 and 5.

Radiation therapy:	180 cGy/day for 5 days per week (total dose, 5,040 cGy)

Followed by surgical resection and then adjuvant chemotherapy with 5-FU at 500 mg/m² IV for 5 days every 28 days for a total of 4 cycles [223].

Infusion 5-FU + Radiation Therapy

5-Fluorouracil:	225 mg/m²/day IV continuous infusion throughout entire course of radiation therapy
Radiation therapy:	180 cGy/day for 5 days per week (total dose, 5,040 cGy)

Followed by surgical resection and then adjuvant chemotherapy with capecitabine, 5-FU/LV, or FOLFOX4 for a total of 4 months [224].

Capecitabine + Radiation Therapy

Capecitabine:	825 mg/m² PO bid throughout the entire course of radiation therapy or 900–1,000 mg/m² PO bid on days 1–5 of each week of radiation therapy
Radiation therapy:	180 cGy/day for 5 days per week (total dose, 5,040 cGy)

Followed by surgical resection and then adjuvant chemotherapy with capecitabine, 5-FU, or 5-FU/LV for a total of 4 cycles [225].

5-FU/LV Oxaliplatin + Radiation Therapy

5-Fluorouracil:	200 mg/m²/day IV continuous infusion throughout entire course of radiation therapy
Oxaliplatin:	60 mg/m² IV on days 1, 8, 15, 22, 29, and 36
Radiation therapy:	180 cGy/day for 5 days each week (total dose, 5,040 cGy)

Followed by surgical resection 4–6 weeks after completion of chemoradiotherapy and then adjuvant chemotherapy [226].

XELOX + Radiation Therapy

Capecitabine:	825 mg/m^2 PO bid on days 1–14 and 22–35
Oxaliplatin:	50 mg/m^2 IV on days 1, 8, 22, and 29
Radiation therapy:	180 cGy/day for 5 days per week (total dose, 5,040 cGy)

Followed by surgical resection and then adjuvant chemotherapy with

Capecitabine:	1,000 mg/m^2 PO bid on days 1–14
Oxaliplatin:	130 mg/m^2 IV on day 1

Repeat cycle every 3 weeks for 4 cycles [227].

Adjuvant Therapy

Combination Regimens

5-Fluorouracil + Leucovorin (weekly schedule, high dose)

5-Fluorouracil:	500 mg/m^2 IV weekly for 6 weeks
Leucovorin:	500 mg/m^2 IV over 2 hours weekly for 6 weeks, administered before 5-fluorouracil

Repeat cycle every 8 weeks for a total of 4 cycles (32 weeks total) [228].

5-Fluorouracil + Leucovorin (weekly schedule, low dose)

5-Fluorouracil:	500 mg/m^2 IV weekly for 6 weeks
Leucovorin:	20 mg/m^2 IV weekly for 6 weeks, administered before 5-fluorouracil

Repeat cycle every 8 weeks for a total of 4 or 6 cycles (32 or 48 weeks total) [229].

Oxaliplatin + 5-Fluorouracil + Leucovorin (FOLFOX4)

Oxaliplatin:	85 mg/m^2 IV on day 1
5-Fluorouracil:	400 mg/m^2 IV bolus, followed by 600 mg/m^2 IV continuous infusion for 22 hours on days 1 and 2
Leucovorin:	200 mg/m^2 IV on days 1 and 2 as a 2-hour infusion before 5-fluorouracil

Repeat cycle every 2 weeks for a total of 12 cycles (6 months total) [230].

Oxaliplatin + 5-Fluorouracil + Leucovorin (mFOLFOX7)

Oxaliplatin:	100 mg/m^2 IV on day 1
5-Fluorouracil:	3,000 mg/m^2 IV continuous infusion on days 1 and 2 for 46 hours

| Leucovorin: | 200 mg/m^2 IV on day 1 as a 2-hour infusion before 5-fluorouracil |

Repeat cycle every 2 weeks for a total of 12 cycles (6 months total) [231].

Oxaliplatin + Capecitabine (XELOX)

| Oxaliplatin: | 130 mg/m^2 IV on day 1 |
| Capecitabine: | 1,000 mg/m^2 PO bid on days 1–14 |

Repeat cycle every 3 weeks for a total of 8 cycles (6 months total) [232]. Dose may be decreased to 850 mg/m^2 PO bid days 1–14 to reduce risk of toxicity without compromising efficacy.

LV5FU2 (deGramont regimen)

| 5-Fluorouracil: | 400 mg/m^2 IV bolus, followed by 600 mg/m^2 IV continuous infusion for 22 hours on days 1 and 2 |
| Leucovorin: | 200 mg/m^2 IV on days 1 and 2 as a 2-hour infusion before 5-fluorouracil |

or

| L-Leucovorin: | 100 mg/m^2 IV on days 1 and 2 as a 2-hour infusion before 5-fluorouracil |

Repeat cycle every 2 weeks for a total of 12 cycles [230].

Capecitabine

| Capecitabine: | 1,250 mg/m^2 PO bid on days 1–14 |

Repeat cycle every 21 days for a total of 8 cycles [233]. Dose may be decreased to 850–1,000 mg/m^2 PO bid on days 1–14 to reduce risk of toxicity without compromising clinical efficacy.

Metastatic Disease

Combination Regimens

Irinotecan + 5-Fluorouracil + Leucovorin (Modified IFL Saltz regimen)

Irinotecan:	125 mg/m^2 IV over 90 minutes weekly for 2 weeks
5-Fluorouracil:	500 mg/m^2 IV weekly for 2 weeks
Leucovorin:	20 mg/m^2 IV weekly for 2 weeks

Repeat cycle every 3 weeks [234].

Irinotecan + 5-Fluorouracil + Leucovorin (Douillard regimen)

| Irinotecan: | 180 mg/m^2 IV on day 1 |
| 5-Fluorouracil: | 400 mg/m^2 IV bolus, followed by 600 g/m^2 IV continuous infusion for 22 hours on days 1 and 2 |

Leucovorin: 200 mg/m^2 IV on days 1 and 2 as a 2-hour infusion prior to 5-fluorouracil

Repeat cycle every 2 weeks [235].

Irinotecan + 5-Fluorouracil + Leucovorin (FOLFIRI regimen)

Irinotecan: 180 mg/m^2 IV on day 1

5-Fluorouracil: 400 mg/m^2 IV bolus on day 1, followed by 2,400 mg/m^2 IV continuous infusion for 46 hours

Leucovorin: 200 mg/m^2 IV on day 1 as a 2-hour infusion prior to 5-fluorouracil

Repeat cycle every 2 weeks [236].

Oxaliplatin + 5-Fluorouracil + Leucovorin (FOLFOX4)

Oxaliplatin: 85 mg/m^2 IV on day 1

5-Fluorouracil: 400 mg/m^2 IV bolus, followed by 600 mg/m^2 IV continuous infusion for 22 hours on days 1 and 2

Leucovorin: 200 mg/m^2 IV on days 1 and 2 as a 2-hour infusion before 5-fluorouracil

or

L-Leucovorin: 100 mg/m^2 IV on days 1 and 2 as a 2-hour infusion before 5-fluorouracil

Repeat cycle every 2 weeks [237].

Oxaliplatin + 5-Fluorouracil + Leucovorin (FOLFOX6)

Oxaliplatin: 100 mg/m^2 IV on day 1

5-Fluorouracil: 400 mg/m^2 IV bolus on day 1, followed by 2,400 mg/m^2 IV continuous infusion for 46 hours

Leucovorin: 400 mg/m^2 IV on day 1 as a 2-hour infusion before 5-fluorouracil

Repeat cycle every 2 weeks [238].

Oxaliplatin + 5-Fluorouracil + Leucovorin (FOLFOX7)

Oxaliplatin: 130 mg/m^2 IV on day 1

5-Fluorouracil: 2,400 mg/m^2 IV continuous infusion on days 1 and 2 for 46 hours

Leucovorin: 400 mg/m^2 IV on day 1 as a 2-hour infusion before 5-fluorouracil

or

| L-Leucovorin: | 200 mg/m^2 IV on days 1 and 2 as a 2-hour infusion before 5-fluorouracil |

Repeat cycle every 2 weeks [239].

Oxaliplatin + 5-Fluorouracil + Leucovorin (mFOLFOX7)

Oxaliplatin:	100 mg/m^2 IV on day 1
5-Fluorouracil:	3,000 mg/m^2 IV continuous infusion on days 1 and 2 for 46 hours
Leucovorin:	200 mg/m^2 IV on day 1 as a 2-hour infusion before 5-fluorouracil

Repeat cycle every 2 weeks [240].

FOLFOXIRI

Irinotecan:	165 mg/m^2 IV on day 1
Oxaliplatin:	85 mg/m^2 IV on day 1
5-Fluorouracil:	3,200 mg/m^2 IV continuous infusion for 46 hours on days 1 and 2
Leucovorin:	200 mg/m^2 IV on day 1 as a 2-hour infusion prior to 5-fluorouracil

Repeat cycle every 2 weeks for a total of 12 cycles [241].

FOLFOXIRI + Bevacizumab

Irinotecan:	165 mg/m^2 IV on day 1
Oxaliplatin:	85 mg/m^2 IV on day 1
5-Fluorouracil:	3,200 mg/m^2 IV continuous infusion for 46 hours on days 1 and 2
Leucovorin:	200 mg/m^2 IV on day 1 as a 2-hour infusion prior to 5-fluorouracil
Bevacizumab:	5 mg/kg IV on day 1

Repeat cycle every 2 weeks [242].

FOLFOXIRI + Panitumumab

Irinotecan:	150 mg/m^2 IV on day 1
Oxaliplatin:	85 mg/m^2 IV on day 1
5-Fluorouracil:	3,000 mg/m^2 IV continuous infusion for 46 hours on days 1 and 2
Leucovorin:	200 mg/m^2 IV on day 1 as a 2-hour infusion prior to 5-fluorouracil
Panitumumab:	6 mg/kg IV on day 1

Repeat cycle every 2 weeks [243].

Cetuximab + Irinotecan

Cetuximab:

400 mg/m^2 IV loading dose, then 250 mg/m^2 IV weekly

Irinotecan:

350 mg/m^2 IV on day 1

Repeat cycle every 21 days [244].

or

Cetuximab:

400 mg/m^2 IV loading dose, then 250 mg/m^2 IV weekly

Irinotecan:

180 mg/m^2 IV on day 1

Repeat cycle every 14 days [244].

Capecitabine + Oxaliplatin (XELOX)

Capecitabine:

1,000 mg/m^2 PO bid on days 1–14

Oxaliplatin:

130 mg/m^2 IV on day 1

Repeat cycle every 21 days [245]. May decrease dose of capecitabine to 850 mg/m^2 PO bid and dose of oxaliplatin to 100 mg/m^2 IV to reduce risk of toxicity without compromising clinical efficacy.

or

Capecitabine:

1,750 mg/m^2 PO bid on days 1–7

Oxaliplatin:

85 mg/m^2 IV on day 1

Repeat cycle every 14 days [245]. May decrease dose of capecitabine to 1,000–1,250 mg/m^2 PO bid to reduce risk of toxicity without compromising clinical efficacy.

Capecitabine + Irinotecan (XELIRI)

Capecitabine:

1,000 mg/m^2 PO bid on days 1–14

Irinotecan:

250 mg/m^2 IV on day 1

Repeat cycle every 21 days [246]. May decrease dose of capecitabine to 850 mg/m^2 PO bid and dose of irinotecan to 200 mg/m^2 IV to reduce risk of toxicity without compromising clinical efficacy.

or

Capecitabine:

1,500 mg/m^2 PO bid on days 2–8

Irinotecan:

150 mg/m^2 IV on day 1

Repeat cycle every 14 days [247].

Capecitabine + Mitomycin-C

Capecitabine:

1,000 mg/m^2 PO bid on days 1–14

Mitomycin-C:

7 mg/m^2 IV on day 1

Repeat capecitabine every 3 weeks and mitomycin-C every 6 weeks [248].

Oxaliplatin + Irinotecan (IROX regimen)

Oxaliplatin:	85 mg/m^2 IV on day 1
Irinotecan:	200 mg/m^2 IV on day 1

Repeat cycle every 3 weeks [249].

5-Fluorouracil + Leucovorin (Roswell Park schedule, high dose)

5-Fluorouracil:	500 mg/m^2 IV weekly for 6 weeks
Leucovorin:	500 mg/m^2 IV weekly for 6 weeks, administered before 5-fluorouracil.

Repeat cycle every 8 weeks [250].

5-Fluorouracil + Leucovorin + Bevacizumab

5-Fluorouracil:	500 mg/m^2 IV weekly for 6 weeks
Leucovorin:	500 mg/m^2 IV weekly for 6 weeks, administered before 5-fluorouracil.
Bevacizumab:	5 mg/kg IV every 2 weeks

Repeat cycle every 8 weeks [251].

TAS-102 + Bevacizumab

TAS-102:	35 mg/m^2 PO bid on days 1–5 and 8–12
Bevacizumab:	5 mg/kg IV on days 1 and 15

Repeat cycle every 28 days [252].

5-Fluorouracil + Leucovorin (German schedule, low dose)

5-Fluorouracil:	600 mg/m^2 IV weekly for 6 weeks
Leucovorin:	20 mg/m^2 IV weekly for 6 weeks, administered before 5-fluorouracil.

Repeat cycle every 8 weeks [253].

5-Fluorouracil + Leucovorin (de Gramont regimen)

5-Fluorouracil:	400 mg/m^2 IV and then 600 mg/m^2 IV for 22 hours on days 1 and 2
Leucovorin:	200 mg/m^2 IV on days 1 and 2 as a 2-hour infusion before 5-fluorouracil

Repeat cycle every 2 weeks [254].

FOLFOX4 + Bevacizumab

Oxaliplatin:	85 mg/m^2 IV on day 1
5-Fluorouracil:	400 mg/m^2 IV bolus, followed by 600 mg/m^2 IV continuous infusion on days 1 and 2

Leucovorin: 200 mg/m^2 IV on days 1 and 2 as a 2-hour infusion before 5-fluorouracil

Bevacizumab: 10 mg/kg IV every 2 weeks
Repeat cycle every 2 weeks [255].

LV5FU2 + Mitomycin-C

5-Fluorouracil: 400 mg/m^2 IV bolus, followed by 600 mg/m^2 IV continuous infusion on days 1 and 2

Leucovorin: 200 mg/m^2 IV on days 1 and 2 as a 2-hour infusion before 5-fluorouracil

Mitomycin-C 7 mg/m^2 IV on day 1
Repeat 5-FU/LV every 2 weeks and mitomycin-C every 4 weeks [256].

Capecitabine + Oxaliplatin (XELOX) + Bevacizumab

Capecitabine: 850 mg/m^2 PO bid on days 1–14
Oxaliplatin: 130 mg/m^2 IV on day 1
Bevacizumab: 7.5 mg/kg every 3 weeks
Repeat cycle every 21 days [257].

Cetuximab + Bevacizumab + Irinotecan

Cetuximab: 400 mg/m^2 IV loading dose, then 250 mg/m^2 IV weekly

Bevacizumab: 5 mg/kg IV every 2 weeks
Irinotecan: 180 mg/m^2 IV on day 1
Repeat cycle every 2 weeks [258].

Cetuximab + Bevacizumab

Cetuximab: 400 mg/m^2 IV loading dose, then 250 mg/m^2 IV weekly

Bevacizumab: 5 mg/kg IV every 2 weeks
Repeat cycle every 2 weeks [258].

Irinotecan + Cetuximab

Irinotecan: 125 mg/m^2 IV weekly for 4 weeks
Cetuximab: 400 mg/m^2 IV loading dose, then 250 mg/m^2 IV weekly

Repeat cycle every 6 weeks [259, 260].
or
Irinotecan: 350 mg/m^2 IV on day 1
Cetuximab: 400 mg/m^2 IV loading dose, then 250 mg/m^2 IV weekly

Repeat cycle every 3 weeks [261].

FOLFIRI + Cetuximab

Irinotecan:	180 mg/m^2 IV on day 1
5-Fluorouracil:	400 mg/m^2 IV bolus followed by 2,400 mg/m^2 IV continuous infusion for 46 hours on days 1 and 2
Leucovorin:	400 mg/m^2 IV on day 1 as a 2-hour infusion prior to 5-fluorouracil
Cetuximab:	400 mg/m^2 IV loading dose, then 250 mg/m^2 IV weekly

Repeat cycle every 2 weeks [262].

FOLFOX4 + Cetuximab

Oxaliplatin:	85 mg/m^2 IV on day 1
5-Fluorouracil:	400 mg/m^2 IV bolus followed by 600 mg/m^2 IV continuous infusion for 22 hours on days 1 and 2
Leucovorin:	200 mg/m^2 IV on days 1 and 2 as a 2-hour infusion prior to 5-fluorouracil
Cetuximab:	400 mg/m^2 IV loading dose, then 250 mg/m^2 IV weekly

Repeat cycle every 2 weeks [263].

FOLFOX6 + Cetuximab

Oxaliplatin:	85 mg/m^2 IV on day 1
5-Fluorouracil:	400 mg/m^2 IV bolus on day 1, followed by 2,400 mg/m^2 IV continuous infusion over 46 hours on days 1 and 2
Leucovorin:	400 mg/m^2 IV on day 1 as a 2-hour infusion before 5-fluorouracil
Cetuximab:	400 mg/m^2 IV loading dose and then 250 mg/m^2 IV weekly

Repeat cycle every 2 weeks [264].

FOLFOX4 + Panitumumab

Oxaliplatin:	85 mg/m^2 IV on day 1
5-Fluorouracil:	400 mg/m^2 IV bolus followed by 600 mg/m^2 IV continuous infusion for 22 hours on days 1 and 2
Leucovorin:	200 mg/m^2 IV on days 1 and 2 as a 2-hour infusion before 5-fluorouracil
Panitumumab:	6 mg/kg IV on day 1

Repeat cycle every 2 weeks [265].

FOLFIRI + Panitumumab

Irinotecan:	180 mg/m^2 IV on day 1
5-Fluorouracil:	400 mg/m^2 IV bolus on day 1, followed by 2,400 mg/m^2 IV continuous infusion for 46 hours on days 1 and 2
Leucovorin:	400 mg/m^2 IV on day 1 as a 2-hour infusion before 5-fluorouracil
Panitumumab:	6 mg/kg IV on day 1

Repeat cycle every 2 weeks [266].

FOLFIRI + Bevacizumab

Irinotecan:	180 mg/m^2 IV on day 1
5-Fluorouracil:	400 mg/m^2 IV bolus on day 1, followed by 2,400 mg/m^2 IV continuous infusion for 46 hours on days 1 and 2
Leucovorin:	400 mg/m^2 IV on day 1 as a 2-hour infusion prior to 5-fluorouracil
Bevacizumab:	5 mg/kg IV every 2 weeks

Repeat cycle every 2 weeks [267].

XELIRI + Bevacizumab

Irinotecan:	200 mg/m^2 IV on day 1
Capecitabine:	800 mg/m^2 PO on days 1–14
Bevacizumab:	7.5 mg/kg IV on day 1

Repeat cycle every 3 weeks [268].

FOLFIRI + Ziv-aflibercept

Irinotecan:	180 mg/m^2 IV on day 1
5-Fluorouracil:	400 mg/m^2 IV bolus on day 1, followed by 2,400 mg/m^2 IV continuous infusion for 46 hours on days 1 and 2
Leucovorin:	400 mg/m^2 IV on day 1 as a 2-hour infusion prior to 5-fluorouracil
Ziv-aflibercept:	4 mg/kg IV on day 1

Repeat cycle every 2 weeks [269].

FOLFIRI + Ramucirumab

Irinotecan:	180 mg/m^2 IV on day 1
5-Fluorouracil:	400 mg/m^2 IV bolus on day 1, followed by 2,400 mg/m^2 IV continuous infusion for 46 hours on days 1 and 2

Leucovorin:	400 mg/m^2 IV on day 1 as a 2-hour infusion prior to 5-fluorouracil
Ramucirumab:	8 mg/kg IV on day 1

Repeat cycle every 2 weeks [270].

Vemurafenib + Irinotecan + Cetuximab (VIC) (BRAF:V600E mutation)

Vemurafenib:	960 mg PO bid
Irinotecan:	180 mg/m^2 IV on day 1
Cetuximab:	500 mg/m^2 IV on day 1

Repeat cycle every 2 weeks [271]. Used only for patients with BRAF V600E-mutant mCRC.

Binimetinib + Encorafenib + Cetuximab (BEC) (BRAF:V600E mutation)

Binimetinib:	45 mg PO bid
Encorafenib:	300 mg PO daily
Cetuximab:	400 mg/m^2 IV loading dose, then 250 mg/m^2 IV weekly

Continue treatment until disease progression [272]. Used only for patients with BRAF V600E-mutant mCRC.

Encorafenib + Cetuximab (EC) (BRAF:V600E mutation)

Encorafenib:	300 mg PO daily
Cetuximab:	400 mg/m^2 IV loading dose, then 250 mg/m^2 IV weekly

Continue treatment until disease progression [273]. Used only for patients with BRAF V600E-mutant mCRC.

Encorafenib + Panitumumab (EP) (BRAF:V600E mutation)

Encorafenib:	300 mg PO daily
Panitumumab:	6 mg/kg IV on day 1

Continue treatment until disease progression [274]. Used only for patients with BRAF V600E-mutant mCRC.

Nivolumab + Ipilimumab (MSI-H/dMMR)

Nivolumab:	3 mg/kg IV on day 1
Ipilimumab:	1 mg/kg IV on day 1

Repeat cycle every 21 days for 4 cycles and then treat with nivolumab 240 mg IV every 2 weeks or 480 mg every 4 weeks [275]. Used only for MSI-H/dMMR and TMB-H disease.

Trastuzumab + Lapatinib

Trastuzumab:

4 mg/kg IV on day 1 for first cycle and then 2 mg/kg IV on day 1 for subsequent cycles

Lapatinib:

1,000 mg PO daily

Repeat cycle every 21 days [276]. Use only in setting of HER2-amplified disease and wild-type RAS/BRAF.

Trastuzumab + Tucatinib

Trastuzumab:

8 mg/kg IV on day 1 of first cycle and then 6 mg/kg IV every 3 weeks

Tucatinib:

300 mg PO bid

Repeat cycle every 21 days [277]. Use only in setting of HER2-amplified disease and wild-type RAS/BRAF.

Trastuzumab + Pertuzumab

Trastuzumab:

8 mg/kg IV loading dose on day 1 and then 6 mg/kg IV every 3 weeks

Pertuzumab:

840 mg IV loading dose on day 1 and then 420 mg IV every 3 weeks

Repeat cycle every 21 days [278]. Used only for patients with HER2-positive disease and wild-type RAS/BRAF.

Hepatic Artery Infusion

Floxuridine

Floxuridine (FUDR):

0.3 mg/kg/day HAI on days 1–14

Dexamethasone:

20 mg HAI on days 1–14

Heparin:

50,000 U HAI on days 1–14

Repeat cycle every 14 days [279].

Single-Agent Regimens

Capecitabine

Capecitabine:

$1,250 mg/m^2$ PO bid on days 1–14

Repeat cycle every 21 days [280]. Dose may be decreased to $850–1,000 mg/m^2$ PO bid on days 1–14 to reduce risk of toxicity without compromising clinical efficacy.

CPT-11 (weekly schedule)

CPT-11:

$125 mg/m^2$ IV over 90 minutes weekly for 4 weeks

Repeat cycle every 6 weeks [281].

or

CPT-11:

$125 mg/m^2$ IV over 90 minutes weekly for 2 weeks

Repeat cycle every 3 weeks.
or
CPT-11:   175 mg/m^2 IV on days 1 and 10
Repeat cycle every 3 weeks [282].

CPT-11 (monthly schedule)
CPT-11:   350 mg/m^2 IV on day 1
Repeat cycle every 3 weeks [283].

Cetuximab
Cetuximab: 400 mg/m^2 IV loading dose, then
                                 250 mg/m^2 IV weekly

Repeat cycle on a weekly basis [284].
or
Cetuximab: 500 mg/m^2 IV every 2 weeks (no
                                 loading dose is necessary)

Repeat cycle every 2 weeks [285].

Panitumumab
Panitumumab: 6 mg/kg IV every 2 weeks
Repeat cycle every 2 weeks [286].

5-Fluorouracil (continuous infusion)
5-Fluorouracil: 2,600 mg/m^2 IV over 24 hours weekly
Repeat cycle weekly for 4 weeks [287].
or
5-Fluorouracil: 1,000 mg/m^2/day IV continuous
                                 infusion on days 1–4

Repeat cycle every 21–28 days [288].
or
5-Fluorouracil: 200 mg/m^2/day IV continuous infusion
                                 on days 1–4

L-Leucovorin: 5 mg/m^2/day IV on days 1–4
Repeat cycle every 28 days [289].

Trastuzumab deruxtecan-nxki
Trastuzumab deruxtecan: 6.4 mg/kg IV on day 1
Repeat cycle every 21 days [290]. Used only for patients with HER2-positive disease and wild-type RAS/BRAF.

Regorafenib

Regorafenib: 160 mg PO daily on days 1–21
Repeat cycle every 28 days [291].
or
Regorafenib: 80 mg PO daily on days 1–7
Increase by 40 mg PO daily every week until target dosing of 160 mg is reached depending on tolerability
Repeat cycle every 28 days [292].

TAS-102

TAS-102: 35 mg/m^2 PO bid on days 1–5
                                            and 8–12
Repeat cycle every 28 days [293].

Pembrolizumab (MSI-H/dMMR)

Pembrolizumab: 200 mg IV on day 1
Repeat cycle every 3 weeks [294]. May also administer 400 mg IV every 6 weeks.

Nivolumab (MSI-H/dMMR)

Nivolumab: 3 mg/kg IV day on 1
Repeat cycle every 2 weeks [295]. May also administer using a fixed dose of 240 mg IV on every 2 weeks or 480 mg IV every 4 weeks.

Larotrectinib (NTRK fusion)

Larotrectinib: 100 mg PO bid
Repeat cycle every 28 days [296].

Entrectinib (NTRK fusion)

Entrectinib: 600 mg PO once daily
Repeat cycle every 28 days [297].

ENDOMETRIAL CANCER

Combination Regimens

Paclitaxel + Carboplatin

Paclitaxel: 175 mg/m^2 IV over 3 hours on day 1
Carboplatin: AUC of 5, IV on day 1
Repeat cycle every 28 days [298].

Dostarlimab + Paclitaxel + Carboplatin

Dostarlimab: 500 mg IV on day 1
Paclitaxel: 175 mg/m^2 IV on day 1
Carboplatin: AUC of 5, IV on day 1

Repeat cycle every 28 days for 6 cycles followed by dostarlimab (1,000 mg IV) every 6 weeks for up to 3 years [299].

AC

Doxorubicin: 60 mg/m^2 IV on day 1
Cyclophosphamide: 500 mg/m^2 IV on day 1

Repeat cycle every 21 days [300].

AP

Doxorubicin: 50 mg/m^2 IV on day 1
Cisplatin: 50 mg/m^2 IV on day 1

Repeat cycle every 21 days [301].

Doxorubicin + Paclitaxel

Doxorubicin: 50 mg/m^2 IV on day 1
Paclitaxel: 150 mg/m^2 IV on day 1

Repeat cycle every 21 days [302].

Cisplatin + Doxorubicin + Paclitaxel

Cisplatin: 50 mg/m^2 IV on day 1
Doxorubicin: 45 mg/m^2 IV on day 1
Paclitaxel: 160 mg/m^2 IV over 3 hours on day 2
Filgrastim: 5 µg/kg SC on days 3–12

Repeat cycle every 21 days [303].

CAP

Cyclophosphamide: 500 mg/m^2 IV on day 1
Doxorubicin: 50 mg/m^2 IV on day 1
Cisplatin: 50 mg/m^2 IV on day 1

Repeat cycle every 21 days [304].

Carboplatin + Doxorubicin liposome

Carboplatin: AUC of 5, IV on day 1
Doxorubicin liposome: 40 mg/m^2 IV on day 1

Repeat cycle every 28 days [305].

Paclitaxel + Carboplatin + Bevacizumab

Paclitaxel:	175 mg/m^2 IV over 3 hours on day 1
Carboplatin:	AUC of 5, IV on day 1
Bevacizumab:	15 mg/kg IV on day 1

Repeat cycle every 21 days [306].

Paclitaxel + Ifosfamide (carcinosarcoma)

Paclitaxel:	135 mg/m^2 IV over 3 hours on day 1
Ifosfamide:	1,600 mg/m^2/day IV on days 1–3

Repeat cycle every 21 days for up to 8 cycles [307]. Mesna to be given as either IV or PO. G-CSF support at 5 µg/kg/day SC to be started on day 4.

Cisplatin + Ifosfamide (carcinosarcoma)

Cisplatin:	20 mg/m^2/day IV on days 1–4
Ifosfamide:	1,500 mg/m^2/day IV on day 1
Mesna:	120 mg/m^2 IV (loading dose) followed by 1,500 mg/m^2/day for 24 hours

Repeat cycle every 21 days for 3 cycles [308].

Gemcitabine + Docetaxel

Gemcitabine:	900 mg/m^2 IV on days 1 and 8
Docetaxel:	100 mg/m^2 IV on day 8

Repeat cycle every 21 days [309].

Pembrolizumab + Lenvatinib

Pembrolizumab:	200 mg IV on day 1
Lenvatinib:	20 mg PO daily

Repeat cycle every 3 weeks [310]. Can also give pembrolizumab at 400 mg IV every 6 weeks.

Single-Agent Regimens

Doxorubicin

Doxorubicin:	60 mg/m^2 IV on day 1

Repeat cycle every 21 days [311].

Megestrol

Megestrol:	160 mg PO daily

Continue until disease progression or undue toxicity [312].

Paclitaxel

Paclitaxel: $200 \ mg/m^2$ IV over 3 hours on day 1

Repeat cycle every 21 days [313]. Reduce dose to $175 \ mg/m^2$ IV for patients with prior pelvic radiation therapy.

Topotecan

Topotecan: $1.0 \ mg/m^2/day$ IV on days 1–5

Repeat cycle every 21 days [314]. Reduce dose to $0.8 \ mg/m^2/day$ IV on days 1–3 in patients with prior radiation therapy.

Temsirolimus

Temsirolimus: 25 mg IV on day 1

Repeat cycle every 28 days [315].

Dostarlimab (MSI-H/dMMR)

Dostarlimab: 500 mg IV on day 1

Repeat cycle every 21 days for 4 cycles and then 1,000 mg IV every 6 weeks [316].

Pembrolizumab (MSI-H/dMMR)

Pembrolizumab: 200 mg IV on day 1

Repeat cycle every 21 days for up to 2 years [317].

ESOPHAGEAL CANCER

Neoadjuvant Combined Modality Therapy

Paclitaxel + Carboplatin + Radiation Therapy (CROSS regimen)

Paclitaxel: $50 \ mg/m^2$ IV on days 1, 8, 15, 22, and 29

Carboplatin: AUC of 2 IV on days 1, 8, 15, 22, and 29

Chemotherapy concurrently with radiation therapy of 1.8 Gy in 23 fractions for total dose of 41.4 Gy over 5 weeks [318].

5-Fluorouracil + Cisplatin + Radiation Therapy (PRODIGE5/ACCORD17)

5-Fluorouracil: $1,000 \ mg/m^2/day$ IV continuous infusion on days 1–4

Cisplatin: $75 \ mg/m^2$ IV on day 1

Repeat cycle every 28 days for a total of 2 cycles given concurrently with radiation therapy. Two additional cycles are given every 21 days after completion of the combined modality therapy [319].

Radiation therapy: 200 cGy/day for 5 days per week to a total dose of 5,000 cGy over 5 weeks

FOLFOX + Radiation Therapy (PRODIGE5/ACCORD17)

Oxaliplatin: 85 mg/m^2 IV on day 1

5-Fluorouracil: 400 mg/m^2 IV bolus on day 1, followed by 1,600 mg/m^2 IV continuous infusion for 46 hours

Leucovorin: 200 mg/m^2 IV on day 1 as a 2-hour infusion before the bolus 5-fluorouracil dose

Radiation therapy: 200 cGy/day for 5 days per week to a total dose of 5,000 cGy over 5 weeks

Repeat cycle every 2 weeks for a total of 6 cycles with the first 3 cycles given concurrently with radiation therapy [319].

CAPOX + Radiation Therapy

Oxaliplatin: 85 mg/m^2 IV on days 1, 15, and 29

Capecitabine: 625 mg/m^2 PO bid on days 1–5 for 5 weeks

Radiation therapy: 180 cGy/day for 5 days per week to a total dose of 5,400 cGy

Chemotherapy is given concurrently with radiation therapy, followed by surgical resection [320].

5-Fluorouracil + Cisplatin + Radiation Therapy (FFD French regimen)

5-Fluorouracil: 800 mg/m^2/day IV continuous infusion on days 1–5

Cisplatin: 15 mg/m^2 IV on days 1–5. Administer on days 1, 22, 43, 64, and 92

Radiation therapy: 200 cGy/day for 5 days per week to a total dose of 6,600 cGy over 6.5 weeks

Chemotherapy is given concurrently with radiation therapy, followed by surgical resection [321].

5-Fluorouracil + Cisplatin + Radiation Therapy (Hopkins/Yale regimen)

5-Fluorouracil: 225 mg/m^2/day IV continuous infusion on days 1–30

Cisplatin: 20 mg/m^2/day IV on days 1–5 and 26–30

| Radiation therapy: | 200 cGy/day to a total dose of 4,400 cGy |

Chemotherapy is given concurrently with radiation therapy [322], followed by esophagectomy and then adjuvant chemotherapy in patients who had total gross removal of disease with negative margins.

Adjuvant Chemotherapy

| Paclitaxel: | 135 mg/m^2 IV for 24 hours on day 1 |
| Cisplatin: | 75 mg/m^2 IV on day 2 |

Adjuvant chemotherapy is given 8–12 weeks after esophagectomy, and each cycle is given every 21 days for a total of 3 cycles [322].

MAGIC Trial

Preoperative ECF Chemotherapy

Epirubicin:	50 mg/m^2 IV on day 1
Cisplatin:	60 mg/m^2 IV on day 1
5-Fluorouracil:	200 mg/m^2/day IV continuous infusion on days 1–21

Repeat cycle every 21 days for 3 cycles [323].

Followed by esophagectomy and then adjuvant chemotherapy in patients who had total gross removal of disease with negative margins.

Adjuvant Chemotherapy

Epirubicin:	50 mg/m^2 IV on day 1
Cisplatin:	60 mg/m^2 IV on day 1
5-Fluorouracil:	200 mg/m^2/day IV continuous infusion on days 1–21

Repeat cycle every 21 days for 3 cycles [323].

FLO Trial

Preoperative FLO Chemotherapy

Oxaliplatin:	85 mg/m^2 IV on day 1
Leucovorin:	200 mg/m^2 IV on day 1
5-Fluorouracil:	2,600 mg/m^2 IV continuous infusion over 24 hours on day 1

Repeat cycle every 2 weeks for 4 cycles [324]. Followed by surgical resection and then adjuvant chemotherapy in patients who had total gross removal of disease with negative margins.

Adjuvant Chemotherapy

Oxaliplatin:	85 mg/m^2 IV on day 1
Leucovorin:	200 mg/m^2 IV on day 1
5-Fluorouracil:	2,600 mg/m^2 IV continuous infusion over 24 hours on day 1

Repeat cycle every 2 weeks for 4 cycles [324].

FLOT4 Trial

Preoperative FLOT Chemotherapy

Docetaxel:	50 mg/m^2 IV on day 1
Oxaliplatin:	85 mg/m^2 IV on day 1
Leucovorin:	200 mg/m^2 IV on day 1
5-Fluorouracil:	2,600 mg/m^2 IV continuous infusion over 24 hours on day 1

Repeat cycle every 2 weeks for 4 cycles [325]. Followed by esophagectomy and then adjuvant chemotherapy in patients who had total gross removal of disease with negative margins.

Adjuvant Chemotherapy

Docetaxel:	50 mg/m^2 IV on day 1
Oxaliplatin:	85 mg/m^2 IV on day 1
Leucovorin:	200 mg/m^2 IV on day 1
5-Fluorouracil:	2,600 mg/m^2 IV continuous infusion over 24 hours on day 1

Repeat cycle every 2 weeks for 4 cycles. Note that only patients with resectable gastric or GE junction tumors were included in this trial [325].

Metastatic Disease

Note: All tumors should be tested for HER2 and MSS prior to first-linetherapy. Essentially any regimen can have trastuzumab added if the tumor is HER2 positive using the following schedule:

Trastuzumab:	8 mg/kg IV on day 1 of cycle, followed by 6 mg/kg IV every 3 weeks [326]

Combination Regimens

5-Fluorouracil + Cisplatin

5-Fluorouracil:	1,000 mg/m^2/day IV continuous infusion on days 1–5
Cisplatin:	100 mg/m^2 IV on day 1

Repeat cycle on weeks 1, 5, 8, and 11 [327].

FOLFOX

5-Fluorouracil:	400 mg/m^2 IV bolus on day 1 followed by 2,400 mg/m^2 IV continuous infusion over 46 hours
Leucovorin:	400 mg/m^2 IV on day 1
Oxaliplatin:	400 mg/m^2 IV on day 1

Repeat cycle every 14 days [324].

Paclitaxel + Cisplatin

Paclitaxel:	200 mg/m^2 IV over 24 hours on day 1
Cisplatin:	75 mg/m^2 IV on day 2

Repeat cycle every 21 days [328]. G-CSF support is recommended.

Capecitabine + Oxaliplatin

Capecitabine:	1,000 mg/m^2 PO bid on days 1–14
Oxaliplatin:	130 mg/m^2 IV on day 1

Repeat cycle every 21 days [329].

ECF

Epirubicin:	50 mg/m^2 IV on day 1
Cisplatin:	60 mg/m^2 IV on day 1
5-Fluorouracil:	200 mg/m^2/day IV continuous infusion

Repeat cycle every 21 days [330].

EOF

Epirubicin:	50 mg/m^2 IV on day 1
Oxaliplatin:	130 mg/m^2 IV on day 1
5-Fluorouracil:	200 mg/m^2/day IV continuous infusion

Repeat cycle every 21 days [330].

ECX

Epirubicin:	50 mg/m^2 IV on day 1
Cisplatin:	60 mg/m^2 IV on day 1
Capecitabine:	625 mg/m^2 PO bid continuously

Repeat cycle every 21 days [330].

EOX

Epirubicin:	50 mg/m^2 IV on day 1
Oxaliplatin:	130 mg/m^2 IV on day 1
Capecitabine:	625 mg/m^2 PO bid continuously

Repeat cycle every 21 days [330].

Pembrolizumab + Cisplatin + 5-Fluorouracil

Pembrolizumab:	200 mg IV on day 1
Cisplatin:	80 mg/m^2 IV on day 1
5-Fluorouracil:	800 mg/m^2 IV on days 1–5

Repeat cycle every 3 weeks up to 6 cycles followed by pembrolizumab monotherapy for up to 35 cycles [331].

Nivolumab + Cisplatin + 5-Fluorouracil

Nivolumab:	240 mg IV on days 1 and 15
Cisplatin:	80 mg/m^2 IV on day 1
5-Fluorouracil:	800 mg/m^2 IV on days 1–5

Repeat cycle every 28 days [332].

Nivolumab + Ipilimumab

Nivolumab:	360 mg IV every 2 weeks
Ipilimumab:	1 mg/kg IV on day 1

Repeat cycle every 42 days up to 2 years [332].

Nivolumab + FOLFOX6

Nivolumab:	240 mg IV on day 1
Oxaliplatin:	85 mg/m^2 IV on day 1
5-Fluorouracil:	400 mg/m^2 IV bolus on day 1, followed by 2,400 mg/m^2 IV continuous infusion over 46 hours on days 1 and 2
Leucovorin:	400 mg/m^2 IV on day 1 as a 2-hour infusion before 5-fluorouracil.

Repeat cycle every 2 weeks [333].

Nivolumab + CAPOX

Nivolumab:	360 mg IV on day 1
Capecitabine:	1,000 mg/m^2 PO bid on days 1–14
Oxaliplatin:	130 mg/m^2 IV on day 1

Repeat cycle every 21 days [333].

Pembrolizumab + Trastuzumab + CAPOX (HER-2 positive disease)

Pembrolizumab:	200 mg IV on day 1
Trastuzumab:	8 mg/kg IV on day 1 loading dose and 6 mg/kg with all subsequent cycles
Capecitabine:	850 mg/m^2 PO bid on days 1–14
Oxaliplatin:	130 mg/m^2 IV on day 1

Repeat cycle every 21 days [334].

Pembrolizumab + Trastuzumab + 5-Fluorouracil + Cisplatin (HER-2 positive disease)

Pembrolizumab: 200 mg IV on day 1

Trastuzumab: 8 mg/kg IV on day 1 loading dose and 6 mg/kg with all subsequent cycles

5-Fluorouracil: 800 mg/m^2 IV continuous infusion on days 1–5

Cisplatin: 80 mg/m^2 IV on day 1

Repeat cycle every 21 days [334].

Single-Agent Regimens

Paclitaxel

Paclitaxel: 250 mg/m^2 IV over 24 hours on day 1

Repeat cycle every 21 days [335]. G-CSF support is recommended.

Docetaxel

Docetaxel: 100 mg/m^2 IV on day 1

Repeat cycle every 21 days. [336].

TAS-102

TAS-102:   35 mg/m^2 PO bid on days 1–5 and 8–12

Repeat cycle every 28 days [337].

Pembrolizumab

Pembrolizumab: 200 mg IV on day 1

Repeat cycle every 3 weeks [338]. May also administer 400 mg IV every 6 weeks.

Nivolumab

Nivolumab: 240 mg IV on day 1

Repeat cycle every 2 weeks or can administer 480 mg IV every 4 weeks [339].

Trastuzumab deruxtecan-nxki

Trastuzumab deruxtecan: 6.4 mg/kg IV on day 1

Repeat cycle every 21 days [340]. Used only for patients with HER2-positive disease and wild-type RAS and BRAF.

GASTRIC CANCER

Perioperative Chemotherapy

FLOT4 Trial

Preoperative FLOT Chemotherapy

Docetaxel:	50 mg/m^2 IV on day 1
Oxaliplatin:	85 mg/m^2 IV on day 1
Leucovorin:	200 mg/m^2 IV on day 1
5-Fluorouracil:	2,600 mg/m^2 IV continuous infusion over 24 hours on day 1

Repeat cycle every 2 weeks for 4 cycles [325]. Followed by gastrectomy and then adjuvant chemotherapy in patients who had total gross removal of disease with negative margins.

Adjuvant Chemotherapy

Docetaxel:	50 mg/m^2 IV on day 1
Oxaliplatin:	85 mg/m^2 IV on day 1
Leucovorin:	200 mg/m^2 IV on day 1
5-Fluorouracil:	2,600 mg/m^2 IV continuous infusion over 24 hours on day 1

Repeat cycle every 2 weeks for 4 cycles [325].

Preoperative FLO Chemotherapy

Oxaliplatin:	85 mg/m^2 IV on day 1
Leucovorin:	200 mg/m^2 IV on day 1
5-Fluorouracil:	2,600 mg/m^2 IV continuous infusion over 24 hours on day 1

Repeat cycle every 2 weeks for 3 cycles [324]. Followed by gastrectomy and then adjuvant chemotherapy in patients who had total gross removal of disease with negative margins.

Adjuvant Chemotherapy

Oxaliplatin:	85 mg/m^2 IV on day 1
Leucovorin:	200 mg/m^2 IV on day 1
5-Fluorouracil:	2,600 mg/m^2 IV continuous infusion over 24 hours on day 1

Repeat cycle every 2 weeks for 3 cycles [324].

Adjuvant Therapy

5-Fluorouracil+ Leucovorin + RT

One cycle of chemotherapy is administered as follows:

5-Fluorouracil:	425 mg/m^2 IV on days 1–5
Leucovorin:	20 mg/m^2 IV on days 1–5

Chemoradiotherapy is then started 28 days after the start of the initial cycle of chemotherapy as follows:

Radiation therapy:	180 cGy/day to a total dose of 4,500 cGy, starting on day 28
5-Fluorouracil:	400 mg/m^2 IV on days 1–4 and days 23–25 of radiation therapy
Leucovorin:	20 mg/m^2 IV on days 1–4 and days 23–25 of radiation therapy

Chemoradiotherapy is followed by 2 cycles of chemotherapy that are given 1 month apart and include [341]:

5-Fluorouracil:	425 mg/m^2 IV on days 1–5
Leucovorin:	20 mg/m^2 IV on days 1–5

Capecitabine + RT

One cycle of chemotherapy is administered as follows:

Capecitabine:	1,000 mg/m^2 PO bid on days 1–14

Chemoradiotherapy is then started 21 days after the start of the initial cycle of chemotherapy as follows:

Radiation therapy:	180 cGy/day to a total dose of 4,500 cGy, starting on day 28
Capecitabine:	825 mg/m^2 PO on Monday to Friday

Chemoradiotherapy is followed by 2 cycles of chemotherapy that are given 3 weeks apart and include [342]:

Capecitabine:	1,000 mg/m^2 PO on days 1–14

Capecitabine + Oxaliplatin

Capecitabine:	1,000 mg/m^2 PO bid on days 1–14
Oxaliplatin:	130 mg/m^2 IV on day 1

Repeat cycle every 21 days for 6 months [343].

Metastatic Disease

Combination Regimens

DCF

Docetaxel:	75 mg/m^2 IV on day 1
Cisplatin:	75 mg/m^2 IV on day 1

| 5-Fluorouracil: | 750 mg/m^2/day IV continuous infusion on days 1–5 |

Repeat cycle every 21 days [344].

CF

| Cisplatin: | 100 mg/m^2 IV on day 1 |
| 5-Fluorouracil: | 1,000 mg/m^2/day IV continuous infusion on days 1–5 |

Repeat cycle every 28 days [345].

ECF

Epirubicin:	50 mg/m^2 IV on day 1
Cisplatin:	60 mg/m^2 IV on day 1
5-Fluorouracil:	200 mg/m^2/day IV continuous infusion

Repeat cycle every 21 days [330].

EOF

Epirubicin:	50 mg/m^2 IV on day 1
Oxaliplatin:	130 mg/m^2 IV on day 1
5-Fluorouracil:	200 mg/m^2/day IV continuous infusion

Repeat cycle every 21 days [330].

ECX

Epirubucin:	50 mg/m^2 IV on day 1
Cisplatin:	60 mg/m^2 IV on day 1
Capecitabine:	625 mg/m^2 PO bid continuously

Repeat cycle every 21 days [330].

EOX

Epirubicin:	50 mg/m^2 IV on day 1
Oxaliplatin:	130 mg/m^2 IV on day 1
Capecitabine:	625 mg/m^2 PO bid continuously

Repeat cycle every 21 days [330].

Docetaxel + Cisplatin

| Docetaxel: | 85 mg/m^2 IV on day 1 |
| Cisplatin: | 75 mg/m^2 IV on day 1 |

Repeat cycle every 21 days [346].

Capecitabine + Cisplatin

Capecitabine:	1,000 mg/m^2 PO bid on days 1–14
Cisplatin:	80 mg/m^2 IV on day 1

Repeat cycle every 21 days [347].

XP + Trastuzumab

Capecitabine:	1,000 mg/m^2 PO bid on days 1–14
Cisplatin:	80 mg/m^2 IV on day 1
Trastuzumab:	8 mg/kg IV loading dose, then 6 mg/kg IV every 3 weeks

Repeat cycle every 21 days [348]. Used only for HER2-overexpressing adenocarcinoma. May consider adding pembrolizumab, regardless of PD-L1 CPS, at a dose of 200 mg IV on day 1 with cycles repeated every 3 weeks.

FP + Trastuzumab

5-Fluorouracil:	800 mg/m^2 IV continuous infusion on days 1–5
Cisplatin:	80 mg/m^2 IV on day 1
Trastuzumab:	8 mg/kg IV loading dose, then 6 mg/kg IV every 3 weeks

Repeat cycle every 21 days [348]. Used only for HER2-overexpressing adenocarcinoma. May consider adding pembrolizumab, regardless of PD-L1 CPS, at a dose of 200 mg IV on day 1 with cycles repeated every 3 weeks.

FLO

5-Fluorouracil:	2,600 mg/m^2 IV on day 1 as a continuous infusion over 24 hours
Leucovorin:	200 mg/m^2 IV on day 1 as a 2-hour infusion
Oxaliplatin:	85 mg/m^2 IV on day 1

Repeat cycle every 14 days [349].

FOLFOX

Oxaliplatin:	85 mg/m^2 IV on day 1
5-Fluorouracil:	400 mg/m^2 IV bolus on day 1 followed by 2,400 mg/m^2 IV continuous infusion over 46 hours on days 1–3
Leucovorin:	400 mg/m^2 IV on day 1

Repeat cycle every 2 weeks [350].

Paclitaxel + Ramucirumab

Paclitaxel:	80 mg/m^2 IV on days 1, 8, and 15
Ramucirumab:	8 mg/kg IV on days 1 and 15

Repeat cycle every 28 days [351].

FOLFIRI + Ramucirumab

Irinotecan:	180 mg/m^2 IV on day 1
5-Fluorouracil:	400 mg/m^2 IV bolus on day 1, followed by 2,400 mg/m^2 IV continuous infusion for 46 hours on days 1 and 2
Leucovorin:	400 mg/m^2 IV on day 1 as a 2-hour infusion prior to 5-fluorouracil
Ramucirumab:	8 mg/kg IV on day 1

Repeat cycle every 2 weeks [352].

Irinotecan + Ramucirumab

Irinotecan:	150 mg/m^2 IV on day 1
Ramucirumab:	8 mg/kg IV on day 1

Repeat cycle every 2 weeks [353].

Pembrolizumab + Cisplatin + 5-Fluorouracil

Pembrolizumab:	200 mg IV on day 1
Cisplatin:	80 mg/m^2 IV on day 1
5-Fluorouracil:	800 mg/m^2 IV on day 1

Repeat cycle every 3 weeks up to 6 cycles followed by pembrolizumab as monotherapy for up to 35 cycles [331].

Nivolumab + FOLFOX6

Nivolumab:	240 mg IV on day 1
Oxaliplatin:	85 mg/m^2 IV on day 1
5-Fluorouracil:	400 mg/m^2 IV bolus on day 1, followed by 2,400 mg/m^2 IV continuous infusion over 46 hours on days 1 and 2
Leucovorin:	400 mg/m^2 IV on day 1 as a 2-hour infusion before 5-fluorouracil.

Repeat cycle every 2 weeks [333].

Nivolumab + CAPOX

Nivolumab:	360 mg IV on day 1
Capecitabine:	850 mg/m^2 PO bid on days 1–14

| Oxaliplatin: | 130 mg/m^2 IV on day 1 |
| Bevacizumab: | 7.5 mg/kg every 3 weeks |

Repeat cycle every 21 days [333].

Nivolumab + Ipilimumab

| Nivolumab: | 3 mg/kg IV on day 1 every 2 weeks |
| Ipilimumab: | 1 mg/kg IV on day 1 every 6 weeks |

Continue nivolumab every 2 weeks and ipilimumab every 6 weeks. Used in first-line setting in metastatic or locally advanced unresectable esophageal squamous cell carcinoma regardless of PD-L1 status [354].

Pembrolizumab + Trastuzumab + CAPOX (HER-2 positive disease)

Pembrolizumab:	200 mg IV on day 1
Trastuzumab:	8 mg/kg IV on day 1 in first infusion and 6 mg/kg for all subsequent cycles
Capecitabine:	850 mg/m^2 PO bid on days 1–14
Oxaliplatin:	130 mg/m^2 IV on day 1

Repeat cycle every 21 days [334].

Pembrolizumab + Trastuzumab + 5-Fluorouracil + Cisplatin (HER-2 positive disease)

Pembrolizumab:	200 mg IV on day 1
Trastuzumab:	8 mg/kg IV on day 1 in first infusion and 6 mg/kg for all subsequent cycles
5-Fluorouracil:	800 mg/m^2 IV continuous infusion on days 1–5
Cisplatin:	80 mg/m^2 IV on day 1

Repeat cycle every 21 days [334].

Single-Agent Regimens

5-Fluorouracil

| 5-Fluorouracil: | 500 mg/m^2 IV on days 1–5 |

Repeat cycle every 28 days [355].

5-Fluorouracil + Leucovorin

| 5-Fluorouracil: | 370 mg/m^2 IV on days 1–5 |
| Leucovorin: | 200 mg/m^2 IV on days 1–5 |

Repeat cycle every 21 days [356].

Paclitaxel

Paclitaxel: 250 mg/m^2 IV on day 1

Repeat cycle every 21 days [357].

or

Paclitaxel: 80 mg/m^2 IV on days 1, 8, and 15

Repeat cycle every 28 days [358].

Docetaxel

Docetaxel: 100 mg/m^2 IV on day 1

Repeat cycle every 21 days [359].

or

Docetaxel: 36 mg/m^2 IV weekly for 6 weeks

Repeat cycle every 8 weeks [360].

Irinotecan

Irinotecan: 250 mg/m^2 IV on day 1

Repeat cycle every 3 weeks [361]. Dose of irinotecan can be increased to 350 mg/m^2 based on toxicity.

Ramucirumab

Ramucirumab: 8 mg/kg IV on day 1

Repeat cycle every 14 days [362].

Pembrolizumab

Pembrolizumab: 200 mg IV on day 1

Repeat cycle every 3 weeks [363]. May also administer 400 mg IV every 6 weeks.

Nivolumab

Nivolumab: 240 mg IV on day 1

Repeat cycle every 2 weeks or can administer 480 mg IV every 4 weeks. Used for MSS/pMMR esophageal squamous cell carcinoma after prior fluoropyrimidine- and platinum-based chemotherapy and for MSI-H/dMMR disease [339].

Dostarlimab (MSI-H/dMMR)

Dostarlimab: 500 mg IV on day 1 every 3 weeks for 4 doses followed by 1,000 mg IV on day 1 every 6 weeks

Repeat cycle every 3 weeks for 4 doses, followed by 1,000 mg IV on day 1 every 6 weeks [364].

Trastuzumab deruxtecan-nxki

Trastuzumab deruxtecan: 6.4 mg/kg IV on day 1

Repeat cycle every 21 days [365]. Used only for patients with HER2-positive disease and wild-type RAS and BRAF.

TAS-102

TAS-102:   35 mg/m^2 PO bid on days 1–5 and 8–12

Repeat cycle every 28 days [366].

GASTROINTESTINAL STROMAL TUMOR (GIST)

Adjuvant Therapy

Imatinib

Imatinib: 400 mg/day PO

Continue treatment for a total of 3 years [367]. Use for patients with intermediate or high risk of recurrence after complete gross resection.

Metastatic Disease

Single-Agent Regimens

Imatinib

Imatinib: 400 mg/day PO

Continue treatment until disease progression [368]. May increase dose to 600 mg/day if no response is seen. In patients with KIT exon 9 (or exon 11) mutation, use dose of 800 mg/day (400 mg bid).

Nilotinib

Nilotinib: 400 mg PO bid

Continue treatment until disease progression [369].

Dasatinib

Dasatinib: 50 mg PO bid for 1 week followed by 70 mg PO bid

Continue treatment until disease progression [370].

Sunitinib

Sunitinib: 50 mg/day PO for 4 weeks

Repeat cycle every 6 weeks [371].

Sorafenib

Sorafenib: 400 mg/day PO bid

Continue treatment until disease progression [372].

Regorafenib

Regorafenib: 160 mg/day PO for 21 days

Repeat cycle every 28 days [373].

Ripretinib

Ripretinib: 150 mg PO daily

Repeat cycle every 28 days [374]. Consider increasing dose to 150 mg PO bid if progression on once daily dosing.

Avapritinib

Avapritinib: 300 mg PO daily

Repeat cycle every 28 days [375]. Preferred frontline regimen for PDGFRA exon 18 D842V mutation, which confers primary resistance to imatinib and sunitinib.

Cabozantinib

Cabozantinib: 60 mg PO daily

Repeat cycle every 28 days [376].

HEAD AND NECK CANCER

Combined Modality Therapy

Cetuximab + Radiation Therapy

Cetuximab: 400 mg/m^2 IV loading dose, 1 week before radiation therapy, then 250 mg/m^2 IV weekly

Radiation therapy: 200 cGy/day for 5 days per week (total dose, 7,000 cGy)

Cetuximab is given concurrently with radiation therapy [377].

TPF Induction Chemotherapy Followed by Carboplatin + Radiation Therapy

Docetaxel: 75 mg/m^2 IV on day 1

Cisplatin: $75–100 \text{ mg/m}^2$ IV on day 1

5-Fluorouracil: $1,000 \text{ mg/m}^2$/day IV continuous infusion on days 1–4

Repeat cycle every 3 weeks for 3 cycles followed by:

| Carboplatin: | AUC of 1.5, IV weekly for 7 weeks during radiation therapy |
| Radiation therapy: | 200 cGy/day to a total dose of 7,400 cGy |

At the completion of chemoradiotherapy, surgical resection as indicated [378].

Combination Regimens

TIP

Paclitaxel:	175 mg/m² IV over 3 hours on day 1
Ifosfamide:	1,000 mg/m² IV on days 1–3
Mesna:	600 mg/m² IV on days 1–3 before ifosfamide
Cisplatin:	60 mg/m² IV on day 1

Repeat cycle every 21–28 days [379].

TPF

Docetaxel:	75 mg/m² IV on day 1
Cisplatin:	75–100 mg/m² IV over 24 hours on day 1
5-Fluorouracil:	1,000 mg/m² over 24 hours on days 1–4

Repeat cycle every 21 days [380].

TIC

Paclitaxel:	175 mg/m² IV over 3 hours on day 1
Ifosfamide:	1,000 mg/m² IV over 2 hours on days 1–3
Mesna:	400 mg/m² IV before ifosfamide and 200 mg/m² IV, 4 hours after ifosfamide
Carboplatin:	AUC of 6, IV on day 1

Repeat cycle every 21–28 days [381].

Paclitaxel + Carboplatin

| Paclitaxel: | 175 mg/m² IV over 3 hours on day 1 |
| Carboplatin: | AUC of 6, IV on day 1 |

Repeat cycle every 21 days [382].

Paclitaxel + Cisplatin

Paclitaxel:	175 mg/m² IV over 3 hours on day 1
Cisplatin:	75 mg/m² IV on day 2
G-CSF:	5 µg/kg/day SC on days 4–10

Repeat cycle every 21 days [383].

PF

Cisplatin:	100 mg/m^2 IV on day 1
5-Fluorouracil:	1,000 mg/m^2/day IV continuous infusion on days 1–5

Repeat cycle every 21–28 days [384].

Carboplatin + 5-FU

Carboplatin:	AUC of 5, IV on day 1
5-Fluorouracil:	1,000 mg/m^2/day IV continuous infusion on days 1–4

Repeat cycle every 21 days [385].

Pembrolizumab + Carboplatin + 5-FU

Pembrolizumab:	200 mg IV on day 1
Carboplatin:	AUC of 5, IV on day 1
5-Fluorouracil:	1,000 mg/m^2/day IV continuous infusion on days 1–4

Repeat cycle every 21 days for 4 cycles followed by pembrolizumab monotherapy at 200 mg IV on day 1 every 3 weeks for up to 35 cycles [386].

Pembrolizumab + Cisplatin + 5-FU

Pembrolizumab:	200 mg IV on day 1
Cisplatin:	100 mg IV on day 1
5-Fluorouracil:	1,000 mg/m^2/day IV continuous infusion on days 1–4

Repeat cycle every 21 days for 4 cycles followed by pembrolizumab monotherapy at 200 mg IV on day 1 every 3 weeks for up to 35 cycles [386].

PF + Cetuximab

Cisplatin:	100 mg/m^2 IV on day 1
5-Fluorouracil:	1,000 mg/m^2/day IV continuous infusion on days 1–4
Cetuximab:	400 mg/m^2 IV loading dose, then 250 mg/m^2 IV weekly

Repeat cycle every 21 days for up to 6 cycles. If no evidence of disease progression at the end of 6 cycles, can continue with weekly cetuximab [387].

Carboplatin + 5-FU + Cetuximab

Carboplatin:	AUC of 5, IV on day 1
5-Fluorouracil:	1,000 mg/m^2/day IV continuous infusion on days 1–4

Cetuximab: 400 mg/m^2 IV loading dose, then
                            250 mg/m^2 IV weekly

Repeat cycle every 21 days for up to 6 cycles. If no evidence of disease progression at the end of 6 cycles, can continue with weekly cetuximab [387].

Cisplatin + Cetuximab

Cisplatin: 100 mg/m^2 IV on day 1
Cetuximab: 400 mg/m^2 IV loading dose, then
                            250 mg/m^2 IV weekly

Repeat cycle every 21 days [388].

PF-Larynx Preservation

Cisplatin: 100 mg/m^2 IV on day 1
5-Fluorouracil: 1,000 mg/m^2/day IV continuous
                            infusion on days 1–5
Radiation therapy: 6,600–7,600 cGy in 180–200 cGy
                            fractions

Repeat cycle every 21–28 days for 3 cycles [389].

Concurrent Chemoradiation Therapy for Laryngeal Preservation

Cisplatin: 100 mg/m^2 IV on days 1, 22, and 43
Radiation therapy: 7,000 cGy in 200 cGy fractions

Administer cisplatin concurrently with radiation therapy [390].

Chemoradiotherapy for Nasopharyngeal Cancer

Cisplatin: 100 mg/m^2 IV on days 1, 22, and 43
                            during radiotherapy
Radiation therapy: Total dose of 7,000 cGy in 180–200 cGy
                            fractions

At the completion of chemoradiotherapy, chemotherapy is administered as follows:

Cisplatin: 80 mg/m^2 IV on day 1
5-Fluorouracil: 1,000 mg/m^2/day IV continuous
                            infusion on days 1–4

Repeat cycle every 28 days for a total of 3 cycles [391].

VP

Vinorelbine: 25 mg/m^2 IV on days 1 and 8
Cisplatin: 80 mg/m^2 IV on day 1

Repeat cycle every 21 days [392].

Single-Agent Regimens

Docetaxel

Docetaxel: 100 mg/m^2 IV on day 1

Repeat cycle every 21 days [393].

Paclitaxel

Paclitaxel: 250 mg/m^2 IV over 24 hours on day 1

Repeat cycle every 21 days [394].

or

Paclitaxel: 137–175 mg/m^2 IV over 3 hours on day 1

Repeat cycle every 21 days [395].

Vinorelbine

Vinorelbine: 30 mg/m^2 IV weekly

Repeat cycle every week [395].

Cetuximab

Cetuximab: 400 mg/m^2 IV loading dose, then 250 mg/m^2 IV weekly

Repeat cycle every week [396].

Pembrolizumab

Pembrolizumab: 200 mg IV on day 1

Repeat cycle every 3 weeks [397]. May also administer 400 mg IV every 6 weeks.

Nivolumab

Nivolumab: 240 mg IV on day 1

Repeat cycle every 14 days [398].

HEPATOCELLULAR CANCER

Combination Regimens

FOLFOX4

Oxaliplatin: 85 mg/m^2 IV on day 1

5-Fluorouracil: 400 mg/m^2 IV bolus, followed by 600 mg/m^2 IV continuous infusion for 22 hours on days 1 and 2

Leucovorin: 200 mg/m^2 IV on days 1 and 2 as a 2-hour infusion before 5-fluorouracil

Repeat cycle every 2 weeks [399].

Atezolizumab + Bevacizumab

Atezolizumab:	1,200 mg IV on day 1
Bevacizumab:	15 mg/kg IV on day 1

Repeat cycle every 21 days [400].

Ipilimumab + Nivolumab

Ipilimumab:	3 mg/kg IV on day 1
Nivolumab:	1 mg/kg IV on day 1

Repeat cycle every 21 days for 4 cycles followed by

Nivolumab:	240 mg IV on day 1

Repeat cycle every 2 weeks [401]. May also administer 480 mg IV on day 1 every 4 weeks.

Durvalumab + Tremelimumab

For weight >30 kg

Durvalumab:	1,500 mg IV on day 1
Tremelimumab:	300 mg IV on day 1 of first cycle only

Repeat durvalumab every 28 days [402].

For weight <30 kg

Durvalumab:	20 mg/kg IV on day 1
Tremelimumab:	4 mg/kg IV on day 1

Repeat durvalumab every 4 weeks [402].

Single-Agent Regimens

Sorafenib

Sorafenib:	400 mg PO bid

Continue until disease progression [403]. Dose may be reduced to 400 mg once daily or 400 mg every 2 days.

Lenvatinib

Lenvatinib:	12 mg PO daily if body weight >60 kg, or 8 mg PO daily if body weight <60 kg

Continue until disease progression [404]. Dose may be reduced to 4 mg daily or 4 mg every other day depending on toxicity.

Cabozantinib

Cabozantinib:	60 mg PO daily

Continue until disease progression [405]. Dose may be reduced to 40 mg daily and 20 mg daily depending on toxicity.

Regorafenib

Regorafenib: 160 mg PO daily for 21 days

Repeat cycle every 28 days [406].

Nivolumab

Nivolumab: 240 mg IV on day 1

Repeat cycle every 2 weeks [407]. May also give 480 mg IV on day 1 every 4 weeks

Pembrolizumab

Pembrolizumab: 10 mg/kg IV on day 1

Repeat cycle every 14 days [408]. May also administer 200 mg IV every 3 weeks or 400 mg IV every 6 weeks.

Ramucirumab

Ramucirumab: 8 mg/kg IV on day 1

Repeat cycle every 14 days [409]. Use only if AFP≥400 ng/mL.

KAPOSI'S SARCOMA

Combination Regimens

BV

Bleomycin: 10 U/m^2 IV on days 1 and 15

Vincristine: 1.4 mg/m^2 IV on days 1 and 15 (maximum, 2 mg)

Repeat cycle every 2 weeks [410].

ABV

Doxorubicin: 40 mg/m^2 IV on day 1

Bleomycin: 15 U/m^2 IV on days 1 and 15

Vinblastine: 6 mg/m^2 IV on day 1

Repeat cycle every 28 days [411].

Single-Agent Regimens

Daunorubicin liposome

Daunorubicin liposome: 40 mg/m^2 IV on day 1

Repeat cycle every 14 days [412].

Doxorubicin liposome

Doxorubicin liposome: 20 mg/m^2 IV on day 1

Repeat cycle every 21 days [413]

Paclitaxel

Paclitaxel:
Repeat cycle every 21 days [414].

135 mg/m^2 IV over 3 hours on day 1

or

Paclitaxel:
Repeat cycle every 2 weeks [415].

100 mg/m^2 IV over 3 hours on day 1

Docetaxel

Docetaxel:

25 mg/m^2 IV weekly for 8 weeks, then every other week

Continue until disease progression [416].

Etoposide

Etoposide:
Repeat cycle every 2 weeks [417].

50 mg PO daily on days 1–7

Vinorelbine

Vinorelbine:
Repeat cycle every 2 weeks [418].

30 mg/m^2 IV on day 1

Interferon-α

Interferon α-2a:

36 million IU/m^2 SC or IM, daily for 8–12 weeks [419]

Interferon α-2b:

30 million IU/m^2 SC or IM, 3 times weekly [420]

Pomalidomide

Pomalidomide:
Repeat cycle every 28 days [421].

5 mg PO daily for 21 days

LEUKEMIA

Acute Lymphocytic Leukemia

Induction Therapy

Linker Regimen [422, 423]

Daunorubicin:

50 mg/m^2 IV every 24 hours on days 1–3

Vincristine:

2 mg IV on days 1, 8, 15, and 22

| Prednisone: | 60 mg/m^2 PO divided into 3 doses on days 1–28 |
| L-Asparaginase: | 6,000 U/m^2 IM on days 17 28 |

If bone marrow on day 14 is positive for residual leukemia,

| Daunorubicin: | 50 mg/m^2 IV on day 15 |

If bone marrow on day 28 is positive for residual leukemia,

Daunorubicin:	50 mg/m^2 IV on days 29 and 30
Vincristine:	2 mg IV on days 29 and 36
Prednisone:	60 mg/m^2 PO on days 29–42
L-Asparaginase:	6,000 U/m^2 IM on days 29–35

Consolidation Therapy
Linker Regimen [422, 423]
Treatment A (cycles 1, 3, 5, and 7)

Daunorubicin:	50 mg/m^2 IV on days 1 and 2
Vincristine:	2 mg IV on days 1 and 8
Prednisone:	60 mg/m^2 PO on days 1–14
L-Asparaginase:	12,000 U/m^2 on days 2, 4, 7, 9, 11, and 14

Treatment B (cycles 2, 4, 6, and 8)

| Teniposide: | 165 mg/m^2 IV on days 1, 4, 8, and 11 |
| Cytarabine: | 300 mg/m^2 IV on days 1, 4, 8, and 11 |

Treatment C (cycle 9)

| Methotrexate: | 690 mg/m^2 IV over 42 hours |
| Leucovorin: | 15 mg/m^2 IV every 6 hours for 12 doses beginning at 42 hours |

Maintenance Therapy
Linker Regimen [422, 423]

| Methotrexate: | 20 mg/m^2 PO weekly |
| 6-Mercaptopurine: | 75 mg/m^2 PO daily |

Continue for a total of 30 months of complete response.

CNS Prophylaxis

| Cranial irradiation: | 1,800 cGy in 10 fractions over 12–14 days |
| Methotrexate: | 12 mg IT weekly for 6 weeks |

Begin within 1 week of complete response.

In patients with documented CNS involvement at time of diagnosis, intrathecal chemotherapy should begin during induction chemotherapy.

Methotrexate:	12 mg IT weekly for 10 doses
Cranial irradiation:	2,800 cGy

Induction Therapy
Larson Regimen [424]
Induction (weeks 1–4)

Induction (weeks 1–4):	1,200 mg/m^2 IV on day 1
Daunorubicin:	45 mg/m^2 IV on days 1–3
Vincristine:	2 mg IV on days 1, 8, 15, and 22
Prednisone:	60 mg/m^2/day PO on days 1–21
L-Asparaginase:	6,000 U/m^2 SC on days 5, 8, 11, 15, 18, 22

Early Intensification (weeks 5–12)

Methotrexate:	15 mg IT on day 1
Cyclophosphamide:	1,000 mg/m^2 IV on day 1
6-Mercaptopurine:	60 mg/m^2/day PO on days 1–14
Cytarabine:	75 mg/m^2 IV on days 1–4 and 8–11
Vincristine:	2 mg IV on days 15 and 22
L-Asparaginase:	6,000 U/m^2 SC on days 15, 18, 22, and 25

Repeat the early intensification cycle once.

CNS Prophylaxis and Interim Maintenance (weeks 13–25)

Cranial irradiation:	2,400 cGy on days 1–12
Methotrexate:	15 mg IT on days 1, 8, 15, 22, and 29
6-Mercaptopurine:	60 mg/m^2/day PO on days 1–70
Methotrexate:	20 mg/m^2 PO on days 36, 43, 50, 57, and 64

Late Intensification (weeks 26–33)

Doxorubicin:	30 mg/m^2 IV on days 1, 8, and 15
Vincristine:	2 mg IV on days 1, 8, and 15
Dexamethasone:	10 mg/m^2/day PO on days 1–14
Cyclophosphamide:	1,000 mg/m^2 IV on day 29
6-Thioguanine:	60 mg/m^2/day PO on days 29–42
Cytarabine:	75 mg/m^2 on days 29, 32, 36–39

Prolonged Maintenance (continue until 24 months after diagnosis)

Vincristine:	2 mg IV on day 1
Prednisone:	60 mg/m^2/day PO on days 1–5
Methotrexate:	20 mg/m^2 PO on days 1, 8, 15, and 22
6-Mercaptopurine:	80 mg/m^2/day PO on days 1–28

Repeat maintenance cycle every 28 days.

Hyper-CVAD Regimen

Cyclophosphamide:	300 mg/m^2 IV every 12 hours for 6 doses on days 1–3
Mesna:	600 mg/m^2 IV over 24 hours on days 1–3 ending 6 hours after the last dose of cyclophosphamide
Vincristine:	2 mg IV on days 4 and 11
Doxorubicin:	50 mg/m^2 IV on day 4
Dexamethasone:	40 mg PO or IV on days 1–4 and 11–14

Alternate cycles every 21 days with the following:

Methotrexate:	200 mg/m^2 IV over 2 hours, followed by 800 mg/m^2 IV over 24 hours on day 1
Leucovorin:	15 mg IV every 6 hours for 8 doses, starting 24 hours after completion of methotrexate infusion
Cytaribine:	3,000 mg/m^2 IV every 12 hours for 4 doses on days 2–3
Methylprednisolone:	50 mg IV bid on days 1–3

Alternate 4 cycles of hyper-CVAD with 4 cycles of high-dose methotrexate and cytarabine therapy [425].

CNS Prophylaxis

Methotrexate:	12 mg IT on day 2
Cytarabine:	100 mg IT on day 8

Repeat with each cycle of chemotherapy, depending on the risk of CNS disease.

Supportive Care

Ciprofloxacin:	500 mg PO bid
Fluconazole:	200 mg/day PO
Acyclovir:	200 mg PO bid
G-CSF:	10 µg/kg/day starting 24 hours after the end of chemotherapy (i.e., on day 5 of hyper-CVAD therapy and on day 4 of high-dose methotrexate and cytarabine therapy)

Single-Agent Regimens

Clofarabine
Clofarabine: $52 \ mg/m^2$ IV for 5 days

Repeat cycle every 2–6 weeks [426].

Nelarabine
Nelarabine: $1.5 \ g/m^2/day$ IV on days 1, 3, and 5

Repeat cycle every 28 days up to a total of 4 cycles [426a].

Imatinib
Imatinib: 600 mg PO daily

Continue until disease progression [427].

Dasatinib
Dasatinib: 70 mg PO bid

Continue until disease progression [428].

Nilotinib
Nilotinib: 400–600 mg PO bid

Continue until disease progression [429].

Brexucabtagene autoleucel [430]
Cyclophosphamide: $900 \ mg/m^2$ IV on day 2

Fludarabine: $25 \ mg/m^2$ IV on days 4, 3, and 2

Brexucabtagene autoleucel: 1.0×10^6 CAR-positive T cells/kg (maximum, 1×10^8 cells) IV on day 1

Tisagenlecleucel [431]
Cyclophosphamide: $250 \ mg/m^2$ IV on days 5, 4, and 3

Fludarabine: $25 \ mg/m^2$ IV on days 5, 4, and 3

Tisagenlecleucel: 0.2–5.0×10^8 CAR-positive T cells per kg IV on day 1 (patients 50 kg or less)

0.1–2.5×10^8 CAR-positive T cells IV on day 1 (patients >50 kg)

Blinatumomab
Blinatumomab: $9 \ \mu g$ IV on days 1–7 and $28 \ \mu g$ IV on days 8–28 on cycle 1; $28 \ \mu g$ on days 1–28 on all subsequent cycles

Repeat cycle every 42 days [432].

Inotuzumab

Inotuzumab: 0.8 mg/m^2 IV on days 1, 8, and 15
Repeat cycle every 21 days (433).
For patients who achieve CR or CRi:
Inotuzumab: 0.5 mg/m^2 IV on days 1, 8, and 15
Repeat cycle every 28 days (433).
For patients who do not achieve CR or CRi:
Inotuzumab: 0.8 mg/m^2 IV on day 1
0.5 mg/m^2 IV on days 8 and 15
Repeat cycle every 28 days (433).

Acute Myelogenous Leukemia

Induction Regimens

Ara-C + Daunorubicin (7 + 3) [434]

Cytarabine: $100 \text{ mg/m}^2\text{/day}$ IV continuous infusion on days 1–7

Daunorubicin: 45 mg/m^2 IV on days 1–3

Liposomal Daunorubicin and Cytarabine **[435]**

Lip daunorubicin/cytarabine: 100 U/m^2 (44 mg/m^2 daunorubicin and 100 mg/m^2 cytarabine) IV on days 1, 3, and 5

A second induction course and up to 2 cycles of consolidation therapy can be given [391].

Ara-C + Daunorubicin + Gemtuzumab

Cytarabine: 200 mg/m^2 IV on days 1–7
Daunorubicin: 60 mg/m^2 IV on days 1–3
Gemtuzumab: 3 mg/m^2 IV on days 1, 4, and 7

In patients with a complete remission after induction therapy, they should then receive 2 cycles of consolidation therapy with cytarabine and daunorubicin administered using the dosing schedule as above and gemtuzumab at 3 mg/m^2 IV on day 1 [436].

Ara-C + Idarubicin [437]

Cytarabine: $100 \text{ mg/m}^2\text{/day}$ IV continuous infusion on days 1–7

Idarubicin: 12 mg/m^2 IV on days 1–3

Ara-C + Daunorubicin + Quizartinib

Cytarabine: $100 \text{ mg/m}^2\text{/day}$ IV continuous infusion on days 1–7

| Daunorubicin: | 60 mg/m² IV on days 1–3 |
| Quizartinib: | 40 mg PO daily starting on day 8 for 14 days |

In patients with a complete remission after induction therapy, they should then receive consolidation therapy with high-dose cytarabine plus quizartinib 40 mg PO daily [438].

Quizartinib + Ara-C + Idarubicin

Cytarabine:	100 mg/m²/day IV continuous infusion on days 1–7
Idarubicin:	12 mg/m² IV on days 1–3
Quizartinib:	40 mg PO daily starting on day 8 for 14 days

In patients with a complete remission after induction therapy, they should then receive consolidation therapy with high-dose cytarabine plus quizartinib 40 mg PO daily [438].

Ara-C + Doxorubicin [439]

| Cytarabine: | 100 mg/m²/day IV continuous infusion on days 1–7 |
| Doxorubicin: | 30 mg/m² IV on days 1–3 |

Ara-C + Clofarabine

| Clofarabine: | 40 mg/m² IV over 1 hour on days 2–6 |
| Cytarabine: | 1,000 mg/m² IV over 2 hours on days 1–5 |

Repeat cycles every 4–6 weeks for up to a total of 3 cycles [440].

Ara-C + Daunorubicin + Midostaurin

Cytarabine:	200 mg/m² IV on days 1–7
Daunorubicin:	60 mg/m² IV on days 1–3
Midostaurin:	50 mg/m² PO bid on days 8–21

In patients who achieve a complete remission after induction therapy, they should then receive consolidation therapy.

Consolidation

| Cytarabine: | 3,000 mg/m² IV every 12 hours on days 1, 3, and 5 |
| Midostaurin: | 50 mg/m² PO bid on days 8–21 |

Repeat cycle every 28 days for a total of 4 cycles of consolidation therapy.

In patients who remain in complete remission after completion of consolidation therapy, they then receive maintenance therapy.

Maintenance

Midostaurin:	50 mg/m^2 PO bid

Repeat cycle every 28 days for a total of 12 cycles [441].

AIDA (acute promyelocytic leukemia only) [442]

ATRA:	45 mg/m^2 PO daily
Idarubicin:	12 mg/m^2 IV on days 2, 4, 6, and 8

Tretinoin + Daunorubicin + Cytarabine (acute promyelocytic leukemia) [443]

ATRA:	45 mg/m^2 PO daily
Daunorubicin:	60 mg/m^2 IV on days 1–3
Cytarabine:	200 mg/m^2 IV on days 1–7

Tretinoin + Arsenic trioxide (acute promyelocytic leukemia)

ATRA:	45 mg/m^2 PO daily
Arsenic trioxide:	0.15 mg/kg/day IV starting on day 10

Continue treatment until CR [444]. Once in CR, patients receive the following:

ATRA:	45 mg/m^2 PO daily on weeks 1–2, 5–6, 9–10, 13–14, 17–18, 21–22, and 25–26
Arsenic trioxide:	0.15 mg/kg/day IV on Monday–Friday on weeks 1–4, 9–12, 17–20, and 25–28

Therapy should be terminated 28 weeks after the CR date.

Mitoxantrone + Etoposide (salvage regimen) [445]

Mitoxantrone:	10 mg/m^2/day IV on days 1–5
Etoposide:	100 mg/m^2/day IV on days 1–5

FLAG

Fludarabine:	30 mg/m^2 IV on days 1–5
Cytarabine:	2,000 mg/m^2/day IV over 4 hours on days 1–5 starting 3.5 hours after fludarabine
G-CSF:	5 µg/kg/day SC starting 24 hours before chemotherapy

An additional cycle may be given in the setting of a partial response [446].

Consolidation Regimens

Ara-C + Daunorubicin (5 + 2) [447]

Cytarabine:	100 mg/m^2/day IV continuous infusion on days 1–5
Daunorubicin:	45 mg/m^2 IV on days 1 and 2

Liposomal Daunorubicin and Cytarabine [435]

Lip daunorubicin/cytarabine: 29 mg/m^2 daunorubicin and 65 mg/m^2 cytarabine on days 1 and 3

Ara-C + Idarubicin [448]

Cytarabine: 100 mg/m^2 IV continuous infusion on days 1–5

Idarubicin: 13 mg/m^2 IV on days 1 and 2

Repeat cycle every 21–28 days.

Glasdegib + Cytarabine

Glasdegib: 100 mg PO daily

Cytarabine: 20 mg SC BID on days 1–10

Repeat cycle every 28 days [449].

Venetoclax + Azacitidine (or Decitabine)

Venetoclax: 20 mg ramp up to 400 mg PO daily

Azacitidine: 75 mg/m^2 IV on days 1–7

Repeat cycle every 28 days [450].

or

Venetoclax: 20 mg ramp up to 400 mg PO daily

Decitabine: 20 mg/m^2 IV on days 1–5

Repeat cycle every 28 days [450].

Ivosidenib + Azacitidine (IDH1 mutation)

Ivosidenib: 500 mg PO daily

Azacitidine: 75 mg/m^2 IV on days 1–7

Repeat cycle every 28 days [451].

Single-Agent Regimens

Cladribine [452]

Cladribine: 0.1 mg/kg/day IV continuous infusion on days 1–7

High-Dose Cytarabine

Cytarabine: 1,500–3,000 mg/m2 IV over 3 hours, every 12 hours on days 1, 3, and 5

Repeat cycle every 28 days [453].

Clofarabine

Clofarabine: 40 mg/m^2 IV on days 1–5
Repeat cycle every 3–6 weeks [454].

Tretinoin (acute promyelocytic leukemia only) [455]

Tretinoin: 45 mg/m^2 PO daily in 1–2 divided doses

Arsenic trioxide (acute promyelocytic leukemia only)

Arsenic trioxide: 0.15 mg/kg IV daily

Continue until bone marrow remission up to a maximum of 60 doses [456].
Patients who meet the criteria for clinical CR can receive an additional course
of arsenic trioxide as consolidation beginning 3–4 weeks after completion of
induction therapy up to a cumulative total of 25 doses [457].

Sorafenib

Sorafenib: 200–400 mg PO bid

Continue until disease progression or stem cell transplant [458].

Azacitidine

Azacitidine: 75 mg/m^2 SC daily for 7 days
Repeat cycle every 28 days for at least 6 cycles [459].

Azacitidine (maintenance therapy)

Azacitidine: 300 mg PO daily for 14 days
Repeat cycle every 28 days until relapse [460].

Decitabine

Decitabine: 20 mg/m^2 IV on days 1–5
Repeat cycle every 4 weeks [461].

Enasidenib (IDH2 mutation)

Enasidenib: 100 mg PO daily
Repeat cycle every 28 days [462].

Ivosidenib (IDH1 mutation)

Ivosidenib: 500 mg PO daily

Continue until disease progression or toxicity [463]. Treat for a minimum of
6 months to allow time for clinical response.

Olutasidenib (IDH1 mutation)

Olutasidenib: 150 mg PO bid

Continue until disease progression or toxicity [464].

Gilteritinib (FLT3 mutation)

Gilteritinib: 120 mg PO daily

Repeat cycle every 28 days [465].

Chronic Lymphocytic Leukemia

Combination Regimens

CVP

Cyclophosphamide: 400 mg/m^2 PO on days 1–5 (or 800 mg/m^2 IV on day 1)

Vincristine: 1.4 mg/m2 IV on day 1 (maximum dose, 2 mg)

Prednisone: 100 mg/m^2 PO on days 1–5

Repeat cycle every 21 days [466].

CF

Cyclophosphamide: 1,000 mg/m^2 IV on day 1

Fludarabine: 20 mg/m^2 IV on days 1–5

Trimethoprim/sulfamethoxazole
(Bactrim DS): 1 tablet PO bid

Repeat cycle every 21–28 days [467].

FP

Fludarabine: 30 mg/m^2 IV on days 1–5

Prednisone: 30 mg/m^2 IV on days 1–5

Repeat cycle every 28 days [468].

CP

Chlorambucil: 30 mg/m^2 PO on day 1

Prednisone: 80 mg PO on days 1–5

Repeat cycle every 28 days [466].

FR

Fludarabine: 25 mg/m^2 IV on days 1–5

Rituximab: 375 mg/m^2 IV on days 1 and 4 of cycle 1 and then on day 1 with all subsequent cycles

Repeat cycle every 28 days for 6 cycles [469, 470].

FCR

Fludarabine:	25 mg/m^2 IV on days 1–3
Cyclophosphamide:	250 mg/m^2 IV on days 1–3
Rituximab:	375 mg/m^2 IV on day 1

Repeat cycle every 28 days for 6 cycles [471]. On cycles 2–6, rituximab is given at 500 mg/m^2.

PCR

Pentostatin:	2 mg/m^2 IV on day 1
Cyclophosphamide:	600 mg/m^2 IV on day 1
Rituximab:	375 mg/m^2 IV on day 1

Repeat cycle every 21 days [472].

Bendamustine + Rituximab

Bendamustine:	90 mg/m^2 IV on days 1 and 2
Rituximab:	375 mg/m^2 IV on day 0 of cycle 1, then 500 mg/m^2 IV on day 1 of cycles 2–6

Repeat cycle every 28 days for up to 6 cycles [473].

Venetoclax + Rituximab

Venetoclax:	20 mg/day PO on days 1–7
	50 mg/day PO on days 8–14
	100 mg/day PO on days 15–21
	200 mg/day PO on days 22–28 and then 400 mg/day PO daily
Rituximab:	375 mg/m^2 IV on day 1 of cycle 1, then 500 mg/m^2 IV on day 1 of cycles 2–6

Repeat cycle every 28 days for up to 6 cycles [474]. After cycle 6, venetoclax is continued at 400 mg PO daily for up to 2 years.

Idelasib + Rituximab [475]

Idelasib:	150 mg PO bid
Rituximab:	375 mg/m^2 IV on day 1, then 500 mg/m^2 IV every 2 weeks for 4 doses and then every 4 weeks for 3 doses for a total of 8 doses

Obinutuzumab + Chlorambucil

Obinutuzumab:	100 mg IV on day 1, cycle 1; 900 mg IV on day 2, cycle 1; 1,000 mg IV on days 8 and 15 of cycle 1; 1,000 mg IV on day 1 of cycles 2–6

Chlorambucil: 0.5 mg/kg PO on days 1 and 15
Repeat cycle every 28 days for up to 6 cycles [476].

Obinutuzumab + Venetoclax

Obinutuzumab: 100 mg IV on day 1 and 900 mg IV on day 2 (or 1,000 mg on day 1), 1,000 mg on day 8 and 1,000 mg on day 15 of cycle 1, and subsequently 1,000 mg on day 1 of cycles 2 through 6.

Venetoclax: Start on day 22 of cycle 1 with a 5-week dose ramp-up (1 week each of 20, 50, 100, and 200 mg PO, then 400 mg PO daily for 1 week), thereafter at 400 mg PO daily until completion of cycle 12

Repeat cycle every 28 days for up to 6 cycles with obinutuzumab and 12 cycles with venetoclax [477].

Acalabrutinib + Obinutuzumab

Acalabrutinib: 100 mg PO bid

Obinutuzumab: 100 mg IV on day 1 and 900 mg IV on day 2 (or 1,000 mg on day 1), 1,000 mg on day 8, and 1,000 mg on day 15 of cycle 1, and subsequently 1,000 mg on day 1 of cycles 2 through 6.

Repeat cycle every 28 days for up to 6 cycles with obinutuzumab [478].

Ibrutinib + Rituximab

Ibrutinib: 420 mg PO daily

Rituximab: 50 mg/m^2 IV on day 1 of cycle 2

325 mg/m^2 IV on day 2 of cycle 2

500 mg/m^2 IV on day 1 of cycles 3 through 7

Repeat cycle every 28 days [479].

Single-Agent Regimens

Alemtuzumab

Alemtuzumab: 30 mg/day IV, 3 times per week

Repeat weekly for up to a maximum of 23 weeks [480]. Premedicate with diphenhydramine 50 mg PO and acetaminophen 625 mg PO 30 minutes before drug infusion. Patients should be placed on trimethoprim/sulfamethoxazole (Bactrim DS) PO bid and famciclovir 250 mg PO bid from day 8 through 2 months following completion of therapy.

Chlorambucil

Chlorambucil: 6–14 mg/day PO as induction therapy and then 0.7 mg/kg PO for 2–4 days

Repeat cycle every 21 days [481].

Cladribine

Cladribine: 0.09 mg/kg/day IV continuous infusion on days 1–7

Repeat cycle every 28–35 days [482].

Fludarabine

Fludarabine: 20–30 mg/m^2 IV on days 1–5

Repeat cycle every 28 days [483].

Prednisone

Prednisone: 20–30 mg/m^2/day PO for 1–3 weeks [484].

Rituximab

Rituximab: 375 mg/m^2 IV weekly for 4 weeks

Repeat cycle every 6 months for a total of 4 courses [485].

Ofatumumab

Ofatumumab: 300 mg IV initial dose followed 1 week later by 2,000 mg IV weekly dose for 7 doses, followed 4 weeks later by 2,000 mg IV every 4 weeks for 4 doses.

A total of 12 doses is recommended [486].

Pentostatin

Pentostatin: 4 mg/m^2 IV on day 1

Repeat cycle every 14 days [487].

Bendamustine

Bendamustine: 100 mg/m^2 IV on days 1 and 2

Repeat cycle every 28 days for up to 6 cycles [488].

or

Bendamustine: 60 mg/m^2 IV on days 1–5

Repeat cycle every 28 days [489]. In patients >70 years, use dose of 50 mg/m^2.

Lenalidomide

Lenalidomide: 10 mg PO daily on days 1–28

Increase dose by 5 mg every 28 days up to a maximum of 25 mg daily until disease progression or toxicity [490].

Ibrutinib

Ibrutinib: 560 mg PO daily

Continue treatment until disease progression [491].

Acalabrutinib

Acalabrutinib: 100 mg PO bid

Continue treatment until disease progression [491].

Zanubrutinib

Zanubrutinib: 160 mg PO bid

Continue treatment until disease progression [492].

Venetoclax

Venetoclax: 20 mg/day PO on days 1–7

                                              50 mg/day PO on days 8–14

                                              100 mg/day PO on days 15–21

                                              200 mg/day PO on days 22–28 and then 400 mg/day PO daily

Continue treatment until disease progression [493].

Duvelisib

Duvelisib: 25 mg PO bid

Repeat cycle every 28 days [494].

Chronic Myelogenous Leukemia

Combination Regimens

Interferon + Cytarabine

Interferon α-2b: 5 million U/m^2 SC daily

Cytarabine: 20 mg/m^2 SC daily for 10 days

Repeat cytarabine on a monthly basis [495]. The dose of interferon should be reduced by 50% when the neutrophil count drops below 1,500/mm^3, the platelet count drops below 100,000/m^3, or both. Interferon and cytarabine should both be discontinued when the neutrophil count drops below 1,000/mm^3, platelet count drops below 50,000/mm^3, or both.

Single-Agent Regimens

Imatinib

Imatinib:	400 mg/day PO (chronic phase); 600 mg/day PO (accelerated phase blast crisis) [496]

Dasatinib

Dasatinib:	70 mg PO bid [497]
or	
Dasatinib:	100 mg PO daily [498]

Nilotinib

Nilotinib:	400 mg PO bid [499]
or	
Nilotinib:	300 mg PO bid [500]

Bosutinib

Bosutinib:	500 mg PO daily [501]

Ponatinib

Ponatinib:	45 mg PO daily [502]

Asciminib (Ph+CML in CP)

Asciminib:	80 mg PO daily or 40 mg PO bid [503]

Asciminib (Ph+CML in CP with the T315I mutation)

Asciminib:	200 mg PO bid [504]

Busulfan

Busulfan:	1.8 mg/m^2/day PO [505]

Hydroxyurea

Hydroxyurea:	1–5 g/day PO [506]

Interferon α-2a

Interferon α-2a:	3 million U/day SC for the first 2 weeks, then 6 million U/day SC for the next 2 weeks, and 9 million U/day SC thereafter [507]

Omacetaxine

Omacetaxine: 1.25 mg/m² SC bid on days 1–14 for first cycle and induction phase followed by 1.25 mg/m² SC bid on days 1–7 as maintenance phase

Repeat cycle every 28 days [508].

Hairy Cell Leukemia

Combination Regimens

Cladribine + Rituximab

Cladribine: 0.15 mg/kg IV continuous infusion on days 1–5

Rituximab: 375 mg/m² IV on day 1

Administer weekly rituximab for 8 weeks [509]

Single-Agent Regimens

Moxetumomab pasudotox-tdfk

Moxetumomab pasudotox-tdfk: 0.04 mg/kg IV on days 1, 3, and 5

Repeat cycle every 28 days for 6 cycles [510].

Cladribine

Cladribine: 0.09 mg/kg/day IV continuous infusion on days 1–7

Administer one cycle [511].

Pentostatin

Pentostatin: 4 mg/m² IV on day 1

Repeat cycle every 14 days for 6 cycles [512].

Interferon α-2a

Interferon α-2a: 3 million U SC or IM, 3 times per week

Continue treatment for up to 1 to 1.5 years [513].

LUNG CANCER

Non–Small Cell Lung Cancer

Neoadjuvant Therapy

Nivolumab + Carboplatin + Pemetrexed (non-squamous histology)

Nivolumab: 360 mg IV on day 1

Carboplatin: AUC of 5, IV on day 1

Pemetrexed: 500 mg/m² on day 1

Repeat cycle every 21 days for 3 cycles to be followed by surgery [514]. After surgery, up to 4 cycles of adjuvant chemotherapy, radiotherapy, or both could be given.

Nivolumab + Cisplatin + Pemetrexed (non-squamous histology)

Nivolumab:	360 mg IV on day 1
Cisplatin:	75 mg/m^2 IV on day 1
Pemetrexed:	500 mg/m^2 IV on day 1.

Repeat cycle every 21 days for 3 cycles to be followed by surgery [514]. After surgery, up to 4 cycles of adjuvant chemotherapy, radiotherapy, or both could be given.

Nivolumab + Paclitaxel + Carboplatin

Nivolumab:	360 mg IV on day 1
Paclitaxel:	175 mg/m^2 IV over 3 hours on day 1
Carboplatin:	AUC of 6, IV on day 1

Repeat cycle every 21 days for 3 cycles to be followed by surgery [514].

Nivolumab + Paclitaxel + Cisplatin

Nivolumab:	360 mg IV on day 1
Paclitaxel:	175 mg/m^2 IV over 3 hours on day 1
Cisplatin:	80 mg/m^2 IV on day 1

Repeat cycle every 21 days for 3 cycles to be followed by surgery [514]. After surgery, up to 4 cycles of adjuvant chemotherapy, radiotherapy, or both could be given.

Pembrolizumab + Cisplatin + Gemcitabine (non-squamous histology)

Pembrolizumab:	200 mg IV on day 1
Cisplatin:	80 mg/m^2 IV on day 1
Gemcitabine:	1,000 mg/m^2 on days 1 and 8

Repeat cycle every 21 days for 4 cycles to be followed by surgery and adjuvant chemotherapy plus pembrolizumab [515]. Adjuvant pembrolizumab to be given for up to 13 cycles.

Pembrolizumab + Cisplatin + Pemetrexed

Pembrolizumab:	200 mg IV on day 1
Cisplatin:	75 mg/m^2 IV on day 1
Pemetrexed:	500 mg/m^2 on day 1.

Repeat cycle every 21 days for 4 cycles to be followed by surgery and adjuvant chemotherapy plus pembrolizumab [515]. Adjuvant pembrolizumab to be given for up to 13 cycles.

Combined Modality Therapy

Cisplatin + Etoposide + Radiation Therapy

Cisplatin:	50 mg/m^2 IV on days 1, 8, 29, and 36
Etoposide:	50 mg/m^2 IV on days 1–5 and 29–33
Radiation therapy:	180 cGy/day for a total dose of 4,500 cGy

Chemotherapy is given concurrently with radiation therapy [516].

Weekly Paclitaxel + Carboplatin + Radiation Therapy

Paclitaxel:	45 mg/m^2 IV weekly for 7 weeks
Carboplatin:	AUC of 2, IV weekly for 7 weeks
Radiation therapy:	200 cGy/day for a total dose of 6,300 cGy over 7 weeks

Chemotherapy is given concurrently with radiation therapy [517]. Three to 4 weeks after the completion of chemoradiotherapy, 2 additional cycles of the following chemotherapy are given:

Paclitaxel:	200 mg/m^2 IV on day 1
Carboplatin:	AUC of 6, IV on day 1

Repeat cycle every 21 days for 2 cycles.

Adjuvant Therapy

Combination Regimens

Paclitaxel + Carboplatin

Paclitaxel:	200 mg/m^2 IV over 3 hours on day 1
Carboplatin:	AUC of 6, IV on day 1

Repeat cycle every 21 days for 4 cycles [518].

Vinorelbine + Cisplatin

Vinorelbine:	25 mg/m^2 IV weekly for 16 weeks
Cisplatin:	50 mg/m^2 IV on days 1 and 8

Repeat cycle every 28 days for 4 cycles [519].

Cisplatin + Vinblastine

Cisplatin:	100 mg/m^2 IV on day 1
Vinblastine:	4 mg/m^2 IV on days 1, 8, 15, 22, and 29, then every 2 weeks after day 43

Repeat cycle every 28 days for 4 cycles [520].

Etoposide + Cisplatin

Etoposide: 100 mg/m^2 IV on days 1–3

Cisplatin: 100 mg/m^2 IV on day 1

Repeat cycle every 28 days for 4 cycles [520].

Pemetrexed + Cisplatin

Pemetrexed: 500 mg/m^2 IV on day 1

Cisplatin: 80 mg/m^2 IV on day 1

Repeat cycle every 21 days for 6 cycles [521]. Folic acid at 350–1,000 µg PO q day beginning 1 week prior to therapy and vitamin B12 at 1,000 µg IM beginning 1–2 weeks prior to first dose of therapy and repeated every 9 weeks. Dexamethasone at 4 mg PO bid on the day before, the day of, and the day after pemetrexed.

Single-Agent Regimens

Atezolizumab

Atezolizumab: 1,200 mg IV on day 1.

Repeat cycle every 21 days for 16 cycles or 1 year [522]. Atezolizumab is to be given after adjuvant platinum-based chemotherapy (1–4 cycles). May also be given 840 mg IV every 2 weeks or 1,680 mg IV every 4 weeks.

Osimertinib

Osimertinib: 80 mg/day PO

Continue treatment for 3 years or until evidence of disease recurrence [523].

Metastatic Disease

Combination Regimens

Carboplatin + Paclitaxel (PC)

Carboplatin: AUC of 6, IV on day 1

Paclitaxel: 200 mg/m^2 IV over 3 hours on day 1

Repeat cycle every 21 days [524].

Carboplatin + Nab-Paclitaxel

Carboplatin: AUC of 6, IV on day 1

Nab-Paclitaxel: 100 mg/m^2 IV weekly on days 1, 8, and 15

Repeat cycle every 21 days [525].

Carboplatin + Paclitaxel (weekly regimen)

Carboplatin: AUC of 6, IV on day 1

Paclitaxel: 100 mg/m^2 IV weekly for 3 weeks

Repeat cycle every 4 weeks up to 4 cycles [526]. If response or stable disease, may then treat with maintenance chemotherapy of:

Paclitaxel: 70 mg/m^2 IV weekly for 3 weeks
Continue until disease progression.

Carboplatin + Paclitaxel + Bevacizumab (PCB)
Carboplatin: AUC of 6, IV on day 1
Paclitaxel: 200 mg/m^2 IV on day 1
Bevacizumab: 15 mg/kg IV on day 1
Repeat cycle every 21 days [524].

Gemcitabine + Cisplatin + Bevacizumab (GCB)
Gemcitabine: 1,250 mg/m^2 IV on days 1 and 8
Cisplatin: 80 mg/m^2 IV on day 1
Bevacizumab: 7.5 or 15 mg/kg IV on day 1
Repeat cycle every 21 days for a total of 6 cycles [527].

Cisplatin + Paclitaxel
Cisplatin: 80 mg/m^2 IV on day 1
Paclitaxel: 175 mg/m^2 IV over 3 hours on day 1
Repeat cycle every 21 days [528].

Docetaxel + Carboplatin
Docetaxel: 75 mg/m^2 IV on day 1
Carboplatin: AUC of 6, IV on day 1
Repeat cycle every 21 days [529].

Docetaxel + Cisplatin
Docetaxel: 75 mg/m^2 IV on day 1
Cisplatin: 75 mg/m^2 IV on day 1
Repeat cycle every 21 days [530].

Docetaxel + Gemcitabine
Docetaxel: 100 mg/m^2 IV on day 8
Gemcitabine: 1,100 mg/m^2 IV on days 1 and 8
Repeat cycle every 21 days [531]. G-CSF support is required from day 9 to day 15.

Gemcitabine + Cisplatin
Gemcitabine: 1,000 mg/m^2 IV on days 1, 8, and 15
Cisplatin: 100 mg/m^2 IV on day 1
Repeat cycle every 21 days [532].

Gemcitabine + Carboplatin

Gemcitabine: 1,000 mg/m^2 IV on days 1 and 8
Carboplatin: AUC of 5, IV on day 1
Repeat cycle every 21 days [533].

Gemcitabine + Vinorelbine

Gemcitabine: 1,200 mg/m^2 IV on days 1 and 8
Vinorelbine: 30 mg/m^2 IV on days 1 and 8
Repeat cycle every 21 days [534].

Vinorelbine + Cisplatin

Vinorelbine: 30 mg/m^2 IV on days 1, 8, and 15
Cisplatin: 120 mg/m^2 IV on day 1
Repeat cycle every 28 days [535].

Vinorelbine + Cisplatin + Cetuximab

Vinorelbine: 25 mg/m^2 IV on days 1 and 8
Cisplatin: 80 mg/m^2 IV on day 1
Cetuximab: 400 mg/m^2 IV loading dose, then
                                      250 mg/m^2 IV weekly
Repeat cycle every 3 weeks up to 6 cycles [536].

Vinorelbine + Carboplatin

Vinorelbine: 25 mg/m^2 IV on days 1 and 8
Carboplatin: AUC of 6, IV on day 1
Repeat cycle every 28 days [537].

Pemetrexed + Cisplatin

Pemetrexed: 500 mg/m^2 IV on day 1
Cisplatin: 75 mg/m^2 IV on day 1
Repeat cycle every 21 days up to 6 cycles [538]. Folic acid at 350–1,000 μg PO q day beginning 1 week prior to therapy and vitamin B12 at 1,000 μg IM beginning 1–2 weeks prior to first dose of therapy and repeated every 9 weeks. Dexamethasone at 4 mg PO bid on the day before, the day of, and the day after pemetrexed.

Pemetrexed + Carboplatin

Pemetrexed: 500 mg/m^2 IV on day 1
Carboplatin: AUC of 5, IV on day 1
Repeat cycle every 21 days up to 6 cycles [539]. Folic acid at 350–1,000 μg PO q day beginning 1 week prior to therapy and vitamin B12 at 1,000 μg IM beginning 1–2 weeks prior to first dose of therapy and repeated every 9 weeks. Dexamethasone at 4 mg PO bid on the day before, the day of, and the day after pemetrexed.

EP

Etoposide:	120 mg/m^2 IV on days 1–3
Cisplatin:	60 mg/m^2 IV on day 1

Repeat cycle every 21–28 days [540].

EP + Docetaxel

Etoposide:	50 mg/m^2 IV on days 1–5 and 29–33
Cisplatin:	50 mg/m^2 IV on days 1, 8, 29, and 36

Administer concurrent thoracic radiotherapy, followed 4–6 weeks after the completion of combined modality therapy by

Docetaxel:	75 mg/m^2 IV on day 1

Repeat cycle every 21 days for 3 cycles [541]. Dose of docetaxel can be escalated to 100 mg/m^2 IV on subsequent cycles in the absence of toxicity.

Docetaxel + Bevacizumab

Docetaxel:	75 mg/m^2 IV on day 1
Bevacizumab:	15 mg/kg IV on day 1

Repeat cycle every 21 days [542].

Pemetrexed + Carboplatin + Bevacizumab

Pemetrexed:	500 mg/m^2 IV on day 1
Carboplatin:	AUC of 6, IV on day 1
Bevacizumab:	15 mg/kg IV on day 1

Repeat cycle every 21 days up to 6 cycles [543]. Folic acid at 350–1,000 μg PO q day beginning 1 week prior to therapy and vitamin B12 at 1,000 μg IM beginning 1–2 weeks prior to first dose of therapy and repeated every 9 weeks. Dexamethasone at 4 mg PO bid on the day before, the day of, and the day after pemetrexed.

Pemetrexed + Carboplatin + Pembrolizumab

Pemetrexed:	500 mg/m^2 IV on day 1
Carboplatin:	AUC of 5, IV on day 1
Pembrolizumab:	200 mg IV on day 1

Repeat cycle every 21 days up to 4 cycles [544]. Followed by pembrolizumab maintenance therapy up to a total of 35 cycles and pemetrexed maintenance.

Folic acid at 350–1,000 μg PO q day beginning 1 week prior to therapy and vitamin B12 at 1,000 μg IM beginning 1–2 weeks prior to first dose of therapy and repeated every 9 weeks. Dexamethasone at 4 mg PO bid on the day before, the day of, and the day after pemetrexed.

Pemetrexed + Cisplatin + Pembrolizumab

Pemetrexed:	500 mg/m^2 IV on day 1
Cisplatin:	75 mg/m^2 IV on day 1
Pembrolizumab:	200 mg IV on day 1

Repeat cycle every 21 days up to 4 cycles [544]. Followed by pembrolizumab maintenance therapy up to a total of 35 cycles and pemetrexed maintenance.

Folic acid at 350–1,000 µg PO q day beginning 1 week prior to therapy and vitamin B12 at 1,000 µg IM beginning 1–2 weeks prior to first dose of therapy and repeated every 9 weeks. Dexamethasone at 4 mg PO bid on the day before, the day of, and the day after pemetrexed.

Cisplatin + Vinorelbine + Cetuximab

Cisplatin:	80 mg/m^2 IV on day 1
Vinorelbine:	25 mg/m^2 IV continuous on days 1 and 8
Cetuximab:	400 mg/m^2 IV loading dose, then 250 mg/m^2 IV weekly

Repeat cycle every 21 days up to 6 cycles [545].

Platinum-Based Chemotherapy + Maintenance Pemetrexed (non-squamous histology)

Platinum-based chemotherapy × 4 cycles, followed by:

Pemetrexed:	500 mg/m^2 IV on day 1

Repeat cycle every 21 days until disease progression [546]. Folic acid at 350–1,000 µg PO q day beginning 1 week prior to therapy and vitamin B12 at 1,000 µg IM beginning 1–2 weeks prior to first dose of therapy and repeated every 9 weeks. Dexamethasone at 4 mg PO bid on the day before, the day of, and the day after pemetrexed.

Nab-Paclitaxel + Carboplatin

Nab-Paclitaxel:	100 mg/m^2 IV on days 1, 8, and 15
Carboplatin:	AUC of 6, IV on day 1

Repeat cycle every 21 days [547].

Docetaxel + Ramucirumab

Docetaxel:	75 mg/m^2 IV on day 1
Ramucirumab:	10 mg/kg IV on day 1

Repeat cycle every 21 days [548].

Gemcitabine + Cisplatin + Necitumumab

Gemcitabine:	1,250 mg/m^2 IV on days 1 and 8
Cisplatin:	75 mg/m^2 IV on day 1

Necitumumab: 800 mg IV on days 1 and 8
Repeat cycle every 21 days [549].

Dabrafenib + Trametinib (BRAF:V600E mutation)
Dabrafenib: 150 mg PO bid
Trametinib: 2 mg PO daily
Continue treatment until disease progression [550].

Carboplatin + Paclitaxel + Pembrolizumab
Carboplatin: AUC of 6, IV on day 1
Paclitaxel: 200 mg/m^2 IV on day 1
Pembrolizumab: 200 mg IV on day 1
Repeat cycle every 21 days for 4 cycles followed by pembrolizumab for up to a total of 35 treatments [551].

Carboplatin + Nab-Paclitaxel + Pembrolizumab
Carboplatin: AUC of 6, IV on day 1
Nab-Paclitaxel: 100 mg/m^2 IV weekly on days 1, 8, and 15
Pembrolizumab: 200 mg IV on day 1
Repeat cycle every 21 days for 4 cycles followed by pembrolizumab for up to a total of 35 treatments [551].

Atezolizumab + Bevacizumab + Paclitaxel + Carboplatin (non-squamous)
Atezolizumab: 1,200 mg IV on day 1
Bevacizumab: 15 mg/kg IV on day 1
Paclitaxel: 200 mg/m^2 IV on day 1
Carboplatin: AUC of 6, IV on day 1
Repeat cycle every 21 days for up to 6 cycles followed by atezolizumab and bevacizumab until disease progression or toxicity [552].

Atezolizumab + Nab-Paclitaxel + Carboplatin (non-squamous)
Atezolizumab: 1,200 mg IV on day 1
Nab-Paclitaxel: 200 mg/m^2 IV on day 1
Carboplatin: AUC of 6, IV on day 1
Repeat cycle every 21 days for up to 6 cycles followed by atezolizumab until disease progression or toxicity [552].

Ramucirumab + Erlotinib
Ramucirumab: 10 mg/kg IV on day 1
Erlotinib: 150 mg PO daily
Repeat cycle every 14 days [553].

Ipilimumab + Nivolumab

Ipilumumab: 1 mg/kg on day 1

Nivolumab: 360 mg IV on days 1 and 21, along
                                         with two cycles of platinum-based
                                         chemotherapy.

Repeat cycle every 6 weeks [554].

Durvalumab + Tremelimumab + Platinum-Based Chemotherapy

Weight >30 kg

Durvalumab: 1,500 mg IV on day 1

Tremelimumab: 75 mg IV on day 1 along with
                                         platinum-based chemotherapy

Repeat cycle every 3 weeks for 4 cycles and then administer durvalumab 1,500 mg
IV every 4 weeks as a single agent with histology-based pemetrexed maintenance
therapy every 4 weeks, and a fifth dose of tremelimumab 75 mg IV in combination
with durvalumab dose 6 at week 16 [555].

For weight <30 kg

Durvalumab: 20 mg/kg IV on day 1

Tremelimumab: 1 mg/kg IV on day 1 along with
                                         platinum-based chemotherapy

Repeat cycle every 3 weeks for 4 cycles and then administer durvalumab 20 mg/kg
IV every 4 weeks as a single agent with histology-based pemetrexed maintenance
therapy every 4 weeks, and a fifth dose of tremelimumab 1 mg/kg IV in
combination with durvalumab dose 6 at week 16 [555].

Cemiplimab + Platinum-Based Chemotherapy

Cemiplimab: 350 mg IV on day 1 along with
                                         platinum-based chemotherapy

Repeat cycle every 21 days for up to 108 weeks in combination with
platinum-doublet chemotherapy followed by pemetrexed maintenance as
indicated for both squamous and non-squamous histologies [556].

Single-Agent Regimens

Paclitaxel

Paclitaxel: 225 mg/m^2 IV over 3 hours on day 1

Repeat cycle every 21 days [557].

or

Paclitaxel: 80–100 mg/m^2 IV weekly for 3 weeks

Repeat cycle every 28 days after 1-week rest [558].

Nab-Paclitaxel

Nab-Paclitaxel: 125 mg/m^2 IV on days 1, 8, and 15

Repeat cycle every 28 days [559].

Docetaxel

Docetaxel: $75 \ mg/m^2$ IV on day 1

Repeat cycle every 21 days [560].

or

Docetaxel: $36 \ mg/m^2$ IV weekly for 6 weeks

Repeat cycle every 8 weeks after 2-week rest [561]. Premedicate with dexamethasone 8 mg PO at 12 hours and immediately before docetaxel infusion and 12 hours after each dose.

Pemetrexed

Pemetrexed: $500 \ mg/m^2$ IV on day 1

Repeat cycle every 21 days [562]. Folic acid at 350–1,000 µg PO q day beginning 1 week prior to therapy and vitamin B12 at 1,000 µg IM beginning 1–2 weeks prior to first dose of therapy and repeated every 3 cycles.

Gemcitabine

Gemcitabine: $1,000 \ mg/m^2$ IV on days 1, 8, and 15

Repeat cycle every 28 days [563].

Vinorelbine

Vinorelbine: $25 \ mg/m^2$ IV on day 1

Repeat cycle every 7 days [564].

Gefitinib (EGFR exon19 deletions, exon 21 L858R mutations)

Gefitinib: 250 mg/day PO

Continue treatment until disease progression [565].

Erlotinib (EGFR exon19 deletions, exon 21 L858R mutations)

Erlotinib: 150 mg/day PO

Continue treatment until disease progression [566].

Afatinib (EGFR exon19 deletions, exon 21 L858R mutations)

Afatinib: 40 mg/day PO

Continue treatment until disease progression [567].

Dacomitinib (EGFR exon19 deletions, exon 21 L858R mutations)

Dacomitinib: 45 mg/day PO

Continue treatment until disease progression [568].

Sunitinib

Sunitinib: 50 mg/day PO for 4 weeks

Repeat cycle every 6 weeks [569].

Cetuximab

Cetuximab: 400 mg/m² IV loading dose, then 250 mg/m² IV weekly

Repeat cycle every week [570].

Amivantamab (EGFR exon 20 insertion mutations)

Amivantamab: 1,050 mg IV once weekly for the first 4 weeks, then every 2 weeks at week 5

For patients >80 kg, a dose of 1,400 mg should be administered

Repeat cycle every 2 weeks starting at week 5 [571].

Mobocertinib (EGFR exon 20 insertion mutations)

Mobocertinib: 160 mg PO daily

Continue until disease progression or toxicity [572].

Nivolumab

Nivolumab: 240 mg IV on day 1

Repeat cycle every 2 weeks [573]. May also administer 480 mg IV on day 1 with cycles every 4 weeks.

Crizotinib (ALK or ROS1 positive)

Crizotinib: 250 mg PO bid

Continue treatment until disease progression [574].

Ceritinib (ALK or ROS1 positive)

Ceritinib: 750 mg/day PO

Continue treatment until disease progression [575].

Alectinib (ALK rearrangements)

Alectinib: 600 mg PO bid

Continue treatment until disease progression [576].

Brigatinib (ALK rearrangements)

Brigatinib: 90 mg PO daily for first 7 days and then 180 mg PO daily

Continue treatment until disease progression [577].

Lorlatinib (ALK rearrangements, ROS1)

Lorlatinib: 100 mg PO daily

Continue treatment until disease progression [578].

Entrectinib (NTRK fusions)

Entrectinib: 600 mg PO daily

Continue until disease progression [579]

Osimertinib (EGFR exon19 deletions, exon 21 L858R mutations, or T790M mutation)

Osimertinib: 80 mg/day PO

Continue treatment until disease progression [580].

Selpercatinib (RET fusion-positive)

Selpercatinib:
120 mg PO bid for patients < 50 kg
160 mg PO bid for patients >50 kg

Repeat cycle every 21 days [581].

Pralsetinib (RET fusion-positive)

Pralsetinib: 400 mg/day PO

Continue treatment until disease progression [582].

Capmatinib (MET exon 14 skipping)

Capmatinib: 400 mg PO bid

Repeat cycle every 28 days [583].

Tepotinib (MET exon 14 skipping)

Tepotinib: 450 mg PO daily

Continue treatment until disease progression [584].

Sotorasib (KRAS:G12C mutation)

Sotorasib: 960 mg PO daily

Continue treatment until disease progression [585].

Adagrasib (KRAS:G12C mutation)

Adagrasib: 600 mg PO bid

Continue treatment until disease progression [586].

Pembrolizumab

Pembrolizumab: 200 mg IV on day 1

Repeat cycle every 3 weeks [587]. May also administer 400 mg IV every 6 weeks.

Nivolumab

Nivolumab: 3 mg/kg IV on day 1

Repeat cycle every 14 days [588]. May also administer 240 mg IV every 2 weeks or 480 mg IV every 4 weeks.

Durvalumab

| Durvalumab: | 10 mg/kg IV on day 1 |

Repeat cycle every 14 days [589].

Atezolizumab

| Atezolizumab: | 1,200 mg IV on day 1 |

Repeat cycle every 21 days [590].

Cemiplimab

| Cemiplimab: | 350 mg IV on day 1 |

Repeat cycle every 21 days [591].

Trastuzumab deruxtecan (HER2 mutation)

| Trastuzumab deruxtecan: | 5.4 mg/kg IV on day 1 |

Repeat cycle every 21 days [592].

Small Cell Lung Cancer

Combination Regimens

Atezolizumab + Carboplatin + Etoposide

Atezolizumab:	1,200 mg IV on day 1
Carboplatin:	AUC of 5, IV on day 1
Etoposide:	100 mg/m^2 IV on days 1–3

Repeat cycle every 3 weeks for 4 cycles followed by

| Atezolizumab: | 1,200 mg IV on day 1 |

Repeat cycle every 3 weeks [593]. May also give atezolizumab at 840 mg IV every 2 weeks or 1,680 mg IV every 4 weeks.

Durvalumab + Carboplatin + Etoposide

Durvalumab:	1,500 mg IV on day 1
Carboplatin:	AUC of 5, IV on day 1
Etoposide:	100 mg/m^2 IV on days 1–3

Repeat cycle every 3 weeks for 4 cycles. Durvalumab is then given at 1,500 mg IV on day 1 every 4 weeks as a single agent [594].

EP

| Etoposide: | 80 mg/m^2 IV on days 1–3 |
| Cisplatin: | 80 mg/m^2 IV on day 1 |

Repeat cycle every 21 days [595].

EC

Etoposide: 100 mg/m^2 IV on days 1–3
Carboplatin: AUC of 6, IV on day 1
Repeat cycle every 28 days [596].

Irinotecan + Cisplatin

Irinotecan: 60 mg/m^2 IV on days 1, 8, and 15
Cisplatin: 60 mg/m^2 IV on day 1
Repeat cycle every 28 days [597].

Topotecan + Cisplatin

Topotecan: 1.7 mg/m^2/day PO on days 1–5
Cisplatin: 60 mg/m^2 IV on day 5
Repeat cycle every 21 days up to 4 cycles or 2 cycles beyond best response [598].

Carboplatin + Paclitaxel + Etoposide

Carboplatin: AUC of 6, IV on day 1
Paclitaxel.   200 mg/m^2 IV over 1 hour on day 1
Etoposide: 50 mg alternating with 100 mg PO on days 1–10

Repeat cycle every 21 days [599].

Carboplatin + Paclitaxel

Carboplatin: AUC of 2, IV on days 1, 8, and 15
Paclitaxel: 80 mg/m^2 IV on days 1, 8, and 15
Repeat cycle every 28 days for 6 cycles [600].

CAV

Cyclophosphamide: 1,000 mg/m^2 IV on day 1
Doxorubicin: 40 mg/m^2 IV on day 1
Vincristine: 1 mg/m^2 IV on day 1 (maximum, 2 mg)
Repeat cycle every 21 days [601].

CAE

Cyclophosphamide: 1,000 mg/m^2 IV on day 1
Doxorubicin: 45 mg/m^2 IV on day 1
Etoposide: 50 mg/m^2 IV on days 1–5
Repeat cycle every 21 days [602].

Single-Agent Regimens

Etoposide

Etoposide:	160 mg/m^2 PO on days 1–5

Repeat cycle every 28 days [603].

or

Etoposide:	50 mg/m^2/day PO on days 1–21

Repeat cycle as tolerated [604].

Paclitaxel

Paclitaxel:	80–100 mg/m^2 IV weekly for 3 weeks

Repeat cycle every 28 days [605].

Topotecan

Topotecan:	1.5 mg/m^2 IV on days 1–5

Repeat cycle every 21 days [606].

Gemcitabine

Gemcitabine:	1,000 mg/m^2 PO on days 1, 8, and 15

Repeat cycle every 28 days [607].

Nivolumab

Nivolumab:	240 mg IV on day 1

Repeat cycle every 14 days [608]. May also administer 480 mg IV every 4 weeks.

Pembrolizumab

Pembrolizumab:	200 mg IV on day 1

Repeat cycle every 21 days [609]. May also administer 400 mg IV every 6 weeks.

Lurbinectedin

Lurbinectedin:	3.2 mg/m^2 IV on day 1

Repeat cycle every 21 days [610].

LYMPHOMA

Cutaneous T-cell Lymphoma

Single-Agent Regimens

Mogamulizumab-kpkc

Mogamulizumab-kpkc:	1 mg/kg IV on days 1, 8, 15, and 22 of cycle 1 and then on days 1 and 15 of all subsequent cyles

Repeat cycle every 28 days [611].

Vorinostat

Vorinostat:	400 mg PO daily

Continue therapy until disease progression [612].

Romidepsin

Romidepsin:	14 mg/m^2 IV on days 1, 8, and 15

Repeat cycle every 28 days [613].

Belinostat

Belinostat:	1,000 mg/m^2 IV on days 1–5

Repeat cycle every 21 days [614].

Hodgkin's Lymphoma

Combination Regimens

ABVD

Doxorubicin:	25 mg/m^2 IV on days 1 and 15
Bleomycin:	10 U/m^2 IV on days 1 and 15
Vinblastine:	6 mg/m^2 IV on days 1 and 15
Dacarbazine:	375 mg/m^2 IV on days 1 and 15

Repeat cycle every 28 days [615].

B + AVD

Brentuximab:	1.2 mg/kg IV on days 1 and 15
Doxorubicin:	25 mg/m^2 IV on days 1 and 15
Vinblastine:	6 mg/m^2 IV on days 1 and 15
Dacarbazine:	375 mg/m^2 IV on days 1 and 15

Repeat cycle every 28 days [616].

MOPP

Nitrogen mustard:	6 mg/m^2 IV on days 1 and 8
Vincristine:	1.4 mg/m^2 IV on days 1 and 8
Procarbazine:	100 mg/m^2 PO on days 1–14
Prednisone:	40 mg/m^2 PO on days 1–14

Repeat cycle every 28 days [617].

MOPP/ABVD Hybrid

Nitrogen mustard:	6 mg/m^2 IV on days 1 and 8
Vincristine:	1.4 mg/m^2 IV on day 1 (maximum dose, 2 mg)
Procarbazine:	100 mg/m^2 PO on days 1–14

Prednisone:	40 mg/m^2 PO on days 1–14
Doxorubicin:	35 mg/m^2 IV on day 8
Bleomycin:	10 U/m^2 IV on day 8
Hydrocortisone:	100 mg IV given before bleomycin
Vinblastine:	6 mg/m^2 IV on day 8

Repeat cycle every 28 days [618].

MOPP Alternating with ABVD
See MOPP and ABVD regimens outlined above.

Stanford V
Nitrogen mustard:	6 mg/m^2 IV on day 1
Doxorubicin:	25 mg/m^2 IV on days 1 and 15
Vinblastine:	6 mg/m^2 IV on days 1 and 15
Vincristine:	1.4 mg/m^2 IV on days 8 and 22
Bleomycin:	5 U/m^2 IV on days 8 and 22
Etoposide:	60 mg/m^2 IV on days 15 and 16
Prednisone:	40 mg PO every other day

Repeat cycle every 28 days [619]. In patients >50 years of age, vinblastine dose reduced to 4 mg/m^2 and vincristine dose reduced to 1 mg/m^2 on weeks 9 and 12. Dose of prednisone tapered starting on week 10. Patient should be placed on prophylactic trimethoprim/sulfamethoxazole (Bactrim DS) PO bid and acyclovir 200 mg PO tid.

EVA
Etoposide:	100 mg/m^2 IV on days 1–3
Vinblastine:	6 mg/m^2 IV on day 1
Doxorubicin:	50 mg/m^2 IV on day 1

Repeat cycle every 28 days for up to 6 cycles [620].

EVAP
Etoposide:	120 mg/m^2 IV on days 1, 8, and 15
Vinblastine:	4 mg/m^2 IV on days 1, 8, and 15
Cytarabine:	30 mg/m^2 IV on days 1, 8, and 15
Cisplatin:	40 mg/m^2 IV on days 1, 8, and 15

Repeat cycle every 28 days [621].

Mini-BEAM
Carmustine:	60 mg/m^2 IV on day 1
Etoposide:	75 mg/m^2 IV on days 2–5

| Ara-C: | 100 mg/m^2 IV every 12 hours on days 2–5 |
| Melphalan: | 30 mg/m^2 IV on day 6 |

Repeat cycle every 4–6 weeks [622].

BEACOPP

Bleomycin:	10 mg/m^2 IV on day 8
Etoposide:	100 mg/m^2 IV on days 1–3
Doxorubicin:	25 mg/m^2 IV on day 1
Cyclophosphamide:	650 mg/m^2 IV on day 1
Vincristine:	1.4 mg/m^2 IV on day 8 (maximum, 2 mg)
Procarbazine:	100 mg/m^2 PO on days 1–7
Prednisone:	40 mg/m^2 PO on days 1–14

Repeat cycle every 21 days [623].

BEACOPP Escalated

Bleomycin:	10 mg/m^2 IV on day 8
Etoposide:	200 mg/m^2 IV on days 1–3
Doxorubicin:	35 mg/m^2 IV on day 1
Cyclophosphamide:	1,200 mg/m^2 IV on day 1
Vincristine:	1.4 mg/m^2 IV on day 8 (maximum dose, 2 mg)
Procarbazine:	100 mg/m^2 PO on days 1–7
Prednisone:	40 mg/m^2 PO on days 1–14

Repeat cycle every 21 days [624]. G-CSF support, at dose of 5 µg/kg/day SC, starting on day 8 and continuing until neutrophil recovery.

GVD

For transplant-naïve patients:

Gemcitabine:	1,000 mg/m^2 IV on days 1 and 8
Vinorelbine:	20 mg/m^2 IV on days 1 and 8
Doxil:	15 mg/m^2 IV on days 1 and 8

Repeat cycle every 21 days [625].

or

For post-transplant patients:

Gemcitabine:	800 mg/m^2 IV on days 1 and 8
Vinorelbine:	15 mg/m^2 IV on days 1 and 8
Doxil:	10 mg/m^2 IV on days 1 and 8

Repeat cycle every 21 days [625].

Single-Agent Regimens

Gemcitabine

Gemcitabine.	1,250 mg/m^2 IV on days 1, 8, and 15

Repeat cycle every 28 days [626].

Rituximab

Rituximab:	375 mg/m^2 IV on day 1

Repeat weekly for 4 weeks [627].

Brentuximab

Brentuximab:	1.8 mg/kg IV on day 1

Repeat cycle every 3 weeks for up to 16 cycles [628].

Nivolumab

Nivolumab:	240 mg IV on day 1

Repeat cycle every 2 weeks [629]. May also administer 480 mg IV every 4 weeks.

Pembrolizumab

Pembrolizumab:	200 mg IV on day 1

Repeat cycle every 21 days [630]. May also administer 400 mg IV every 6 weeks.

Bendamustine

Bendamustine:	70–120 mg/m^2 IV on days 1 and 2

Repeat weekly for 4 weeks [631].

Everolimus

Everolimus:	10 mg PO daily

Continue until disease progression [632].

Lenalidomide

Lenalidomide:	25 mg PO daily

Continue until disease progression [633].

Non-Hodgkin's Lymphoma

Low-Grade Lymphoma

Combination Regimens

CVP

Cyclophosphamide:	400 mg/m^2 PO on days 1–5 (or 800 mg/m^2 IV on day 1)
Vincristine:	1.4 mg/m^2 IV on day 1 (maximum, 2 mg)

Prednisone: 100 mg/m² PO on days 1–5
Repeat cycle every 21 days [634].

CHOP

Cyclophosphamide: 750 mg/m² IV on day 1
Doxorubicin: 50 mg/m² IV on day 1
Vincristine: 1.4 mg/m² IV on day 1 (maximum, 2 mg)
Prednisone: 100 mg/m² PO on days 1–5
Repeat cycle every 21 days [635].

CNOP

Cyclophosphamide: 750 mg/m² IV on day 1
Mitoxantrone: 10 mg/m² IV on day 1
Vincristine: 1.4 mg/m² IV on day 1 (maximum, 2 mg)
Prednisone: 50 mg/m² PO on days 1–5
Repeat cycle every 21 days [636].

FND

Fludarabine: 25 mg/m² IV on days 1–3
Mitoxantrone: 10 mg/m² IV on day 1
Dexamethasone: 20 mg PO on days 1–5
Bactrim DS: 1 tablet PO bid, 3 times per week
Repeat cycle every 21 days [637].

FC

Fludarabine: 20 mg/m² IV on days 1–5
Cyclophosphamide: 1,000 mg/m² IV on day 1
Bactrim DS: 1 tablet PO bid
Repeat cycle every 21–28 days [638].

FCR

Fludarabine: 25 mg/m² IV on days 1–3
Cyclophosphamide: 300 mg/m² IV on days 1–3
Rituximab: 375 mg/m² IV on day 1
Repeat cycle every 21 days for 4 cycles [639].

R-CHOP

Cyclophosphamide: 750 mg/m2 IV on day 1
Doxorubicin: 50 mg/m² IV on day 1

| Vincristine: | 1.4 mg/m^2 IV on day 1 (maximum, 2 mg) |
| Prednisone: | 100 mg/day PO on days 1–5 |

Repeat cycle every 21 days up to 6 cycles [640]. Patients who experience a response to therapy can then receive maintenance therapy with

| Rituximab: | 375 mg/m^2 IV on day 1 |

Repeat cycle every 3 months up to a maximum of 2 years.

R-FCM

Rituximab:	375 mg/m^2 IV on day 0
Fludarabine:	25 mg/m^2 IV on days 1–3
Cyclophosphamide:	200 mg/m^2 IV on days 1–3
Mitoxantrone:	8 mg/m^2 IV on day 1

Repeat cycle every 4 weeks for a total of 4 cycles [641]. Patients who experience a response can then receive maintenance therapy at 3 and 9 months after completion of therapy with

| Rituximab: | 375 mg/m^2 IV weekly for 4 weeks |

Bendamustine + Rituximab

| Bendamustine: | 90 mg/m^2 IV on days 1 and 2 |
| Rituximab: | 375 mg/m^2 IV on day 1 |

Repeat cycle every 28 days for 4 cycles [642].

or

| Rituximab: | 375 mg/m^2 IV on day 1 |
| Bendamustine: | 90 mg/m^2 IV on days 2 and 3 |

Repeat cycle every 28 days for 4–6 cycles [643]. An additional dose of rituximab is administered 1 week prior to the first cycle and 4 weeks after the last cycle.

Polatuzumab vedotin + Bendamustine + Rituximab

Polatuzumab vedotin:	1.8 mg/kg IV on day 2 of cycle 1 and on day 1 of subsequent cycles
Bendamustine:	90 mg/m^2 IV on days 2 and 3 of cycle 1 and on days 1 and 2 of subsequent cycles
Rituximab:	375 mg/m^2 IV on day 1

Repeat cycle every 21 days for up to 6 cycles [644].

Lenalidomide + Rituximab

| Lenalidomide: | 20 mg/day PO on days 1–21 |
| Rituximab: | 375 mg/m^2 IV on days 1, 8, 15, and 22 of cycle 1 and on day 1 of cycles 2–5 |

Repeat cycle every 28 days [645].

Bortezomib (mantle cell lymphoma)

Bortezomib: 1.3 mg/m² IV or SC on days 1, 4, 8, and 11

Repeat cycle every 21 days for up to 17 cycles [646].

Ibrutinib (mantle cell lymphoma)

Ibrutinib: 560 mg/day PO

Continue treatment until disease progression [647].

Acalabrutinib (mantle cell lymphoma)

Acalabrutinib: 100 mg PO bid

Continue treatment until disease progression [648].

Zanubrutinib (mantle cell lymphoma)

Zanubrutinib: 160 mg PO bid

Repeat cycle every 28 days [649].

Pirtobrutinib (mantle cell lymphoma)

Pirtobrutinib: 200 mg/day PO

Continue treatment until disease progression [650].

Copanlisib

Copanlisib: 60 mg IV on days 1, 8, and 15

Repeat cycle every 28 days [651].

Bendamustine + Obinutuzumab

Bendamustine: 90 mg/m² IV on days 1 and 2
Obinutuzumab: 1,000 mg IV on days 1, 8, and 15

First cycle is administered over 28 days followed by

Bendamustine: 90 mg/m² IV on days 1 and 2
Obinutuzumab: 1,000 mg IV on day 1

Repeat cycle every 28 days for a total of 5 cycles [652].

Tazemetostat (EZH2 mutant)

Tazemetostat: 800 mg PO bid

Repeat cycle every 28 days [653].

Revlimid + Rituximab

Revlimid: 20 mg PO daily on days 1–21
Rituximab: 375 mg/m² IV on days 1, 8, 15, and 22 of cycle 1 and on day 1 of cycles 2–5

Repeat cycle every 28 days [654].

Mosunetuzumab

Mosunetuzumab: 1 mg IV on day 1, 2 mg IV on day 8, 60 mg IV on day 15 of cycle; 60 mg IV on day 1 of cycle 2; 30 mg IV on day 1 of cycle 3 thereafter

Repeat cycle every 21 days. Patients with a complete response should stop therapy after 8 cycles. For patients with a partial response or stable disease, continue treatment for up to 17 cycles [655].

Brexucabtagene autoleucel [mantle cell lymphoma; 656]

Cyclophosphamide: 250 mg/m^2 IV on days 5, 4, and 3

Fludarabine: 25 mg/m^2 IV on days 5, 4, and 3

Brexucabtagene autoleucel: 2.0×10^6 CAR-positive T cells/kg (maximum, 2×10^8 cells) IV on day 1

Tisagenlecleucel [657]

Cyclophosphamide: 250 mg/m^2 IV on days 5, 4, and 3

Fludarabine: 25 mg/m^2 IV on days 5, 4, and 3

Tisagenlecleucel: $0.6–6.0 \times 10^8$ CAR-positive T cells IV on day 1

Intermediate-Grade Lymphoma

CHOP

Cyclophosphamide: 750 mg/m^2 IV on day 1

Doxorubicin: 50 mg/m^2 IV on day 1

Vincristine: 1.4 mg/m^2 IV on day 1 (maximum, 2 mg)

Prednisone: 100 mg PO on days 1–5

Repeat cycle every 21 days [658].

CHOP + Rituximab

Cyclophosphamide: 750 mg/m^2 IV on day 1

Doxorubicin: 50 mg/m^2 IV on day 1

Vincristine: 1.4 mg/m^2 IV on day 1 (maximum, 2 mg)

Prednisone: 40 mg/m^2 PO on days 1–5

Rituximab: 375 mg/m^2 IV on day 1

Repeat cycle every 21 days [659]. Rituximab is to be administered first, followed by cyclophosphamide, doxorubicin, and vincristine.

or

R-CHOP-14

Cyclophosphamide:	750 mg/m^2 IV on day 1
Doxorubicin:	50 mg/m^2 IV on day 1
Vincristine:	1.4 mg/m^2 IV on day 1 (maximum, 2 mg)
Prednisone:	100 mg/day PO on days 1–5
Rituximab:	375 mg/m^2 IV on day 1

Repeat cycle every 2 weeks up to 6 cycles [660]. G-CSF support to start on day 4 of each cycle.

CNOP

Cyclophosphamide:	750 mg/m^2 IV on day 1
Mitoxantrone:	10 mg/m^2 IV on day 1
Vincristine:	1.4 mg/m^2 IV on day 1 (maximum, 2 mg)
Prednisone:	100 mg PO on days 1–5

Repeat cycle every 21 days [661].

EPOCH

Etoposide:	50 mg/m^2/day IV continuous infusion on days 1–4
Prednisone:	60 mg/m^2 PO on days 1–5
Vincristine:	0.4 mg/m^2/day IV continuous infusion on days 1–4
Cyclophosphamide:	750 mg/m^2 IV on day 5, beginning after infusion
Doxorubicin:	10 mg/m^2/day IV continuous infusion on days 1–4

Repeat cycle every 21 days [662]. Prophylaxis with trimethoprim/sulfamethoxazole (Bactrim DS) 1 tablet PO bid, 3 times per week to reduce the risk of PJP infection.

EPOCH + Rituximab

Etoposide:	50 mg/m^2/day IV continuous infusion on days 1–4
Prednisone:	60 mg/m^2 PO bid on days 1–5
Vincristine:	0.4 mg/m^2/day IV continuous infusion on days 1–4
Cyclophosphamide:	750 mg/m^2 IV on day 5, beginning after infusion
Doxorubicin:	10 mg/m^2/day IV continuous infusion on days 1–4
Rituximab:	375 mg/m^2 IV on day 1

Repeat cycle every 21 days [663]. Rituximab is to be administered first followed by infusions of etoposide, doxorubicin, and vincristine. Prophylaxis with trimethoprim/sulfamethoxazole (Bactrim DS) 1 tablet PO bid, 3 times per week to reduce the risk of PJP infection.

MACOP-B

Methotrexate:	400 mg/m^2 IV on weeks 2, 6, and 10
Leucovorin:	15 mg/m^2 PO every 6 hours for 6 doses, beginning 24 hours after methotrexate
Doxorubicin:	50 mg/m^2 IV on weeks 1, 3, 5, 7, 9, and 11
Cyclophosphamide:	350 mg/m^2 IV on weeks 1, 3, 5, 7, 9, and 11
Vincristine:	1.4 mg/m^2 IV on weeks 2, 4, 6, 8, 10, and 12
Prednisone:	75 mg/day PO for 12 weeks with taper over the last 2 weeks
Bleomycin:	10 U/m2 IV on weeks 4, 8, and 12
Bactrim DS:	1 tablet PO bid
Ketoconazole:	200 mg/day PO

Administer one cycle [664].

m-BACOD

Methotrexate:	200 mg/m^2 IV on days 8 and 15
Leucovorin:	10 mg/m^2 PO every 6 hours for 8 doses, beginning 24 hours after methotrexate
Bleomycin:	4 U/m^2 IV on day 1
Doxorubicin:	45 mg/m^2 IV on day 1
Cyclophosphamide:	600 mg/m^2 IV on day 1
Vincristine:	1 mg/m^2 IV on day 1 (maximum, 2 mg)
Dexamethasone:	6 mg/m^2 PO on days 1–5

Repeat cycle every 21 days [665].

ProMACE/CytaBOM

Prednisone:	60 mg/m^2 PO on days 1–14
Doxorubicin:	25 mg/m^2 IV on day 1
Cyclophosphamide:	650 mg/m^2 IV on day 1
Etoposide:	120 mg/m^2 IV on day 1
Cytarabine:	300 mg/m^2 IV on day 8

Bleomycin:	5 U/m² IV on day 8
Vincristine:	1.4 mg/m² IV on day 8
Methotrexate:	120 mg/m² IV on day 8
Leucovorin rescue:	25 mg/m² PO every 6 hours for 6 doses, beginning 24 hours after methotrexate

Repeat cycle every 21 days [666]. Prophylaxis with trimethoprim/sulfamethoxazole (Bactrim DS) 1 tablet PO bid on days 1-21 to reduce the risk of PJP infection.

ESHAP (salvage regimen)

Etoposide:	40 mg/m² IV on days 1–4
Methylprednisolone:	500 mg IV on days 1–4
Cisplatin:	25 mg/m²/day IV continuous infusion on days 1–4
Cytarabine:	2,000 mg/m² IV on day 5 after completion of cisplatin and etoposide

Repeat cycle every 21 days [667].

DHAP (salvage regimen)

Cisplatin:	100 mg/m² IV continuous infusion over 24 hours on day 1
Cytarabine:	2,000 mg/m² IV over 3 hours every 12 hours for 2 doses on day 2 after completion of cisplatin infusion
Dexamethasone:	40 mg PO or IV on days 1–4

Repeat cycle every 3–4 weeks [668].

ICE (salvage regimen)

Ifosfamide:	5,000 mg/m² IV continuous infusion for 24 hours on day 2
Etoposide:	100 mg/m² IV on days 1–3
Carboplatin:	AUC of 5, IV on day 2
Mesna:	5,000 mg/m² IV in combination with ifosfamide dose

Repeat cycle every 14 days [669]. G-CSF support is administered at 5 µg/kg/day on days 5–12.

RICE (salvage regimen)

Rituximab:	375 mg/m² IV on day 1
Ifosfamide:	5,000 mg/m² IV continuous infusion for 24 hours on day 4
Etoposide:	100 mg/m² IV on days 3–5

| Carboplatin: | AUC of 5, IV on day 4 |
| Mesna: | 5,000 mg/m^2 IV in combination with ifosfamide dose |

Repeat cycle every 14 days [670]. Rituximab is also given at 48 hours before the start of the first cycle. G-CSF is administered at 5 μg/kg/day SC on days 7–14 after the first 2 cycles and at 10 μg/kg/day SC after the third cycle.

MINE (salvage regimen)

Mesna:	1,330 mg/m^2 IV administered at same time as ifosfamide on days 1–3, then 500 mg IV 4 hours after ifosfamide on days 1–3
Ifosfamide:	1,330 mg/m^2 IV on days 1–3
Mitoxantrone:	8 mg/m^2 IV on day 1
Etoposide:	65 mg/m^2 IV on days 1–3

Repeat cycle every 21 days [671].

R-GemOx

Rituximab:	375 mg/m^2 IV on day 1
Gemcitabine:	1,000 mg/m^2 IV on day 2
Oxaliplatin:	50 mg/m^2 IV on day 2

Repeat cycle every 2 weeks for a total of 8 cycles [672].

or

Rituximab:	375 mg/m^2 IV on day 0
Gemcitabine:	1,000 mg/m^2 IV on day 1
Oxaliplatin:	100 mg/m^2 IV on day 1

Repeat cycle every 2 weeks for a total of 6 cycles [673].

Polatuzumab vedotin + Bendamustine + Rituximab (PBR)

Polatuzumab vedotin:	1.8 mg/kg IV on day 2 of cycle 1 and on day 1 of subsequent cycles
Bendamustine:	90 mg/m^2 IV on days 2 and 3 of cycle 1 and on days 1 and 2 of subsequent cycles
Rituximab:	375 mg/m^2 IV on day 1

Repeat cycle every 21 days for up to 6 cycles [674].

Pola + R-CHP

Polatuzumab:	1.8 mg/kg IV on day 1
Rituximab:	375 mg/m^2 IV on day 1
Cyclophosphamide:	750 mg/m^2 IV on day 1

| Doxorubicin: | 50 mg/m^2 IV on day 1 |
| Prednisone: | 100 mg PO on days 1-5 |

Repeat cycle every 21 days for up to 6 cycles. Administer rituximab monotherapy for cycles 7 and 8 [675].

Tafasitamab-cxix + Lenalidomide

| Tafasitamab-cxix: | 12 mg/kg IV on days 1, 4, 8, 15, and 22 on cycle 1; 12 mg/kg IV on days 1, 8, 15, and 22 on cycles 2 and 3; 12 mg/kg IV on days 1 and 15 on cycles 4 and beyond |
| Lenalidomide: | 25 mg/day PO |

Repeat cycle every 28 days for up to 12 cycles, followed by tafasitamab monotherapy until disease progression [676].

Glofitamab + Obinutuzumab

| Glofitamab: | 2.5 mg IV on day 8 and 10 mg IV on day 15 on cycle 1; 30 mg IV on day 1 of all subsequent cycles |
| Obinutuzumab: | 1,000 mg IV on day 1 |

Repeat cycle every 21 days for up to 12 cycles [677].

Loncastuximab

| Loncastuximab: | 0.15 mg/kg IV on day 1 on cycles 1 and 2; 0.075 mg/kg IV on day 1 on cycle 3 and beyond |

Repeat cycle every 3 weeks [678].

Epcoritamab

| Epcoritamab: | 0.16 mg SC on day 1; 0.8 mg SC on day 8; and 48 mg SC on days 15 and 22 of cycle 1. |
| | 48 mg SC weekly on cycle 2 and 3 followed by 48 mg SC every other week on cycles 4–9. |

Repeat cycle every 28 days from cycle 10 [679].

Selinexor

| Selinexor: | 60 mg PO on days 1 and 3 |

Repeat cycle every 7 days [680].

Umbralisib

| Umbralisib: | 800 mg PO daily |

Continue until disease progression [681].

Axicabtagene ciloleucel [682]

Cyclophosphamide:	500 mg/m^2 IV on days 5, 4, and 3
Fludarabine:	30 mg/m^2 IV on days 5, 4, and 3
Axicabtagene ciloleucel:	2 × 10^6 CAR-positive T cells/kg body weight IV on day 1

Lisocabtagene maraleucel [683]

Cyclophosphamide:	300 mg/m^2 IV on days 5, 4, and 3
Fludarabine:	30 mg/m^2 IV on days 5, 4, and 3
Lisocabtagene maraleucel:	50–110 × 10^6 CAR-positive T cells IV on day 1

Tisagenlecleucel [684]

Cyclophosphamide:	250 mg/m^{2}IV on days 5, 4, and 3
Fludarabine:	25 mg/m^2 IV on days 5, 4, and 3
Tisagenlecleucel:	0.6–6.0 × 10^8 CAR-positive T cells IV on day 1

High-Grade Lymphoma

Magrath Protocol (Burkitt's lymphoma)

Cyclophosphamide:	1,200 mg/m^2 IV on day 1
Doxorubicin:	40 mg/m^2 IV on day 1
Vincristine:	1.4 mg/m^2 IV on day 1 (maximum, 2 mg)
Prednisone:	40 mg/m^2 PO on days 1–5
Methotrexate:	300 mg/m^2 IV on day 10 for 1 hour, then 60 mg/m^2 IV on days 10 and 11 for 41 hours
Leucovorin rescue:	15 mg/m^2 IV every 6 hours for 8 doses, starting 24 hours after methotrexate on day 12
Intrathecal ara-C:	30 mg/m^2 IT on day 7, cycle 1 only; 45 mg/m^2 IT on day 7, all subsequent cycles
Intrathecal methotrexate:	12.5 mg IT on day 10, all cycles

Repeat cycle every 28 days [685].

or

Regimen A (CODOX-M) [686]

Cyclophosphamide:	800 mg/m^2 IV on day 1 and 200 mg/m^2 IV on days 2–5

Doxorubicin:	40 mg/m^2 IV on day 1
Vincristine:	1.5 mg/m^2 IV on days 1 and 8 in cycle 1 and on days 1, 8, and 15 in cycle 3
Methotrexate:	1,200 mg/m^2 IV over 1 hour, followed by 240 mg/m2/hour for the next 23 hours on day 10
Leucovorin:	192 mg/m^2 IV starting at hour 36 after the start of the infusion and 12 mg/m^2 IV every 6 hours thereafter until serum methotrexate levels <50 nM

CNS Prophylaxis

| Cytarabine: | 70 mg IT on days 1 and 3 |
| Methotrexate: | 12 mg IT on day 15 |

Regimen B (IVAC)

Ifosfamide:	1,500 mg/m^2 IV on days 1–5
Etoposide:	60 mg/m^2 IV on days 1–5
Cytarabine:	2 g/m^2 IV every 12 hours on days 1 and 2 for a total of 4 doses
Methotrexate:	12 mg IT on day 5

Stanford Regimen (small noncleaved cell and Burkitt's lymphoma)

Cyclophosphamide:	1,200 mg/m^2 IV on day 1
Doxorubicin:	40 mg/m^2 IV on day 1
Vincristine:	1.4 mg/m^2 IV on day 1 (maximum, 2 mg)
Prednisone:	40 mg/m^2 PO on days 1–5
Methotrexate:	3 g/m^2 IV over 6 hours on day 10
Leucovorin rescue:	25 mg/m^2 IV or PO every 6 hours for 12 doses, beginning 24 hours after methotrexate
Intrathecal methotrexate:	12 mg IT on days 1 and 10

Repeat cycle every 21 days [687].

Hyper-CVAD/Methotrexate-Ara-C

| Cyclophosphamide: | 300 mg/m^2 IV every 12 hours for 6 doses on days 1–3 |
| Mesna: | 600 mg/m^2/day continuous infusion on days 1–3 to start 1 hour before cyclophosphamide until 12 hours after completion of cyclophosphamide |

Vincristine:	2 mg IV on days 4 and 11
Doxorubicin:	50 mg/m^2 IV over 24 hours on day 4
Dexamethasone:	40 mg PO or IV on days 1–4 and days 11–14
Methotrexate:	200 mg/m^2 IV over 2 hours followed by 800 mg/m^2 continuous infusion over 22 hours on day 1
Cytarabine:	3,000 mg/m^2 IV over 2 hours every 12 hours for 4 doses on days 2–3 (1,000 mg/m^2 for patients >60 years old)
Leucovorin:	50 mg IV every 6 hours starting 12 hours after completion of methotrexate until methotrexate level <50 nM. Administer every 3–4 weeks on cycles 1, 3, 5, and 7 [688].

Administer every 3–4 weeks on cycles 2, 4, 6, and 8

Intrathecal Chemotherapy Prophylaxis

Methotrexate:	12 mg IT on day 2 of each cycle for a total of 3–4 treatments
Cytarabine:	100 mg IT on day 8 of each cycle for a total of 3–4 treatments
Intrathecal chemotherapy:	Administer intrathecal chemotherapy twice a week with methotrexate 12 mg and cytarabine 100 mg, respectively, until no more cancer cells in CSF, then decrease intrathecal chemotherapy to once a week for 4 weeks, followed by methotrexate 12 mg on day 2 and cytarabine 100 mg on day 8 for the remaining chemotherapy cycles.

Single-Agent Regimens
Rituximab

Rituximab:	375 mg/m^2 IV on days 1, 8, 15, and 22

Repeat one additional cycle [689].
or

Rituximab:	375 mg/m^2 IV on days 1, 8, 15, and 22, followed by 375 mg/m^2 IV at week 12 and at months 5, 7, and 9 [690]

Ibritumomab Tiuxetan Regimen

Rituximab:	250 mg/m^2 IV on days 1 and 8

| 111In-Ibritumomab tiuxetan: | 5 mCi of 111In, 1.6 mg of ibritumomab tiuxetan IV on day 1 |
| 90Y-Ibritumomab tiuxetan: | 0.4 mCi/kg IV over 10 min on day 8 after the day 8 rituximab dose |

Dose of ^{90}Y-ibritumomab tiuxetan is capped at 32 mCi [691].

Fludarabine

| Fludarabine: | 25 mg/m^2 IV on days 1–5 |

Repeat cycle every 28 days [692].

Cladribine

| Cladribine: | 0.5–0.7 mg/kg SC on days 1–5 or 0.1 mg/kg IV on days 1–7 |

Repeat cycle every 28 days [693].

Bendamustine

| Bendamustine: | 120 mg/m^2 IV on days 1 and 2 |

Repeat cycle every 21 days up to 8 cycles [694].

Vorinostat (peripheral T-cell lymphoma)

| Vorinostat: | 400 mg PO daily |

Continue therapy until disease progression [695]. If toxicity is observed, dose may be reduced to 300 mg PO daily.

Pralatrexate

| Pralatrexate: | 30 mg/m^2 IV weekly for 6 weeks |

Repeat cycle every 7 weeks [696]. Folic acid at 1–1.25 mg PO q day beginning 10 days prior to therapy and vitamin B12 at 1 mg IM beginning no more than 10 weeks prior to first dose of therapy and repeated every 8–10 weeks.

Brentuximab

| Brentuximab: | 1.8 mg/kg IV on day 1 |

Repeat cycle every 3 weeks for up to 16 cycles [697].

Romidepsin (peripheral T-cell lymphoma)

| Romidepsin: | 14 mg/m^2 IV on days 1, 8, and 15 |

Repeat cycle every 28 days [698].

Belinostat (peripheral T-cell lymphoma)

| Belinostat: | 1,000 mg/m^2 IV on days 1–5 |

Repeat cycle every 21 days [699].

Bortezomib *(mantle cell lymphoma)*

Bortezomib:	1.3–1.5 mg/m^2 IV on days 1, 4, 8, and 11

Repeat cycle every 21 days [700].

Lenalidomide *(mantle cell lymphoma)*

Lenalidomide:	25 mg/day PO on days 1–21

Repeat cycle every 28 days for up to 52 weeks [701].

Pembrolizumab

Pembrolizumab:	200 mg IV on day 1

Repeat cycle every 3 weeks [702]. May also administer 400 mg IV every 6 weeks.

Primary CNS Lymphoma

Combination Regimens

Methotrexate:	3,500 mg/m^2 IV over 2 hours every other week for 5 doses
Intrathecal methotrexate:	12 mg IT weekly every other week after IV methotrexate
Leucovorin:	10 mg IV every 6 hours for 12 doses starting 24 hours after IV methotrexate; 10 mg IV every 12 hours for 8 doses starting 24 hours after IT methotrexate
Vincristine:	1.4 mg/m^2 IV every other week along with IV methotrexate
Procarbazine:	100 mg/m^2/day PO for 7 days on first, third, and fifth cycle of IV methotrexate

Once chemotherapy is completed, whole-brain radiation therapy is administered to a total dose of 45 cGy [703].

R-MPV + Radiation Therapy + Cytarabine

Rituximab:	500 mg/m^2 IV on day 1
Methotrexate:	3,500 mg/m^2 IV on day 2
Leucovorin:	20–25 mg every 6 hours starting 24 hours after methotrexate infusion for 72 hours or until serum methotrexate level, 1 × 10^{-8} mg/dL

Increase leucovorin to 40 mg every 4 hours IV if methotrexate level > 1 × 10^{-8} mg/dL at 48 hours or >1 × 10^{-8} mg/dL at 72 hours.

Vincristine:	1.4 mg/m^2 (maximum, 2.8 mg) IV on day 2
Procarbazine:	100 mg/m^2 PO on days 1–7 of odd-numbered cycles only

If positive CSF cytology, administer 12 mg methotrexate IT between days 5 and 12 of each cycle.

Repeat cycle every 2 weeks for 5 cycles [704].

After 5 cycles of R-MPV:

If CR, whole-brain radiotherapy (WBRT) 180 cGy/day for 13 days to a total of 2,340 cGy beginning 3–5 weeks after the completion of R-MPV.

If PR, administer 2 additional cycles of R-MPV. If CR is achieved after 7 cycles of R-MPV, administer WBRT 180 cGy/day $\times$ 13 days to a total of 2,340 cGy beginning 3–5 weeks after completion of R-MPV.

If persistent disease exists after 7 cycles of R-MPV, administer WBRT 180 cGy/day $\times$ 25 days to a total of 4,500 cGy beginning 3–5 weeks after the completion of R-MPV.

If stable or progressive disease after 5 cycles of R-MPV, administer WBRT 180 cGy/day for 25 days to a total of 4,500 cGy beginning 3–5 weeks after the completion of R-MPV. Three weeks after the completion of WBRT, consolidation therapy is given with cytarabine 3 g/m^2/day (maximum, 6 g) IV over 3 hours for 2 days. A second cycle of cytarabine is given 1 month later.

Single-Agent Regimens

High-Dose Methotrexate

Methotrexate:	8,000 mg/m^2 IV on day 1

Repeat cycle every 2 weeks up to 8 cycles, followed by 8,000 mg/m^2 IV on day 1 every month up to 100 months [705].

Temozolomide

Temozolomide:	150 mg/m^2/day PO on days 1–5

Repeat cycle every 4 weeks [706].

Topotecan

Topotecan:	1.5 mg/m^2 IV on days 1–5

Repeat cycle every 3 weeks [707].

MALIGNANT MELANOMA

Adjuvant Therapy

Combination Regimens

Dabrafenib + Trametinib

Dabrafenib:	150 mg PO bid
Trametinib:	2 mg PO daily

Continue treatment for up to 12 months [708].

Single-Agent Regimens

Interferon α-2b

Interferon α-2b: 20 million U/m^2 IV, 5 times weekly for 4 weeks, then 10 million IU/m^2 SC, 3 times weekly for 48 weeks

Treatment is for a total of 1 year [709].

Peg-Interferon α-2b

Peg-Interferon α-2b: 6 µg/kg SC weekly for 8 weeks, then
3 µg/kg SC weekly for up to 5 years
Treatment is for up to a total of 5 years [710].

Nivolumab

Nivolumab: 240 mg IV on day 1

Repeat cycle every 2 weeks [711]. May also administer 480 mg IV every 4 weeks.

Ipilimumab

Ipilimumab: 10 mg/kg IV on day 1

Repeat cycle every 3 weeks for 4 doses followed by 10 mg/kg IV on day 1 every 12 weeks for up to 3 years [712].

Pembrolizumab

Pembrolizumab: 200 mg IV on day 1

Repeat cycle every 3 weeks [713]. May also administer 400 mg IV every 6 weeks.

Metastatic Disease

Combination Regimens

Dacarbazine + Carmustine + Cisplatin

Dacarbazine: 220 mg/m^2 IV on days 1–3
Carmustine: 150 mg/m^2 IV on day 1
Cisplatin: 25 mg/m^2 IV on days 1–3

Repeat cycle with dacarbazine and cisplatin every 21 days and carmustine every 42 days [714].

IFN + Dacarbazine

Interferon α-2b: 15 million IU/m^2 IV on days 1–5, 8–12, and 15–19 as induction therapy

Interferon α-2b: 10 million IU/m^2 SC 3 times weekly after induction therapy

Dacarbazine: 200 mg/m^2 IV on days 22–26
Repeat cycle every 28 days [715].

Temozolomide + Thalidomide

Temozolomide:	75 mg/m^2/day PO for 6 weeks
Thalidomide:	200 mg/day PO for 6 weeks

Repeat cycle every 8 weeks [716]. Consider dose escalation to 400 mg/day for patients <70 years and starting at a lower dose of 100 mg/day with dose escalation to 250 mg/day for patient >70 years.

Dabrafenib + Trametinib

Dabrafenib:	150 mg PO bid
Trametinib:	2 mg PO daily

Continue treatment until disease progression [717].

Cobimetinib + Vemurafenib

Cobimetinib:	60 mg/day PO on days 1–21
Vemurafenib:	960 mg PO bid

Repeat cycle every 28 days [718].

Atezolizumab + Cobimetinib + Vemurafenib

Atezolizumab:	840 mg IV on day 1
Cobimetinib:	60 mg/day PO on days 1–21
Vemurafenib:	720 mg PO bid

Repeat cycle every 28 days [719].

Binimetinib + Encorafenib

Binimetinib:	45 mg PO bid
Encorafenib:	300 mg PO daily

Continue treatment until disease progression [720].

Nivolumab + Ipilimumab

Ipilimumab:	3 mg/kg IV on day 1
Nivolumab:	1 mg/kg IV on day 1

Repeat cycle every 21 days for 4 cycles followed by

Nivolumab:	240 mg IV on day 1

Repeat cycle every 2 weeks until disease progression [721]. May also administer 480 mg IV every 4 weeks.

Nivolumab + Relatlimab

Nivolumab:	480 mg IV on day 1
Relatlimab:	160 mg IV on day 1

Repeat cycle every 28 days [722].

Single-Agent Regimens

Dacarbazine

Dacarbazine: 250 mg/m^2 IV on days 1–5

Repeat cycle every 21 days [723].

or

Dacarbazine: 850 mg/m^2 IV on day 1

Repeat cycle every 3–6 weeks [724].

Interferon α-2b

Interferon α-2b: 20 million IU/m^2 IM, 3 times weekly
                                                for 12 weeks [725].

Aldesleukin

Aldesleukin (IL-2):   720,000 IU/kg IV every 8 hours on
                                                days 1–5 and 15–19

Repeat cycle in 6- to 12-week intervals [726].

or

Aldesleukin (IL-2):   100,000 IU/kg IV every 4 hours on
                                                days 1–5 and 15–19

Repeat cycle in 12-week intervals up to a total of 3 cycles [727].

or

Aldesleukin (IL-2):   720,000 IU/kg IV at 8 am and 6 pm on
                                                days 1–5 and 15–19

Treat up to a maximum of 8 total doses on days 1–5 and repeat on days 15–19.
Repeat cycle in 8- to 12-week intervals [728].

Ipilimumab

Ipilimumab: 3 mg/kg IV on day 1

Repeat cycle every 3 weeks for a total of 4 doses [729].

Pembrolizumab

Pembrolizumab: 200 mg IV on day 1

Repeat cycle every 3 weeks [730]. May also administer 400 mg IV every 6 weeks.

Nivolumab

Nivolumab: 240 mg IV on day 1

Repeat cycle every 2 weeks [731]. May also administer 480 mg IV every 4 weeks.

Tebentafusp-tebn

Tebentafusp: 20 μg IV on day 1; 30 μg IV on day 8;
                                                68 μg IV on day 15; and then 68 μg IV
                                                weekly thereafter

Repeat cycle every week [732].

Temozolomide
Temozolomide: $\qquad$ 150 mg/m^2 PO on days 1–5

Repeat cycle every 28 days [733]. If tolerated, can increase dose to 200 mg/m^2 PO on days 1–5.

Vemurafenib
Vemurafenib: $\qquad$ 960 mg PO bid

Continue treatment until disease progression [734].

Dabrafenib
Dabrafenib: $\qquad$ 150 mg PO bid

Continue treatment until disease progression [735].

Trametinib
Trametinib: $\qquad$ 2 mg PO daily

Continue treatment until disease progression [736].

MALIGNANT MESOTHELIOMA

Combination Regimens

Doxorubicin + Cisplatin
Doxorubicin: $\qquad$ 60 mg/m^2 IV on day 1

Cisplatin: $\qquad$ 60 mg/m^2 IV on day 1

Repeat cycle every 21–28 days [737].

CAP
Cyclophosphamide: $\qquad$ 500 mg/m^2 IV on day 1

Doxorubicin: $\qquad$ 50 mg/m^2 IV on day 1

Cisplatin: $\qquad$ 80 mg/m^2 IV on day 1

Repeat cycle every 21 days [738].

Gemcitabine + Cisplatin
Gemcitabine: $\qquad$ 1,000 mg/m^2 IV on days 1, 8, and 15

Cisplatin: $\qquad$ 100 mg/m^2 IV on day 1

Repeat cycle every 28 days [739].

Gemcitabine + Carboplatin

Gemcitabine: 1,000 mg/m^2 IV on days 1, 8, and 15
Carboplatin: AUC of 5, IV on day 1
Repeat cycle every 28 days [740].

Pemetrexed + Cisplatin

Pemetrexed: 500 mg/m^2 IV on day 1
Cisplatin: 75 mg/m^2 IV on day 1
Repeat cycle every 21 days [741]. Folic acid at 350–1,000 μg PO q day beginning 1 week prior to therapy and vitamin B12 at 1,000 μg IM to start 1–2 weeks prior to first dose of therapy and repeated every 3 cycles.

Gemcitabine + Vinorelbine

Gemcitabine: 1,000 mg/m^2 IV on days 1 and 8
Vinorelbine: 25 mg/m^2 IV on days 1 and 8
Repeat cycle every 21 days [742].

Pemetrexed + Gemcitabine

Pemetrexed: 500 mg/m^2 IV on day 8
Gemcitabine: 1,250 mg/m^2 IV on days 1 and 8
Repeat cycle every 21 days [743]. Folic acid at 350–1,000 μg PO q day beginning 1–2 weeks prior to therapy and vitamin B12 at 1,000 μg IM to start 1–2 weeks prior to first dose of therapy and repeated every 3 cycles.

Nivolumab + Ipilimumab

Nivolumab: 360 mg IV on day 1 every 3 weeks
Ipilimumab: 1 mg/kg IV on day 1 every 6 weeks
Continue treatment for up to 2 years [744].

Single-Agent Regimens

Pemetrexed

Pemetrexed: 500 mg/m^2 IV on day 1
Repeat cycle every 21 days [745]. Folic acid at 350–1,000 μg PO q day beginning 1 week prior to therapy and vitamin B12 at 1,000 μg IM to start 1–2 weeks prior to first dose of therapy and repeated every 3 cycles.

Dexamethasone 4 mg PO bid on the day before, day of, and day after each dose of pemetrexed.

Vinorelbine

Vinorelbine: 30 mg/m^2 IV weekly
One cycle consists of 6 weekly injections. Continue until disease progression [746].

Gemcitabine

Gemcitabine: $1,250 \text{ mg/m}^2$ IV on days 1, 8, and 15
Repeat cycle every 28 days up to a total of 10 cycles [747].

Pembrolizumab

Pembrolizumab: 10 mg/kg IV on day 1
Repeat cycle every 14 days [748].

Nivolumab

Nivolumab: 3 mg/kg IV on day 1
Repeat cycle every 14 days [749].

MERKEL CELL CANCER

Combination Regimens

EP

Etoposide: 80 mg/m^2 IV on days 1–3
Cisplatin: 80 mg/m^2 IV on day 1
Repeat cycle every 21 days [594].

EC

Etoposide: 100 mg/m^2 IV on days 1–3
Carboplatin: AUC of 6, IV on day 1
Repeat cycle every 28 days [595].

CAV

Cyclophosphamide: $1,000 \text{ mg/m}^2$ IV on day 1
Doxorubicin: 40 mg/m^2 IV on day 1
Vincristine: 1 mg/m^2 IV on day 1 (maximum, 2 mg)
Repeat cycle every 21 days [601].

Single-Agent Regimens

Avelumab

Avelumab: 10 mg/kg IV on day 1
Repeat cycle every 2 weeks [750].

Pembrolizumab

Pembrolizumab: 200 mg IV on day 1
Repeat cycle every 3 weeks [751]. May also administer 400 mg IV every 6 weeks.

Nivolumab

Nivolumab: 240 mg IV on day 1

Repeat cycle every 2 weeks [752]. May also administer 480 mg IV every 4 weeks.

Retifanlimab

Retifanlimab: 500 mg IV on day 1

Repeat cycle every 4 weeks up to 2 years [753].

MULTIPLE MYELOMA

Combination Regimens

MP

Melphalan:	8–10 mg/m^2 PO on days 1–4
Prednisone:	60 mg/m^2 on days 1–4

Repeat cycle every 42 days [754].

MPT

Melphalan:	0.25 mg/kg PO on days 1–4
Prednisone:	1.5 mg/kg PO on days 1–4
Thalidomide:	50–100 mg/day PO q day

Repeat cycle every 28 days [755].

or

Melphalan:	0.20 mg/kg/day PO on days 1–4
Prednisone:	2 mg/kg/day PO on days 1–4
Thalidomide:	100 mg PO q day

Repeat cycle every 42 days (patients older than 75) [756].

MPL

Melphalan:	0.18 mg/kg PO on days 1–4
Prednisone:	2 mg/kg PO on days 1–4
Lenalidomide:	10 mg/day PO on days 1–21

Repeat cycle every 28 days [757].

VAD

Vincristine:	0.4 mg/day IV continuous infusion on days 1–4
Doxorubicin:	9 mg/m^2/day IV continuous infusion on days 1–4
Dexamethasone:	40 mg PO on days 1–4, 9–12, and 17–20

Repeat cycle every 28 days [758].

Thalidomide + Dexamethasone

Thalidomide:	200 mg/day PO
Dexamethasone:	40 mg/day PO on days 1–4, 9–12, and 17–20 for first 4 cycles and then 40 mg/day PO on days 1–4

Repeat cycle every 28 days [759].

Lenalidomide + Dexamethasone

Lenalidomide:	25 mg/day PO on days 1–21
Dexamethasone:	40 mg/day PO on days 1–4, 9–12, and 17–20 (first 4 cycles) and then 40 mg/day PO on days 1–4 with future cycles

Repeat cycles every 28 days [760].

or

Lenalidomide:	25 mg/day PO on days 1–21
Dexamethasone:	40 mg/m^2/day PO on days 1, 8, 15, and 22

Repeat cycle every 28 days [761].

RVD

Lenalidomide:	25 mg/day PO on days 1–14
Bortezomib:	1.3 mg/m^2 IV or SC on days 1, 4, 8, and 11
Dexamethasone:	20 mg/day PO on days 1, 2, 4, 5, 8, 9, 11, and 12

Repeat cycle every 21 days for 8 cycles [762].

Panobinostat + Bortezomib + Dexamethasone

Panobinostat:	20 mg/day PO on days 1, 3, 5, 8, 10, and 12
Bortezomib:	1.3 mg/m^2 IV on days 1, 4, 8, and 11
Dexamethasone:	20 mg/day PO on days 1, 2, 4, 5, 8, 9, 11, and 12

Repeat cycle every 21 days [763].

PD

Pomalidomide:	4 mg/day PO on days 1–21
Dexamethasone:	40 mg/day PO on day 1

Repeat cycle every 28 days [764].

or

| Pomalidomide: | 2 mg/day PO on days 1–21 |
| Dexamethasone: | 40 mg/day PO on days 1, 8, 15, and 22 |

Repeat cycle every 28 days [765].

DVD

Doxorubicin liposome:	40 mg/m^2 IV on day 1
Vincristine:	2 mg IV on day 1
Dexamethasone:	40 mg PO on days 1–4

Repeat cycles every 28 days [766].

Bortezomib + Doxorubicin liposome

| Bortezomib: | 1.3 mg/m^2 IV or SC on days 1, 4, 8, and 11 |
| Doxorubicin liposome: | 30 mg/m^2 IV infusion on day 4 |

Repeat cycle every 21 days [767].

Bortezomib + Melphalan

| Bortezomib: | 1.0 mg/m^2 IV or SC on days 1, 4, 8, and 11 |
| Melphalan: | 0.10 mg/kg PO on days 1–4 |

Repeat cycle every 28 days up to 8 cycles [768].

BMP

Bortezomib:	1.3 mg/m^2 IV or SC on days 1, 4, 8, 11, 22, 25, 29, and 32
Melphalan:	9 mg/m^2 PO on days 1–4
Prednisone:	60 mg/m^2 PO on days 1–4

Repeat cycle every 6 weeks for 4 cycles [769], then

Bortezomib:	1.3 mg/m^2 IV on days 1, 8, 22, and 29
Melphalan:	9 mg/m^2 PO on days 1–4
Prednisone:	60 mg/m^2 PO on days 1–4

Repeat cycle every 6 weeks for 5 cycles [769].

BMPT

Bortezomib:	1–1.3 mg/m^2 IV or SC on days 1, 4, 15, and 22
Melphalan:	6 mg/m^2 PO on days 1–5
Prednisone:	60 mg/m^2 PO on days 1–5
Thalidomide:	50 mg PO daily

Repeat cycle every 5 weeks for 6 cycles [770].

RMPT

Lenalidomide:	10 mg PO on days 1–21
Melphalan:	0.18 mg/kg PO on days 1–4
Prednisone:	2 mg/kg PO on days 1–4
Thalidomide:	50 mg PO daily on days 1–28

Repeat cycle every 28 days for 6 cycles followed by maintenance lenalidomide 10 mg PO on days 1–21 until progression or toxicity [771].

Carfilzomib + Lenalidomide + Dexamethasone (CLD)

Carfilzomib:	20 mg/m^2 IV on days 1 and 2 of cycle 1, and if tolerated, then 27 mg/m^2 IV on days 8, 9, 15, and 16 during cycles 1 through 12, and 27 mg/m^2 IV on days 1, 2, 15, and 16 during cycles 13 through 18, after which carfilzomib is discontinued
Lenalidomide:	25 mg PO on days 1–21
Dexamethasone:	40 mg PO on days 1, 8, 15, and 22

Repeat cycle every 28 days for up to 9 cycles [772].

Carfilzomib + Dexamethasone (CD)

Carfilzomib:	20 mg/m^2 IV on days 1, 8, and 15 of cycle 1, and then 70 mg/m^2 IV on days 1, 8, and 15 for all subsequent cycles
Dexamethasone:	40 mg PO on days 1, 8, and 15 for all cycles 40 mg PO on days 1, 8, 15, and 22 (cycles 1–9 only)

Repeat cycle every 28 days [773].

Lenalidomide + Dexamethasone + Ixazomib

Lenalidomide:	25 mg/day PO on days 1–21
Dexamethasone:	40 mg/day PO on days 1, 8, 15, and 22
Ixazomib:	4 mg/day PO on days 1, 8, and 15

Repeat cycle every 28 days until disease progression [774].

Daratumumab + Bortezomib + Dexamethasone

Daratumumab:	16 mg/kg IV weekly on cycles 1–3
	16 mg/kg IV on day 1 of cycles 4–8
	16 mg/kg IV on day 1 of cycles 9+
Bortezomib:	1.3 mg/m^2 IV on days 1, 4, 8, and 11 on cycles 1–8

Dexamethasone: 20 mg PO on days 1, 2, 4, 5, 8, 9, 11,
                                        and 12 on cycles 1–8

Continue treatment until disease progression or toxicity [775].

Elotuzumab + Lenalidomide + Dexamethasone

Elotuzumab: 10 mg/kg IV on days 1, 8, 15, and 22

Lenalidomide: 25 mg PO on days 1–21

Dexamethasone: 8 mg IV prior to elotuzumab infusion
                                        and 28 mg PO on days 1, 8, 15, and 22
                                        and 40 mg PO on day 28

Repeat cycle every 28 days for two cycles followed by:

Elotuzumab: 10 mg/kg IV on days 1 and 15

Lenalidomide: 25 mg PO on days 1–21

Dexamethasone: 8 mg IV prior to elotuzumab infusion
                                        and 28 mg PO on days 1 and 15, and
                                        40 mg PO on days 22 and 28

Repeat cycle every 28 days until disease progression [776].

Selinexor + Dexamethasone

Selinexor: 80 mg PO on days 1 and 3

Dexamethasone: 20 mg PO on days 1 and 3

Continue treatment until disease progression [777].

Isatuximab + Pomalidomide + Dexamethasone

Isatuximab: 10 mg/kg IV on days 1, 8, 15, and 22
                                        of cycle 1 followed by 10 mg/kg IV
                                        on days 1 and 15 on all subsequent
                                        cycles

Pomalidomide: 4 mg PO daily on days 1–21

Dexamethasone: 40 mg PO weekly on days 1, 8, 15,
                                        and 22

Repeat cycle every 28 days [778].

Daratumumab + Bortezomib + Thalidomide + Dexamethasone

Daratumumab: 16 mg/kg IV on days 1, 8, 15, 22, 29,
                                        36, 42, and 49, followed by once every
                                        2 weeks for 16 weeks, followed by
                                        once every 4 weeks

Bortezomib: 1.3 mg/m^2 IV or SC on days 1, 4, 8,
                                        and 11

Thalidomide: 200–800 mg PO daily

Dexamethasone: 40 mg PO on days 1, 8, 15, and 22

Administer for 4 cycles followed by autologous stem cell transplant, followed by 2 cycles of consolidation therapy [779].

Daratumumab + Lenalidomide + Dexamethasone

Daratumumab:	16 mg/kg IV weekly during cycles 1 and 2, every 2 weeks during cycles 3 through 6, and every 4 weeks thereafter
Lenalidomide:	25 mg PO on days 1–21
Dexamethasone:	40 mg PO days 1, 8, 15, and 22

Repeat cycle every 28 days [780].

Melphalan Flufenamide + Dexamethasone

Melphalan flufenamide:	40 mg IV on day 1
Dexamethasone:	40 mg PO on days 1, 8, 15, and 22

Repeat cycle every 28 days [781].

Single-Agent Regimens

Dexamethasone

Dexamethasone: 40 mg IV or PO on days 1–4, 9–12, and 17–20

Repeat cycle every 21 days [782].

Melphalan

Melphalan: 90–140 mg/m^2 IV on day 1

Repeat cycle every 28–42 days [783].

Thalidomide

Thalidomide: 200–800 mg PO daily

Continue treatment until disease progression or undue toxicity [784].

Lenalidomide

Lenalidomide: 30 mg PO daily on days 1–21

Repeat cycle every 28 days until disease progression or undue toxicity [785].

or

Lenalidomide

Lenalidomide: 10 mg PO daily on days 1–21

For maintenance therapy after autologous stem-cell transplantation, repeat cycle every 28 days until disease progression or undue toxicity [786].

Bortezomib

Bortezomib: 1.3 mg/m^2 IV or SC on days 1, 4, 8, and 11

Repeat cycle every 21 days [787].

Carfilzomib

Carfilzomib: 20 mg/m^2 IV on days 1, 2, 8, 9, 15, and 16. After cycle 1, increase dose to 27 mg/m^2 IV

Repeat cycle every 28 days for up to 12 cycles [788].

Daratumumab

Daratumumab: 16 mg/kg IV on days 1, 8, 15, 22, 29, 36, 42, and 49 followed by once every 2 weeks for 16 weeks, followed by once every 4 weeks

Continue treatment until disease progression [789].

Daratumumab + Hyaluronidase

Daratumumab: 1,800 mg daratumumab SC and 30,000 units hyaluronidase administered SC once weekly (cycles 1–2), every 2 weeks (cycles 3–6), and every 4 weeks thereafter (28-day cycles)

Continue treatment until disease progression [790].

Ibrutinib

Ibrutinib: 420 mg/day PO daily

Continue treatment until disease progression [791].

Belantamab mafodotin-blmf

Belantamab mafodotin: 2.5 mg/kg IV on day 1

Repeat cycle every 3 weeks [792].

Teclistamab-cqyv

Teclistamab-cqyv: 1.5 mg/kg IV on day 1

Repeat cycle once weekly [793].

Talquetamab-tgvs

Talquetamab-tgvs: 0.01 mg/kg SC on day 1; 0.06 mg/kg SC on day 4; 0.4 mg/kg SC on day 7; and then 0.4 mg/kg SC weekly thereafter

Repeat cycle every week [794].

Idecabtagene vicleucel [795]

Cyclophosphamide:	300 mg/m^2 IV on days 5, 4, and 3
Fludarabine:	30 mg/m^2 IV on days 5, 4, and 3
Idecabtagene vicleucel:	300–460 × 10^6 CAR-positive T cells IV on day 1

Ciltacabtagene vicleucel [796]

Cyclophosphamide:	300 mg/m^2 IV on days 5, 4, and 3
Fludarabine:	30 mg/m^2 IV on days 5, 4, and 3
Ciltacabtagene vicleucel:	0.75 × 10^6 CAR-positive T cells IV on day 1

MYELODYSPLASTIC SYNDROME

Combination Regimens

Cedazuridine + Decitabine

Cedazuridine:	100 mg PO on days 1–5
Decitabine:	35 mg PO on days 1–5

Repeat cycle every 28 days [797].

Single-Agent Regimens

Azacitidine

Azacitidine:	75 mg/m^2 SC daily for 7 days

Repeat cycle every 4 weeks. Patients should be treated for at least 4 cycles [798].

Decitabine

Decitabine:	15 mg/m^2 IV continuous infusion over 3 hours every 8 hours for 3 days

Repeat cycle every 4 weeks. Patients should be treated for at least 4 cycles [799].

or

Decitabine:	20 mg/m^2 IV continuous infusion over 1 hour for 5 days

Repeat cycle every 4–6 weeks. Patients should be treated for at least 4 cycles [800].

Lenalidomide

Lenalidomide:	10 mg PO daily

Continue until disease progression [801].

or

Lenalidomide:	10 mg PO daily for 21 days

Repeat cycle every 28 days [801].

Imatinib

Imatinib:	400 mg PO daily

Continue until disease progression [802].

Luspatercept

Luspatercept:	1 mg/kg SC on day 1

Repeat cycle every 21 days [803]. May receive increasing dose to 1.33 mg/kg SC and then up to 1.75 mg/kg SC.

Antithymocyte globulin (ATG) + Cyclosporine

ATG:	15 mg/kg IV on days 1–5
Cyclosporine:	5–6 mg/kg PO bid

Adjust cyclosporine dose to maintain blood levels between 100 and 300 ng/mL [804].

NTRK GENE FUSION CANCER

Single-Agent Regimens

Larotrectinib

Larotrectinib:	100 mg PO bid

Repeat cycle every 21 days [805].

Entrectinib

Entrectinib:	600 mg PO daily

Continue until disease progression [806].

OSTEOGENIC SARCOMA

Combination Regimens

Etoposide + Ifosfamide

Etoposide:	100 mg/m^2/day IV on days 1–5
Ifosfamide:	3,500 mg/m^2/day IV on days 1–5

| Mesna: | 700 mg/m^2 IV with first ifosfamide dose, then 3, 6, and 9 hours later on days 1–5 |

Repeat cycle every 21 days for 2 cycles [807]. G-CSF support at 5 μg/kg/day SC to start on day 6, followed by surgical resection of primary tumor and then intensive maintenance chemotherapy.

| Methotrexate: | 1,200 mg/m^2 IV on weeks 1, 2, 6, 7, 11, 12, 16, 17, 30, and 31 |

| Leucovorin: | 15 mg IV every 6 hours for 10 doses starting 24 hours after start of high-dose methotrexate |

or

| L-Leucovorin: | 7.5 mg IV every 6 hours for 10 doses starting 24 hours after start of high-dose methotrexate |

| Doxorubicin: | 37.5 mg/m^2/day IV on days 1 and 2 on weeks 3, 13, 21, 27, and 32 |

| Cisplatin: | 60 mg/m^2/day IV on days 1 and 2 on weeks 3, 13, 21, and 27 |

| Ifosfamide: | 2,400 mg/m^2/day IV on days 1–5 on weeks 8, 18, and 24 |

Administer G-CSF support at 5 μg/kg/day SC on weeks 8, 18, and 24.

Cisplatin + Doxorubicin + High-Dose Methotrexate

| Doxorubicin: | 25 mg/m^2/day IV on days 1–3 on weeks 0 and 5 |

| Cisplatin: | 120 mg/m^2 IV on day 1 on weeks 0 and 5 |

| Methotrexate: | 1,200 mg/m^2 IV on day 1 on weeks 3, 4, 8, and 9 |

| Leucovorin: | 10 mg IV every 6 hours for 10 doses starting 24 hours after start of high-dose methotrexate |

or

| L-Leucovorin: | 7.5 mg IV every 6 hours for 10 doses starting 24 hours after start of high-dose methotrexate |

Induction chemotherapy is followed by surgical resection of primary tumor and then maintenance chemotherapy to begin on week 12 and continuing until week 31 [808].

| Doxorubicin: | 25 mg/m^2/day IV on days 1–3 on weeks 12, 17, 22, and 27 |

| Cisplatin: | 120 mg/m^2 IV on day 1 on weeks 12 and 17 |

Methotrexate:	1,200 mg/m^2 IV on day 1 on weeks 15, 16, 20, 21, 25, 26, 30, and 31
Leucovorin:	10 mg IV every 6 hours for 10 doses starting 24 hours after start of high-dose methotrexate
or	
L-Leucovorin:	7.5 mg IV every 6 hours for 10 doses starting 24 hours after start of high-dose methotrexate

OVARIAN CANCER (EPITHELIAL)

Combination Regimens

CC
Carboplatin:	300 mg/m^2 IV on day 1
Cyclophosphamide:	600 mg/m^2 IV on day 1

Repeat cycle every 28 days [809].

CC
Cisplatin:	100 mg/m^2 IV on day 1
Cyclophosphamide:	600 mg/m^2 IV on day 1

Repeat cycle every 28 days [810].

CP
Cisplatin:	75 mg/m^2 IV on day 2
Paclitaxel:	135 mg/m^2 IV over 24 hours on day 1

Repeat cycle every 21 days [811].

Carboplatin + Paclitaxel
Carboplatin:	AUC of 6–7.5, IV on day 1
Paclitaxel:	175 mg/m^2 IV over 3 hours on day 1

Repeat cycle every 21 days [812].
or
Carboplatin:	AUC of 2, IV on days 1, 8, and 15
Paclitaxel:	60 mg/m^2 IV on days 1, 8, and 15

Repeat cycle every 28 days [813].

Carboplatin + Paclitaxel + Bevacizumab

Carboplatin:	AUC of 6, IV on day 1
Paclitaxel:	175 mg/m^2 IV over 3 hours on day 1
Bevacizumab:	15 mg/kg IV on day 1

Repeat cycle every 21 days for 6 cycles, then maintenance bevacizumab for cycles 7–22 [814].

Carboplatin + Docetaxel

Carboplatin:	AUC of 6, IV on day 1
Docetaxel:	60 mg/m^2 IV on day 1

Repeat cycle every 21 days [815].

Carboplatin + Doxorubicin liposome

Carboplatin:	AUC of 5, IV on day 1
Doxorubicin liposome:	30 mg/m^2 IV on day 1

Repeat cycle every 28 days [816].

Gemcitabine + Doxorubicin liposome

Gemcitabine:	1,000 mg/m^2 IV on days 1 and 8
Doxorubicin liposome:	30 mg/m^2 IV on day 1

Repeat cycle every 21 days [817].

Gemcitabine + Cisplatin

Gemcitabine:	800–1,000 mg/m^{2}IV on days 1 and 8
Cisplatin:	30 mg/m^2 IV on days 1 and 8

Repeat cycle every 21 days [818].

Gemcitabine + Carboplatin

Gemcitabine:	1,000 mg/m^2 IV on days 1 and 8
Carboplatin:	AUC of 4, IV on day 1

Repeat cycle every 21 days [819].

Paclitaxel + IP Cisplatin + IP Paclitaxel

Paclitaxel:	135 mg/m^2 IV over 24 hours on day 1
Cisplatin:	100 mg/m^2 IP on day 2
Paclitaxel:	60 mg/m^2 IP on day 8

Repeat cycle every 21 days up to 6 cycles [820].

Pemetrexed + Carboplatin

Pemetrexed: 500 mg/m^2 IV on day 1

Carboplatin: AUC of 5, IV on day 1

Repeat cycle every 21 days [821]. Folic acid at 350–1,000 µg PO q day beginning
1–2 weeks prior to therapy and vitamin B12 at 1,000 µg IM to start 1–2 weeks prior
to first dose of therapy and repeated every 3 cycles. Dexamethasone 4 mg PO bid
on the day before, day of, and day after each dose of pemetrexed.

Olaparib + Bevacizumab

Olaparib: 300 mg PO bid

Bevacizumab: 15 mg IV on day 1

Repeat cycle every 21 days [822].

Niraparib + Bevacizumab

Niraparib: 300 mg PO daily

Bevacizumab: 15 mg IV on day 1

Repeat cycle every 21 days [823].

Single-Agent Regimens

Mirvetuximab soravtansine-gynx

Mirvetuximab: 6 mg/kg IV on day 1

Repeat cycle every 3 weeks [824].

Altretamine

Altretamine: 260 mg/m^2/day PO in 4 divided doses
                                              after meals and at bedtime

Repeat cycle every 14–21 days [825].

Doxorubicin liposome

Doxorubicin liposome: 40–50 mg/m^2 IV over 1 hour on day 1

Repeat cycle every 28 days [826].

Paclitaxel

Paclitaxel: 135 mg/m^2 IV over 3 hours on day 1

Repeat cycle every 21 days [827].

Ixabepilone

Ixabepilone: 20 mg/m^2 IV on days 1, 8, and 15

Repeat cycle every 28 days [828].

Topotecan

Topotecan: 1.5 mg/m^2 IV on days 1–5

Repeat cycle every 21 days [829].

Gemcitabine

Gemcitabine: 800 mg/m^2 IV weekly for 3 weeks

Repeat cycle every 4 weeks [830].

Etoposide

Etoposide: 50 mg/m^2/day PO on days 1–21

Repeat cycle every 28 days [831].

Vinorelbine

Vinorelbine: 30 mg/m^2 IV on days 1 and 8

Repeat cycle every 21 days [832].

Pemetrexed

Pemetrexed: 900 mg/m^2 IV on day 1

Repeat cycle every 21 days [833]. Folic acid at 350–1,000 μg PO q day beginning 1 week prior to therapy and vitamin B12 at 1,000 μg IM to start 1–2 weeks prior to first dose of therapy and repeated every 3 cycles. Dexamethasone 4 mg PO bid on the day before, day of, and day after each dose of pemetrexed.

Bevacizumab

Bevacizumab: 15 mg/kg IV on day 1

Repeat cycle every 21 days [834].

Capecitabine

Capecitabine: 1,000 mg/m^2 PO bid on days 1–14

Repeat cycle every 21 days [835].

Olaparib

Olaparib: 400 mg PO bid

Repeat cycle every 28 days [836].

Olaparib (maintenance after first-line chemotherapy)

Olaparib: 300 mg PO bid

Repeat cycle every 28 days [837].

Rucaparib

Rucaparib: 600 mg PO daily

Repeat cycle every 28 days [838].

Niraparib

Niraparib: 300 mg PO daily

Repeat cycle every 28 days [839].

Niraparib

Niraparib: 200 mg PO daily for body weight <77 kg, platelet count <150,000, or both

Repeat cycle every 28 days for 36 months or until disease progression [840].

OVARIAN CANCER (GERM CELL)

Combination Regimens
BEP

Bleomycin: 30 U IV on days 2, 9, and 16

Etoposide: 100 mg/m^2 IV on days 1–5

Cisplatin: 20 mg/m^2 IV on days 1–5

Repeat cycle every 21 days [841].

PANCREATIC CANCER

Adjuvant Therapy

Combination Regimens
Gemcitabine + Capecitabine (GEM-CAP)

Gemcitabine: 1,000 mg/m^2 IV on days 1, 8, and 15

Capecitabine: 830 mg/m^2 PO bid on days 1–21

Repeat cycle every 28 days for a total of 6 cycles [842].

mFOLFIRINOX

Oxaliplatin: 85 mg/m^2 IV on day 1

Irinotecan: 150 mg/m^2 IV on day 1

Leucovorin: 400 mg/m^2 IV on day 1

5-Fluorouracil: 2,400 mg/m^2 IV continuous infusion over 46 hours on days 1 and 2

Repeat cycle every 2 weeks for a total of 12 cycles [843].

Single-Agent Regimens
5-Fluorouracil + Leucovorin

5-Fluorouracil: 425 mg/m^2 IV on days 1–5

Leucovorin: 20 mg/m^2 IV on days 1–5

Repeat cycle every 28 days for a total of 6 cycles [844].

Capecitabine

Capecitabine:	1,000–1,250 mg/m^2 PO on days 1–14

Repeat cycle every 21 days for a total of 6 cycles [845].

Gemcitabine

Gemcitabine:	1,000 mg/m^2 IV on days 1, 8, and 15

Repeat cycle every 28 days for a total of 6 cycles [846].

Locally Advanced Disease

Combination Regimens

RTOG Chemoradiation Regimen

Gemcitabine:	1,000 mg/m^2 IV on days 1, 8, and 15

Followed by concurrent chemoradiation:

5-Fluorouracil:	250 mg/m^2/day IV continuous infusion during radiation therapy
Radiation therapy:	180 cGy/day to a total dose of 5,040 cGy

Chemotherapy and radiation therapy started on the same day and given concurrently.

After chemoradiation:

Gemcitabine:	1,000 mg/m^2 IV on days 1, 8, and 15

Repeat cycle every 4 weeks for a total of 3 cycles [847]. Adjuvant chemotherapy is given to patients with complete gross total resection of pancreatic adenocarcinoma.

Gemcitabine + Radiation Therapy (ECOG regimen)

Gemcitabine:	600 mg/m^2 IV weekly for 6 weeks
Radiation therapy:	180 cGy/day to a total dose of 5,040 cGy. Chemotherapy and radiation therapy started on the same day and given concurrently.

Four weeks after the completion of chemoradiation:

Gemcitabine:	1,000 mg/m^2 IV on days 1, 8, and 15

Repeat cycle every 4 weeks for a total of 5 cycles [848]. For patients with locally advanced unresectable pancreatic adenocarcinoma.

Capecitabine-Based Chemoradiotherapy (SCALOP regimen)

Gemcitabine:	1,000 mg/m^2 IV on days 1, 8, and 15
Capecitabine:	830 mg/m^2 PO bid on days 1–21

Repeat cycle every 28 days for 3 cycles [849]. Patients with stable or responding disease receive one additional cycle, followed by concurrent chemoradiation:

| Capecitabine: | 830 mg/m^2 PO bid Monday–Friday for 6 weeks |
| Radiation therapy: | 180 cGy/day to a total dose of 5,040 cGy. |

Chemotherapy and radiation therapy started on the same day and given concurrently [849].

Metastatic Disease

Combination Regimens

5-Fluorouracil + Leucovorin

| 5-Fluorouracil: | 425 mg/m^2 IV on days 1–5 |
| Leucovorin: | 20 mg/m^2 IV on days 1–5 |

Repeat cycle every 28 days [850].

Gemcitabine + Capecitabine (GEM-CAP)

| Gemcitabine: | 1,000 mg/m^2 IV on days 1 and 8 |
| Capecitabine: | 650 mg/m^2 PO bid on days 1–14 |

Repeat cycle every 21 days [851].

or

| Gemcitabine: | 1,000 mg/m^2 IV on days 1, 8, and 15 |
| Capecitabine: | 830 mg/m^2 PO bid on days 1–21 |

Repeat cycle every 28 days [852].

Gemcitabine + Docetaxel + Capecitabine (GTX)

Gemcitabine:	750 mg/m^2 IV over 75 minutes on days 4 and 11
Docetaxel:	30 mg/m^2 IV on days 4 and 11
Capecitabine:	750 mg/m^2 PO bid on days 1–14

Repeat cycle every 3 weeks [853].

Gemcitabine + Cisplatin

| Gemcitabine: | 1,000 mg/m^2 IV over 100 minutes on days 1, 8, and 15 |
| Cisplatin: | 50 mg/m^2 on days 1 and 8 |

Repeat cycle every 4 weeks [854].

Gemcitabine + Oxaliplatin

| Gemcitabine: | 1,000 mg/m^2 IV over 100 minutes on day 1 |
| Oxaliplatin: | 100 mg/m^2 over 2 hours on day 2 |

Repeat cycle every 2 weeks [855].

or

Gemcitabine:	1,000 mg/m^2 IV over 100 minutes on day 1
Oxaliplatin:	100 mg/m^2 over 2 hours on day 1

Repeat cycle every 2 weeks [856].

Gemcitabine + Erlotinib

Gemcitabine:	1,000 mg/m^2 IV weekly for 7 weeks, then 1-week rest; subsequent cycles 1,000 mg/m^2 IV weekly for 3 weeks with 1-week rest
Erlotinib:	100 mg PO daily

Repeat 3-week cycles every 28 days [857].

Capecitabine + Erlotinib

Capecitabine:	1,000 mg/m^2 PO bid on days 1–14
Erlotinib:	150 mg PO daily

Repeat cycle every 21 days [858].

FOLFIRINOX

Oxaliplatin:	85 mg/m^2 IV on day 1
Irinotecan:	180 mg/m^2 IV on day 1
Leucovorin:	400 mg/m^2 IV on day 1
5-Fluorouracil:	400 mg/m^2 IV on day 1
5-Fluorouracil:	2,400 mg/m^2 IV continuous infusion over 46 hours on days 1 and 2

Repeat cycle every 2 weeks [859].

Nab-Paclitaxel + Gemcitabine

Nab-Paclitaxel:	125 mg/m^2 IV on days 1, 8, and 15
Gemcitabine:	1,000 mg/m^2 IV on days 1, 8, and 15

Repeat cycle every 28 days [860].
or

Nab-Paclitaxel:	125 mg/m^2 IV on days 1 and 15
Gemcitabine:	1,000 mg/m^2 IV on days 1 and 15

Repeat cycle every 28 days [861].

Liposomal Irinotecan + 5-Fluorouracil + Leucovorin

Liposomal Irinotecan:	70 mg/m^2 IV on day 1
5-Fluorouracil:	2,400 mg/m^2 IV continuous infusion over 46 hours on days 1 and 2

| Leucovorin: | 400 mg/m^2 IV on day 1 |

Repeat cycle every 2 weeks [862].

Single-Agent Regimens

Pembrolizumab

| Pembrolizumab: | 200 mg IV on day 1 |

Repeat cycle every 3 weeks [863]. Used only in setting of MSI-H/dMMR disease.

Olaparib

| Olaparib: | 300 mg PO bid |

Continue therapy until evidence of disease progression [864]. Patients must have germline BRCA1/2 mutation and have received at least 16 weeks of platinum-based chemotherapy.

Gemcitabine

| Gemcitabine: | 1,000 mg/m^2 IV weekly for 7 weeks, then 1-week rest; subsequent cycles 1,000 mg/m^2 IV weekly for 3 weeks with 1-week rest |

Repeat 3-week cycle every 28 days [865].
or

| Gemcitabine: | 1,000 mg/m^2 IV over 100 min at 10 mg/m^2/min on days 1, 8, and 15 |

Repeat cycle every 28 days [866].

Capecitabine

| Capecitabine: | 1,250 mg/m^2 PO bid on days 1–14 |

May decrease dose to 850–1,000 mg/m^2 PO bid on days 1–14 to reduce the risk of toxicity without compromising clinical efficacy.

Repeat cycle every 21 days [867].

PROSTATE CANCER

Combination Regimens

Flutamide + Leuprolide [868]

| Flutamide: | 250 mg PO tid |
| Leuprolide: | 7.5 mg IM every 28 days or 22.5 mg IM every 12 weeks |

Flutamide + Goserelin [869]

| Flutamide: | 250 mg PO tid |
| Goserelin: | 10.8 mg SC every 12 weeks |

Estramustine + Etoposide

Estramustine:	15 mg/kg/day PO in 4 divided doses on days 1–21
Etoposide:	50 mg/m^2/day PO in 2 divided doses on days 1–21

Repeat cycle every 28 days [870].

Estramustine + Vinblastine

Estramustine:	600 mg/m^2 PO daily on days 1–42
Vinblastine:	4 mg/m^2 IV weekly for 6 weeks

Repeat cycle every 8 weeks [871].

Paclitaxel + Estramustine

Paclitaxel:	120 mg/m^2 IV continuous infusion on days 1–4
Estramustine:	600 mg/m^2 PO daily, starting 24 hours before paclitaxel

Repeat cycle every 21 days [872].
or

Paclitaxel:	90 mg/m^2 IV weekly for 3 weeks
Estramustine:	140 mg PO tid, starting day before, day of, and day after paclitaxel

Repeat cycle every 28 days [873].

Mitoxantrone + Prednisone

Mitoxantrone:	12 mg/m^2 IV on day 1
Prednisone:	5 mg PO bid daily

Repeat cycle every 21 days [874].

Docetaxel + Estramustine

Docetaxel:	35 mg/m^2 IV on day 2 of weeks 1 and 2
Estramustine:	420 mg PO for the first 4 doses and 280 mg PO for the next 5 doses on days 1–3 of weeks 1 and 2

Repeat cycle every 21 days [875]. Dexamethasone is administered at 4 mg PO bid on days 1–3 of weeks 1 and 2.
or

Docetaxel:	60 mg/m^2 IV on day 2
Estramustine:	280 mg PO tid on days 1–5

Repeat cycle every 21 days [876].

Docetaxel + Prednisone

Docetaxel: 75 mg/m^2 IV on day 1
Prednisone: 5 mg PO bid
Repeat cycle every 21 days for up to a total of 10 cycles [877].

Docetaxel + Prednisone + Bevacizumab

Docetaxel: 75 mg/m^2 IV on day 1
Prednisone: 5 mg PO bid
Bevacizumab: 15 mg/kg IV on day 1
Repeat cycle every 21 days [878].

Cabazitaxel + Prednisone

Cabazitaxel: 25 mg/m^2 IV on day 1
Prednisone: 10 mg PO daily
Repeat cycle every 21 days [879].
or
Cabazitaxel: 20 mg/m^2 IV on day 1
Prednisone: 10 mg PO daily
Repeat cycle every 21 days [880].
or
Cabazitaxel: 10 mg/m^2 IV on days 1, 8, 15, and 22
Prednisone: 5 mg PO bid
Repeat cycle every 5 weeks [881].

Cabazitaxel + Carboplatin

Cabazitaxel: 20 mg/m^2 IV on day 1
Carboplatin: AUC of 4, IV on day 1
Repeat cycle every 21 days [882].

Abiraterone + Prednisone

Abiraterone: 1,000 mg PO daily
Prednisone: 5 mg PO bid
Continue until disease progression [883].

Niraparib + Abiraterone + Prednisone

Niraparib: 200 mg PO daily
Abiraterone: 1,000 mg PO daily
Prednisone: 5 mg PO bid
Repeat cycle every 28 days [884].

Olaparib + Abiraterone + Prednisone

Olaparib:	300 mg PO daily
Abiraterone:	1,000 mg PO daily
Prednisone:	5 mg PO bid

Continue until disease progression [885].

Talazoparib + Enzalutamide

Talazoparib:	0.5 mg PO daily
Enzalutamide:	160 mg PO daily
Prednisone:	5 mg PO bid

Repeat cycle every 28 days [886].

Docetaxel + Leuprolide

Docetaxel:	75 mg/m^2 IV on day 1
Leuprolide:	7.5 mg IM on day 1

Repeat cycle every 21 days for 6 cycles [887].

Single-Agent Regimens

Paclitaxel

Paclitaxel:	135–170 mg/m^2 IV as a 24-hour infusion on day 1

Repeat cycle every 3 weeks [888].
or

Paclitaxel:	100 mg/m^2 IV on days 1, 8, and 15

Repeat cycle every 4 weeks [889].

Docetaxel

Docetaxel:	75 mg/m^2 IV on day 1

Repeat cycle every 21 days [890].
or

Docetaxel:	20–40 mg/m^2 weekly for 3 weeks

Repeat cycle every 4 weeks [891].

Estramustine

Estramustine:	14 mg/kg/day PO in 3–4 divided doses [892]

Goserelin

Goserelin:	3.6 mg SC on day 1

Repeat cycle every 28 days [893].
or

Goserelin: 10.8 mg SC on day 1
Repeat cycle every 12 weeks [894].

Goserelin (adjuvant therapy)
Goserelin: 3.6 mg SC on day 1
Repeat cycle every 28 days for 24 months [895].

Degarelix
Degarelix: 240 mg SC starting dose followed
                                             28 days later by the first maintenance
                                             dose of 80 mg SC
Repeat maintenance dose every 28 days [896].

Relugolix
Relugolix: Loading dose of 360 mg PO on
                                             day 1 followed by 120 mg PO daily
Continue until evidence of disease progression [897].

Leuprolide
Leuprolide: 7.5 mg SC on day 1
Repeat cycle every 28 days [898].
or
Leuprolide: 22.5 mg SC on day 1
Repeat cycle every 12 weeks [899].
or
Leuprolide: 30 mg SC on day 1
Repeat cycle every 16 weeks [900].

Bicalutamide
Bicalutamide: 50 mg PO daily
In patients refractory to other anti-androgen agents, may start with a higher dose
of 150 mg PO daily [901].

Flutamide
Flutamide: 250 mg PO tid [902]

Nilutamide
Nilutamide: 300 mg PO on days 1–30, then 150 mg
                                             PO daily [903]

Apalutamide
Apalutamide: 240 mg PO daily [904]

Darolutamide
Darolutamide: 600 mg PO bid [905]

Prednisone
Prednisone: 5 mg PO bid [906]

or

Prednisone: 5 mg PO qid [907]

Ketoconazole
Ketoconazole: 1,200 mg PO daily [908]

Aminoglutethimide
Aminoglutethimide: 250 mg PO qid, if tolerated may increase to 500 mg PO qid [909]

Sipuleucel-T
Sipuleucel-T: Administer contents of infusion bag IV over 60 minutes on day 1

Repeat cycle every 2 weeks for a total of 3 doses [910].

Enzalutamide
Enzalutamide: 160 mg PO daily [911]

Olaparib (germline or somatic HRR gene-mutated mCRPC)
Olaparib: 300 mg PO bid

Repeat cycle every 28 days [912].

Rucaparib (germline or somatic BRCA mutation)
Rucaparib: 600 mg PO bid

Repeat cycle every 28 days [913].

Pembrolizumab
Pembrolizumab: 200 mg IV on day 1

Repeat cycle every 3 weeks [914]. May also administer pembrolizumab 400 mg IV every 6 weeks.

RENAL CELL CANCER

Adjuvant Therapy

Single-Agent Regimens

Sunitinib

Sunitinib:	50 mg PO daily for 4 weeks

Repeat cycle every 6 weeks [915].

Pembrolizumab

Pembrolizumab:	200 mg IV on day 1

Repeat cycle every 21 days for up to 17 cycles [916]. May also administer 400 mg IV on day 1 every 42 days.

Metastatic Disease

Combination Regimens

Bevacizumab + Interferon α-2a

Bevacizumab:	10 mg/kg IV every 2 weeks
Interferon α-2a:	9 million U SC, 3 times per week, for 1 year

Continue treatment until disease progression [917].

Interferon-α + IL-2

Interferon α-2a:	9 million U SC on days 1–4, weeks 1–4
Interleukin-2:	12 million U SC on days 1–4, weeks 1–4

Repeat cycle every 6 weeks [918].

Lenvatinib + Everolimus

Lenvatinib:	18 mg/day PO daily
Everolimus:	5 mg/day PO daily

Continue treatment until disease progression [919].

Ipilimumab + Nivolumab

Ipilimumab:	1 mg/kg IV on day 1
Nivolumab:	3 mg/kg IV on day 1

Repeat cycle every 21 days for 4 cycles followed by

Nivolumab:	240 mg IV on day 1

Repeat cycle every 14 days until disease progression [920]. May also administer 480 mg IV on day 1 every 28 days.

Bevacizumab + Everolimus

Bevacizumab:	10 mg/kg IV on day 1
Everolimus:	10 mg/day PO daily

Repeat cycle every 14 days [921].

Pembrolizumab + Axitinib

Pembrolizumab:	200 mg IV on day 1
Axitinib:	5 mg PO bid

Repeat cycle every 3 weeks [922]. May also administer pembrolizumab 400 mg IV every 6 weeks.

Pembrolizumab + Lenvatinib

Pembrolizumab:	200 mg IV on day 1
Lenvatinib:	20 mg PO daily

Repeat cycle every 3 weeks [923]. May also administer pembrolizumab 400 mg IV every 6 weeks.

Avelumab + Axitinib

Avelumab:	10 mg/kg IV on day 1
Axitinib:	5 mg PO bid

Repeat cycle every 2 weeks [924].

Nivolumab + Cabozantinib

Nivolumab:	240 mg IV on day 1
Cabozantinib:	40 mg PO daily

Repeat cycle every 2 weeks [925]. May also administer nivolumab 480 mg IV every 4 weeks.

Single-Agent Regimens

Bevacizumab

Bevacizumab:	10 mg/kg IV on day 1

Repeat cycle every 2 weeks [926].

Sunitinib

Sunitinib:	50 mg PO daily for 4 weeks

Repeat cycle every 6 weeks [927].
or

Sunitinib:	50 mg PO daily for 2 weeks

Repeat cycle every 3 weeks [928].
or

Sunitinib:	37.5 mg PO daily

Repeat cycle every 3 weeks [929].

Sorafenib

Sorafenib: 400 mg PO bid

Continue treatment until disease progression [930].

Pazopanib

Pazopanib: 800 mg PO daily

Continue treatment until disease progression [931].

Axitinib

Axitinib: 5 mg PO bid; after 2 weeks may increase dose to 7 mg PO bid; after 2 weeks may increase dose to 10 mg PO bid

Continue cycle every 6 weeks [932].

Temsirolimus

Temsirolimus: 25 mg IV weekly

Continue treatment disease progression [933].

Everolimus

Everolimus: 10 mg PO daily

Continue treatment until disease progression [934].

Interleukin-2

Interleukin-2:   720,000 IU/kg IV every 8 hours on days 1–5 and 15–19

Repeat cycles in 6- to 12-week intervals up to a total of 3 cycles [935].

or

Interleukin-2:   720,000 IU/kg IV at 8 am and 6 pm on days 1–5 and 15–19

Treat up to a maximum of 8 total doses on days 1–5 and repeat on days 15–19. Repeat cycles in 8- to 12-week intervals [728].

Interferon-α

Interferon α-2a: 5–15 million U SC daily or 3–5 times per week

Continue treatment until disease progression [936].

Cabozantinib

Cabozantinib: 60 mg PO daily

Continue treatment until disease progression [937].

Nivolumab

Nivolumab: 240 mg IV on day 1

Repeat cycle every 2 weeks [938]. May also administer 480 mg IV every 4 weeks.

Tivozanib

Tivozanib: 1.34 mg PO on days 1–21

Repeat cycle every 28 days [939].

SOFT TISSUE SARCOMAS

Combination Regimens

AD

Doxorubicin: 15 mg/m^2/day IV continuous infusion on days 1–4

Dacarbazine: 250 mg/m^2/day IV continuous infusion on days 1–4

Repeat cycle every 21 days [940].

AI

Doxorubicin: 20 mg/m^2/day IV continuous infusion on days 1–3

Ifosfamide: 1,500 mg/m^2/day IV continuous infusion on days 1–4

Mesna: 225 mg/m^2 IV over 1 hour before ifosfamide and at 4 and 8 hours after ifosfamide

Repeat cycle every 21 days [941]. On day 5, G-CSF support should be started at 5 µg/kg/day for 10 days.

MAID

Mesna: 2,500 mg/m^2/day IV continuous infusion on days 1–4

Doxorubicin: 20 mg/m^2/day IV continuous infusion on days 1–3

Ifosfamide: 2,500 mg/m^2/day IV continuous infusion on days 1–3

Dacarbazine: 300 mg/m^2/day IV continuous infusion on days 1–3

Repeat cycle every 21 days [942].

CYVADIC

Cyclophosphamide:	500 mg/m^2 IV on day 1
Vincristine:	1.5 mg/m^2 IV on day 1 (maximum, 2 mg)
Doxorubicin:	50 mg/m^2 IV on day 1
Dacarbazine:	750 mg/m^2 IV on day 1

Repeat cycle every 21 days [943].

Gemcitabine + Docetaxel

Gemcitabine:	900 mg/m^2 IV over 90 minutes on days 1 and 8
Docetaxel:	100 mg/m^2 IV on day 8

Repeat cycle every 21 days [944].

Gemcitabine + Navelbine

Gemcitabine:	800 mg/m^2 IV over 90 minutes on days 1 and 8
Vinorelbine:	25 mg/m^2 IV on days 1 and 8

Repeat cycle every 21 days [945].

CAV Alternating with IE (Ewing's Sarcoma)

Cyclophosphamide:	1,200 mg/m^2 IV on day 1
Doxorubicin:	75 mg/m^2 IV on day 1
Vincristine:	2 mg IV on day 1
Ifosfamide:	1,800 mg/m^2 IV on days 1–5
Etoposide:	100 mg/m^2 IV on days 1–5

Alternate CAV with IE every 21 days for a total of 17 cycles [946]. When the cumulative dose of doxorubicin reaches 375 mg/m^2, switch to dactinomycin at 1.25 mg/m^2.

Single-Agent Regimens

Atezolizumab

Atezolizumab:	1,200 mg IV on day 1

Repeat cycle every 21 days [947]. May also administer 840 mg IV every 2 weeks or 1,680 mg IV every 4 weeks.

Doxorubicin

Doxorubicin:	75 mg/m^2 IV on day 1

Repeat cycle every 21 days [943].

Gemcitabine

Gemcitabine: 1,200 mg/m^2 IV on days 1 and 8
Repeat cycle every 21 days [944].

Ifosfamide

Ifosfamide: 3,000 mg/m^2/day IV on days 1–3
Repeat cycle every 21 days [948].

Doxorubicin Liposome

Doxorubicin liposome: 50 mg/m^2 IV on day 1
Repeat cycle every 28 days [949].

Pazopanib

Pazopanib: 800 mg PO daily
Continue treatment until disease progression [950].

Trabectedin

Trabectedin: 1.5 mg/kg IV on day 1
Repeat cycles every 21 days [951].

Eribulin

Eribulin: 1.4 mg/m^2 IV on days 1 and 8
Repeat cycles every 21 days [952].

Tazemetostat

Tazemetostat: 800 mg PO bid
Continue treatment until disease progression [953]. Effective in advanced epithelioid sarcoma with loss of INI1/SMARCB1.

Pexidartinib

Pexidartinib: 400 mg PO bid
Continue treatment until disease progression [954].

SQUAMOUS CELL CANCER OF THE SKIN

Single-Agent Regimens

Cemiplimab-rwlc

Cemiplimab-rwlc: 350 mg IV on day 1
Repeat cycle every 21 days [955].

Pembrolizumab

Pembrolizumab: 200 mg IV on day 1

Repeat cycle every 3 weeks [956]. May also administer 400 mg IV every 6 weeks.

TESTICULAR CANCER

Adjuvant Therapy

PEB

Cisplatin: 20 mg/m^2/day IV on days 1–5

Etoposide: 100 mg/m^2/day IV on days 1–5

Bleomycin: 30 U IV on days 2, 9, and 16

Repeat cycle every 28 days for a total of 2 cycles [957]. Adjuvant therapy of stage II testicular cancer treated with orchiectomy and retroperitoneal lymph node dissection.

Carboplatin

Carboplatin: AUC of 7, IV on day 1

Administer one dose for adjuvant therapy of stage I seminoma [958].

Metastatic Disease

Combination Regimens

BEP

Bleomycin: 30 U IV on days 1, 8, and 15

Etoposide: 100 mg/m^2/day IV on days 1–5

Cisplatin: 20 mg/m^2/day IV on days 1–5

Repeat cycle every 21 days [959].

EP

Etoposide: 100 mg/m^2/day IV on days 1–5

Cisplatin: 20 mg/m^2/day IV on days 1–5

Repeat cycle every 21 days [960].

PVB

Cisplatin: 20 mg/m^2/day IV on days 1–5

Vinblastine: 0.15 mg/kg IV on days 1 and 2

Bleomycin: 30 U IV on days 2, 9, and 16

Repeat cycle every 21 days [961].

VAB-6

Vinblastine:	4 mg/m^2 IV on day 1
Dactinomycin:	1 mg/m^2 IV on day 1
Bleomycin:	30 U IV on day 1, then 20 U/m^2 continuous infusion on days 1–3
Cisplatin:	20 mg/m^2 IV on day 4
Cyclophosphamide:	600 mg/m^2 IV on day 1

Repeat cycle every 21 days [962].

VeIP (salvage regimen)

Vinblastine:	0.11 mg/kg IV on days 1 and 2
Ifosfamide:	1,200 mg/m^2/day IV on days 1–5
Cisplatin:	20 mg/m^2/day IV on days 1–5
Mesna:	400 mg/m^2 IV, given 15 minutes before first ifosfamide dose, then 1,200 mg/m^2/day IV continuous infusion for 5 days

Repeat cycle every 21 days [963].

VIP (salvage regimen)

Etoposide (VP-16):	75 mg/m^2/day IV on days 1–5
Ifosfamide:	1,200 mg/m^2/day IV on days 1–5
Cisplatin:	20 mg/m^2/day IV on days 1–5
Mesna:	400 mg/m^2 IV, given 15 minutes before first ifosfamide dose, then 1,200 mg/m^2/day IV continuous infusion for 5 days

Repeat cycle every 21 days [963].

TIP (salvage regimen)

Paclitaxel:	250 mg/m^2 IV over 24 hours on day 1
Ifosfamide:	1,500 mg/m^2/day IV on days 2–5
Cisplatin:	25 mg/m^2/day IV on days 1–5
Mesna:	500 mg/m^2 IV, given before ifosfamide dose, and at 4 and 8 hours after ifosfamide on days 2–5

Repeat cycle every 21 days for a total of 4 cycles [964]. G-CSF support at 5 µg/kg/day SC should be given on days 7–18.

Paclitaxel + Gemcitabine

Paclitaxel: 100 mg/m^2 IV on days 1, 8, and 15
Gemcitabine: 1,000 mg/m^2 IV on days 1, 8, and 15
Repeat cycle every 28 days for a total of 6 cycles [965].

Paclitaxel + Gemcitabine + Oxaliplatin

Paclitaxel: 80 mg/m^2 IV on days 1 and 8
Gemcitabine: 800 mg/m^2 IV on days 1 and 8
Oxaliplatin: 130 mg/m^2 IV on day 1
Repeat cycle every 21 days [966].

Single-Agent Regimens

Etoposide

Etoposide: 50 mg/m^2 q day PO
Repeat cycle every 14–21 days [967].

THYMOMA

Combination Regimens

CAP

Cyclophosphamide: 500 mg/m^2 IV on day 1
Doxorubicin: 50 mg/m^2 IV on day 1
Cisplatin: 50 mg/m^2 IV on day 1
Repeat cycle every 21 days [968].

Cisplatin + Etoposide

Cisplatin: 60 mg/m^2 IV on day 1
Etoposide: 120 mg/m^2 IV on days 1–3
Repeat cycle every 21 days [969].

ADOC

Cisplatin: 50 mg/m^2 IV on day 1
Doxorubicin: 40 mg/m^2 IV on day 1
Vincristine: 0.6 mg/m^2 IV on day 3
Cyclophosphamide: 700 mg/m^2 IV on day 4
Repeat cycle every 28 days [970].

VIP

Etoposide:	75 mg/m^2 IV on days 1–4
Ifosfamide:	1,200 mg/m^2 IV on days 1–4
Cisplatin:	20 mg/m^2 IV on days 1–4
Mesna:	240 mg/m^2 IV before first ifosfamide dose, then 4 and 8 hours later on days 1–4

Repeat cycle every 21 days for a total of 4 cycles [971]. G-CSF support at 5 µg/kg/day should be given on days 5–15.

Gemcitabine + Topotecan

Gemcitabine:	1,000 mg/m^2 IV on days 1, 8, and 15
Topotecan:	0.75–1.5 mg/m^2 IV on days 1, 8, and 15

Repeat cycle every 21 days [972].

Carboplatin + Paclitaxel

Carboplatin:	AUC of 6, IV on day 1
Paclitaxel:	225 mg/m^2 IV on day 1

Repeat cycle every 21 days [973].

Single-Agent Regimens

Pembrolizumab

Pembrolizumab:	200 mg IV on day 1

Repeat cycle every 21 days [974]. May also pembrolizumab 400 mg IV every 6 weeks.

THYROID CANCER

Combination Regimens

Doxorubicin + Cisplatin

Doxorubicin:	60 mg/m^2 IV on day 1
Cisplatin:	40 mg/m^2 IV on day 1

Repeat cycle every 21 days [975].

Single-Agent Regimens

Doxorubicin

Doxorubicin:	60 mg/m^2 IV on day 1

Repeat cycle every 21 days [975].

Sorafenib

Sorafenib: 400 mg PO bid

Continue treatment until disease progression [976].

Sunitinib

Sunitinib: 37.5 mg PO daily

Continue treatment until disease progression [977].

or

Sunitinib: 50 mg PO daily for 4 weeks

Repeat cycle every 6 weeks [978].

Pazopanib

Pazopanib: 800 mg PO daily

Continue treatment until disease progression [979].

Vandetanib (medullary carcinoma of the thyroid)

Vandetanib: 300 mg PO daily

Continue treatment until disease progression [980].

Cabozantinib

Cabozantinib: 60 mg PO daily

Continue treatment until disease progression [981].

Lenvatinib

Lenvatinib: 24 mg PO daily

Continue treatment until disease progression [982].

Selpercatinib

Selpercatinib: 120 mg PO bid (if <50 kg)

160 mg PO bid (if >50 kg)

Repeat cycle every 28 days [983].

Pralsetinib

Pralsetinib: 400 mg PO daily

Repeat cycle every 28 days [984].

VON HIPPEL-LANDAU ASSOCIATED CANCERS

Single-Agent Regimens

Belzutifan

Belzutifan: 120 mg PO daily

Continue treatment until disease progression [985].

WALDENSTRÖM'S MACROGLOBULINEMIA

Combination Regimens

Bortezomib + Dexamethasone + Rituximab (BDR)

Bortezomib: 1.3 mg/m^2 IV on days 1, 4, 8, and 11

Dexamethasone: 40 mg IV on days 1, 4, 8, and 11

Rituxumab: 375 mg/m^2 IV on day 11

Repeat for 4 cycles as induction therapy followed by a 12-week break and then 4 additional cycles, each given 12 weeks apart [986].

Rituximab + Dexamethasone + Cyclophosphamide

Rituxumab: 375 mg/m^2 IV on day 1

Dexamethasone: 20 mg IV on day 1

Cyclophosphamide: 100 mg/m^2 PO bid

Repeat cycle every 21 days [987].

Carfilzomib + Dexamethasone + Rituximab (CDR)

Carfilzomib: 20 mg/m^2 IV on days 1, 2, 8, and 9 in cycle 1 and then 36 mg/m^2 IV on days 1, 2, 8, and 9 in cycles 2–6

Dexamethasone: 20 mg IV on days 1, 2, 8, and 9

Rituxumab: 375 mg/m^2 IV on days 2 and 9

Repeat cycle every 21 days for up to 6 induction cycles, followed by an 8-week break, and then 8 additional cycles of maintenance therapy as follows [988]:

Carfilzomib: 36 mg/m^2 IV on days 1 and 2 in cycle 1 and then 36 mg/m^2 IV on days 1, 2, 8, and 9 in cycles 2–6

Dexamethasone: 20 mg IV on days 1 and 2

Rituxumab: 375 mg/m^2 IV on day 2

Repeat cycle every 8 weeks for up to 8 cycles.

Ixazomib + Dexamethasone + Rituximab (IDR)

Ixazomib: 4 mg/day PO on days 1, 8, and 15
Dexamethasone: 20 mg/day PO on days 1, 8, 15, and 22
Rituximab: 375 mg/m^2 IV on day 1
Repeat cycle every 28 days for up to 6 cycles of induction [989].

Bendamustine + Rituximab

Bendamustine: 90 mg/m^2 IV on days 1 and 2
Rituxumab: 375 mg/m^2 IV on day 1
Repeat cycle every 28 days for 4 cycles [990].

Single-Agent Regimens

Dexamethasone

Dexamethasone: 40 mg IV or PO on days 1–4, 9–12, and 17–20

Repeat cycle every 21 days [782].

Ibrutinib

Ibrutinib: 420 mg/day PO
Continue treatment until disease progression [991].

Zanubrutinib

Zanubrutinib: 160 mg PO bid
Repeat cycle every 28 days [991].

References

1.   M Fassnacht, et al. N Engl J Med 2012;366:2189–2197.
2.   M Flam, et al. J Clin Oncol 1996;14:2527–2539.
3.   JF Bosset, et al. Eur J Cancer 2003;39:45–51.
4.   KA Goodman, et al. Int J Radiat Oncol Biol Phys 2017; 98:1087–1095.
5.   JA Ajani, et al. JAMA 2008;2997:1914–1921.
6.   C Eng, et al. Clin Colorectal Cancer 2019;187:301-306.
7.   C Faivre, et al. Bull Cancer 1999;86:861–865.
8.   C Eng, et al. Oncotarget 2014;5:11133–11142.
9.   M Matsunaga, et al. Case Rep Oncol 2016;9:249–254.
10. S Mondaca, et al. Clin Colorectal Cancer 2019;18:e39–e52.
11. PA Ott, et al. Ann Oncol 2017;28:1036–1041.
12. VK Morris, et al. Lancet Oncol 2017;18:446–453.

13. A Seklulic, et al. N Engl J Med 2012;366:2171–2179.
14. MR Migden, et al. Lancet Oncol 2015;16:716–728.
15. A Stratigos, et al. Lancet Oncol 2021;22:848–857.
16. JN Primrose, et al. Lancet Oncol 2019;20:663–673.
17. E Ben-Joseph, et al. J Clin Oncol 2015;33:2617–2622.
18. DY Oh, et al. J Clin Oncol 2022;40:Abstract 378]
19. S Thongprasert, et al. Ann Oncol 2005;16:279–281.
20. JW Valle, et al. N Engl J Med 2010;362:1273–1281.
21. RT Shroff, et al. JAMA Oncol 2019;5:824–830.
22. JJ Knox, et al. J Clin Oncol 2005;23:2332–2338.
23. T Andre, et al. Ann Oncol 2004;15:1339–1343.
24. J Taieb, et al. Ann Oncol 2002;13:1192–1196.
25. S Qin, et al. J Clin Oncol 2013:3501–3508.
26. YS Hong, et al. Cancer Chemother Pharmacol 2007;60:321–328.
27. O Nehls, et al. Br J Cancer 2008;98:309–315.
28. V Sahai, et al. JAMA Oncol 2018;4:1707–1712.
29. V Subbiah, et al. Lancet Oncol. 2020; doi:10.1016/S1470-2045 (20) 30321-1.
30. YZ Patt, et al. Cancer 2004;101:578–586.
31. DT Le, et al. N Engl J Med 2015;372:2509–2520.
32. JS Park, et al. Jpn J Clin Oncol 2005;35:68–73.
33. GK Abou-Alfa, et al. Lancet Oncol 2020;21:796–807.
34. GK Abou-Alfa, et al. Lancet Oncol 2020; 21:671–684.
35. F Meric-Berenstam, et al. Cancer Discov 2022;12:402–415.
36. M Javle, et al. J Clin Oncol 2020;36:276–282.
37. DF Bajorin, et al. N Engl J Med 2021;384:2102-2114.
38. DF Bajorin, et al. Cancer 2000;88:1671–1678.
39. G Iyer, et al. J Clin Oncol 2018. doi: 10.1200/JCO.2017.75.0158.
40. D Kaufman, et al. J Clin Oncol 2000;18:1921–1927.
41. H Linardou, et al. Urology 2004;64:479–484.
42. AA Meluch, et al. J Clin Oncol 2001;19:3018–3024.
43. CN Sternberg, et al. Cancer 2001;92:2993–2998.
44. BJ Gitlitz, et al. Cancer 2003;98:1863–1869.
45. CN Sternberg, et al. Cancer 1989;64:2448–2458.
46. WG Harker, et al. J Clin Oncol 1985;3:1463–1470.
47. MD Santis, et al. J Clin Oncol 2009;27:5634–5638.
48. X Garcia del Muro, et al. Br J Cancer 2002;86:326–330.
49. D Vaughn, et al. Cancer 2002;95:1022–1027.
50. R Dreicer, et al. J Clin Oncol 2000;18:1058–1061.
51. ND James, et al. N Engl J Med 2012;366:1477–1488.
52. CJ Hoimes, et al. J Clin Oncol;41:22-31.
53. MJ Moore, et al. J Clin Oncol 1997;15:3441–3445.

54. BJ Roth, et al. J Clin Oncol 1994;12:2264–2270.

55. D Vaughn, et al. J Clin Oncol 2002;20:937–940.

56. CJ Sweeney, et al. J Clin Oncol 2006;24:3451–3457.

57. JE Rosenberg, et al. Lancet 2016;387:1909–1920.

58. T Powles, et al. Ann Oncol 2016;27 (suppl 6):842.

59. C Massard, et al. J Clin Oncol 2016;34:3199–3125.

60. P Sharma, et al. Lancet Oncol 2017;18:312–322.

61. MS Farina, et al. Drugs 2017;77:1077–1089.

62. AO Siefker-Radtke, et al. Lancet Oncol 2022; 23:248-258.

63. JE Rosenberg, et al. J Clin Oncol 2019; 37:2592–2600.

64. ST Tagawa, et al. J Clin Oncol 202. doi: 10.1200/JCO.20.03489.

65. N Kleinmann, et al. Lancet Oncol 2020;21:776–785.

66. SA Boorjian, et al. Lancet Oncol 2021;22:107-117.

66a. N Pemmaraju, et al. N Engl J Med 2019;860:1628-1637.

67. R Stupp, et al. N Engl J Med 2005;352:987–995.

68. VA Levin, et al. Int J Radiat Oncol Biol Phys 1990;18:321–324.

69. LM DeAngelis, et al. Ann Neurol 1998;44:691–695.

70. JC Buckner, et al. J Clin Oncol 2003;21:251–255.

71. JJ Vredenburgh, et al. J Clin Oncol 2007;25:4722–4729.

72. MA Badruddoja, et al. Cancer Chemother Pharmacol 2017;80:715-721.

73. DA Reardon, et al. Cancer 2011;26:188–193.

74. M Glas, et al. J Clin Oncol, 2009;27:1257–1261.

75. A Yung, et al. Proc Am Soc Clin Oncol 1999;18:139a.

76. A Yung, et al. J Clin Oncol 1999;17:2762–2771.

77. E Raymond, et al. Ann Oncol 2003;14:603–614.

78. H Friedman, et al. J Clin Oncol 1999;17:1516–1525.

79. K Beal, et al. Radiat Oncol 2011;6:2–15.

80. H Bear, et al. J Clin Oncol 2003;21:4165–4174.

81. A Schneeweiss, et al. Ann Oncol 2013;24:2278–2284.

82. B Fisher, et al. J Clin Oncol 2000;8:1483–1496.

83. C Hudis, et al. J Clin Oncol 1999;17:93–100.

84. JA Sparano, et al. N Engl J Med 2008;358:1663–1671.

85. JA Sparano, et al. San Antonio Breast Cancer Symposium 2014 (abstract 53-03).

86. S Jones, et al. J Clin Oncol 2006;24:5381–5387.

87. M Martin, et al. N Engl J Med 2005;352:2302–2313.

88. DR Budman, et al. J Natl Cancer Inst 1998;90:1205–1211.

89. RB Weiss, et al. Am J Med 1987;83:455–463.

90. CJ Poole, et al. N Engl J Med 2006;355:1851–1862.

91. RC Coombes, et al. J Clin Oncol 1996;14:35–45.

92. H Roche, et al. J Clin Oncol 2006;24:5664–5671.

93. HJ Burstein, et al. J Clin Oncol 2005;23:8340–8347.

94. M Citron, et al. J Clin Oncol 2003;21:1431–1439.

95. S Puhalla, et al. J Clin Oncol 2008;26:1691–1697.

96. EH Romond, et al. N Engl J Med. 2005;353:1673–1684.

97. C Dang, et al. J Clin Oncol 2006;24:17S (abstract 582).

98. D Slamon, et al. N Engl J Med 2011;365:1273–1283.

99. H Joensuu, et al. N Engl J Med 2006;354:809–820.

100. J Baselga, et al. N Engl J Med 2012;366:109–119.

101. A Chan, et al. Lancet Oncol 2016;17:367–377.

102. GV Minckwitz, et al. N Engl J Med 2019;380:617–628.

103. B Fisher, et al. J Natl Cancer Inst 1997;89:1673–1682.

104. A Howell, et al. Lancet 2005;365:60–62.

105. BIG I-98 Collaborative Group, et al. N Engl J Med 2009;361:766–776.

106. PE Goss, et al. J Natl Cancer Inst 2005;97:1262–1271.

107. RC Coombes, et al. N Engl J Med 2004;350:1081–1092.

108. M Gnant, et al. N Engl J Med 2009;360:679–691.

109. ANJ Tutt, et al. N Engl J Med 2021;384:2394–2405.

110. SRD Johnston, et al. J Clin Oncol 2020;38:3987–3998.

111. M Martin, et al. JAMA Oncol 2022;8:1190-1194.

112. J Baselga, et al. N Engl J Med 2012,366:520 529.

113. GE Sledge, et al. J Clin Oncol 2003;21:588–592.

114. MN Levine, et al. J Clin Oncol 1998;16:2651–2658.

115. J O'Shaughnessy, et al. J Clin Oncol 2002;20:2812–2823.

116. L Biganzoli, et al. Oncologist 2002;7 (suppl):29–35.

117. ES Thomas, et al. J Clin Oncol 2007;25:5210–5217.

118. V Dieras. Oncology 1997;11:31–33.

119. G Brufman, et al. Ann Oncol 1997;8:155–162.

120. JA Sparano, et al. J Clin Oncol 2001;19:3117–3125.

121. The French Epirubicin Study Group. J Clin Oncol 1991;9:305–312.

122. KS Albain, et al. J Clin Oncol 2008;26:3950–3957.

123. EA Perez, et al. Cancer 2000;88:124–131.

124. V Fitch, et al. Proc Am Soc Clin Oncol 2003;22:23 (abstract 90).

125. K Miller, et al. N Engl J Med 2007;35:2666–2676.

126. P Schmid, et al. J Clin Oncol 2019;37 (15 suppl) abstract 1003.

127. DJ Slamon, et al. N Engl J Med 2001;344:783–792.

128. MM Goldenberg, et al. Clin Ther 1999;21:309–318.

129. E Francisco, et al. J Clin Oncol 2002;20:1800–1808.

130. M Pegram, et al. Proc Am Soc Clin Oncol 2007;25 (LBA1008).

131. D Loesch, et al. Clin Breast Cancer 2008;8:178–186.

132. HJ Burstein, et al. J Clin Oncol 2001;19:2722–2730.

133. J O'Shaughnessy, et al. Clin Breast Cancer 2004;5:142–147.

134. G Schaller, et al. J Clin Oncol 2007;25:3246–3250.

135. R Bartsch, et al. J Clin Oncol 2007;25:3853–3858.

136. KL Blackwell, et al. J Clin Oncol 2010;28:1124–1130.

137. CE Geyer, et al. N Engl J Med 2006;355:2733–2743.

138. RA Freedman, et al. J Clin Oncol 2019;37:1081–1089.

139. RK Murthy, et al. N Engl J Med 2020;382:597–609.

140. HS Rugo, et al. JAMA Oncol 2021;7:1–12.

141. RS Finn, et al. Lancet Oncol 2015;16:25–35.

142. GN Hortobagyi, et al. N Engl J Med 2016;375:1738–1748.

143. NC Turner, et al. N Engl J Med 2015;373:209–219.

144. GW Sledge, et al. J Clin Oncol 2017;35:2875–2884.

145. F Andre, et al. N Engl J Med 2019;380:1929–1940.

146. MP Goetz, et al. J Clin Oncol 2017;35:3638–3646.

147. IA Jaiyesimi, et al. J Clin Oncol 1995;13:513–529.

148. DF Hayes, et al. J Clin Oncol 1995;13:2556–2566.

149. PE Lonning, et al. J Clin Oncol 2000;18:2234–2244.

150. A Buzdar, et al. J Clin Oncol 1996;14:2000–2011.

151. P Dombernowsky, et al. J Clin Oncol 1998;16:453–461.

152. A. Howell. Clin Cancer Res 2001;7 (suppl 12):4402s–4410s.

153. A Di Leo, et al. J Clin Oncol 2010;28:4594–4600.

154. FC Bidard, et al. J Clin Oncol 2022;40:3246-3256.

155. GG Kimmick, et al. Cancer Treat Res 1998;94:231–254.

156. J Baselga, et al. Semin Oncol 1999;26 (suppl 12):78–83.

157. PH Hsieh, et al. npj Breast Cancer 2022;8:32.

158. HS Rugo, et al. JAMA Oncol 2021;7:573–584.

159. YA Leo and YY Syed. Target Oncol 2019;14:749–758.

160. S Verma, et al. N Engl J Med 2012;367:1783–1791.

161. S Modi, et al. N Engl J Med 2020;382:610–621.

162. JL Blum, et al. J Clin Oncol 1999;17:485–493.

163. S Chan. Oncology 1997;11 (Suppl 8):19–24.

164. J Baselga, et al. Oncologist 2001;6 (suppl 3):26–29.

165. FA Holmes, et al. J Natl Cancer Inst 1991;83:1797–1805.

166. EA Perez. Oncologist 1998;3:373–389.

167. EA Perez, et al. J Clin Oncol 2007;25:3407–3414.

168. P Fumoleau, et al. Semin Oncol 1995;22 (suppl 5):22–28.

169. FM Torti, et al. Ann Intern Med 1983;99:745–749.

170. J Carmichael, et al. Semin Oncol 1996;23 (suppl 10):77–81.

171. SE Al-Batran, et al. Oncol 2006;70:141–146.

172. JL Blum, et al. Clin Breast Cancer 2007;7:850-856.

173. JA O'Shaughnessy, et al. Breast Cancer Res Treat 2004;88:Suppl 1 (abstract 1070).

174. J Cortes, et al. Lancet 2011;377:914–923.

175. M Robson, et al. N Engl J Med 2017;377:523–533.

176.	JK Litton, et al. N Engl J Med 2018;379:753–763.

177.	A Bardia, et al. N Engl J Med 2019;380:743–751.

178.	MN Dickler, et al. Clin Cancer Res 2017. doi:10.1158/1078-0432.

179.	JD Hainsworth, et al. J Clin Oncol 1997;15:2385–2393.

180.	E Longeval, et al. Cancer 1982;50:2751–2756.

181.	JD Hainsworth, et al. J Clin Oncol 1992;10:912–922.

182.	FA Greco, et al. J Clin Oncol 2002;20:1651–1656.

183.	AK Moller, et al. Acta Oncol 2010;49:423–430.

184.	JD Hainsworth, et al. Cancer J 2010;16:70–75.

185.	JD Hainsworth, et al. Cancer 2010;116:2448–2454.

186.	JD Hainsworth, et al. J Clin Oncol 2007;25:1747–1752.

187.	A Naing, et al. J Immunother Cancer 2020;8:e000347.	doi 10 1136.

188.	CG Moertel, et al. N Engl J Med 1992;326:519–526.

189.	CG Moertel, et al. Cancer 1991;68:227–232.

190.	ME Pavel, et al. Lancet 2011;378:2005–2012.

191.	JR Strosberg, et al. Cancer 2011;117:268–275.

192.	L Saltz, et al. Cancer 1993;72:244.

193.	ME Coplin, et al. N Engl J Med 2014;371:224–233.

194.	MH Kulke, et al. J Clin Oncol 2008;26:3403–3410.

195.	JC Yao, et al. N Engl J Med 2011;364:514–523.

196.	J Strosberg, et al. N Engl J Med 2017;376:125–135.

197.	PG Rose, et al. N Engl J Med 1995;15:1144.

198.	M Morris, et al. N Engl J Med 1999;340:1137–1143.

199.	J Fiorica, et al. Gynecol Oncol 2002;85:89–94.

200.	KS Tewari, et al. J Clin Oncol 2013;31:Suppl (abstract 3).

201.	RT Penson, et al. Lancet Oncol 2015;16:301–311.

202.	EJ Buxton, et al. J Natl Cancer Inst 1989;81:359–361.

203.	AM Murad, et al. J Clin Oncol 1994;12:55–59.

204.	CW Whitney, et al. J Clin Oncol 1999;17:1339–1348.

205.	S Pignata, et al. J Clin Oncol 1999;17:756–760.

206.	I Chitapanarux, et al. Gynecol Oncol 2003;89:402–407.

207.	BJ Monk, et al. Proc Am Soc Clin Oncol 2008;26:(LBA5504).

208.	CA Brewer, et al. Gynecol Oncol 2006;100:385–388.

209.	S Nagao, et al. Gynecol Oncol 2005;96:805–809.

210.	DS Miller, et al. J Clin Oncol 2014;32:2744–2749.

211.	N Colombo, et al. N Engl J Med 2021;385:1856–1867.

212.	T Levy, et al. Proc Am Soc Clin Oncol 1996;15:292a.

213.	T Thigpen, et al. Semin Oncol 1997;24 (suppl 2):41–46.

214.	CF Verschraegen, et al. J Clin Oncol 1997;15:625–631.

215.	LI Muderspach, et al. Gynecol Oncol 2001;81:213–215.

216.	D Lorusso, et al. Ann Oncol 2010;21:61–66.

217. RJ Schilder, et al. Gynecol Oncol 2005;95:103–107.

218. RL Coleman, et al. Lancet Oncol 2021;22:609–619.

219. JHM Schellens, et al. J Clin Oncol 2017;35 (Suppl: abstr 5514).

220. A Cercek, et al. JAMA Oncol 2018;4:e180071.

221. J Garcia-Aguilar, et al. J Clin Oncol 2022;40:2546-2556.

222. A Cercek, et al. N Engl J Med 2022;386:2363–2376.

223. R Sauer, et al. N Engl J Med 2004;351:1731–1740.

224. BD Minsky. Oncology 1994;6:53–58.

225. BD Minsky. Clin Colorectal Cancer 2004;4 (Suppl 1):S29–36.

226. DP Ryan, et al. J Clin Oncol 2006;24:2557–2562.

227. C Rodel, et al. J Clin Oncol 2007;25:110–117.

228. N Wolmark, et al. J Clin Oncol 1993;11:1879–1887.

229. AB Benson, et al. Oncology 2000;14:203–212.

230. T Andre, et al. N Engl J Med 2004;350:2343–2351.

231. KY Chung and LB Saltz. Cancer J 2007;13:192–197.

232. HJ Schmoll, et al. J Clin Oncol 2007;25:102–109.

233. C Twelves, et al. N Engl J Med 2005;352:2696–2704.

234. JJ Hwang, et al. Am J Oncol Rev 2003;2 (Suppl 5):15–25.

235. JY Douillard, et al. Lancet 2000;355:1041–1047.

236. T Andre, et al. Eur J Cancer 1999;35:1343–1347.

237. A de Gramont, et al. J Clin Oncol 2000;18:2938–2947.

238. C Tournigand, et al. J Clin Oncol 2004;22:229–237.

239. T Andre, et al. Proc Am Soc Clin Oncol 2003;22:253 (abstract 1016).

240. F Maindrault-Goebel, et al. J Clin Oncol 2006;24 (June 20 Supplement):3504.

241. A Falcone, et al. J Clin Oncol 2007;25:1670–1676.

242. F Loupakis, et al. N Engl J Med 2014;371:1609–1618.

243. L Fornaro, et al. Ann Oncol 2013;24:2062–2067.

244. D Cunningham, et al. N Engl J Med 2004;351:337–345.

245. W Scheithauer, et al. J Clin Oncol 2003;21:1307–1312.

246. D. Kerr. Oncology 2002;16 (Suppl 14):12–15.

247. MM Borner, et al. Ann Oncol 2005;16:282–288.

248. DH Lim, et al. Cancer Chemother Pharmacol 2005;56:10–14.

249. RM Goldberg, et al. J Clin Oncol 2004;22:23–30.

250. N Petrelli, et al. J Clin Oncol 1989;7:1419–1426.

251. F Kabbinavar, et al. J Clin Oncol 2005;23:3697–3705.

252. GW Prager, et al. N Engl J Med 2023;388:1657-1667.

253. E Jager, et al. J Clin Oncol 1996;14:2274–2279.

254. A de Gramont, et al. J Clin Oncol 1997;15:808–815.

255. BJ Giantonio, et al. J Clin Oncol 2007;25:1539–1544.

256. A Dimou, et al. Expert Opin Investing Drugs 2010;19:723–735.

257. HS Hochster, et al. J Clin Oncol 2008;26:3523–3529.

258. L Saltz, et al. J Clin Oncol 2007;22:4557–4561.

259. AC Buziad, et al. Clin Colorectal Cancer 2010;9:282–289.

260. D Cunningham, et al. N Engl J Med 2004;351:537–545.

261. AF Sobrero, et al. J Clin Oncol 2008;26:2311–2319.

262. E van Cutsem, et al. N Engl J Med 2009;360:1408–1417.

263. C Bokemeyer, et al. J Clin Oncol 2009;27:663–671.

264. J Scott, et al. J Clin Oncol 2005;23:16S (abstract 3705).

265. JY Doullard, et al. J Clin Oncol 2010;28:4697–4705.

266. M Peeters, et al. J Clin Oncol 2010;28:4706–4713.

267. C Cremolini, et al. Lancet Oncol 2015;16:1306-1315.

268. RH Xu, et al. Lancet Oncol 2019;25:660–671.

269. E van Cutsem, et al. J Clin Oncol 2012;30:3499–3506.

270. J Tabernero, et al. Lancet Oncol 2015;16:499–508.

271. DS Hong, et al. Cancer Discov 2016;6:1352–1365.

272. E Van Cutsem, et al. J Clin Oncol 2019;37:1460–1469.

273. S Kopetz, et al. N Engl J Med 2019; 381:1632–1643.

274. S Kopetz, et al. J Clin Oncol 2020; 38(suppl 4;abstr 8).

275. MJ Overman, et al. J Clin Oncol 2018;36:773–779.

276. A Sartore-Bianchi, et al. Lancet Oncol 2016;17:738–746.

277. JH Strickler, et al. J Clin Oncol 2021;39 (suppl 3): TPS153.

278. F Meric-Bernstam, et al. Lancet Oncol 2019;20:518–530.

279. N Kemeny, et al. J Clin Oncol 1994;12:2288–2295.

280. P Hoff, et al. J Clin Oncol 2001;15:2282–2292.

281. HC Pitot, et al. J Clin Oncol 1997;15:2910–2919.

282. H Ulrich-Pur, et al. Ann Oncol 2001;12:1269–1272.

283. P Rougier, et al. J Clin Oncol 1997;15:251–260.

284. LB Saltz, et al. J Clin Oncol 2004;22:1201–1208.

285. J Tabernero, et al. J Clin Oncol 2006;24:18S (abstract 3085).

286. E van Cutsem, et al. J Clin Oncol 2007;25:1658–1664.

287. CG Leichman, et al. J Clin Oncol 1995;13:1303–1311.

288. CG Leichman. Oncology 1999;13 (suppl 3):26–32.

289. A Falcone, et al. Cancer Chemother Pharmacol 1999;44:159–163.

290. S Siena, et al. Lancet Oncol 2021;22:779–789.

291. A Grothey, et al. Lancet 2013;381:303–312.

292. TS Bekaii-Saab, et al. Lancet Oncol 2019;20:1070–1082.

293. RJ Mayer, et al. N Engl J Med 2015;20:1909–1919.

294. D Le, et al. N Engl J Med 2015;372:2509–2520.

295. MJ Overman, et al. Lancet Oncol 2017;18:1182–1191.

296. A Drilon, et al. N Engl J Med 2018;378:731–739.

297. RC Doebele, et al. Lancet Oncol 2020;21:271–282.

298. PJ Hoskins, et al. J Clin Oncol 2001;19:4048–4053.

299. MR Mirza, et al. N Engl J Med 2023;388:2145-2158.

300. JT Thigpen, et al. J Clin Oncol 1994;12:1408-1414.

301. G Deppe, et al. Eur J Gynecol Oncol 1994;15:263-266.

302. JV Fiorica. Oncologist 2002;7 (suppl 5):36-45.

303. GF Fleming, et al. J Clin Oncol 2004;22:2159-2165.

304. TW Burke, et al. Gynecol Oncol 1994;55:47-50.

305. S Pignata, et al. Br J Cancer 2007;96:1639-1643.

306. F Simpkins, et al. Gynecol Oncol 2015;136:240-245.

307. HD Homesley, et al. J Clin Oncol 2007;25:526-531.

308. AH Wolfson, et al. J Clin Oncol 2006;24(18S):5001.

309. ML Hensley, et al. Gynecol Oncol 2008;109:329-334.

310. V Makker, et al. Lancet Oncol 2019;20:711-718.

311. HB Muss. Semin Oncol 1994;21:107-113.

312. JT Thigpen, et al. J Clin Oncol 1999;17:1736-1744.

313. H Ball, et al. Gynecol Oncol 1996;62:278-282.

314. S Wadler, et al. J Clin Oncol 2003;21:2110-2114.

315. AM Oza, et al. J Clin Oncol 2011;29:3278-3285.

316. A Oaknin, et al. JAMA Oncol 2020;6:1766-1772.

317. DM O'Malley, et al. J Clin Oncol 2022;40:752-761.

318. P Van Hagen, et al. N Engl J Med 2012;366:2074-2084.

319. T Conroy, et al. Lancet Oncol 2014;15:305-314.

320. MM Javle, et al. Cancer Invest 2009;27:193-200.

321. L Bedenne, et al. J Clin Oncol 2007;25:1160-1168.

322. Heath El, et al. J Clin Oncol 2000;18:868-876.

323. D Cunningham, et al. N Engl J Med 2006;355:11-20.

324. SE Al-Batran, et al. J Clin Oncol 2008;26:1435-1442.

325. SE Al-Batran, et al. Lancet 2019;393:1948-1957.

326. YJ Bang, et al. Lancet 2010;376:687-697.

327. MS Kies, et al. Cancer 1987;60:2156-2160.

328. DH Ilson, et al. J Clin Oncol 1998;16:1826-1834.

329. E van Meerten, et al. Br J Cancer 2007;96:1348-1352.

330. D Cunningham, et al. N Engl J Med 2008;358:36-46.

331. JM Sun, et al. Lancet 2021;398:759-771.

332. Y Duki, et al. N Engl J Med 2022;386:449-462.

333. YY Janjigian, et al. Lancet 2021;398:27-40.

334. YY Janjigian, et al. Lancet Oncol 2020:21:821-831.

335. JA Ajani, et al. Semin Oncol 1995;22 (Suppl 6):35-40.

336. HR Ford, et al. Lancet Oncol 2013;15:78-86.

337. K Shitara, et al. Lancet Oncol 2018;19:1437-1448.

338. M Shah, et al. JAMA Oncol 2019;5;546-550.

339. K Kato, et al. Lancet Oncol 2019;20;1506-1517.

340. K Shitara, et al. N Engl J Med 2020;382:2419–2430.

341. JS MacDonald, et al. N Engl J Med 2001;345:725–730.

342. EP Jansen, et al. Int J Radiat Oncol Phys 2007;69:1424–1428.

343. Y Bang, et al. Lancet 2012;379:315-321.

344. JA Ajani, et al. J Clin Oncol 2007;25:3205–3209.

345. M Wilke, et al. J Clin Oncol 1989;7:1318–1326.

346. JA Ajani, et al. Proc Am Soc Clin Oncol 2000;20:165a (abstract 657).

347. F Lordick, et al. Lancet Oncol 2013;14:490-499.

348. E van Cutsem, et al. J Clin Oncol 2009;27:18s (LBA4509).

349. SE Al-Batran, et al. J Clin Oncol 2008;26:1435–1442.

350. PC Enzinger, et al. J Clin Oncol 2017;34:2736–2742.

351. H Wilke, et al. Lancet Oncol 2014;11;1224–1235.

352. J Tabernero, et al. Lancet Oncol 2015;16:499–508.

353. Y Kawamoto, et al. Oncologist 2022;27:e642–e649.

354. Y Doki, et al. N Engl J Med 2022;386:449–462.

355. SA Cullinan, et al. J Clin Oncol 1994;12:412–416.

356. S Cascinu, et al. J Chemother 1992;4:185–188.

357. EA Eisenhauer, et al. J Clin Oncol 1994;12:2654–2666.

358. S Hironaka, et al. J Clin Oncol 2013;31:4438–4441.

359. MJ O'Connell. J Clin Oncol 1985;3:1032–1039.

360. JA Ajani. Oncology 2002;16 (suppl 6):89–96.

361. PC Thuss-Patience, et al. Eur J Cancer 2011;47:2306–2314.

362. CS Fuchs, et al. Lancet 2014;383:31–39.

363. CS Fuchs, et al. JAMA Oncol 2018;4:e180013.

364. A Patnaik, et al. Cancer Chemother Pharmacol 2022;89:93–103.

365. K Shitara, et al. N Engl J Med 2020;382:2419–2430.

366. K Shitara, et al. Lancet Oncol 2018;19:1437–1448.

367. H Joensu, et al. J Clin Oncol 2011;29:18S (LBA1).

367. GD Demetri, et al. N Engl J Med 2002;347:472–480.

369. M Montemurro, et al. Eur J Cancer 2009;45:2293–2297.

370. Y Zhou, et al. Cancer Med 2020;9:6225–6233.

371. S Bauer, et al. J Clin Oncol 2022;40:3918-3928.

372. A Italiano, et al. Ann Surg Oncol 2012;19:1551–1559.

373. GD Demetri, et al. Lancet 2013;381:295–302.

374. JY Blay, et al. Lancet Oncol 2020;21:7:923–934.

375. MC Heinrich, et al. J Clin Oncol 2020 (suppl 4;abstr 826).

376. P Schoffski, et al. Eur J Can 2020;134:62–74.

377. JA Bonner, et al. N Engl J Med 2006;354:567–578.

378. MR Posner, et al. N Engl J Med 2007;357:1705–1715.

379. DS Shin, et al. J Clin Oncol 1998;16:1325–1330.

380. M Posner, et al. J Clin Oncol 2001;19:1096–1104.

381. DM Shin, et al. Cancer 1999;91:1316–1323.

382. G Fountzilas, et al. Semin Oncol 1997;24 (Suppl 2):65–67.

383. R Hitt, et al. Semin Oncol 1995;22 (Suppl 15):50–54.

384. JA Kish, et al. Cancer 1984;53:1819–1824.

385. EE Vokes, et al. Cancer 1989;63 (Suppl 6):1048–1053.

386. D Rischin, et al. J Clin Oncol 2019;37(15 suppl): abstract 6000.

387. JB Vermorken, et al. N Engl J Med 2008;359:1116–1127.

388. B Burtness, et al. J Clin Oncol 2005;23:8646–8654.

389. Veterans Affairs Laryngeal Cancer Study Group. N Engl J Med 1991;324:1685–1690.

390. AA Forastiere, et al. N Engl J Med 2003;349:2091–2098.

391. M Al-Sarraf, et al. J Clin Oncol 1998;16:1310–1317.

392. V Gebbia, et al. Am J Clin Oncol 1995;18:293–296.

393. Colevas AD and MR Posner. Am J Clin Oncol 1998;21:482–486.

394. AA Forastiere, et al. Ann Oncol 1994;5 (suppl 6):51–54.

395. M Degardin, et al. Ann Oncol 1998;9:1103–1107.

396. JB Vermorken, et al. J Clin Oncol 2007;25:2171–2177.

397. J Bauml, et al. J Clin Oncol 2016;34:abstract 6011.

398. RL Ferris, et al. N Engl J Med 2016;375:1856–1867.

399. S Qin, et al. J Clin Oncol 2010:28; 303S (abstract 408).

400. RS Finn, et al. N Engl J Med 2020;382:1894–1905.

401. T Yau, et al. JAMA Oncol 2020;6:e204564. doi: 10.1001/jamaoncol.2020.4564.

402. RK Kelley, et al. J Clin Oncol 2021;39:2991–3001.

403. J Llovet, et al. N Engl J Med 2008;359:378–390.

404. M Kudo, et al. Lancet 2018;391:1163–1173.

405. GK Abou-Alfa, et al. N Engl J Med 2018;379:54–63.

406. J Bruix, et al. Lancet 2017;389:56–66.

407. AB El-Khoueiry, et al. Lancet 2017;389:2492–2502.

408. AX Zhu, et al. Lancet Oncol 2018. doi: 10.1016/S1470-2045(18)30351-6.

409. AX Zhu, et al. Lancet Oncol 2019;20:282–296.

410. A Ireland-Gill, et al. Semin Oncol 1992;19 (Suppl 5):32–37.

411. LL Laubenstein, et al. J Clin Oncol 1984;2:1115–1120.

412. PS Gill, et al. J Clin Oncol 1996;14:2353–2364.

413. DW Northfelt, et al. J Clin Oncol 1997;15:653–659.

414. PS Gill, et al. J Clin Oncol 1999;17:1876–1880.

415. PS Gill, et al. Cancer 2002;95:147–154.

416. ST Lim, et al. Cancer 2005;103:417–421.

417. SR Evans, et al. J Clin Oncol 2002;20:3236–3241.

418. G Nasti, et al. J Clin Oncol 2000;18:1550–1557.

419. FX Real, et al. J Clin Oncol 1986;4:544–551.

420. JE Groopman, et al. Ann Intern Med 1984;100:671–676.

421. MN Polizzotto, et al. J Clin Oncol 2016;34:4125–4131.

422. CA Linker, et al. Blood 1987;69:1242–1248.

423. CA Linker, et al. Blood 1991;78:2814–2822.

424. R Larson, et al. Blood 1995;85:2025–2037.

425. HM Kantarjian, et al. J Clin Oncol 2000;18:547–561.

426. S Faderl, et al. Cancer 2005;103:1985–1995.

426a. DJ DeAngelo, et al. Blood 2007;109:5136–5142.

427. OG Ottman, et al. Blood 2002;100:1965–1971.

428. M Talpaz, et al. N Engl J Med 2006;354:2531–2541.

429. HM Kantarjian, et al. N Engl J Med 2006;354:2542–2551.

430. BD Shah, et al. Lancet 2021;398:491-502.

431. SL Maude, et al. N Engl J Med 2018;378:439-448.

432. MS Topp, et al. Lancet Oncol 2015;16:57–66.

433. H Kantarjian, et al. N Engl J Med 2016;375:740–753.

434. JW Yates, et al. Cancer Chemother Rep 1973;57:485–488.

435. JE Lancet, et al. Blood 2014;123:3239–3246.

436. J Lambert, et al. Haematologica 2019;104:113–119.

437. H Preisler, et al. Blood 1987;69:1441–1449.

438. HP Erba, et al. Lancet 2023;401:1571-1583.

439. H Preisler, et al. Cancer Treat Rep 1977;61:89–92.

440. S Faderl, et al. Blood 2006;108:45–51.

441. RM Stone, et al. N Engl J Med 2017; doi: 10.1056/NEJMoa1614359.

442. S Amadori, et al. J Clin Oncol;34:972–979.

443. MA Sanz, et al. Blood 2010;115:5137–5146.

444. E Estey, et al. Blood 2006;107:3469–3473.

445. AD Ho, et al. J Clin Oncol 1988;6:213–217.

446. M Montillo, et al. Am J Hematol 1998;58:105–109.

447. PH Wiernik, et al. Blood 1992;79:313–319.

448. MS Tallman, et al. Blood 2005;106:1154–1163.

449. JE Cortes, et al. Leukemia 2019;33:379–389.

450. CD DiNardo, et al. Blood 2019;133:7–17.

451. P Montesinos, et al. N Engl J Med 2022;386:1519-1531.

452. VM Santana, et al. J Clin Oncol 1992;10:364–369.

453. C Gardin, et al. Blood 2007;109:5129–5132.

454. HM Kantarjian, et al. Blood 2003;102:2379–2386.

455. L Degos, et al. Blood 1995;85:2643–2653.

456. SL Soignet, et al. J Clin Oncol 2001;19:3852–3860.

457. H Dombret, et al. Semin Hematol 2002;39 (2 Suppl 1):8–13.

458. CH Man, et al. Blood 2012;119:5133–5143.

459. P Fenaux, et al. J Clin Oncol 2010;28:562–569.

460. AH Wei, et al. American Society of Hematology Annual Meeting 2019;abstract LBA3.

461. HM Kantarjian, et al. J Clin Oncol 2012;30:2670–2677.

462. EM Stein, et al. Blood 2017;130:722–731.

463. CD DiNardo, et al. N Engl J Med 2018;378:2386–2398.

464. JM Watts, et al. Lancet Haematol 2023;10:e46-e58.

465. AE Perl, et al. J Clin Oncol 2017;35: (15 suppl) abstract 7067.

466. B Raphael, et al. J Clin Oncol 1991;9:770–776.

467. MJ Keating, et al. Blood 1998;92:1165–1171.

468. S O'Brien, et al. Blood 1993;82:1695–1700.

469. JC Byrd, et al. Blood 2003;101:6–14

470. JC Byrd, et al. J Clin Oncol 2011;29:1349–1355.

471. M Keating, et al. J Clin Oncol 2005;22:4079–4088.

472. NE Kay, et al. Blood 2004;104 (abstract 339).

473. JC Byrd, et al. J Clin Oncol 2014;32:3039–3047.

474. JF Seymour, et al. N Engl J Med 2018;378:1107–1120.

475. RR Furman, et al. N Engl J Med 2014;370:997–1007.

476. V Goede, et al. N Engl J Med 2014;370:1101–1110.

477. K Fischer, et al. N Engl J Med 2019;380:2225–2236.

478. JP Sharman, et al. Lancet 2020;395:1278–1291.

479. TD Shanafelt, et al. N Engl J Med 2019;381:432–443.

480. A Osterborg, et al. J Clin Oncol 1997;15:1567–1574.

481. G Dighiero, et al. N Engl J Med 1998;338:1506–1514.

482. A Saven, et al. J Clin Oncol 1995;13:570–574.

483. MJ Keating, et al. Blood 1988;92:1165–1171.

484. A Sawitsky, et al. Blood 1977;50:1049.

485. JD Hainsworth, et al. J Clin Oncol 2003;21:1746–1751.

486. WG Wierda, et al. J Clin Oncol 2010;28:1749–1755.

487. MR Grever, et al. J Clin Oncol 1985;3:1196–1201.

488. M Alvado, et al. Semin Oncol 2002;29(4 suppl 13):19–22.

489. R Kath, et al. J Cancer Res Clin Oncol 2001;127:48–54.

490. A Ferrajoli, et al. Blood 2008;111:5291–5297.

491. JC Byrd, et al. Blood 2020;135:1204–1213.

492. CS Tam, et al. Blood 2019;134:851–859.

493. S Stilgenbauer, et al. Lancet Oncol 2016;17:768–778.

494. IW Flinn, et al. Blood 2018;131:877–887.

495. F Guilhot, et al. N Engl J Med 1997;337:223–229.

496. BJ Druker, et al. N Engl J Med 2001;344:1031–1037.

497. HM Kantarjian, et al. Blood 2007;110:3540–3546.

498. HM Kantarjian, et al. N Engl J Med 2010;362:2260–2270.

499. HM Kantarjian, et al. Blood 2007;109:5143–5150.

500. G Saglio, et al. N Engl J Med 2010;362:2251–2259.

501. HJ Khoury, et al. Blood 2012;119:3403–3412.

502. JE Cortes, et al. Blood 2018;132:393-404.

503. D Rea, et al. Blood 2021;138:2031–2041.

504. ED Deeks, Drugs 2022;82:291–226.

505. R Hehlmann, et al. Blood 1993;82:398–407.

506. R Hehlmann, et al. Blood 1994;84:4064–4077.

507. The Italian Cooperative Study Group on Chronic Myelogenous Leukemia. N Engl J Med 1994;330:820–825.

508. J Cortes, et al. Blood 2012;120:2573–2581.

509. D Chihara, et al. J Clin Oncol 2020; 38:1527–1538.

510. S Dhillon, et al. Drugs 2018;78:1–5.

511. A Saven, et al. Blood 1992;79:111–1120.

512. PA Cassileth, et al. J Clin Oncol 1991;9:243–246.

513. MJ Ratain, et al. Blood 1985;65:644–648.

514. PM Forde, et al. N Engl J Med 2022;386:1973–1985.

515. H Wakalee, et al. N Engl J Med 2023;389:491-503.

516. DR Gandara, et al. J Clin Oncol 2003;21:2004–2010.

517. CP Belani, et al. J Clin Oncol 2005;23:5883–5891.

518. GM Strauss, et al. J Clin Oncol 2008;26:5043-5051.

519. T Winton, et al. N Engl J Med 2005;352:2589–2597.

520. R Arriagada, et al. N Engl J Med 2004;350:351–360.

521. M Kreuter, et al. Ann Oncol 2012;24:986–992.

522. E Felip, et al. Lancet 2021;398:1344–1357.

523. YL Wu, et al. N Engl J Med 2020;383:1711–1723.

524. AB Sandler, et al. N Engl J Med 2006;355:2542–2560.

525. ME Socinski, et al. J Clin Oncol 2012; 30:2055–2062.

526. CP Belani, et al. J Clin Oncol 2008;26:468–473.

527. M Reck, et al. J Clin Oncol 2009;27:1227–1234

528. G Giaccone, et al. J Clin Oncol 1998;16:2133–2141.

529. F Fossella, et al. J Clin Oncol 2003;21:3016–3024.

530. CP Belani, et al. Clin Lung Cancer 1999;1:144–150.

531. V Georgoulias, et al. Lancet 2001;357:1478–1484.

532. RP Abratt, et al. J Clin Oncol 1997;15:744–749.

533. CJ Langer, et al. Semin Oncol 1999;26 (suppl 4):12–18.

534. G Frasci, et al. J Clin Oncol 2000;18:2529–2536.

535. TJ Smith, et al. J Clin Oncol 1995;13:2166–2173.

536. R Rosell, et al. Ann Oncol 2008;19:362–369.

537. M Cremonesi, et al. Oncology 2003;64:97–101.

538. GV Scagliotti, et al. J Clin Oncol 2008;21:3543–3551.

539. J Rodrigues-Pereira, et al. J Thorac Oncol 2011;6:1907-1914.

540. E Longeval, et al. Cancer 1982;50:2751–2756.

541. D Gandara, et al. J Clin Oncol 2003;21:2004–2010.

542. RS Herbst, et al. J Clin Oncol 2007;25:4734–4750.

543. JD Patel, et al. J Clin Oncol 2009;27:3284–3289.

544. L Gandhi, et al. N Engl J Med 2018;378:2078–2092.

545. R Pirker, et al. Lancet 2009;373:1525–1531.

546. T Ciuleanu, et al. Lancet 2009;374:1432-1440.

547. MA Socinski, et al. J Clin Oncol 2012;30:2055–2062.

548. EB Garon, et al. Lancet 2014;384:665–673.

549. N Thatcher, et al. Lancet Oncol 2015;16:763–774.

550. D Planchard, et al. Lancet Oncol 2016;17:642–650.

551. LG Paz-Ares, et al. J Clin Oncol 2018;36 (suppl. abstr 105).

552. MA Socinski, et al. N Engl J Med 2018;378:2288–2301.

553. K Nakagawa, et al. Lancet Oncol 2019;20:1655–1669.

554. M Reck, et al. J Clin Oncol 2020; 38 (suppl. abstr 9501).

555. ML Johnson, et al. J Clin Oncol 2022;doi: 10.1200/JCO.22.00975.

556. M Gogishvili, et al. Nat Med 2022;28:2374-2380.

557. RC Lilenbaum, et al. J Clin Oncol 2005;23:190–196.

558. WJ Tester, et al. Cancer 1997;79:724–729.

559. NA Rizvi, et al. J Clin Oncol 2008;26:639–643.

560. VA Miller, et al. Semin Oncol 2000;27 (suppl 3):3–10.

561. JD Hainsworth, et al. Cancer 2000;89:328–333.

562. N Hanna, et al. J Clin Oncol 2004;22:1589–1597.

563. C Manegold, et al. Ann Oncol 1997;8:525–529.

564. K Furuse, et al. Ann Oncol 1996;7:815–820.

565. RS Herbst. Semin Oncol 2003;30 (suppl 1):30–38.

566. FA Shepherd, et al. J Clin Oncol 2004;22 (suppl 1):14S (abstract 7022).

567. LV Sequist, et al. J Clin Oncol 2013;27:3327–3334.

568. TL Wu, et al. Lancet Oncol 2017;18:1454–1466.

569. MA Socinski, et al. J Clin Oncol 2008;26:650–656.

570. N Hanna, et al. J Clin Oncol 2006;24:5253–5258.

571. K Park, et al. J Clin Oncol 2021;JCO2100662.doi: 10.1200/JCO.21.00662.

572. C Zhou, et al. JAMA Oncol 2021;7:e214761.

573. J Brahmer, et al. N Engl J Med 2015;373:123–135.

574. EL Kwak, et al. N Engl J Med 2010;363:1693–1703.

575. AT Shaw, et al. N Engl J Med 2014;370:1189–1197.

576. AT Shaw, et al. Lancet Oncol 2016;17:234–242.

577. DW Kim, et al. J Clin Oncol 2017. doi: 10.1200/JCO.2016.71.5904.

578. BJ Solomon, et al. Lancet Oncol 2018;19:1654–1667.

579. ZT Al-Salama, et al. Drugs 2019. doi: 10.1007/s40265-019-01177-y.

580. J Yang, et al. J Thorac Oncol 2016;11:S152–153.

581. A Drilon, et al. J Thorac Oncol 2019;14(10):S6–S7.

582. V Subbiah, et al. J Clin Oncol 2020;38(suppl):109. doi: 10.1200/JCO.2020.38.15 _suppl.109.

583. J Wolf, et al. Ann Oncol 2018;29 (suppl 8) doi: 10.1093/annonc/mdy424.090.

584. PK Paik, et al. N Engl J Med 2020;383:931–943.

585. DS Hong, et al. N Engl J Med 2020;383:1207–1217.

586. PA Janne, et al. N Engl J Med 2022;387:120–131.

587. T Mok, et al. J Thorac Oncol 2016;11:S142.

588. S Gettinger, et al. J Clin Oncol 2016;34:2980–2987.

589. SJ Antonia, et al. N Engl J Med 2017;377:1919–1929.

590. J Jassem, et al. J Clin Oncol 2020; 38(suppl.): e21623–e21623.

591. A Sezer, et al. Lancet 2021:397:592–604.

592. BT Li, et al. N Engl J Med 2022;386:241-251.

593. L Horn, et al. N Engl J Med 2018;379:2220–2229.

594. L Paz-Ares, et al. Lancet 2019: 394:1929–1939.

595. DC Ihde, et al. J Clin Oncol 1994;12:2022–2034.

596. M Viren, et al. Acta Oncol 1994;33:921–924.

597. K Noda, et al. N Engl J Med 2002;346:85–91.

598. JR Eckardt, et al. J Clin Oncol 2006;24:2044–2051.

599. JD Hainsworth, et al. J Clin Oncol 1997;15:3464–3470.

600. M Neubauer, et al. J Clin Oncol 2004;22:1872–1877.

601. BJ Roth, et al. J Clin Oncol 1992;10:282–291.

602. J Aisner, et al. Semin Oncol 1986;(suppl 3):54–62.

603. DH Johnson. Semin Oncol 1993;20:315–325.

604. DH Johnson, et al. J Clin Oncol 1990;8:1013–1017.

605. JD Hainsworth, et al. Semin Oncol 1999;26 (suppl 2):60–66.

606. A Ardizzoni, et al. J Clin Oncol 1997;15:2090–2096.

607. GA Masters, et al. J Clin Oncol 2003;21:1550–1555.

608. N Ready, et al. J Thor Oncol 2018; 14:237–244.

609. HC Chung, et al. Proc Am Assoc Cancer Res. 2019; abstract CT073.

610. J Trigo, et al. Lancet Oncol 2020;21:645–654.

611. YH Kim, et al. Lancet Oncol 2018;19:1192–1204.

612. L Argnani, et al. Cancer Treat Rev 2017;61:61–69.

613. F Foss, et al. Clin Lymphoma Myeloma Leuk 2016;16:637–643.

614. F Foss, et al. Br J Hematol 2015;168:811–819.

615. G Bonadonna, et al. Cancer 1975;36:252–259.

616. JM Connors, et al. N Engl J Med 2018;378:331–344.

617. VT DeVita Jr, et al. Ann Intern Med 1970;73:881–895.

618. P Klimo, et al. J Clin Oncol 1985;3:1174–1182.

619. NL Bartlett, et al. J Clin Oncol 1995;13:1080–1088.

620. GP Canellos, et al. Ann Oncol 2003;14:268–272.

621. DL Longo. Semin Oncol 1990;17:716–735.

622. R Colwill, et al. J Clin Oncol 1995;13:396–402.

623. V Diehl, et al. J Clin Oncol 1998;16:3810–3821.

624. H Tesch, et al. Blood 1998;15:4560–4567.

625. NL Bartlett, et al. Ann Oncol 2007;18:1071–1079.

626. A Santoro, et al. J Clin Oncol 2000;18:2615–2619.

627. H Schulz, et al. Blood 2008;111:109–111.

628. A Younes, et al. J Clin Oncol 2012;30:2183–2189.

629. SM Ansell, et al. N Engl J Med 2015;372:311–318.

630. P Armand, et al. J Clin Oncol 2016;34:3733–3739.

631. AJ Moskowitz, et al. J Clin Oncol 2013;31:456–460.

632. PB Johnston, et al. Am J Hematol 2010;85:320–324.

633. TA Fehniger, et al. Blood 2011;118:5119–5125.

634. CM Bagley Jr, et al. Ann Intern Med 1972;76:227–234.

635. WJ Urba, et al. J Natl Cancer Inst Monogr 1990;10:29–37.

636. P Sonnevald, et al. J Clin Oncol 1995;13:2530–2539.

637. P McLaughlin, et al. J Clin Oncol 1996;14:1262–1268.

638. H Hochster, et al. Blood 1994;84 (suppl 1):383a.

639. S Sacchi, et al. Cancer 2007;110:121–128.

640. MHJ van Oers, et al. Blood 2006;108:3295–3301.

641. R Forstpointer, et al. Blood 2006;108:4003–4008.

642. MJ Rummel, et al. J Clin Oncol 2005;23:3383–3389.

643. KS Robinson, et al. J Clin Oncol 2008;26:4473–4479.

644. LH Sehn, et al. Blood Adv 2022;6:533-543.

645. J Leonard, et al. J Clin Oncol 2019;37:1188–1199.

646. RI Fisher, et al. J Clin Oncol 2006;24:4867–4874.

647. ML Wang, et al. N Engl J Med 2013;369:507–516.

648. ML Wang, et al. Lancet 2018;391:659–667.

649. Y Song, et al. Clin Cancer Res 2020;26:4216–4224.

650. D Telaraja, et al. Clin Cancer Res 2023;CCR-23-1272. doi: 10.1158/1078-0432.

651. M Dreyling, et al. Ann Oncol 2017;28:2169–2178.

652. LH Sehn, et al. J Clin Oncol 2015;33:LBA8502.

653. F Morschhauser, et al. Blood. 2019; 134(suppl 1):123.

654. JP Leonard, et al. J Clin Oncol 2019;37:1188–1199.

655. LE Budde, et al. Lancet Oncol 2022;23:1055-1065.

656. M Wang, et al. J Clin Oncol 2023;41:555-567.

657. E Bachy, et al. Nat Med 2022;287:2145-2154.

658. P Klimo, et al. J Clin Oncol 1985;3:1174–1182.

659. B Coiffier, et al. N Engl J Med 2002;346:235–242.

660. M Pfreundschuh, et al. Lancet Oncol 2008;9:105–116.

661. JM Vose, et al. Leuk Lymphoma 2002;43:799–804.

662. WH Wilson, et al. J Clin Oncol 1993;11:1573–1582.

663. WH Wilson. Semin Oncol 2000;27(suppl 12):30–36.

664. P Klimo, et al. Ann Intern Med 1985;102:596–602.

665. MA Shipp, et al. Ann Intern Med 1986;104:757–765.

666. DL Longo, et al. J Clin Oncol 1991;9:25–38.

667. WS Velasquez, et al. J Clin Oncol 1994;12:1169–1176.

668. WS Velasquez, et al. Blood 1988;71:117–122.

669. C Moskowitz, et al. J Clin Oncol 1999;17:3776–3785.

670. T Kewairamani, et al. Blood 2004;103; 3684–3688.

671. MA Rodriguez, et al. Ann Oncol 1995;6:609–611.

672. T El Gnaoui, et al. Ann Oncol 2007;18:1363–1368.

673. QD Shen, et al. Lancet Hematol 2018. doi: 10.1016/S2352-3026 (18)30054-1

674. L Sehn, et al. J Clin Oncol 2020;38:155–165.

675. H Tilly, et al. N Engl J Med 2022;386:351-363.

676. G Salles, et al. Lancet Oncol 2020;21:978–988.

677. MJ Dickinson, et al. N Engl J Med 2022;387:2220-2231.

678. M Hamadani, et al. Blood 2021;137:2634–2645.

679. C Thieblemont, et al. J Clin Oncol 2022;41:2238-2247.

680. N Kalakonda, et al. Lancet Hematol 2020;7:e511–522.

681. HA Burris, et al. Lancet Oncol 2018;19:486–496.

682. SS Neelapu, et al. N Engl J Med 2017;377:2531–2544.

683. SJ Schuster, et al. N Engl J Med 2017;377:2545–2554.

684. JS Abramson, et al. Lancet 2020;396:839–852.

685. I Magrath, et al. Blood 1984;63:1102–1111.

686. I Magrath, et al. J Clin Oncol 1996;14:925.

687. JI Berstein, et al. J Clin Oncol 1986;4:847–858.

688. DA Thomas, et al. Blood 2004;104:1624–1630.

689. P McLaughlin, et al. J Clin Oncol 1998;16:2825–2833.

690. M Ghielmini, et al. Blood 2004;103:4416–4423.

691. TE Witzig, et al. J Clin Oncol 2002;20:2453–2463.

692. CI Falkson. Am J Clin Oncol 1996;19:268–270.

693. DC Betticher, et al. J Clin Oncol 1998;16:850–858.

694. JW Friedberg, et al. J Clin Oncol 2008;26:204–210.

695. BS Mann, et al. Oncologist 2007;12:1247–1252.

696. OA O'Connor, et al. J Clin Oncol 2009;27:4357–4364.

697. B Pro, et al. J Clin Oncol 2012;30:2190–2196.

698. RI Piekarz, et al. Blood 2011;117:5827–5834.

699. OA O'Connor, et al. J Clin Oncol 2015;33:2492–2499.

700. SJ Strauss, et al. J Clin Oncol 2006;24:2105–2112.

701. TM Habermann, et al. Br J Haematol 2009;145:344–349.

702. PL Zinzani, et al. Blood 2017;130:267–270.

703. LE Abrey, et al. J Clin Oncol 2002;18:3144–3150.

704. GD Shah, et al. J Clin Oncol 2007;25:4730–4735.

705. T Batchelor, et al. J Clin Oncol 2003;21:1044–1049.

706.   M Reni, et al. Br J Cancer 2007;96:864–867.

707.   L Fischer, et al. Ann Oncol 2006;17:1141–1145.

708.   LA Hauschild, et al. N Engl J Med 2017;377:1813–1823.

709.   JM Kirkwood, et al. J Clin Oncol 1996;14:7–17.

710.   AM Eggermont, et al. Lancet 2008;372:117–126.

711.   J Weber, et al. N Engl J Med 2017;377:1824–1835.

712.   AM Eggermont, et al. Lancet Oncol 2015;16:522–530.

713.   AM Eggermont, et al. N Engl J Med 2018;378:1789–1801.

714.   ET Creagen, et al. J Clin Oncol 1999;17:1884–1890.

715.   CI Falkson, et al. J Clin Oncol 1998;16:1743–1751.

716.   WJ Hwu, et al. J Clin Oncol 2003;21:3351–3356.

717.   KT Flaherty, et al. N Engl J Med 2012;367:1694–1703.

718.   J Larkin, et al. N Engl J Med 2014;371:1867–1876.

719.   R Gutzmer et al, Lancet 2020;395:1835–1844.

720.   R Dummer, et al. Lancet Oncol 2018;19:603–615.

721.   J Larkin, et al. N Engl J Med 2015;373:23–34.

722.   HA Tawbi, et al. N Engl J Med 2022;386:24–34.

723.   JK Luce, et al. Cancer Chemother Rep 1970;54:119–124.

724.   KI Pritchard, et al. Cancer Treat Rep 1980;64:1123–1126.

725.   JM Kirkwood, et al. Semin Oncol 1997;24 (suppl 4):1–48.

726.   MB Atkins, et al. J Clin Oncol 1999;17:2105–2116.

727.   DR Parkinson, et al. J Clin Oncol 1990;8:1650–1656.

728.   N Acquavella, et al. J Immunother 2008;31:569–576.

729.   JD Wolchok, et al. Lancet Oncology 2010;11:155–164.

730.   C Robert, et al. N Engl J Med 2015;372:2521–2532.

731.   JS Weber, et al. Lancet Oncol 2015;16:375–384.

732.   P Nathan, et al. N Engl J Med 2021;385:1196–1206.

733.   MR Middleton, et al. J Clin Oncol 2000;18:158–166.

734.   JA Sosman, et al. N Engl J Med 2012;366:707–714.

735.   GS Falchook, et al. Lancet 2012;379:1893–1901.

736.   KB Kim, et al. J Clin Oncol 2013;31:482–489.

737.   A Ardizzoni, et al. Cancer 1991;67:2984–2987.

738.   DM Shin, et al. Cancer 1995;76:2230–2236.

739.   AK Nowak, et al. Br J Cancer 2002;87:491–496.

740.   AG Favaretto, et al. Cancer 2003;97:2791–2797.

741.   NJ Vogelzang, et al. J Clin Oncol 2003;21:2636–2644.

742.   PA Zucali, et al. Cancer 2008;112:1555–1561.

743.   GR Simon, et al. J Clin Oncol 2008;21:3567–3572.

744.   P Baas, et al. Lancet 2021;397:375–386.

745.   J Jassem, et al. J Clin Oncol 2008;26:1698–1704.

746.   JPC Steele, et al. J Clin Oncol 2000;18:3912–3917.

747. JP van Meerbeeck, et al. Cancer 1999;85:2577–2582.

748. EW Alley, et al. Lancet Oncol 2017;18:623–630.

749. J Quispel-Janssen, et al. J Thorac Oncol 2018. doi: 10.1016/j.jtho.2018.038.

750. HL Kaufman, et al. Lancet Oncol 2016;10:1374–1385.

751. P Nqhiem, et al. J Clin Oncol 2019;37:693–702.

752. SL Topalian, et al. J Clin Oncol 2020;38:2476–2487.

753. C Kang. Drugs 2023;83:731-737.

754. Southwest Oncology Group Study. Arch Intern Med 1975;135:147–152.

755. A Palumbo, et al. Lancet 2006;367:835.

756. A Palumbo, et al, Cancer 2005;104:1428-1433.

757. A Palumbo, et al. J Clin Oncol 2007;25:4459–4465.

758. B Barlogie, et al. N Engl J Med 1984;310:1353–1356.

759. SV Rajkumar, et al. J Clin Oncol 2002;20:4319–4323.

760. PG Richardson, et al. Blood 2006;108:3458–3464.

761. SV Rajkumar, et al. Proc Am Soc Clin Oncol 2007;25 (LBA8025).

762. PG Richardson, et al. Blood 2010;116:679–686.

763. JF San-Miguel, et al. Lancet Oncol 2014;15:1195–1206.

764. X Leleu, et al. Blood 2013;121:1968–1975.

765. MQ Lacy, et al. Blood 2009;27:5008–5014.

766. MA Hussein, et al. Cancer 2002;95:2160–2168.

767. RZ Orlowski, et al. Cancer 2016;122:2050-2056.

768. JR Berenson, et al. J Clin Oncol 2006;24:937–944.

769. JF San Miguel, et al. N Engl J Med 2008;359:906–917.

770. A Palumbo, et al. Blood 2007;109:2757–2762.

771. A Palumbo, et al. Leukemia 2010;24:1037–1042.

772. AK Stewart, et al. N Engl J Med 2015;372:142–152.

773. P Moreau, et al. Lancet Oncol 2018;19:953–964.

774. P Moreau, et al. Blood 2015;126:727.

775. HM Lokhorst, et al. N Engl J Med 2015;373:1207–1219.

776. S Lonial, et al. N Engl J Med 2015;373:621–631.

777. C Chen, et al. Blood 2018 131:855–863.

778. M Attal, et al. Lancet 2019; 394; 2096–2107.

779. P Moreau, et al. Lancet 2019; 394:29–38.

780. T Facon, et al. N Engl J Med 2019; 380:2104–2115.

781. PG Richardson, et al. J Clin Oncol 2021; 39:757–767.

782. R Alexanian, et al. Ann Intern Med 1986;105:8–11.

783. D Cunningham, et al. J Clin Oncol 1994;12:764–768.

784. S Singhal, et al. N Engl J Med 1999;341:1565–1571.

785. PG Richardson, et al. Blood 2006;108:3458–3464.

786. A Palumbo, et al. N Engl J Med 2014;371:895–905.

787. P Moreau, et al. Lancet Oncol 2011;12:431–440.

788. R Vij, et al. Blood 2012;119:5661–5670.
789. S Lonial, et al. Lancet 2016;387:1551–1560.
790. MV Mateos, et al. Lancet Hematol 2020;7:e370-380.
791. SP Treon, et al. N Engl J Med 2015;372:1430–1400.
792. S Lonial, et al. Lancet Oncol 2020;21:207–221.
793. P Moreau, et al. N Engl J Med 2022;387:495–505.
794. A Chari, et al. N Engl J Med 2022;387:2232-2244.
795. NC Munshi, et al. N Engl J Med 2021;384:705–716.
796. JG Berdeja, et al. Lancet 2021;398:314-324.
797. G Garcia-Manero, et al. Blood 2020;136:674–683.
798. LR Silverman, et al. J Clin Oncol 2006;24:3895–3903.
799. HM Kantarjian, et al. Cancer 2006;106:1794–1803.
800. HM Kantarjian, et al. Semin Hematology 2005;32(suppl 2):S17–S22.
801. N Galili, et al. Expert Opin Investig Drugs 2006;15:805–813.
802. M David, et al. Blood 2007;109:61–64.
803. P Fenaux, et al. N Engl J Med 2020;382:140–151.
804. JR Passweg, et al. J Clin Oncol 2011;29:303–309.
805. A Drilon, et al. N Engl J Med 2018;378:731–739.
806. A Drilon, et al. Cancer Discov 2017;7:400–409.
807. A Goorin, et al. Med Pediatr Oncol 1995;24:362–367.
808. PA Meyers, et al. J Clin Oncol 2005;23:2004–2011.
809. K Swenerton, et al. J Clin Oncol 1992;10:718–726.
810. D Alberts, et al. J Clin Oncol 1992;10:706–717.
811. WP McGuire, et al. N Engl J Med 1996;334:1–6.
812. RE Ozols. Semin Oncol 1995;22(suppl 15):1–6.
813. S Pignata, et al. Crit Rev Oncol Hematol 2008;66:229–236.
814. RA Burger, et al. J Clin Oncol 2010:28:946S (LBA1).
815. M Markman, et al. J Clin Oncol 2001;19:1901–1905.
816. S Pignant, et al. J Clin Oncol 2009;27:18S (LBA5509).
817. G D'Agostino, et al. Br J Cancer 2003;89:1180–1184.
818. RA Nagourney, et al. Gynecol Oncol 2003;88:35–39.
819. T. Thigpen. Semin Oncol 2006;33(suppl 6):S26–S32.
820. DK Armstrong, et al. N Engl J Med 2006;354:34–43.
821. UA Matulonis, et al. J Clin Oncol 2008;26:5761–5766.
822. I Ray-Coquard, et al. N Engl J Med 2019; 381:2416–2428.
823. MR Mirza, et al. Lancet 2019;20:1409–1419.
824. KN Moore, et al. Ann Oncol 2021;32:757–765.
825. M Markman. Gynecol Oncol 1998;69:226–229.
826. PG Rose, et al. Gynecol Oncol 2001;82:323–328.
827. WP McGuire, et al. Ann Intern Med 1989;111:273–279.
828. K DeGeest, et al. J Clin Oncol 2010:28:149–153.

829. AP Kudelka, et al. J Clin Oncol 1996;14:1552–1557.

830. B Lund, et al. J Natl Cancer Inst 1994;86:1530–1533.

831. RF Ozols. Drugs 1999;58(suppl 3):43–49.

832. P Sorensen, et al. Gynecol Oncol 2001;81:58–62.

833. DS Miller, et al. J Clin Oncol 2009;27:2686–2691.

834. RA Burger, et al. J Clin Oncol 2007;25:5165–5171.

835. JK Wolf, et al. Gynecol Oncol 2006;102:468–474.

836. J Ledermann, et al. Lancet Oncol 2014;15:852–861.

837. K Moore, et al. N Engl J Med 2018;379:2495–2505.

838. E Swisher, et al. Lancet Oncol 2017;18:75–87.

839. M Mirza, et al. N Engl J Med 2016;375:2154–2164.

840. A Gonzalez-Martin, et al. N Engl J Med 2019;381:2391–2402.

841. MA Dimopoulos, et al. Gynecol Oncol 2004;95:695–700.

842. JP Neoptolemos, et al. Lancet 2017;389:1011–1024.

843. T Conroy, et al. N Engl J Med 2018;379:2395–2406.

844. JP Neoptolemos, et al. JAMA 2012;308:147-156.

845. TH Cartwright, et al. J Clin Oncol 2002;20:160–164.

846. H Oettle, et al. JAMA 2007;297:267–277.

847. WF Regine, et al. J Clin Oncol 2006;25 (abstract 4007).

848. PJ Loehrer, et al. J Clin Oncol 2008;26 (abstract 4506).

849. S Mukherjee, et al. Lancet Oncol 2013;14:317–326.

850. JA DeCaprio, et al. J Clin Oncol 1991;9:2128–2133.

851. V Hess, et al. J Clin Oncol 2003;21:66–68.

852. RA Hubner, et al. Pancreas 2013;42:511–515.

853. RL Fine, et al. Cancer Chemother Pharmacol 2008;61:167–175.

854. V Heinemann, et al. Ann Oncol 2000;11:1399–1403.

855. C Louvet, et al. J Clin Oncol 2002;20:1512–1518.

856. C Louvet, et al. J Clin Oncol 2007;25:18S (abstract 4592).

857. MJ Moore, et al. J Clin Oncol 2005;23:16S (abstract 1).

858. MH Kulke, et al. J Clin Oncol 2007;25:4787–4792.

859. T Conroy, et al. N Engl J Med 2011;364:1817-1825.

860. DD Von Hoff, et al. N Engl J Med 2013;369:1691–1703.

861. H Rehman, et al. Therap Adv Gastroenterol 2020;13:1–7.

862. A Wang-Gilam, et al. Lancet 2016;387:545–557.

863. M Maio, et al. Ann Oncol 2022;33:929–938.

864. T Golan, et al. N Engl J Med 2019;381:317–327.

865. HA Burris, et al. J Clin Oncol 1997;15:2403–2413.

866. R Brand, et al. Invest New Drugs 1997;15:331–341.

867. TH Cartwright, et al. J Clin Oncol 2002;20:160–164.

868. MA Eisenberger, et al. Semin Oncol 1994;21:613–619.

869. CD Jurincic, et al. Semin Oncol 1991;18 (Suppl 6):21–25.

870. KJ Pienta, et al. J Clin Oncol 1994;12:2005–2012.

871. GR Hudes, et al. J Clin Oncol 1992;11:1754–1761.

872. GR Hudes, et al. J Clin Oncol 1997;15:3156–3163.

873. DJ Vaughn, et al. Cancer 2004;100:746–750.

874. IF Tannock, et al. J Clin Oncol 1996;14:1756–1764.

875. MS Copur, et al. Semin Oncol 2001;28:16–21.

876. DP Petrylak, et al. N Engl J Med 2004;351:1513–1520.

877. IF Tannock, et al. N Engl J Med 2004;351:1502–1512.

878. S Halabi, et al. J Clin Oncol 2010;28:951S (LBA 4511).

879. JS DeBono, et al. Lancet 2010;376:1147-1154.

880. M Eisenberger, et al. J Clin Oncol 2017;35:3198–3206.

881. MA Climent, et al. Eur J Cancer 2017;878:30–37.

882. PG Corn, et al. Lancet Oncol 2019;20:1432–1443.

883. JS DeBono, et al. N Engl J Med 2011;364:1995–2005.

884. KN Chi, et al. J Clin Oncol 2023;41:3339-3351.

885. N Clarke, et al. Lancet Oncol 2018:975-986.

886. N Agarwal, et al. Lancet 2023;402:291-303.

887. CE Kyriakopoulos, et al. J Clin Oncol 2018;36:1080-1087.

888. BJ Roth, et al. Cancer 1993;72:2457–2460.

889. WR Berry, et al. Clin Prostate Cancer 2004;3:104-111.

890. DP Petrylak. Semin Oncol 2000;27(suppl 3):24–29.

891. R. Dreicer. Hematol Oncol Clin North Am 2006;20:935–946.

892. G. Hudes. Semin Urol Oncol 1997;15:13–19.

893. GP Murphy, et al. Urology 1984;23:54–63.

894. GA Dijkman, et al. Eur Urol 1995;27:43–46.

895. GE Hanks, et al. J Clin Oncol 2003;21:3972–3978.

896. L Klotz, et al. BJU Int 2008;10:1531–1538.

897. ND Shore, et al. N Engl J Med 2020;382:2187–2196.

898. The Leuprolide Study Group. N Engl J Med 1984;311:1281–1286.

899. R Sharifi, et al. Clin Ther 1996;18:647–657.

900. O Sartor, et al. Urology 2003;62:319–323.

901. PF Schellhammer, et al. Urology 1997;50:330–336.

902. DG McLeod, et al. Cancer 1993;72:3870–3873.

903. RA Janknegt, et al. J Urol 1993;149:77–82.

904. MR Smith, et al. N Engl J Med 2018;378:1408–1418.

905. K Fizaki, et al. N Engl J Med 2019;380:1235–1246.

906. IF Tannock, et al. J Clin Oncol 1989;7:590–597.

907. SD Fossa, et al. J Clin Oncol 2001;19:62–71.

908. DE Johnson, et al. Urology 1988;31:132–134.

909. KA Havlin, et al. Cancer Treat Res 1988;39:83–96.

910. PW Kantoff, et al. N Engl J Med 2010;363:411–422.

911.	HI Scher, et al. N Engl J Med 2012;367:1187–1197.

912.	JS De Bono, et al. N Engl J Med 2020;382:2091–2102.

913.	W Abida, et al. J Clin Oncol 2018;36:6 (suppl. TPS388-TPS388).

914.	ES Antonarakis, et al. J Clin Oncol 2020;38:395–405.

915.	A Ravaud, et al. N Engl J Med 2016;375:2246–2254.

916.	T Powles, et al. Lancet Oncolg 2022;23:1133–1144.

917.	B Escudier, et al. Lancet 2007;370:2103–2111.

918.	J Atzpodien, et al. Semin Oncol 1993;20(suppl 9):22.

919.	RJ Motzer, et al. Lancet Oncol 2015;16:1473–1482.

920.	RJ Motzer, et al. N Engl J Med 2018;378:1277–1290.

921.	MH Voss, et al. J Clin Oncol 2016;34:3846–3853.

922.	BI Rini, et al. N Engl J Med 2019; 380:1116–1127.

923.	RJ Motzer, et al. N Engl J Med 2021;384:1289–1300.

924.	RJ Motzer, et al. N Engl J Med 2019; 380:1103–1115.

925.	TK Choueiri, et al. N Engl J Med 2021;384:829–841.

926.	JC Yang, et al. N Engl J Med 2003;349:427–434.

927.	RJ Motzer, et al. 2006;24:16–24.

928.	YG Najjar, et al. Eur J Cancer 2014;50:1084–1089.

929.	CH Barrios, et al. Cancer 2012;118:1252-1259.

930.	MJ Ratain, et al. J Clin Oncol 2006;24:2505–2512.

931.	CN Sternberg, et al. J Clin Oncol 2010;28:1061–1068.

932.	Rini Bl, et al., et al. Lancet 2011;378:1931–1939.

933.	G Hudes, et al. N Engl J Med 2007;356:2271–2281.

934.	RJ Motzer, et al. Lancet 2008;372:449–456.

935.	G Fyfe, et al. J Clin Oncol 1995;13:688–696.

936.	LM Minasian, et al. J Clin Oncol 1993;11:1368–1375.

937.	TK Choueiri, et al. N Engl J Med 2015;373:1814–1822.

938.	RJ Motzer et al. Lancet Oncol 2015;16:1473–1482.

939.	BI Rini et al. Lancet Oncol 2020;21:95–104.

940.	K Antman, et al. J Clin Oncol 1993;11:1276–1285.

941.	FP Worden, et al. J Clin Oncol 2005;23:105–112.

942.	A Elias, et al. J Clin Oncol 1989;7:1208–1216.

943.	A Santoro, et al. J Clin Oncol 1995;13:1537–1545.

944.	RG Maki, et al. J Clin Oncol 2007;25:2755–2763.

945.	P Dileo, et al. Cancer 2007;109:1863–1869.

946.	E Holcombe, et al. N Engl J Med 2003;348:694–701.

947.	AR Naqash, et al. J Clin Oncol 2021;39:11519.

948.	AT van Oosterom, et al. Eur J Cancer 2002;38:2397–2406.

949.	I Judson, et al. Eur J Cancer 2001;37:870–877.

950.	Graaf van Der, et al. J Clin Oncol 2011;29:18S (LBA 10002).

951.	GD Demetri, et al. J Clin Oncol 2016;34:786–793.

952.   P Schoffski, et al. Lancet 2016;387:1629–1637.

953.   M Gounder, et al. Lancet Oncol 2020;21:1423-1432.

954.   WD Tap, et al. Lancet 2019;94:478–487.

955.   MR Migden, et al. N Engl J Med 2018;379:341–351.

956.   JJ Grob, et al. J Clin Oncol 2020;38:2916–2925.

957.   LH Einhorn, et al. J Clin Oncol 1989;7:387–391.

958.   RT Oliver, et al. Lancet 2005;366:293–300.

959.   CR Nichols, et al. J Clin Oncol 1998;16:1287–1295.

960.   G Bosl, et al. J Clin Oncol 1988;6:1231–1238.

961.   LH Einhorn, et al. Ann Intern Med 1977;87:293–298.

962.   D Vugrin, et al. Ann Intern Med 1981;95:59–61.

963.   PJ Loehrer, et al. Ann Intern Med 1988;109:540–546.

964.   GV Kondagunat, et al. J Clin Oncol 2005;23:6549–6555.

965.   LH Einhorn, et al. J Clin Oncol 2007;25:513–516.

966.   C Bokemeyer, et al. Ann Oncol 2008;19:448–453.

967.   JC Miller, et al. Semin Oncol 1990;17(1 Suppl 2):36–39.

968.   PJ Loehrer, et al. J Clin Oncol 1994;12:1164–1168.

969.   G Giaccone, et al. J Clin Oncol 1996;14:814–820.

970.   A Fornasiero, et al. Cancer 1991;68:30–33.

971.   PJ Loehrer, et al. Cancer 2001;91:2010–2015.

972.   WN William, et al. Am J Clin Oncol 2009;32:15–19.

973.   GL Lemma, et al. J Clin Oncol 2011;29:2060–2065.

974.   N Adra, et al. Ann Oncol 2018;29:209–214.

975.   K Shimaoka, et al. Cancer 1985;56:2155–2160.

976.   V Gupta-Abramson, et al. J Clin Oncol 2008;26:2010–2015.

977.   LL Carr, et al. Clin Cancer Res 2010:16:5260–5268.

978.   A Ravaud, et al. Eur J Cancer 2017;76:110–117.

979.   KC Bible, et al. Lancet Oncol 2010;11:962–972.

980.   SA Wells, et al. J Clin Oncol 2010;28:767–772.

981.   MS Brose, et al. Lancet Oncol 2021;22:1126-1138.

982.   M Schlumberger, et al. N Engl J Med 2015;372:621–630.

983.   MH Shah, et al. J Clin Oncol 2020;38:15 (suppl. 3594-3594).

984.   J Kim, et al. Clin Cancer Res 2021. doi: 10.1158/1078-0432.

985.   E. Jonasch, et al. N Engl J Med 2021;385:2-36-2046.

986.   SP Treon, et al. J Clin Oncol 2009;27:3830–3835.

987.   MA Dimopoulos, et al. J Clin Oncol 2007;25:3344–3349.

988.   SP Treon, et al. Blood 2014;124:503–510.

989.   M Schlumberger, et al. N Engl J Med 2015;372:621–630.

990.   JJ Castillo, et al. Clin Cancer Res 2018. doi: 10.1158/1078-0432.

991.   CS Tam, et al. Blood 2020;136:2038–2050.

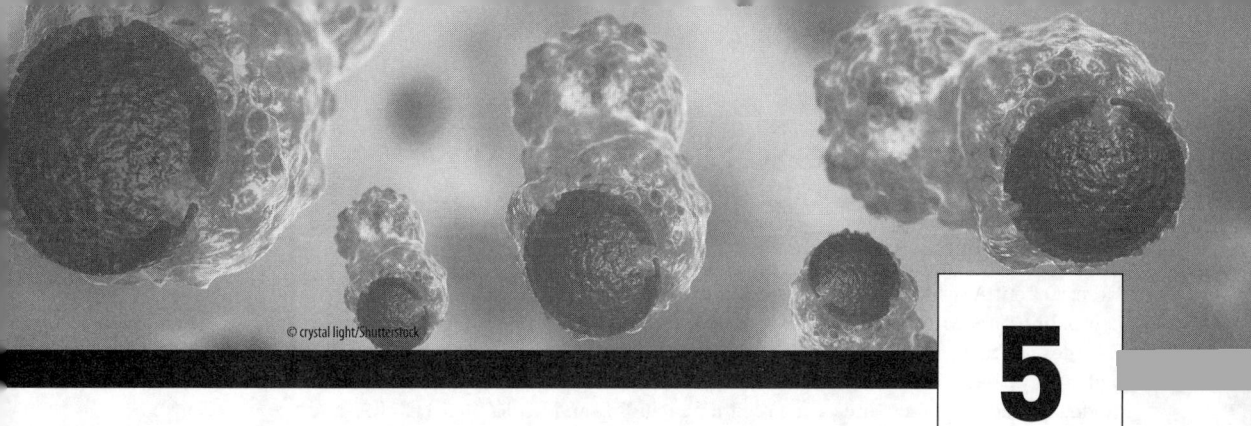

5

Antiemetic Agents for the Treatment of Chemotherapy-Induced Nausea and Vomiting

M. Sitki Copur, Amalia Sofianidi, Laurie J. Harrold, and Edward Chu

This chapter presents an overview of the common regimens for the treatment of chemotherapy-induced nausea and vomiting. These regimens have been selected based on their use in clinical practice in the medical oncology community. It should be emphasized that not all of the drugs and dosages in the regimens have been officially approved by the Food and Drug Administration (FDA). This chapter should serve as a quick reference for physicians and healthcare professionals, and it provides several options for treating both acute and delayed nausea and vomiting. It is not intended to be an all-inclusive review of all the antiemetic treatment regimens, nor is it intended to endorse and/or prioritize any particular antiemetic agent or regimen.

COMMON REGIMENS FOR CHEMOTHERAPY-INDUCED NAUSEA AND VOMITING

Highly Emetogenic Chemotherapy

Note: current ASCO guidelines recommend a four-drug regimen that includes a neurokinin 1 receptor antagonist (NK_1 RA), a serotonin receptor antagonist (5-HT_3 RA), dexamethasone, and olanzapine with dexamethasone and olanzapine continued on days 2–4. These regimens are listed under option "A" below. MASCC/ESMO guidelines recommend a three-drug regimen including an NK_1 RA, a 5-HT_3 RA, and dexamethasone. These regimens are listed under option "B" below. NCCN guidelines include these regimens, as well as a third option of a three-drug regimen that includes olanzapine and omits the NK_1 RA. These regimens are listed under option "C" below. In general, there is no preference for any one of the regimens presented below. NCCN guidelines suggest that if patients experience emesis despite a three-drug regimen or are at particularly high risk for emesis (for example, if using cisplatin or AC-containing chemotherapy regimens), the four-drug regimen (option "A") may be more appropriate. Individual agents in the respective drug classes may be selected based on institutional and/or provider preference.

A. Four-Drug Regimen

Day 1: antiemetic agents are generally given 30 minutes before chemotherapy unless otherwise stated

1. NK_1 RA (choose one):
   a. Aprepitant 125 mg PO once taken 60 minutes before chemotherapy on day 1
   b. Aprepitant injectable emulsion 130 mg IV once (note that this is a different formulation than fosaprepitant)
   c. Fosaprepitant 150 mg IV once
   d. Netupitant 300 mg / palonosetron 0.5 mg (fixed combination product) PO once given 60 min before chemotherapy
   e. Fosnetupitant 235 mg / palonosetron 0.25 mg (fixed combination product) IV once
   f. Rolapitant 180 mg PO once 1–2 hr before chemotherapy (should not be dosed more frequently than every 2 weeks)

2. 5-HT_3 RA (choose one):
   a. Dolasetron 100 mg PO once
   b. Granisetron extended-release formulation 10 mg SQ once, or granisetron 2 mg PO once, or 0.01 mg/kg (max 1 mg) IV once, or 3.1 mg/24-hr transdermal patch applied 24–28 hr prior to first dose of chemotherapy
   c. Ondansetron 16–24 mg PO once, or 8–16 mg IV once
   d. Palonosetron 0.25 mg IV once (or 0.5 mg PO once where available)
   e. If netupitant/palonosetron fixed combination product or fosnetupitant palonosetron fixed combination product are used, no further 5-HT_3 RA is required since these combinations already include palonosetron

3. Olanzapine 5–10 mg PO once (consider 5 mg dose for elderly or oversedated patients)

4. Dexamethasone 12 mg PO/IV once (note: dose can be individualized with both lower and higher doses appropriate in certain situations; for example, steroids should be minimized or avoided in patients receiving cellular therapies or checkpoint inhibitors)

Days 2, 3, 4:

1. Aprepitant 80 mg PO on days 2–3 if aprepitant PO used on day 1

2. Olanzapine 5–10 mg PO daily on days 2, 3, 4

3. Dexamethasone 8 mg PO/IV daily on days 2, 3, 4

B. Three-Drug Regimen without Olanzapine

Day 1: antiemetic agents are generally given 30 min before chemotherapy unless otherwise stated

1. NK_1 RA (choose one):
   a. Aprepitant 125 mg PO once taken 60 min before chemotherapy on day 1
   b. Aprepitant injectable emulsion 130 mg IV once (note that this is a different formulation from fosaprepitant)
   c. Fosaprepitant 150 mg IV once
   d. Netupitant 300 mg / palonosetron 0.5 mg (fixed combination product) PO once given 60 min before chemotherapy
   e. Fosnetupitant 235 mg / palonosetron 0.25 mg (fixed combination product) IV once
   f. Rolapitant 180 mg PO once 1–2 hr before chemotherapy (should not be dosed more frequently than every 2 weeks)

2. $5\text{-}HT_3$ RA (choose one):
   a. Dolasetron 100 mg PO once
   b. Granisetron extended-release formulation 10 mg SQ once, or granisetron 2 mg PO once, or 0.01 mg/kg (max 1 mg) IV once, or 3.1 mg/24-hr transdermal patch applied 24–28 hr prior to first dose of chemotherapy
   c. Ondansetron 16–24 mg PO once, or 8–16 mg IV once
   d. Palonosetron 0.25 mg IV once (or 0.5 mg PO once where available)
   e. If netupitant/palonosetron fixed combination product or fosnetupitant palonosetron fixed combination product are used, no further $5\text{-}HT_3$ RA is required since these combinations already include palonosetron

3. Dexamethasone 12 mg PO/IV once (note: dose can be individualized with both lower and higher doses appropriate in certain situations; for example, steroids should be minimized or avoided in patients receiving cellular therapies or checkpoint inhibitors)

Days 2, 3, 4:

1. Aprepitant 80 mg PO on days 2–3 if aprepitant PO used on day 1
2. Dexamethasone 8 mg PO/IV daily on days 2, 3, 4

C. Three-Drug Regimen without NK$_1$ RA

Day 1: antiemetic agents are generally given 30 minutes before chemotherapy unless otherwise stated

1. 5-HT$_3$ RA:

   Only palonosetron 0.25 mg IV once is so far recommended in this regimen.
2. Olanzapine 5–10 mg PO once (consider 5 mg dose for elderly or oversedated patients)
3. Dexamethasone 12 mg PO/IV once (note: dose can be individualized with both lower and higher doses appropriate in certain situations; for example, steroids should be minimized or avoided in patients getting cellular therapies or checkpoint inhibitors)

Days 2, 3, 4:

1. Olanzapine 5–10 mg PO once (consider 5 mg dose for elderly or oversedated patients)

Note: for anticipatory nausea, can consider adding lorazepam 0.5–2 mg PO to any of these regimens beginning on the night before treatment and then repeating the dose the next day 1–2 hr before chemotherapy begins. Non-pharmacologic methods of prevention may also be helpful.

Moderately Emetogenic Chemotherapy

There is no preference between the different regimens presented below. However, for patients who have failed treatment with 5-HT$_3$ RA plus dexamethasone (option "A") or for those who have additional risk factors for vomiting, the three-drug regimen with 5HT$_3$ RA, NK$_1$ RA, and dexamethasone may be preferable. In addition, for patients treated with option "A" with 5-HT$_3$ RA and dexamethasone but no NK1 RA or olanzapine, NCCN guidelines recommend that granisetron extended-release formulation 10 mg SQ once or palonosetron 0.25 mg IV once may be preferred due to longer half-life and possible reduced risk of delayed nausea/vomiting.

A. Two-Drug Regimen with 5-HT$_3$ RA and Dexamethasone

Day 1: antiemetic agents are generally given 30 min before chemotherapy unless otherwise stated

1. 5-HT$_3$ RA (choose one):
   a. Dolasetron 100 mg PO once
   b. Granisetron extended-release formulation 10 mg SQ once, or granisetron 2 mg PO once, or 0.01 mg/kg (max 1 mg) IV once, or 3.1 mg/24-hr transdermal patch applied 24–28 hr prior to first dose of chemotherapy

    c. Ondansetron 16–24 mg PO once, or 8–16 mg IV once

    d. Palonosetron 0.25 mg IV once (or 0.5 mg PO once where available)

  2. Dexamethasone 12 mg PO/IV once

Days 2 and 3:

  1. Dexamethasone 8 mg PO/IV on day 2, 3

    OR

  2. 5-HT3 RA monotherapy* (choose one):

    a. Granisetron 1–2 mg (total dose) PO daily or 0.01 mg/kg (max 1 mg) IV daily on days 2 and 3

    b. Ondansetron 8 mg PO twice daily or 16 mg PO daily or 8–16 mg IV daily on days 2 and 3

    c. Dolasetron 100 mg PO daily on days 2, 3

*Note: no further 5-HT_3 therapy is required on days 2–3 if palonosetron, granisetron extended-release injection, or granisetron transdermal patch is given on day 1 due to the longer half-life of these formulations

B. Three-Drug Regimen with 5-HT_3 RA, Olanzapine, and Dexamethasone

Day 1: antiemetic agents are generally given 30 min before chemotherapy unless otherwise stated

  1. 5-HT_3 Receptor Antagonist:

    Only palonosetron 0.25 mg IV is recommended as part of this three-drug regimen.

  2. Olanzapine 5–10 mg PO once (consider 5 mg dose for elderly or oversedated patients)

  3. Dexamethasone 12 mg PO/IV once (note: dose can be individualized with both lower and higher doses appropriate in certain situations; for example, steroids should be minimized or avoided in patients getting cellular therapies or checkpoint inhibitors)

Days 2, 3:

  1. Olanzapine 5–10 mg PO once on days 2, 3 (consider 5 mg dose for elderly or oversedated patients)

C. Three-Drug Regimen with NK_1 RA, 5-HT_3 RA, and Dexamethasone

Day 1: antiemetic agents are generally given 30 min before chemotherapy unless otherwise stated

  1. NK_1 RA (choose one):

    a. Aprepitant 125 mg PO once taken 60 min before chemotherapy on day 1

    b. Aprepitant injectable emulsion 130 mg IV once (note that this is a different formulation than fosaprepitant)

    c. Fosaprepitant 150 mg IV once

    d. Netupitant 300 mg / palonosetron 0.5 mg (fixed combination product) PO once given 60 min before chemotherapy

    e. Fosnetupitant 235 mg / palonosetron 0.25 mg (fixed combination product) IV once

    f. Rolapitant 180 mg PO once 1–2 hr before chemotherapy (should not be dosed more frequently than every 2 weeks)

2. 5-HT$_3$ RA (choose one):

    a. Dolasetron 100 mg PO once

    b. Granisetron extended-release formulation 10 mg SQ once, or granisetron 2 mg PO once, or 0.01 mg/kg (max 1 mg) IV once, or 3.1 mg/24-hr transdermal patch applied 24–28 hr prior to first dose of chemotherapy

    c. Ondansetron 16–24 mg PO once, or 8–16 mg IV once

    d. Palonosetron 0.25 mg IV once (or 0.5 mg PO once where available)

    e. If netupitant/palonosetron fixed combination product or fosnetupitant palonosetron fixed combination product are used, no further 5-HT$_3$ RA is required since these combinations already include palonosetron

3. Dexamethasone 12 mg PO/IV once (note: dose can be individualized with both lower and higher doses appropriate in certain situations; for example, steroids should be minimized or avoided in patients getting cellular therapies or checkpoint inhibitors)

Days 2, 3:

1. Aprepitant 80 mg PO on days 2–3 if aprepitant PO used on day 1

2. Dexamethasone 8 mg PO/IV daily on days 2, 3

D. Miscellaneous Regimens not Included Above

1. Dexamethasone 4–8 mg PO or 10–20 mg IV for one dose before chemotherapy; lorazepam 1.5 mg/m^2 IV before chemotherapy; and prochlorperazine 5–25 mg PO or IV before chemotherapy

2. Palonosetron 0.25 mg IV given 30 min before chemotherapy

3. Granisetron transdermal patch (34.3 mg of granisetron) applied to the upper outer arm at a minimum of 24 hr before chemotherapy. The patch should be removed a minimum of 24 hr after the completion of chemotherapy and may be worn for up to 7 days depending on the duration of the chemotherapy regimen.

Note: for anticipatory nausea, can consider adding lorazepam 0.5–2 mg PO to any of these regimens beginning on the night before treatment and then repeating the same dose the next day 1–2 hr before chemotherapy begins. Non-pharmacologic methods of prevention may also be helpful.

Low to Mildly Emetogenic Chemotherapy

1. Prochlorperazine 10–25 mg PO, 5–25 mg IV, or 25 mg PR before chemotherapy and then 10–25 mg PO every 4–6 hr as needed

2. Thiethylperazine 10 mg PO, 10 mg IM, or 10 mg PR every 4–6 hr as needed

3. Ondansetron 8 mg PO bid, with the first dose 30 min before the start of chemotherapy and a subsequent dose 8 hr after the first dose

4. Dexamethasone 4–8 mg PO or 10–20 mg IV before chemotherapy and every 4–6 hr as needed

5. Prochlorperazine 10–25 mg PO, 5–25 mg IV, or 25 mg PR before chemotherapy and then 10–25 mg PO every 6 hr as needed; dexamethasone 4 mg PO or 10–20 mg IV before chemotherapy and continue with 4 mg PO every 6 hr up to a total of four doses as needed

6. Prochlorperazine 10–25 mg PO, 5–25 mg IV, or 25 mg PR before chemotherapy and then 10–25 mg PO every 6 hr as needed; dexamethasone 4 mg PO or 10–20 mg IV before chemotherapy and continue with 4 mg PO every 6 hr up to a total of four doses as needed; and lorazepam 1.5 mg/m^2 IV administered 45 min before chemotherapy

7. Metoclopramide 20–40 mg PO and diphenhydramine 25–50 mg PO every 4–6 hr as needed

8. Metoclopramide 1–2 mg/kg IV and diphenhydramine 25–50 mg IV every 4–6 hr as needed

9. Dolasetron 100 mg PO daily

10. Granisetron 1–2 mg (total dose) PO daily

11. Ondansetron 8–16 mg PO daily

12. Lorazepam 0.5–2 mg PO, sublingual, or IV every 6 hr and can also be used in combination with other antiemetic agents.

13. Nabilone 1–2 mg PO bid or tid. The maximum recommended daily dose is 6 mg given in divided doses 2–3 times a day.

14. Dronabinol 5–10 mg PO every 2–4 hr for a total of 4 to 6 doses per day. May increase the dose by 2.5 mg/m^2 increments if the initial dose is ineffective and there are no significant adverse events. Increasing the dose above 7 mg/m^2 is unlikely to provide any additional benefit.

15. Dimenhydrinate 100 mg PO every 12 hr alternating with prochlorperazine 10 mg PO every 12 hr.

COMMON REGIMENS FOR DELAYED AND/OR BREAKTHROUGH NAUSEA AND VOMITING:

Note: as a general rule, it is important to use an antiemetic agent of a different pharmacologic class from what was used in the initial regimen for prevention of nausea/vomiting. If the patient has significant breakthrough nausea/vomiting, should consider modifying the regimen for future cycles.

1. Metoclopramide 40 mg PO every 4–6 hr and dexamethasone 4–8 mg PO every 4–6 hr for 4 days

2. Metoclopramide 40 mg PO every 4–6 hr; dexamethasone 4–8 mg PO every 4–6 hr; and prochlorperazine 10–25 mg PO every 4–6 hr

3. Aprepitant 80 mg PO and dexamethasone 8–12 mg PO once daily on days 2 and 3

4. Aprepitant 80 mg PO daily, dexamethasone 8–12 mg PO daily, and ondansetron 8 mg PO bid on days 2 and 3

5. Aprepitant 80 mg PO daily, dexamethasone 8–12 mg PO daily, and granisetron 1 mg PO bid on days 2 and 3

6. Aprepitant 80 mg PO daily, dexamethasone 8–12 mg PO daily, and dolasetron 100 mg PO daily on days 2 and 3

7. Olanzapine 10 mg PO on day 1, palonosetron 0.25 mg IV on day 1, dexamethasone 20 mg IV on day 1, and olanzapine 10 mg PO on days 2–4

8. Olanzapine 10 mg PO on days 1–4, aprepitant or fosaprepitant, and a 5-HT3 inhibitor

9. Ondansetron 8 mg PO bid for up to 2–3 days after chemotherapy

10. Ondansetron (orally dissolving tablets) 8 mg sublingual every 8 hr as needed

11. Metoclopramide 20–40 mg PO and diphenhydramine 50 mg PO every 3–4 hr

12. Prochlorperazine suppository 25 mg PR every 12 hr

13. Dolasetron 100 mg PO daily

14. Nabilone 1–2 mg PO bid or tid during the course of each cycle of chemotherapy. The maximum recommended daily dose is 6 mg given in divided doses 2–3 times a day.

15. Dronabinol 5–10 mg PO every 2–4 hr for a total of 4 to 6 doses per day. May increase the dose by 2.5 mg/m^2 increments if the initial dose is ineffective and there are no significant adverse events. It is unlikely that increasing the dose above 7 mg/m^2 will provide any additional benefit.

16. Granisetron 1–2 mg PO daily or 1 mg PO bid or 0.01 mg/kg (maximum 1 mg) IV daily or transdermal patch every 7 days

17. Scopolamine transdermal patch every 72 hr

18. Haloperidol 0.5–2 mg PO or IV every 4–6 hr

19. Lorazepam 0.5–2 mg PO, sublingual, or IV every 6 hr

COMMON REGIMENS FOR RADIATION-INDUCED NAUSEA AND VOMITING:

Guidelines have been developed by NCCN, ASCO, and MASCC/ESMO on the management of radiation-induced nausea and vomiting. NCCN cites total body radiation as being associated with the highest emetogenic risk involving more than 90% of patients. For patients who receive upper abdominal radiation, 30%–90% of patients will experience nausea and vomiting, and this is considered moderate risk. ASCO has identified 4 risk categories as high, moderate, low, and minimal. High risk (>90%) is associated with total body radiation; moderate risk (30%–90%) involves radiation to the upper abdomen or craniospinal area; low risk (10%–30%) involves radiation to the brain, head and neck, thorax, and pelvis; and minimal risk (<10%) involves radiation to the extremities and breast. MASCC/ESMO classify radiation-induced nausea and vomiting based on the sites of radiation in the same four categories as ASCO.

The regimens are as follows:

1. Granisetron 2 mg PO daily and dexamethasone 4 mg PO daily
2. Ondansetron 8 mg PO daily or bid and dexamethasone 4 mg PO daily
3. Tropisetron 5 mg PO daily and dexamethasone 4 mg PO daily
4. Prochlorperazine 5–10 mg PO tid or qid as rescue agent
5. Metoclopramide 5–20 mg tid or qid as rescue agent
6. Dexamethasone 4 mg oral or IV

Table 5-1. Emetogenic Potential of Intravenous Chemotherapy Agents

Level	Frequency of Emesis (%)	Agent
High	>90%	AC regimen (anthracycline plus cyclophosphamide)
		Carboplatin AUC $\geq$4
		Carmustine >250 mg/m^2
		Cisplatin
		Cyclophosphamide >1,500 mg/m^2
		Dacarbazine >500 mg/m^2
		Doxorubicin $\geq$60 mg/m^2
		Epirubicin >90 mg/m^2
		Fam-trastuzumab deruxtecan
		Ifosfamide >2,000 mg/m^2 per dose
		Mechlorethamine
		Melphalan $\geq$140 mg/m^2
		Sacituzumab govitecan
		Streptozocin
Moderate	30–90	Aldesleukin >12–15 million IU/m^2
		Bendamustine
		Busulfan
		Carboplatin AUC$\leq$4
		Carmustine $\leq$250 mg/m^2
		Clofarabine
		Cyclophosphamide $\leq$1,500 mg/m^2
		Cytarabine >200 mg/m^2
		Dactinomycin
		Daunorubicin

Table 5-1 (cont.)

Level	Frequency of Emesis (%)	Agent
Moderate	30–90	Daunorubicin and cytarabine liposome
		Dinutuximab
		Doxorubicin <60 mg/m^2
		Epirubicin ≤90 mg/m^2
		Idarubicin
		Ifosfamide <2,000 mg/m^2
		Interferon-α >10 million IU/m^2
		Irinotecan
		Irinotecan liposomal
		Lurbinectedin
		Melphalan (IV) <140 mg/m^2
		Methotrexate ≥250 mg/m^2
		Oxaliplatin
		Romidepsin
		Temozolomide
		Trabectedin
Low	10–30	Ado-trastuzumab emtansine
		Albumin-bound paclitaxel
		Aldesleukin ≤12 million IU/m^2
		Amivantamab
		Arsenic trioxide
		Axicabtagene ciloleucel
		Azacitidine
		Belinostat
		Brentuximab
		Cabazitaxel
		Carfilzomib
		Ciltacabtagene autoleucel
		Copanlisib
		Cytarabine 100–200 mg/m^2
		Docetaxel
		Doxorubicin liposomal
		Enfortumab vedotin
		Eribulin
		Etoposide

Table 5-1 (cont.)

Level	Frequency of Emesis (%)	Agent
Low	10–30	5-Fluorouracil
		Floxuridine
		Gemcitabine
		Gemtuzumab ozogamicin
		Idecabtagene vicleucel
		Inotuzumab ozogamicin
		Interferon-α 5–10 million IU/m^2
		Isatuximab
		Ixabepilone
		Lisocabtagene maraleucel
		Loncastuximab tesirine
		Methotrexate >50 – <250 mg/m^2
		Mitomycin
		Mitomycin pyelocalyceal solution
		Mitoxantrone
		Mogamulizumab
		Moxetumomab pasudotox
		Necitumumab
		Olaratumab
		Omacetaxine
		Paclitaxel
		Paclitaxel-albumin
		Pemetrexed
		Pentostatin
		Polatuzumab vedotin
		Pralatrexate
		Romidepsin
		Tafasitamab
		Tagraxofusp
		Talimogene laherparepvec
		Tebentafusp
		Thiotepa
		Tisagenlecleucel
		Tisotumab vedotin
		Topotecan
		Ziv-aflibercept

Table 5-1 (cont.)

Level	Frequency of Emesis (%)	Agent
Minimal	<10	Alemtuzumab
		Asparaginase
		Atezolizumab
		Avelumab
		Belantamab mafodotin
		Bevacizumab
		Bleomycin
		Blinatumomab
		Bortezomib
		Cemiplimab
		Cetuximab
		Cladribine
		Cytarabine <100 mg/m^2
		Daratumumab
		Daratumumab and hyaluronidase
		Decitabine
		Denileukin difitox
		Dostarlimab
		Durvalumab
		Elotuzumab
		Fludarabine
		Interferon-α <5 million IU/m^2
		Ipilimumab
		Luspatercept
		Margetuximab
		6-Mercaptopurine
		Methotrexate ≤50 mg/m^2
		Nelarabine
		Nivolumab
		Nivolumab/relatlimab
		Obinutuzumab
		Ofatumumab
		Panitumumab
		Pegaspargase
		Peg-interferon

Table 5-1 (cont.)

Level	Frequency of Emesis (%)	Agent
Minimal	<10	Pembrolizumab
		Pertuzumab
		Pertuzumab/trastuzumab and hyaluronidase
		Ramucirumab
		Rituximab
		Rituximab and hyaluronidase
		Teclistamab
		Temsirolimus
		Trastuzumab
		Trastuzumab and hyaluronidase
		Tremelimumab
		Vinblastine
		Vincristine
		Vincristine liposomal
		Vinorelbine

Table 5-2. Emetogenic Potential of Oral Chemotherapy Agents

Level	Frequency of Emesis (%)	Agent
Moderate to high	>30	Altretamine
		Avapritinib
		Azacitidine
		Binimetinib
		Bosutinib >400 mg/day
		Busulfan ≥4 mg/day
		Cabozantinib
		Capmatinib
		Ceritinib
		Crizotinib
		Cyclophosphamide ≥100 mg/m^2/day
		Dabrafenib
		Enasidenib

Table 5-2 (cont.)

Level	Frequency of Emesis (%)	Agent
Moderate to high	>30	Encorafenib
		Estramustine
		Etoposide
		Fedratinib
		Imatinib >400 mg/day
		Lenvatinib >12 mg/day
		Lomustine
		Midostaurin
		Mitotane
		Mobocertinib
		Niraparib
		Olaparib
		Procarbazine
		Rucaparib
		Selinexor
		Temozolomide >75 mg/m^2/day
Minimal to low	<30	Abemaciclib
		Acalabrutinib
		Afatinib
		Alectinib
		Alpelisib
		Asciminib
		Axitinib
		Belzutifan
		Bexarotene
		Bosutinib <400 mg/day
		Brigatinib
		Busulfan <4 mg/day
		Cabozantinib
		Capecitabine
		Capmatinib
		Chlorambucil
		Cobimetinib
		Crizotinib
		Cyclophosphamide <100 mg/m^2/day
		Dacomitinib

Table 5-2 (cont.)

Level	Frequency of Emesis (%)	Agent
Minimal to low	<30	Dasatinib
		Decitabine and cedazuridine
		Duvelisib
		Entrectinib
		Erdafitinib
		Erlotinib
		Everolimus
		Fludarabine
		Futibatinib
		Gefitinib
		Gilteritinib
		Glasdegib
		Hydroxyurea
		Ibrutinib
		Idelalisib
		Imatinib ≤400 mg/day
		Ivosidenib
		Ixazomib
		Lapatinib
		Larotrectinib
		Lenalidomide
		Lenvatinib ≤12 mg/day
		Lorlatinib
		Melphalan
		Mercaptopurine
		Methotrexate
		Neratinib
		Nilotinib
		Osimertinib
		Pacritinib
		Palbociclib
		Panobinostat
		Pazopanib
		Pemigatinib
		Pexidartinib
		Pomalidomide

Table 5-2 (cont.)

Level	Frequency of Emesis (%)	Agent
Minimal to low	<30	Ponatinib
		Pralsetinib
		Regorafenib
		Ribociclib
		Ripretinib
		Ruxolitinib
		Selpercatinib
		Sonidegib
		Sorafenib
		Sotarasib
		Sunitinib
		Talazoparib
		Tazemetostat
		Temozolomide $\leq$75 mg/m^2/day
		Tepotinib
		Thalidomide
		Thioguanine
		Tivosanib
		Topotecan
		Trametinib
		Tretinoin
		Trifluridine/tipiracil (TAS-102)
		Tucatinib
		Vandetanib
		Vemurafenib
		Venetoclax
		Vismodegib
		Vorinostat
		Zanubrutinib

Data from Hesketh PJ, Kris MG, Basch E, et al. Antiemetics: ASCO Guideline Update [published correction appears in *J Clin Oncol*. 2020 Nov 10;38(32):3825] [published correction appears in *J Clin Oncol*. 2021 Jan 1;39(1):96]. *J Clin Oncol*. 2020;38(24):2782-2797. doi:10.1200/JCO.20.01296; National Comprehensive Cancer Network. NCCN guidelines: treatment by cancer type. https://www.nccn.org/guidelines

Single agents are divided into four different risk levels of emetogenic potential. They are as follows:

1. Minimal: <10% of patients experience acute (<24 hours after chemotherapy) emesis without antiemetic prophylaxis.
2. Low: 10%–30% of patients experience acute emesis without antiemetic prophylaxis.
3. Moderate: 30%–90% of patients experience acute emesis without antiemetic prophylaxis.
4. High: >90% of patients experience acute emesis without antiemetic prophylaxis.

For combination regimens, the emetogenic levels are determined by identifying the most emetogenic agent in the combination and then assessing the relative contribution of the other agents based on the following:

1. Level 1 agents do not contribute to the emetogenic potential of the combination.
2. The addition of one or more level 2 agents increases the emetogenicity of the combination by one level greater than the most emetogenic agent in the combination.
3. The addition of level 3 or 4 agents increases the emetogenicity of the combination by one level per agent.

Index